0100648

AF616099

Mechanisms of Suntanning

Jean-Paul Ortonne
Robert Ballotti

MARTIN DUNITZ

This book is based on the International
Workshop on Molecular Mechanisms of Tanning,
sponsored by L'Oréal Recherche,
held in April 2001, Nice, France.

Publication has been supported by an
educational grant from L'Oréal Recherche.

Mechanisms of Suntanning

Edited by

JEAN-PAUL ORTONNE
Department of Dermatology
Hôpital L'Archet 2
Nice
France

ROBERT BALLOTTI
Laboratory of Biology and Skin Pathophysiology
INSERM U385
Faculty of Medicine
Nice
France

MARTIN DUNITZ

First published in the United Kingdom in 2002
by Martin Dunitz Ltd, The Livery House, 7– 9 Pratt Street, London NW1 0AE

Tel.: +44 (0) 20 74822202
Fax.: +44 (0) 20 72670159
E-mail: info@dunitz.co.uk
Website: http://www.dunitz.co.uk

A CIP record for this book is available from the British Library.

ISBN 1 84184 189 7

Distributed in the USA by
Fulfilment Center
Taylor & Francis
7625 Empire Drive
Florence, KY 41042, USA
Toll Free Tel.: +1 800 634 7064
E-mail: cserve@routledge_ny.com

Distributed in Canada by
Taylor & Francis
74 Rolark Drive
Scarborough, Ontario M1R 4G2, Canada
Toll Free Tel.: +1 877 226 2237
E-mail: tal_fran@istar.ca

Distributed in the rest of the world by
Thomson Publishing Services
Cheriton House
North Way
Andover, Hampshire SP10 5BE, UK
Tel.: +44 (0)1264 332424
E-mail: salesorder.tandf@thomsonpublishingservices.co.uk

Composition by J&L Composition Ltd, Filey, North Yorkshire
Printed and bound in Singapore by Kyodo Printing Co (S'pore) Pte Ltd

Contents

Contributors

Zalfa Abdel-Malek
Associate Professor
University of Cincinnati College of Medicine
Cincinnati OH
USA

Catherine Agapakis-Causse
L'Oréal Recherche
Aulnay
France

Janis Ancans
Department of Biomedical Sciences
University of Bradford
Bradford
UK

Heinz Arnheiter
National Institutes of Health
Bethesda MD
USA

Philippe Bahadoran
Hôpital, L'Archet 2
Nice
France

Robert Ballotti
Laboratory of Biology and Skin Pathophysiology
INSERM U385
Faculty of Medicine
Nice
France

Janusz Z. Beer
Center for Devices and Radiological Health
Food & Drug Administration
Rockville MD
USA

Jean-Philippe Belaidi
L'Oréal Recherche
Aulnay
France

Carola Berking
Department of Dermatology
Ludwig-Maximilians-University
Munich
Germany

Corine Bertolotto
Université de Nice Sophia Antipolis
Nice
France

Keren Bismuth
National Institutes of Health
Bethesda MD
USA

Markus Böhm
Department of Dermatology
University of Münster
Münster
Germany

Jean Jacques Bonerandi
Hôpital de la Timone
Marseille
France

Thomas Brzoska
Department of Dermatology
University of Münster
Münster
Germany

Roger Buscà
Laboratory of Biology and Skin Pathophysiology
INSERM U385
Faculty of Medicine
Nice
France

Candice Cabane
Laboratoire de Physiologie Cellulaire et Moléculaire
Université de Nice Sophia Antipolis
Nice
France

Bénédicte Champagne
Division of Neurophysiology
National Institute for Medical Research
London
UK

Alain Chardon
L'Oréal Recherche
Clichy
France

François J. Christiaens
L'Oréal Recherche
Clichy
France

Sylvie G Consoli
Dermatology Unit
Pitié Salpetriere Hospital
Paris
France

Neal G. Copeland
Mouse Cancer Genetics Program
National Cancer Institute at Frederick
Frederick MD
USA

Benoît Dérijard
Laboratoire Physiologie Cellulaire et Moleculaire
Université de Nice Sophia Antipolis
Nice
France

Hélène Dessauvages
Galderma R&D
Sophia Antipolis
France

Nicole M. Le Douarin
Institut d'Embryologie Cellulaire et Moléculaire du CNRS
Nogent sur Marne
France

Elisabeth Dupin
Institut d'Embryologie Cellulaire et Moléculaire du CNRS
Nogent sur Marne
France

Luc Duteil
CPCAD
Hôpital L'Archet 2
Nice
France

Christine Duval
L'Oréal Recherche
Clichy
France

Mark S Eller
Department of Dermatology
Boston University School of Medicine
Boston MA
USA

Tanja Fisbeck
Department of Dermatology
University of Münster
Münster
Germany

David E Fisher
Division of Pediatric Oncology
Dana Farber Cancer Institute
Boston MA
USA

Giuseppina Giglia-Mari
Institut de Recherches sur le Cancer
Villejuif
France

Barbara A. Gilchrest
Department of Dermatology
Boston University School of Medicine
Boston MA
USA

Colin R. Goding
Eukaryotic Transcription Laboratory
Marie Curie Research Institute
Oxted, Surrey
UK

Ina M. Hadshiew
Department of Dermatology
Boston University School of Medicine
Boston MA
USA

Jon H. Halsson
National Institutes of Health
Bethesda MD
USA

Vincent J. Hearing
Chief, Pigment Cell Biology Section
Laboratory of Cell Biology
National Institutes of Health
Bethesda MD
USA

Meenhard Herlyn
The Wistar Institute
Philadelphia PA
USA

Martin J. Hoogduijn
Department of Biomedical Sciences
University of Bradford
Bradford
UK

Ling Hou
National Institutes of Health
Bethesda MD
USA

Shosuke Ito
Fujita Health University
School of Health Sciences
Japan

Nancy A. Jenkins
Mouse Cancer Genetics Program
National Cancer Institute at Frederick
Frederick MD
USA

André Jomard
Galderma R&D
Sophia Antipolis
France

Alice Jouneau
Institut Curie
Orsay
France

Hervé Kempf
INSERM U36
Collège de France
Paris
France

Nobuhiko Kobayashi
National Institutes of Health
Bethesda MD
USA

Jean Krutmanm
Professor of Dermatology and
Environmental Medicine
Heinrich-Heine University
Düsseldorf
Germany

Dagmar Kulms
Department of Dermatology
University of Münster
Münster
Germany

M. Lynn Lamoreux
The Texas Veterinary Medical Center
College Station TX
USA

Lionel Larue
Institut Curie
Orsay
France

Laure Lecoin
Institut Curie
Orsay
France

Melanie Lee
Eukaryotic Transcription Laboratory
Marie Curie Research Institute
Oxted, Surrey
UK

Thomas A. Luger
Professor, Department of Dermatology
University of Münster
Münster
Germany

Ahmed Mansouri
Max-Planck Institute for Biophysical Chemistry
Göttingen
Germany

Laurent Marrot
L'Oréal Recherche
Aulnay
France

Lydia E. Matesic
Postdoctoral fellow
Mouse Cancer Genetics Program
National Cancer Institute at Frederick
Frederick MD
USA

Jean-Roch Meunier
L'Oréal Recherche
Aulnay
France

Sharon A. Miller
Center for Devices and Radiological Health
Food & Drug Administration
Rockville MD
USA

Dominique Moyal
L'Oréal Recherche
Clichy
France

Atsuo Nakayama
Nagoya University School of Medicine
Nagoya
Japan

Minh-Thanh Nguyen
National Institutes of Health
Bethesda MD
USA

James J. Nordlund MD
Department of Dermatology
University of Cincinnati
Cincinnati OH
USA

Hee-Young Park
Department of Dermatology
Boston University School of Medicine
Boston MA
USA

Isabelle Pélisson
Galderma R&D
Sophia Antipolis
France

Philippe Perez
L'Oréal Recherche
Aulnay
France

Patrick Pla
Institut Curie
Orsay
France

Jonathan L. Rees
Grant Chair of Dermatology
Systems Group, Dermatology
University of Edinburgh
Edinburgh
UK

Marcelle Régnier
L'Oréal Recherche
Clichy
France

Alain Sarasin
Institut de Recherches sur le Cancer
Villejuif
France

Meinhard Schiller
Department of Dermatology
University of Münster
Münster
Germany

Rainer Schmidt
L'Oréal Recherche
Clichy
France

Thomas Scholzen
Department of Dermatology
University of Münster
Münster
Germany

Thomas Schwarz
Department of Dermatology
University of Münster
Münster
Germany

Miri Seiberg
Skin Research Center
J&J CPWW
Skillman NJ
USA

Stanley S. Shapiro
Skin Research Center
J&J CPWW
Skillman NJ
USA

Shigeki Shibahara
Department of Molecular Biology
& Applied Physiology
Tohoku University School of Medicine
Japan

Richard A. Spritz
Human Medical Genetics Program
University of Colorado Health Sciences Center
Denver CO
USA

Helger Stege
Department of Dermatology
Heinrich-Heine University
Düsseldorf
Germany

Taketsugu Tadokoro
National Institutes of Health
Bethesda MD
USA

Anthony J Thody
Professor, Department of Biomedical Sciences
University of Bradford
Bradford
UK

Marina Tsatmali
Department of Biomedical Sciences
University of Bradford
Bradford
UK

Kazumasa Wakamatsu
Fujita Health University
School of Health Sciences
Japan

Karen Yeow
Laboratoire de Physiologie Cellulaire et Moléculaire
Université de Nice Sophia Antipolis
Nice
France

Barbara Z. Zmudzka
Center for Devices and Radiological Health
Food & Drug Administration
Rockville MD
USA

Foreword

Ultraviolet (UV) radiation plays a number of important roles with respect to human health, and its influence on the skin is of paramount concern. UV stimulates pigmentation of the skin (commonly known as tanning) but at the same time damages the DNA in epidermal and dermal cells that eventually give rise to various forms of skin cancer. Melanin pigmentation in the skin provides an excellent benefit in minimizing photocarcinogenesis and it is well known that rates of basal and squamous cell carcinomas are 50 times higher in lightly pigmented skin than in darkly pigmented skin. Even rates of malignant melanoma (the transformed phenotype of the melanocyte) are 10 to 15 times higher in lightly pigmented skin than in darkly pigmented skin, even though those cells are much more active in the more pigmented skin.

In April 2001, an international workshop was held in Nice, France that brought together more than 80 of the leading international scientists investigating various aspects of skin pigmentation and responses to UV radiation. That workshop focused on a discussion of the molecular mechanisms involved in the tanning response and the impact this has on human health. This book summarizes the presentations that were made at that meeting, and provides the latest state-of-the-art understanding of melanocyte and skin biology, and the effects (positive and negative) of UV radiation. The topics covered range from factors that influence the development of melanocyte precursors (melanoblasts) in the embryo, to the intracellular signaling and gene regulation of melanocytes exposed to UV radiation. A number of chapters address important aspects of the formation of pigment granules (melanosomes), the composition of their integral components, the mechanisms involved with pigment synthesis and the properties of those melanins. Factors involved in the transport of melanosomes to the dendrites of melanocytes and their subsequent transfer to keratinocytes are also addressed. And finally, mechanisms involved in the transformation of normal melanocytes to malignant melanoma cells are discussed, along with the value of melanin as a sunscreen and as a factor in one's psychological feeling of health. In sum, the scope of the presentations at that meeting and in this book, cover melanocytes from their early development through their various functions in human skin.

It is to be hoped that future developments in this field, to which all laboratories aspire, will enable the optimization of skin pigmentation to afford maximal protection from UV damage, and thus a minimization of photocarcinogenesis. In closing, I would like to congratulate Prof. Jean-Paul Ortonne and Dr. Robert Ballotti, the co-organizers of this meeting, for their efforts in arranging such an important forum for interactions of international experts in the field, and for producing this book which allows others to peruse the results, musings and future plans of the major laboratories active in this critical field.

Vincent J. Hearing
Chief, Laboratory of Cell Biology
National Cancer Institute, Bethesda, USA

1
Sunlight and cutaneous melanocytes: An overview

Robert Ballotti and Jean-Paul Ortonne

Introduction

Melanocytes and melanogenesis

Melanocytes find their embryonic origin at the neural crest where they exist as non-differentiated precursor cells called melanoblasts. From the neural crest, during embryonic development, melanoblasts migrate to reach the basal layer of the epidermis where they differentiate to mature melanocytes possessing the complete machinery to ensure melanin synthesis and distribution.[1] At the basal layer of the epidermis, melanocytes are ready to receive specific signals that will activate the machinery of pigment synthesis and delivery.

Melanins are synthesized in melanosomes that contain the specific enzymes required for proper melanin production. Among them, the most well characterized enzyme is tyrosinase, which catalyses the two initial rate-limiting reactions of the cascade: the hydroxylation of tyrosine giving 3,4-dihydroxyphenylalanine (DOPA), and the oxidation of DOPA to DOPAquinone. Tyrosinase, related protein 1 (Tyrp1) oxidizes 5,6-dihydroxyindole-2-carboxylic acid (DHICA) to indole-5,6-quinone-2-carboxylic acid and DOPAchrome tautomerase (DCT), which isomerizes DOPAchrome to give DHICA. In mammals, two major types of melanins are produced, the eumelanins which are black-brown, and the phaeomelanins which are yellow-red.[2] The ratio between eumelanins and phaeomelanins in the epidermis may vary, and the amount of eumelanins inversely correlates (roughly) with the skin's photosensitivity. Unlike eumelanins that are photoprotective, phaeomelanins are considerably photolabile and, upon photoexcitation, they may produce highly cytotoxic and mitogenic free radicals that might account for an increased sensitivity of individuals to sunburn and skin cancer.[3]

Because of the ability of melanins to absorb and thus eliminate ultraviolet (UV) photons, skin darkening provides photoprotection against the UV-induced damages that would otherwise adversely affect DNA, membrane lipids and other critical cellular components.

Ultraviolet radiation (UVR)

Sun exposure of the skin induces a cascade of cellular and molecular events involving all cell types, including melanocytes. The solar spectrum includes X-rays, /-rays, radiowaves, microwaves, visible light (400–700 nm), infrared (700–2000 nm) and UVR. The UVR component of sunlight is composed of radiation with wavelengths of 200–400 nm and accounts for 8–9% of the total energy emitted by the sun. The UV region of the solar spectrum is further divided into several wavebands: UVA (320–400 nm), [generally divided into UVA-1 or long-wave UVA (340–400 nm) and UVA-II or short-wave UVA (320–340 nm)], UVB (290–320 nm) and UVC (200–290 nm) that do not reach the earth's surface as they are screened off by the upper atmosphere, and does not play any role in cutaneous biology.[4]

The UVA waveband represents approximately 6.3% of the sun's total emission, including direct flux from the sun and atmosphere-scattered rays, UVA is less affected than UVB by sun elevation, altitude and cloud cover, *i.e.* atmospheric filtration. The main portion of UVA radiation is not trapped by standard glass, which fails to protect against UVA as it does for UVB since the short wavelength cut-off of glass is around 320 nm.

The UVB waveband represents about 1.5% of the sun's total energy emission. UVB reaches earth in relatively small amounts. UVB is very efficient in promoting sunburn and sun tanning of human skin. Sites below sea level are relatively poor in the UVB component of solar energy which reaches the earth's surface (*e.g.* the Dead Sea). In contrast, the amount of UVB increases with altitude. The UVB waveband is potentially very damaging to skin in the long term.

The main natural stimulus of human skin pigmentation is sunlight. Constitutive pigmentation is defined as the amount of cutaneous melanin pigmentation generated in accordance with cellular genetic programs in the absence of external influence. Sunlight is the main natural stimulus that increases the basal level of skin pigmentation. This inducible skin colour is called facultative pigmentation.[5] Acute exposure to artificial UV or sunlight induces two types of photobiological reactions of the melanin pigmentary system: a short-lived immediate darkening called immediate pigment darkening (IPD) and delayed tanning which is considered to be a photoprotective mechanism of the skin. Chronic exposure to UV, particularly to sunlight, induces cumulative changes of melanocytes; these changes vary considerably in severity among individuals, and undoubtedly reflect inherent differences in the vulnerability to solar insult, in the efficiency of the natural photoprotective mechanisms and in the repair capacities of the skin.

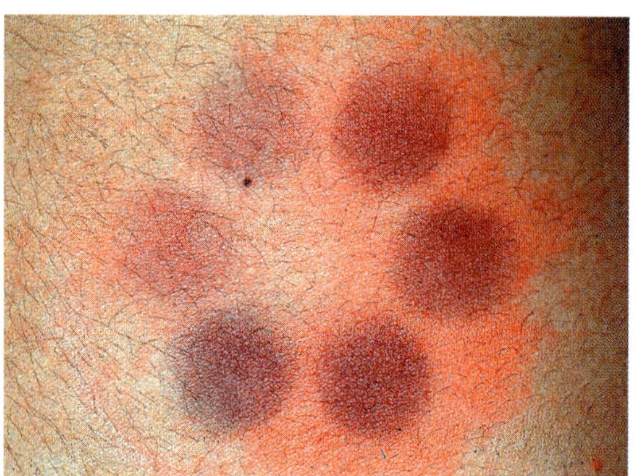

Figure 1.1

Immediate pigment darkening after UVA irradiation.

Acute effects of sunlight on human skin pigmentation

Immediate pigment darkening (IPD)

IPD is a blue-grey pigmentation that develops immediately during exposure of the skin to UVA radiation (320–400 nm) (Fig. 1.1). A partial fading occurs rapidly within 1 hour after the end of exposure. As it decreases, the pigmentation progressively loses its blue component at about 2 hours and beyond, but for high UVA doses a stable residual pigmentation remains, persisting for up to several days. Persistent pigment darkening (PPD), or the stable portion of IPD, is the lasting residual part of IPD. The colour of this residual grey pigmentation must not be confused with that of delayed pigmentation (tanning), since the latter has been shown to occur with a typical brown hue only with high UVA doses or with cumulative sequential exposures and with a delay of about 2–3 days. The action spectra of both IPD and PPD extend throughout the UVA range, from UVB to short visible rays. The response decreases towards long UVA wavelengths and fades away at about 450 nm. IPD is most easily seen in subjects with skin types 3 and 4. It is usually absent or minimal in individuals classified as skin types 1 and 2. IPD is also difficult to visualize in skin types 5 and 6 owing to their constitutive pigmentation. From the results of a large-scale study in which the reaction was studied in over 1300 volunteers, the peak effectiveness was between 320 and 340 nm with the average irradiation doses needed to produce minimal IPD increasing from phototype 1 to phototype 4. A lack of the reaction seemed to correlate well with 'non-brown' eye colour, but did not appear to be related to blonde hair.[6]

The molecular and cellular mechanisms of IPD are still poorly understood. Following biophysical, photochemical and ultrastructural studies, it was concluded that IPD consisted of a combination of photochemical and ultrastructural changes in the melanocytes. Significant modifications in the distribution pattern of microtubules and intermediate filaments from the perinuclear area of the melanocytes to the periphery, associated with the development of prominent dendritic processes, movement of melanosomes from the perikaryon to the dendrites of the melanosomes to the basal keratinocytes were observed.[7, 8] Further studies did not confirm these findings, indicating that IPD is not the result of a transfer of pre-formed melanosomes from the melanocytes to the keratinocytes or a redistribution of the melanosomes.[9] Indeed, disruption of the macrofibrillar and microtubular system by cytochalasin B, colcemid and vincristine does not block IPD.[10] Furthermore, IPD can be elicited in skin damaged by fixation or repeated freezing and thawing, or isolated cadaverous skin, indicating that IPD does not require an active cellular process. In contrast, fading of IPD only occurs in viable skin. IPD is dependent on oxygen concentration. These observations suggest that IPD in non-viable skin is mainly the result of a photo-oxidation of pre-existing melanin which seems to take place through the formation of unstable semiquinone-like free radicals.[11] Another hypothesis proposes that photo-oxidation of semiquinoid to quinoid results in an increase in carbon-oxygen bonds, which causes the darkening of melanins.[12] In viable skin, a spatial rearrangement of melanosomes in melanocytes and/or keratinocytes may also contribute to the skin darkening of IPD.[13] The physiological function of IPD remains unknown. IPD does not protect against UVB-induced erythema or against UVB-induced DNA lesions. Also, IPD is not a light test that discriminates between healthy individuals and melanoma patients.

Delayed tanning (DT)

DT is characterized by a visible brown coloration (Fig. 1.2) in UV-exposed skin which represents an increase in epidermal melanin content. This skin darkening is detectable 3–4 days after irradiation of the skin and is a gradual process. DT is maximally stimulated by exposure to the 'sunburn spectrum', *i.e.* UVB radiation (290–320 nm), and, to a lesser extent, to long-wave UVA and visible radiation (320–700 nm). Histological analysis of irradiated skin shows that multiple exposures to UVA or UVB irradiation induce a marked increase in the number of functional (DOPA-positive) melanocytes, and in their dendricity. Ultrastructural changes include an increase in the number of melanosomes synthesized, an increase in the degree of pigmentation of the melanosomes, and an increase in the number of melanosomes transferred to keratinocytes.[7,8,14,15] In addition, there are distinct changes to the distribution pattern of melanosomes in keratinocytes, probably as a result of a variation in the size of the melanosomes. DT involves synthesis of the new melanosomes, as well as changes in the functional state of melanocytes and keratinocytes. The mechanism underlying these changes in the epidermal melanin unit involves transcriptional responses of the pigmentary genes and post-translational control of the melanin biosynthetic pathway.

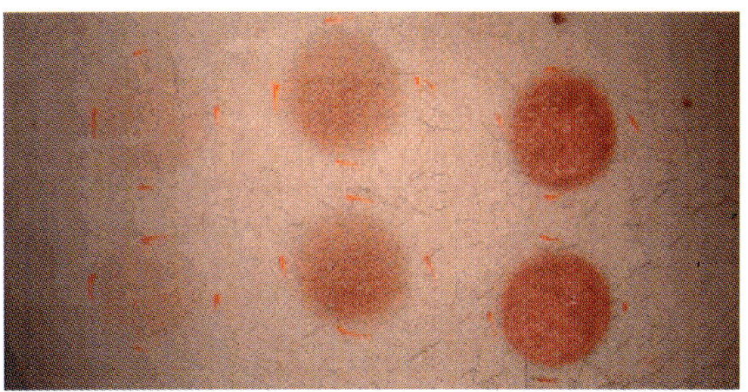

Figure 1.2

Tanning following UVB irradiation.

Few studies of the composition of melanins in photoexposed skin have been performed. It is well established that chronically photoexposed skin contains more melanins than corresponding photoprotected skin and is thus hyperpigmented. Recent findings in Type 5 and 6 photoexposed and photoprotected skin[16] suggest that DHI-eumelanin formation is the dominant pathway for melanogenesis in heavily pigmented skin. Analysis of the relative composition of epidermal melanin in these subjects revealed that DHI-eumelanin is the predominant component (60–70%), followed by DHICA-eumelanin (25–35%), with phaeomelanin being a relatively minor component (2.8%). There was a comparative enrichment of DHI-eumelanin at photoexposed sites with a corresponding decline in the relative contribution from DHICA-eumelanin and pheomelanin. These data suggest that DHI-eumelanin synthesis is the favoured pathway when melanin is increased in chronically photoexposed skin.

UVB-versus UVA-induced tanning

The tanning response induced by UVA alone is 2.3 orders of magnitude less efficient and differs mechanistically from that induced by UVB. The UVA-induced DT requires oxygen at the time of irradiation whereas the UVB response does not. Also, the UVA DT response occurs very rapidly after the immediate pigmentation phase whereas UVB tanning begins only several days after exposure.

Pigmentation following exposure to UVA and UVB shows substantial differences in the time course and distribution of pigment within the epidermis. UVA-induced pigmentation is immediate (IPD) followed by DT (UVA-induced DT) at later time points whereas UVB-induced DT appears only after several days. Histological and ultrastructural examination demonstrate that persistent UVA DT is characterized by a similar melanocytic response to that of UVB irradiation. There is an increase in both melanocyte number and neomelanogenic activity involved in the UVA-induced DT. Thus, although UVA and UVB initiate different photobiological events, they ultimately produce the same melanocytic response.[17]

Striking differences are observed in the melanogenic response of normal human melanocytes to UVA and UVB irradiation depending on culture conditions and the presence of keratinocytes.[18] In culture, keratinocytes play an important role in mediating UVB-induced pigmentation, suggesting that the release of keratinocyte-derived cytokines, growth factors or other mediators is required to induce melanin synthesis. *In vitro*, UVA-induced pigmentation is the result of a rather direct effect on melanocytes; UVA exposure does not cause human keratinocytes to stimulate the secretion of endothelin (ET)-1 and interleukin (IL)-1α.[19] In contrast, the level of granulocyte/macrophage colony-stimulating factor (GM-CSF) is significantly increased in the conditioned medium of human keratinocytes after exposure to UVA.[19] *In vitro*, GM-CSF-containing fractions in UVA-exposed keratinocyte-conditioned medium elicited both mitogenic and melanogenic effects. These observations suggest that GM-CSF is an intrinsic stimulatory component for human melanocytes in UVA-induced melanogenesis.

UVA irradiation exposes cells to oxidative stress by absorption of radiation in endogenous photosensitizers generating reactive oxygen species, notably single oxygen. The oxidative stress induces damage to biomolecules such as lipids, proteins. UVA causes single-strand DNA breaks and 8-hydroxy-2-deoxyguanosine. UVA also induces cyclobutane pyrimidine dimers.[20] UVB causes characteristic lesions such as cyclobutane pyrimidine dimers and pyrimidine 6–4 pyrimidone photoproducts by direct absorption of photons. Experimental data suggest that cyclobutane pyrimidine dimers repair stimulates pigmentation.[21]

Both UVA and UVB are able to stimulate DT. UVB and UVA are both present in the solar spectrum reaching the earth, suggesting that interactions of these wavelengths are likely to occur in the induction of DT after natural sunlight exposure. Indeed, experimental studies show that subthreshold doses of UVA and UVB interact additively in the production of DT in human volunteers.[22] The effect of visible light on human skin pigmentation is poorly characterized.

Visible-light-induced pigmentation

A few studies show that exposure of normal human skin to visible light results in the induction of IPD and DT.[23]

Chronic effects of sunlight on human skin pigmentation

Mottling

Photoaged skin is often characterized by mottled, irregular areas of pigmentation (Figs 1.3 and 1.4), which is paradoxical as the number of epidermal melanocytes in aged skin is decreased compared to the number in young adult skin. This clinical appearance is probably explained by the increased DOPA positivity of melanocytes in the chronically sun-exposed skin and by an irregular distribution of the pigment cells along the dermal–epidermal junction, as well as by an irregular distribution of melanosomes within epidermal keratinocytes.

A morphological and functional heterogeneity of epidermal melanocytes in photoaged skin is well illustrated by electron microscopy (EM) studies. A majority of melanocytes were large, showing changes in hyperactivity. Other pigment cells

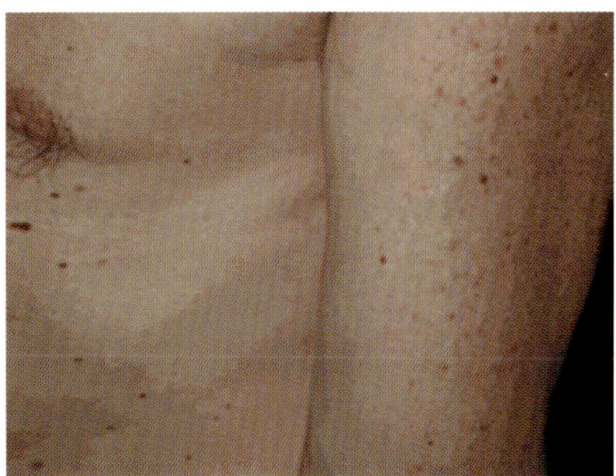

Figure 1.3

Pigmentary abnormalities on the sun-exposed extensor aspect of the arm. Note the sharp limit with the sun-protected skin.

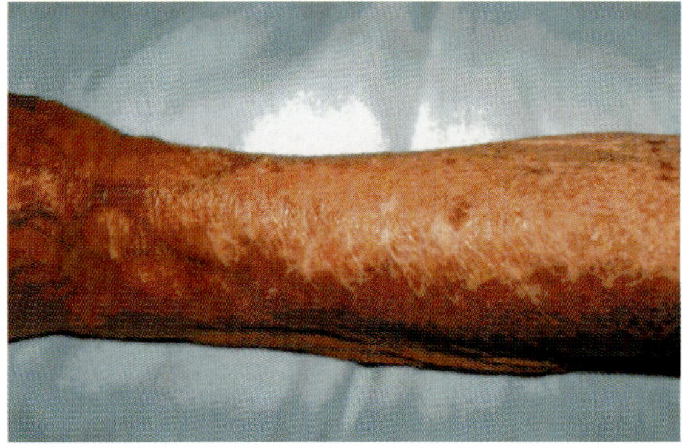

Figure 1.4

Mottling.

exhibited an appearance of having reached the end of an active life cycle. A third group of melanocytes presented a typically inactive appearance.[24]

Ephelides

Ephelides or freckles are small light-brown pigmented macules commonly scattered over sun-exposed skin (Figs 1.5 and 1.6). Usually, they first appear at about the age of 5 years in the Caucasian population, more frequently in fair-skinned individuals with red or light-blond hair and blue eyes, particularly in those of Celtic origin. They increase in number, size and depth of pigmentation during the summer months and are smaller, lighter and fewer in number in the winter. Ephelides partly vanish with age. In freckled individuals, the incidence of melanocytic naevi is increased. Fair skin, red hair and ephelides are indicators for an increased risk of malignant melanoma and non-melanoma skin cancer. With light microscopy, ephelides are characterized by hyperpigmentation of the basal cell layer, without elongation of the rete ridges or an increase in the

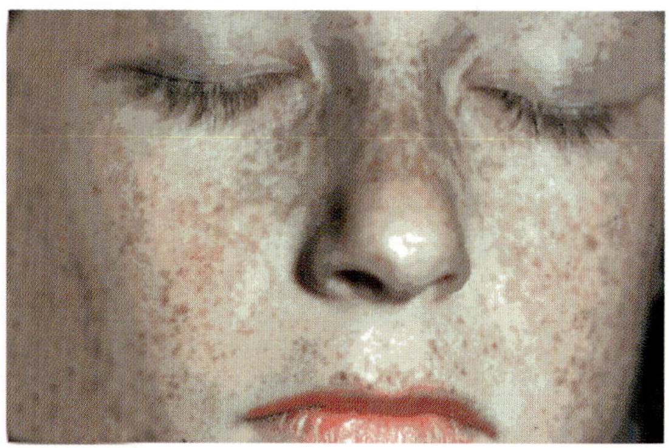

Figure 1.5

Ephelides of the face.

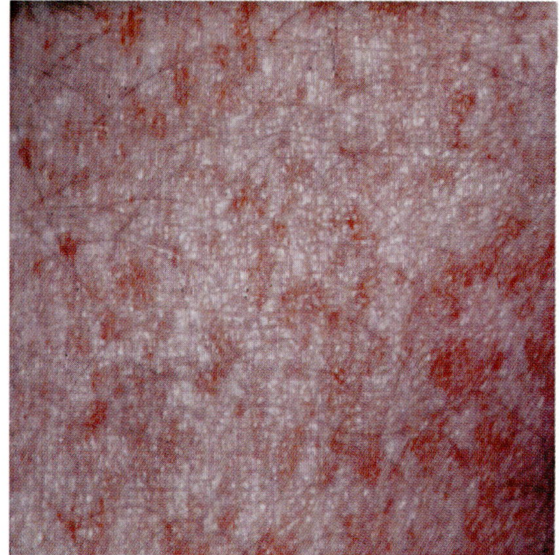

Figure 1.6

Ephelides of the arm.

number of epidermal melanocytes. Freckled skin has significantly fewer DOPA-positive melanocytes per square millimetre than adjacent paler skin, but the melanocytes are larger and are strongly DOPA sensitive.[25] Ultrastructurally, the melanocytes in freckles produce large numbers of mature melanosomes similar to those seen in dark-skinned individuals (long and rod-shaped), but they are different to those of adjacent paler skin, being round with a granular internal structure.[26]

Ephelides in childhood are strongly associated with the presence of melanocortin-1-receptor (MC1R) gene variants independent of skin type and hair colour. The degree of ephelides (freckling) is associated with the number of MC1R gene variants. These observations suggest that MC1R gene is the major ephelides gene.[27] The molecular mechanisms by which MC1R gene variants induce freckling are not yet known. In humans, the MC1R receptor is a key regulator of pigmentation phenotype and sun sensitivity. Melanocytes, which are stimulated by α-melanocyte-stimulating hormone (αMSH) through the MC1R gene, synthesize the black photoprotective eumelanin pigment instead of red phaeomelanin. However, the ratio of eumelanin/phaeomelanin in ephelides is unknown. EM studies demonstrate that ephelide melanocytes produce melanosomes resembling eumelanosomes whereas melanosomes of the phaeomelanic type are present in melanocytes on the surrounding pale skin. MC1R gene variants encoding proteins with altered receptor binding and/or signaling properties are seen to be the most important in determining the risk of ephelides.

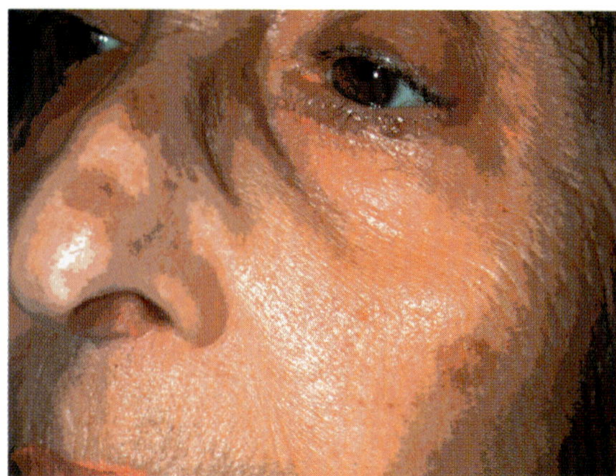

Figure 1.7

Actinic lentigos of the face.

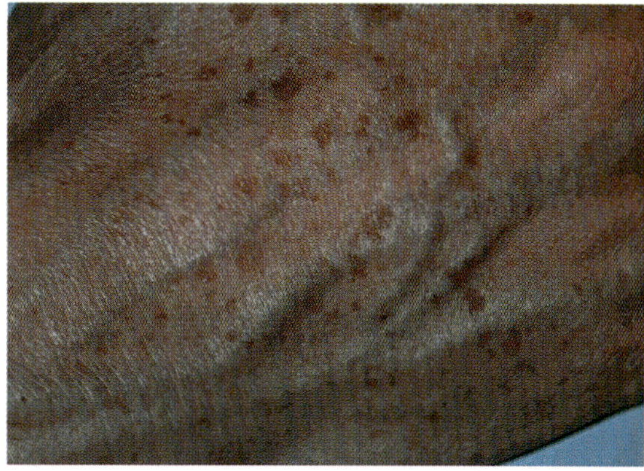

Figure 1.8

Actinic lentigos on the dorsum of the hand.

Actinic lentigo

This condition, also known as senile or solar lentigines, commonly occurs as multiple lesions in areas of skin chronically exposed to the sun (Figs 1.7–1.9).[28] These lentigines, which are benign, hyperpigmented macules, varying in size from a few millimetres to more than 1 cm across, may coalesce and their borders may be regular or irregular. Great variations in the shape have been observed and they are usually dark brown, although yellow, light brown or even black lesions are not uncommon. A mottled appearance, owing to varying degrees of hyperpigmentation, may occur within lesions. There is no scaling, desquamation, hyperkeratosis or infiltration. The incidence of senile lentigines increases with age, being found in more than 90% of Caucasians over 70 years of age; however, the incidence is the same in both sexes and they have been reported to be equally common in subjects with dark or light complexions.

The most prominent histological features include hyperpigmentation of the basal cell layer with a marked increase in the number of epidermal DOPA-positive melanocytes and elongation of the rete ridges, which appear either club-shaped or tortuous with bud-like extensions. When examined using EM,[29] epidermal melanocytes display

Figure 1.9

Diffuse actinic lentiginosis of the back.

increased activity, with nuclei being irregularly shaped and their cytoplasm containing large numbers of melanosomes. There is no pleomorphism of melanosomes and no atypical cytological alterations of melanocytes. The keratinocytes contain increased amounts of melanosomes and melanosome complexes, and melanosomes are also seen in the horny layer, thus suggesting that in addition to the increase in the number of melanocytes and increased melanin synthesis, there is also an abnormality in the lysosomal degradation of pigment granules within the epidermal keratinocytes.

The molecular mechanisms leading to hyperpigmentation of actinic lentigo have been partially dissected.[30] Immunohistochemistry demonstrated that tyrosinase immunopositivity is increased in lesional melanocytes as well as a strong staining for ET-1 along the lower epidermis of actinic lentigo. Accentuated expression of transcripts for ET-1 and for the ET-B receptor in actinic lentigo epidermis was also detected. These observations suggest that an upregulation of the epidermal endothelin cascade plays an important role in the pathogenesis of hypermelanosis of actinic lentigo.

Significant associations between MC1R gene variants and solar lentigines have been found. Although statistically significant, the relationship was weaker compared to the associations between ephelides in childhood and MC1R gene variants.[27] These observations suggest that MC1R gene is involved in the aetiology of solar lentigines but to a lesser extent than for ephelides.

The skin of pigmented hairless mice, once chronically UV irradiated, always develops pigmented spots after a latent period.[31] Histological examination revealed many DOPA-positive epidermal melanocytes and increased melanin granules in the affected epidermis. These observations suggest that these mice represent an animal model of actinic lentigines.[32]

Sunbed (UVA) lentigines

UVA alone or UVA contaminated by small amounts of UVB may induce melanocytic lesions and with the increasing use of sunbeds throughout the year to induce tanning, this problem will probably become more common. Subjects with fair skin who are chronically exposing themselves to UV radiation by using sunbeds should be aware of this potential side-effect since they appear to be most at risk. These lesions, which develop in areas exposed to radiation, are variable in size and are unevenly pigmented with irregular borders; sometimes they have a stellate appearance (Fig. 1.10). Histological examination of the lesions has demonstrated increased numbers of large melanocytes in the epidermal basal layer and a small number of upwardly migrating melanocytes within the epidermis,[32] with some of these cells showing cellular atypia. Ultrastructural examination revealed features similar to other forms of lentigo, with melanosome complexes within melanocytes and keratinocytes containing large numbers of melanosomes.

Sunbed lentigines occur in subjects that have not been using psoralens either topically or orally at the time of UVA irradiation, demonstrating that UVA alone can induce melanocytic lesions resembling those observed in some patients receiving long-term photochemotherapy (see below); both acute and chronic overexposure can apparently induce 'sunbed lentigines'. The long-term behaviour of these lesions is unknown but the occurrence of melanocytic atypia and melanosomal pleomorphism suggests that all patients should be carefully followed up.

Psoralen UVA (PUVA) lentigines

The formation of lentigines is a common side-effect of chronic oral psoralen photochemotherapy.[33,34]

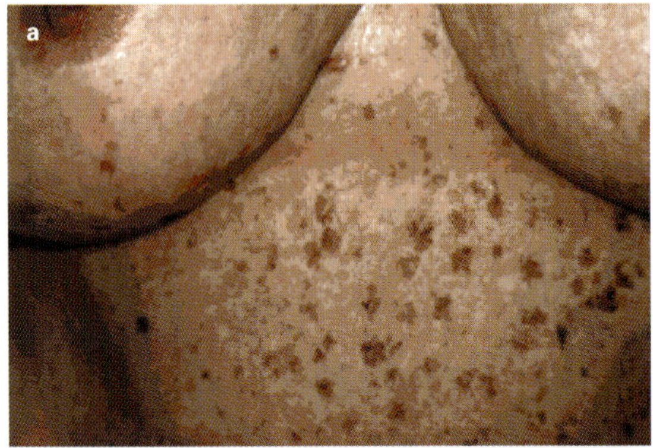

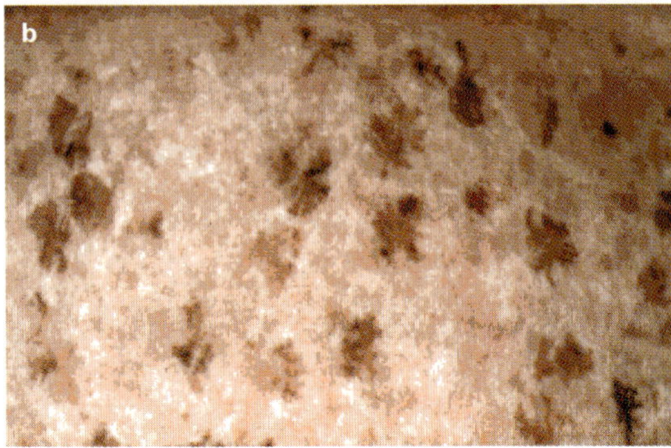

Figure 1.10

UVA lentigos.

Both sexes are equally affected. These lesions, known as PUVA lentigines, which appear after 2–3 years of extensive treatment with PUVA, are clinically slightly different from actinic lentigines. PUVA lentigines are disseminated, hyperpigmented, sharply and irregularly defined macules ranging in size from 2 to 6 mm. They are usually smaller, more numerous and more densely scattered than solar lentigines and can be observed in all PUVA-treated areas, but occur most frequently on the thighs, groin, buttocks, on the shoulders, and the upper back, on the arms and legs and flanks. The most prominent feature of PUVA lentigines is histological elongation of rete ridges with proliferation of functionally active melanocytes. Other features are dyskeratotic cells, enlarged nuclei in keratinocytes and giant keratinocytes. In contrast to actinic lentigines, the melanocytes have highly irregular nuclear contours, occasional prominent nuclei and dendrites that are more numerous and longer. Melanosome alterations are common, including melanosomal pleomorphism and melanin macroglobules.

The mechanism of development of PUVA lentigines is unknown and it has not been established if the melanocyte and keratinocyte abnormalities observed are a reversible effect of PUVA therapy and whether or not these lesions are potentially malignant. A precise follow-up of patients with PUVA lentigines is strongly recommended.

Melanocyte naevogenesis

Studies of melanocytic naevus prevalence have produced evidence implicating the sun in melanocyte naevogenesis. Melanocytic naevi are concentrated on skin surfaces that are exposed to the sun. These lesions are more common among migrants to sunnier climates than among native-born residents. Latitude of residence, and by implication ambient UVR, is strongly related to melanocytic naevus prevalence in Australian children.[35] Increased numbers of melanocytic naevi have been shown to be related to sunburn during childhood. Another study concludes that both acute and chronic exposure to sun is associated with the development of melanocytic naevi.[36] Strong epidemiological evidence supports the hypothesis that the frequency of melanocytic naevi is a good indicator of future development of melanoma. If this is so, the pattern of melanoma risk seems to be established very early in life in children living in sunny countries.

Several animal models of melanocytic naevus have been described, but most of them show a lack of solar-simulated light or UVR in induction protocols. Furthermore, the melanocytic naevi in animals arise from dermal melanocytes rather than the epidermal derivation found in humans. More recently, a guinea-pig model was shown to have some of the essential elements of human melanocytic naevus. Indeed, these naevi are augmented by solar-simulated light, are histologically similar, occupy the same level within the skin and have the same natural history as human naevi.[37]

Melanomagenesis

It is now well established that UVR from the sun is a causal factor in the aetiology of melanoma (Fig. 1.11).[38] Save for lentigo malignant melanoma,

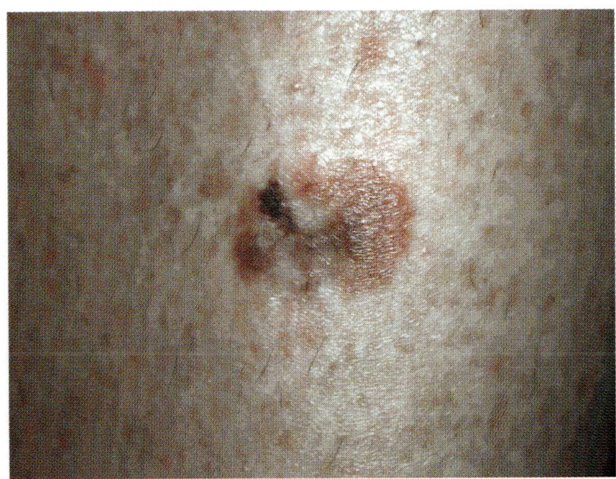

Figure 1.11

Superficial spreading melanoma surrounded by ephelides.

melanoma risk has been linked with intense intermittent exposure to solar radiation as opposed to chronic sun exposure, particularly in young children. The action spectrum for human melanoma itself is unknown. The only action spectrum published for melanoma has been established in the fish model xiphophorus.[39] This action spectrum has a relatively very large component in the UVA region (320–400 nm); however, these findings cannot easily be extrapolated to humans.

One of the most important known phenotypic risk factors for the development of melanoma is an increased total number of melanocytic naevi. Recent studies suggest that the number of melanocyte naevi that develop by the age of 20 years is influenced by cumulative sun exposure from birth as well as severe childhood sunburn and fair-skin phenotype. The melanoma should be preventable by a reduction in sun exposure and by a specific effort to avoid intermittent intense exposure, particularly in early childhood. Experimental support for epidemiological evidence that childhood sunburn is a significant risk of developing malignant melanoma has been reported recently.[40] In a genetically engineered mouse, in which a metallothionein gene promoter forces the overexpression of hepatocyte growth factor/scatter factor (HGF/SF), a single dose of burning UV radiation (UVA + UVB + UVC) to neonates, but not to adults, is necessary and sufficient to induce tumours with high penetrance. These tumours are reminiscent of human melanoma. The neonatal dose roughly corresponded to a sunburning dose of natural sunlight at mid-latitudes in mid-summer. In these irradiated HGF/SF transgenic mice the pigmented tumours were highly interactive with the epidermis and resembled those found in human melanomas. As in human melanomas, molecular analysis demonstrated frequent loss of the ink4a gene. Although it is difficult to extrapolate these observations to sunburn in children, because of striking differences in thickness between mouse and human skin, this animal model is consistent not only with a causal role between childhood sunburn and the development of melanomas, but also with possible promotion by subsequent UV exposure.

Based upon the photoprotective role of melanins, the induction of the capacity to repair DNA by UVR in human skin cells, including melanocytes, and the resistance of melanocytes to UV-induced apoptosis, an interesting hypothesis is that perhaps UV-induced melanomegenesis is not attributable simply to the cumulative dose but rather may be strongly influenced by the dose per exposure and by the pattern of the exposures.[41] In this model, melanocytes would survive, whether damaged extensively by intermittent high-dose exposure to UV radiation, when their melanin content and baseline capacity for DNA repair are low, or damaged slightly during frequent low-dose exposures to UV radiation, when their melanin content and induced capacity to repair DNA are high. Intermittent high-dose exposures are expected to give rise to more melanomas than to frequent low-dose exposures because of the low DNA repair capacity and retention of damaged cells. Thus, responses differ according to the intensity of exposure to UV radiation and whether the exposure occurs under baseline tissue conditions, after long periods of non-exposure, or during the temporary period of increased melanin content and increased DNA repair capacity induced by the most recent exposures.

In contrast with the other types of melanomas, the risk of lentigo maligna (LM), also called Hutchinson's melanotic freckles or Dubreuilh's melanosis, is linked to chronic sunlight exposure. LM is postulated to develop from an abnormal clone of intraepidermal melanocytes on sun-damaged skin. This lesion is commonly observed on the sun-exposed skin of the head and neck, particularly the face, with a predilection for the cheek, in elderly patients (Fig. 1.12).

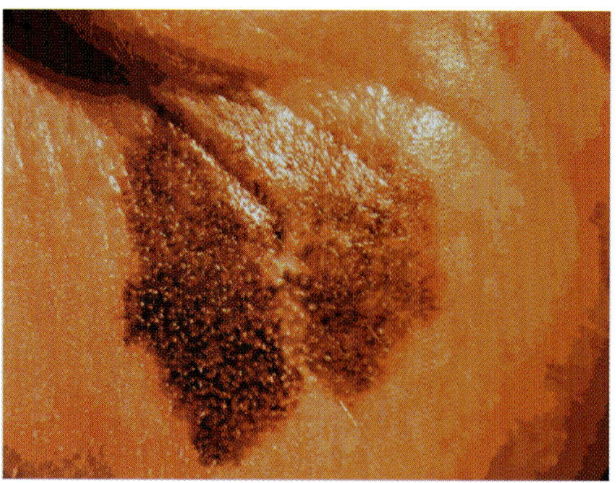

Figure 1.12

Dubreuilh's melanosis.

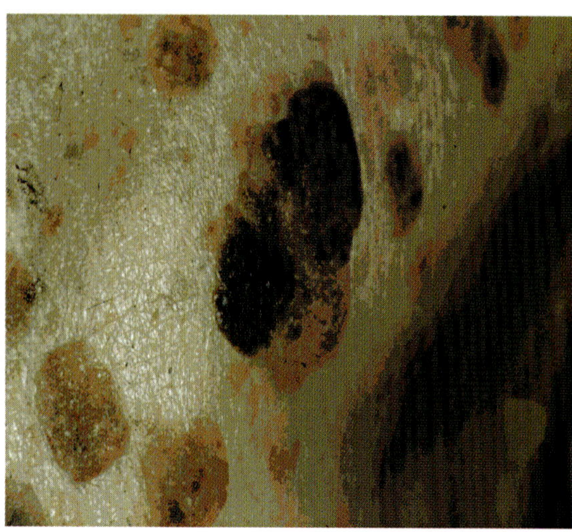

Figure 1.13

Seborrhoeic keratosis.

Benign and malignant pigmented skin epithelial tumours

Seborrhoeic keratoses (SKs) are common skin lesions (Fig. 1.13). They have been shown to occur with increasing age, usually appearing in the fifth decade of life. However, a recent survey demonstrated that SKs are also common lesions in people younger than 30 years. The possible association between sun exposure and SKs has been raised. SKs have a varying degree of melanin pigmentation. A recent study suggests an accentuated secretion of ET-1 by epidermal keratinocytes in SKs is responsible for the hyperpigmentary status of this benign neoplasm.[42]

Correlation between frequent low-dose exposures to sunlight that are cumulatively large over a lifetime and the risk of premalignant actinic keratoses, and non-melanoma skin cancers such as basal cell (BCC) and squamous cell (SCC) carcinomas is universally recognized. Among them, pigmented BCC are the most common, especially in North American black and Hispanic populations, and in Japanese. In these tumours, melanocytes are increased in numbers and interspersed between tumour cells. Most of these pigment cells are in the active phase of melanogenesis.[43] The implication of melanogenic and mitogenic factors in the induction of this increased number and activity of melanocytes is likely but remains to be demonstrated.

Regulation of melanogenesis

As mentioned above, under physiological conditions human skin pigmentation is increased by UVR of solar light. This effect of UV can also be observed in animals including the mouse, guinea pig and Yucatan swine (Chapter 26), and even in the hammerhead shark.[44] Sun-induced skin tanning and particularly delayed skin pigmentation play a key photoprotective role against the carcinogenic effect of UV. Hence, it is crucial to understand the mechanisms of UV-induced melanogenesis, *i.e.* the molecular process accounting for delayed skin tanning. Based on a large number of results and observations gathered in the course of studying UV-induced pigmentation, several hypotheses have been proposed to tentatively explain the melanogenic effect of UV.

Direct effects of UV on melanocytes

In cultured melanocytes or in S91 mouse melanoma cells, UVB radiation induces melanin neosynthesis, thus demonstrating that UV can act directly on melanocytes to induce melanogenesis. UV has been found to increase tyrosinase activity and expression.

One of the first hypotheses to explain this direct effect of UV involves the modification of membrane phospholipids that could activate phospholipase C, therefore releasing diacylglycerol (DAG) that in turn activates protein kinase C (PKC). Numerous observations have reinforced the implication of PKC in the regulation of melanogenesis. Indeed, the addition of oleylacetylglycerol (OAG) to cultured human melanocytes or S91 melanoma cells significantly increases their melanin content.[21,45] Further, OAG stimulates skin pigmentation in the guinea pig.[46] More recently, B. Gilchrest's group has shown that tyrosinase is phosphorylated through a PKC-dependent pathway and that overexpression of PKC-β into non-pigmented melanoma cells leads to the phosphorylation and activation of tyrosinase.[47] However, this hypothesis has not received unanimous approval since several reports have shown clearly that melanogenesis is not affected or even stimulated by the inhibition of PKC.[48]

Direct melanogenic effects of UVR on melanocytes might also involve the production of nitric oxide (NO). NO is a free radical gas synthesized, during the conversion of arginine into L-citrulline, by the enzyme NO synthase, and it is considered to be a major intracellular and intercellular messenger molecule. NO elicits its effects through the activation of a soluble guanylate cyclase, leading to an increase in intracellular cGMP content and the activation of the cGMP-dependent protein kinase. NO and cGMP have been involved in mediation of skin erythema induced by UVB. In human melanocytes, NO donors and cGMP analogues stimulate melanogenesis. Further, UV radiation increases both NO and cGMP production, and the effects of UV on melanogenesis can be blocked by both guanylate cyclase and NO synthase inhibitors.[49] These data strongly suggest that NO and cGMP production are required for UVB-induced melanogenesis.

Additionally, a new concept has emerged from the works of B. Gilchrest's group. These works suggest that DNA damage and DNA repair play a relevant role in the UV-induced melanogenic response on melanocytes. It is known that UV radiation induces DNA damage, mainly characterized by the production of DNA photoproducts such as cyclobutane dipyrimidine (CDP) that are subsequently excised by reparation enzymes. Eller and Gilchrest[50] have shown that thymidine dimers as well as DNA repair enzymes increase melanin content and tyrosinase activity in cultured melanocytes. Similarly, topical daily application of thymidine dinucleotides (for 5 days) to shaved guinea pigs, increased epidermal melanin content. Taken together, these data strengthen the hypothesis that UV light induces melanogenesis at least in part as a direct consequence of its effects on DNA. More recently, the same group has suggested that disruption of telomeres can lead to the stimulation of melanogenesis (Chapter 22).

Besides the suggested role of the above mentioned cellular messengers in melanogenesis, none seems to account for the entire UV melanogenic effects observed *in vivo*. Indeed, the direct melanogenic effects of UV on melanocytes appear to be weak, at least quite under the experimental conditions used so far, and no UV-induced increase in the melanocyte cell number has been observed. Several compelling data have suggested that physiological UV-induced melanocyte activation is the result of an indirect effect of UV through a paracrine regulation process involving keratinocytes.

Indirect effects of UV

Melanocytes cultivated in keratinocyte-conditioned media respond by increasing their growth, melanogenesis and dendricity.[51] These effects are enhanced by keratinocyte exposure to UVR, strongly suggesting that keratinocytes secrete specific factors responsible for melanocyte differentiation. Therefore, keratinocytes seem to be a key cellular component in the physiological tanning response.[52]

Among keratinocyte-secreted factors which induce melanocyte activation, we find prostaglandins PGE2,[53] αMSH and ACTH (Chapters 11 and 12),[54] ET-1,[55, 56] and NO.[49] αMSH, ACTH and PGE2 activate the cAMP pathway in melanocytes, while NO activates the cGMP-dependent signaling events. On the other hand, in response to UV, keratinocytes secrete specific factors that inhibit melanogenesis such as IL-1α, Swope,[56a] tumour necrosis factor-α (TNF-α),[57] interferons[58] and basic fibroblast growth factor (bFGF).[59] The balance between these keratinocyte factors allows a fine-tuning of melanocyte growth and differentiation, thereby controlling skin pigmentation (Fig. 1.14).

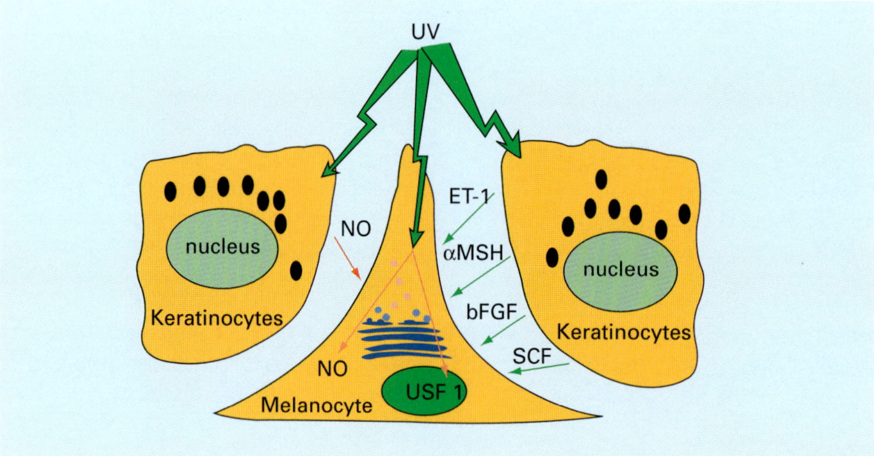

Figure 1.14

Direct and indirect effects of UV on melanogenesis.

Cellular and molecular aspects of skin tanning

Skin tanning involves several cellular processes that allow normal skin pigmentation and the alteration in one of these processes can result in pigmentation defect. Some of these processes are regulated during sun-induced skin tanning. Indeed, UVR of solar light stimulates melanocyte growth and dendricity, and increases melanin synthesis. Melanins are synthesized in specialized intracellular vesicles named melanosomes that are transported to the dendrite tips, and are then transferred to the surrounding keratinocytes to give a uniform skin pigmentation (Fig. 1.15). Although UVR has not been reported to regulate melanosome biogenesis or transport, these steps play a pivotal role in the control of skin pigmentation. Indeed, mutations in genes involved in melanosome biogenesis or transport have been associated with pigmentation disorders found in Hermansky–Pudlak and Griscelli syndromes, respectively. The molecular actors involved in these processes are listed in Table 1.1.

Increased number of active melanocytes

Artificial UV or sun exposure of normal skin is followed by an increase in the number of DOPA-positive epidermal melanocytes (Fig. 1.16).[17,60–62] A similar phenomenon is also observed in laboratory animals. Indeed, this increase in the DOPA-positive melanocyte number may result from: (1) proliferation of pre-existing melanocytes, (2) activation of existing dormant melanocytes with little or no DOPA reactivity, (3) differentiation from melanocyte precursors, and (4) other possibilities such as migration of dermal and/or follicular melanocytes. Pigmented rodents have been used to clarify the cellular mechanisms underlying this biological effect. Several of these studies showed that epidermal melanocytes have mitotic activity and are capable of proliferating in humans and mice. Indeed, mitotic activity of epidermal melanocytes has been observed on the back of UV-irradiated hairless mice.[63] Counting thymidine-labelled DOPA-positive melanocytes after UV irradiation in mice demonstrated that a small proportion of melanocytes divide. Epidermal melanocytes of mice ears exposed to repeated UVB irradiation began to increase 2 days after the first exposure and reached almost saturation at about 14 days.[64] These observations suggest that the UV-induced increase in the number of DOPA-positive epidermal melanocytes is partially due to mitosis. UVB has been demonstrated to act as an independent mitogen for normal human melanocytes in culture,[65] suggesting that melanocyte proliferation results from a direct effect of UVB. A number of investigations have illustrated

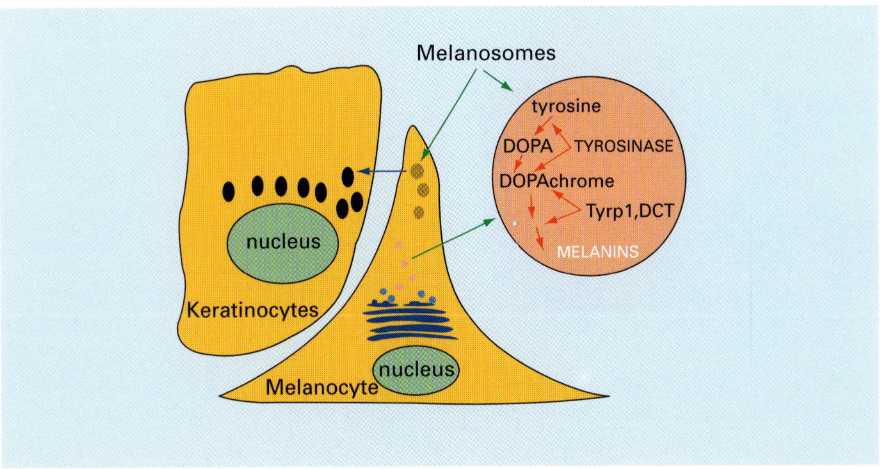

Figure 1.15

Cellular aspects of delayed skin tanning.

Table 1.1 List of the molecular actors involved in the regulation of delayed skin pigmentation.

Growth Factors	*Dendricity*	*Melanosome Transport*	*Melanogenesis*
• bFGF • HGF • SCF • Endothelin-1, -3	• Actin stress fibres • Rho small GTPase • ROCK • Rac	Proximal transport • Tubulin • Kinesin • Dynein	Signaling • PKA • MAPK • P13K, p70S6K, AKT, GSK3
		Distal docking • Myosin Va • Rab27a • Melanophilin	Transcription factors • MITF • SOX10, PAX3 • LEF1, CREB
			Melanin synthesis • Tyrosinase, DCTTrp1 • P, Aim-1

the importance of paracrine control of melanocyte homeostasis by epidermal keratinocytes through UV-induced production and secretion of melanocyte melanogenic factors. ET-1, a potent vasoconstrictive peptide, is also a strong mitogen and melanogen for human melanocytes in culture.[19,66] UVB exposure stimulates autocrine production of ET-1 through IL-1α secretion in keratinocytes. These observations strongly suggest the involvement of ET-1 in the induction of melanocyte proliferation in UVB-induced pigmentation of human skin. Stem cell factor (SCF) has also been reported to stimulate the proliferation of human melanocytes in culture.[19] Recent findings suggest that SCF/c-kit signalling is also involved in the biological mechanism of UVB pigmentation as a mitogen and as a melanogen for human melanocytes.[67] ET-1 may synergistically activate melanocyte functions, probably through the crosstalk mechanisms in the signaling pathway with SCF.[68] Other keratinocyte-derived cytokines that have been documented to be upregulated following UVB irradiation and that can act as melanocyte mitogens include bFGF[69] and αMSH.[70]

The few studies including a quantitative technique to evaluate melanocyte proliferation

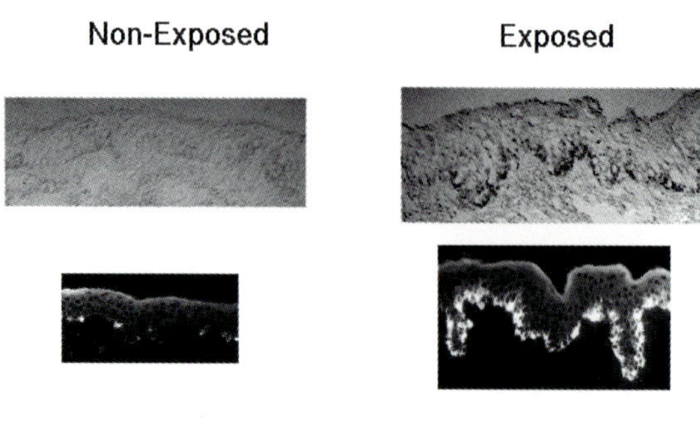

Figure 1.16

UVR increases the number of active melanocytes in human epidermis. Upper panels. Direct light. Note the increase in melanin amount in melanocytes and keratinocytes. Lower panels. Immunofluorescence labelling with anti-Tyrp-1 antibody.

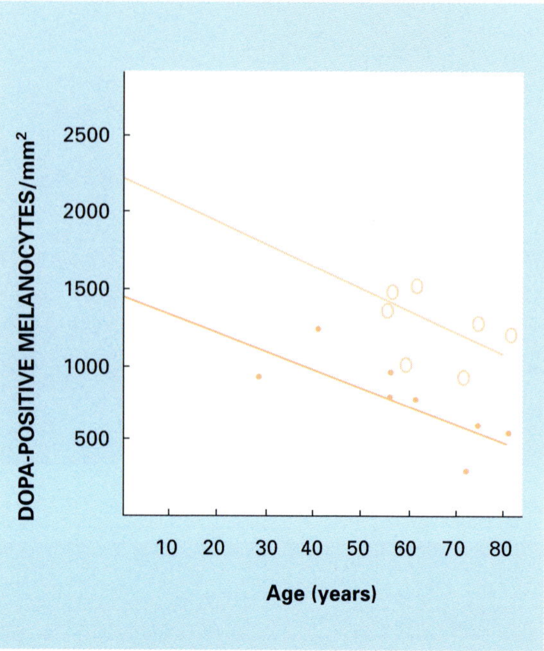

Figure 1.17

Relationship between age and melanocyte density in non-exposed skin (closed dots) and chronically sun-exposed skin (open dots). (Reproduced from B. Gilchrest et al., *J Invest Dermatol* 1979; 79:141–3.)

demonstrated that only a small number of melanocytes divide after UV exposure. The observation that melanocyte proliferation contributes only partially to the increase in the number of DOPA-positive epidermal melanocytes following UV irradiation suggests that other biological mechanisms are involved in this process. Furthermore, a number of investigations indicated that UV irradiation has inhibitory effects on the proliferation of terminally differentiated melanocytes.[71] Although the number of DOPA-positive melanocytes in human skin decreases with age,[72,73] melanocyte density is approximately twofold higher in chronically sun-exposed skin than in protected skin at all ages (Fig. 1.17).[74] This suggests that the principal effect of chronic exposure to the sun on human epidermal melanocytes is not premature ageing but activation and/or proliferation of the exposed melanocytes. The higher numbers of epidermal melanocytes in sun-exposed human skin may be explained by repeated UV exposure irreversibly increasing the number of DOPA-positive melanocytes. On unexposed areas of skin of older subjects, epidermal melanocytes keep their proliferative capacity. Indeed, repeated UV irradiation of non-exposed melanocytes increases the number of melanocytes, even in older subjects.

Recently, the existence of melanocyte precursors in normal skin has been described immunohistochemically in mice. These melanocyte precursors express the kit receptor. A reservoir of these precursors has been described in the lower half of the follicular infundibulum in normal human skin.[75] A recent study in mice demonstrated that these c-kit+ melanocyte precursors, as well Tyrp1+ cells, reside in normal epidermis.[76] kit+ Cells are non-melanotic and DOPA-positive or Tyrp1+ cells in normal murine epidermis are fully differentiated, mature melanocytes. These precursor cells that reside in the skin first differentiate into Mitf+ and DCT+ Tyrp2+ melanocytes by activation of the kit receptor, and then become mature Tyrp1+ melanocytes after UVB exposure.[76] These observations strongly suggest that proliferation of the c-kit+ cells contribute to the UV-induced melanocytogenesis as melanocyte precursors (Fig. 1.18). It remains to be demonstrated that this hypothetical schema of melanocyte proliferation caused by UV exposure also occurs in human skin.

These peptides, which increase the number of active melanocytes, probably act through the

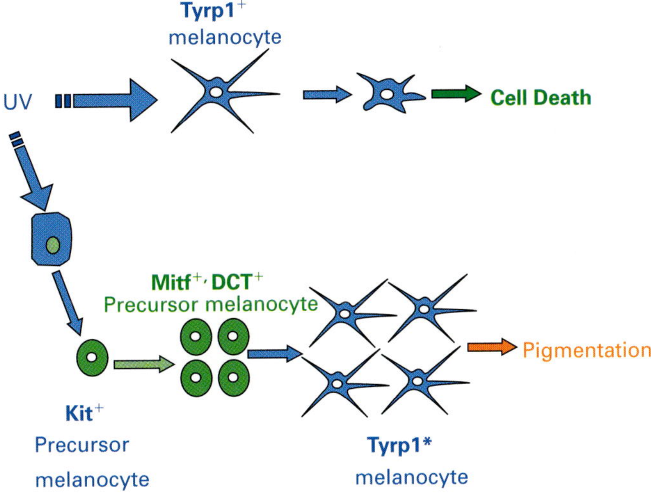

Figure 1.18

Proposed process of UV-induced melanogenesis. (Reproduced from Kawaguchi et al., *J Invest Dermatol* 2001: 116:920–5.)

activation of MAP kinase[77] or PI3 kinase[78] pathways to exert their mitogenic effects. Interestingly, αMSH stimulates p21Ras and ERK, in melanocytes (Chapter 15). The activation of the MAP kinase pathway could explain the mitogenic effects of αMSH on melanocytes.

Melanocyte dendricity

Melanocyte dendricity also plays a pivotal role in skin pigmentation, since dendrites allow the transport and transfer of melanosomes to keratinocytes. In melanocytes, previous studies have shown the involvement of microtubule and actin microfilament networks. *In vitro*, αMSH and cAMP elevating agents strongly stimulate dendricity in melanocyte and melanoma cells. This effect is mediated through the inhibition of the small GTPase, RhoA, and of its target p160 Rho kinase that leads to the disorganization of actin stress fibres and allows dendrite outgrowth.[79] Other small GTPase, *e.g.* RhoG[80] and Rac1,[81] have been involved in dendrite growth in neuronal cells. Interestingly, these GTPase are activated by UV[82] and could participate in UV-induced dendricity.

Melanosome biogenesis, transport and transfer

Melanin synthesis takes place in specialized intracellular vesicles called melanosomes. Melanosomes constitute an integrated system of melanin synthesis, transport and transfer. They are unique organelles related to lysosomes that arise from the early endosomal compartment. Premelanosome, or stage I melanosome, contains Pmel17, the earliest melanosome-specific marker.[83] Tyrosinase and Tyrp1 are targeted from the trans-Golgi network through an adaptator-mediated process that involves the AP3 complex (Chapter 17). Tyrosinase, Tyrp1 and probably DCT are present in stage II melanosomes that contain all the machinery to synthesize melanin.[83] However, additional melanosome-specific proteins such as the P protein[84] and AIM-1[85] play a key role in the regulation of melanogenesis by controlling melanosome pH or mistargeting to lysosomes.

Melanosomes allow the storage and concentration of melanin in impermeable compartments to avoid the toxicity of melanin or of its precursor. Melanosomes are transported to the melanocyte dendrite tips by a biphasic process that involves a ubiquitous long-range transport and a specific short-range transport. The long-range transport is dependent on microtubules and on the molecular motor dynein and kinesin.[86, 87] The short-range transport allows the docking of melanosome to the dendrite tips. Three recently identified proteins, myosin Va, Rab27a and melanophilin, have been involved in this process (Fig. 1.19) (Chapters 18 and 19). Once accumulated at the dendrite tips, melanosomes are transferred to keratinocytes by still undisclosed molecular mechanisms. However, the protease-activated receptor (PAR2) seems to play a role in this process since PAR2 antagonist blocks melanosome transfer and skin pigmentation (Chapter 20). Interestingly, recently it has been shown that the capture of melanosomes by keratinocytes is stimulated by UV and by αMSH.[88]

Transcriptional regulation of melanogenesis enzyme expression

Melanin synthesis is the result of an enzymatic cascade that converts tyrosine to melanin. The expression of tyrosinase, Tyrp1 and DCT, the enzymes that control this process, are tightly regulated during melanocyte differentiation. The complex molecular network that controls the expression of these enzymes upon αMSH stimulation has been thoroughly dissected.

αMSH binds to the MC1R gene. MC1R is coupled to Gαs and activates adenylate cyclase, thereby increasing the intracellular cAMP content. cAMP activates PKA, and PKA phosphorylates and activates CREB which, when activated, binds to the CRE site present in the *MITF* promoter, thereby upregulating its transcription. The increase in MITF expression leads to an augmented MITF binding to the E-box and M-box present in the *tyrosinase* promoter, resulting in an increased tyrosinase expression and the upregulation of melanin synthesis (Chapter 14).

MITF is a basic helix-loop-helix transcription factor containing a leucin-zipper domain involved in melanocyte development and survival (Chapter 4). Indeed, MITF mutations have been detected in patients with type 2 Waardenburg syndrome (WS2A) that presents pigmentary defects in skin, eyes and hair, as well as auditive alterations. More recently, USF1, a transcription factor which shares a significant structural homology with MITF, has been implicated in the stimulation of tyrosinase expression by UVR. Upon UV exposure, USF1 is phosphorylated by the stress-activated kinase p38 (Chapter 10). Then USF1 is able to bind the M-box

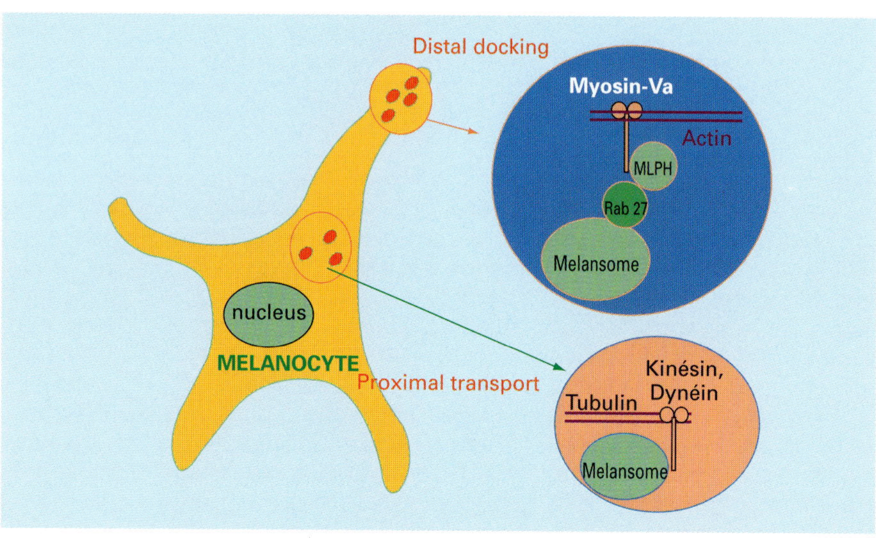

Figure 1.19

Biphasic melanosome transport in melanocytes.

motif of the tyrosinase promoter and to stimulate tyrosinase expression.[89] Thus, the stimulation of melanogenesis gene expression after solar light exposure could be mediated by at least two different transcription factors that act on the same DNA target sequences.

Of note, melanogenic gene expression can be regulated by other transcription factors (Chapter 7). It has been shown that BRN2, a class III POU-domain protein, can inhibit *tyrosinase* promoter activity, probably by competing with MITF binding to the M-box.[90] Recently, TFE3 and TFEB have been reported to stimulate tyrosinase and *Tyrp-1* promoter activities. Brachyury-related transcription factor TBX2 has been shown to inhibit *Tyrp-1* promoter activity through interaction with melanocyte-specific elements.[91] The same element also binds PAX3, a transcription factor containing an homeodomain and a paired domain, encoded by the *Splotch* locus.[92] In humans, PAX3 has been found to be mutated in patients with WS-1 and -3 in which pigmentation defects can be observed. PAX3 binding to these melanocyte-specific elements upregulates *Tyrp-1* promoter activity. The effect of UVR on these transcription factors has not been studied so far.

Regulation of MITF expression

As discussed above, MITF expression is restricted to specific cell types and tissues. The nature of this tissue specificity strongly suggests the existence of specific microphthalmia regulatory partners within the melanocyte lineage. Among the putative candidate molecules, the transcription factors PAX3 and SOX10 have been proposed, since mutations in these factors result, as in the case of MITF mutations, in disruption of neural-crest-derived melanocyte development in mice and humans.[93,94] However, PAX3 is expressed earlier than MITF in the neural crest where melanocytes originate, suggesting that this factor could be susceptible to regulate MITF expression. Watanabe et al.[95] have shown that PAX3 binds and transactivates the MITF promoter and that mutant PAX3 proteins, reproducing the mutations found in WS1 patients, fail to recognize and transactivate the MITF promoter.

SOX10 is a transcription factor expressed in the neural crest at very early stages of embryonic development.[96] *SOX10* mutations in humans are responsible for the WS4, in part characterized by pigmentary defects.[94]

SOX10 has been shown to increase *MITF* promoter activity (Chapter 8). Coexpression of SOX10 and PAX3 has demonstrated a strong activation of *MITF* promoter activity much above the activation induced by PAX3 or SOX10 alone, suggesting a possible synergistic relationship between the action of such factors on MITF expression. A SOX10 deletion construct, corresponding to a mutation found in WS4 patients, blocks SOX10 induction of *MITF* promoter activity, revealing a dominant negative effect of the mutant and the relevant role of SOX10 in MITF expression. These studies indicate that SOX10 and PAX3 function upstream of MITF in the neural crest melanocyte developmental pathway. Further, Wnt-3a, through the transcription factor LEF-1, regulates MITF expression (Chapter 9), and more recently the cut-homeodomain transcription factor Onecut-2 has been shown to bind to the MITF promoter and to stimulate its activity.[97] Finally, MITF is subjected to post-transcriptional regulations such as phosphorylation and ubiquitination that control its stability and activity (Chapter 6).

Conclusions

The dissection of signaling pathways involved in UV-and αMSH-induced melanogenesis is summarized in Figure 1.20. New advances in this direction should help, in the near future, in the development of new treatments for pigmentary disorders. Given the photoprotective role of eumelanins, a better understanding of the mechanisms regulating melanin synthesis could lead to the discovery of topical melanogens inducing melanin production in the absence of UV irradiation, known to induce photoageing and skin cancers.

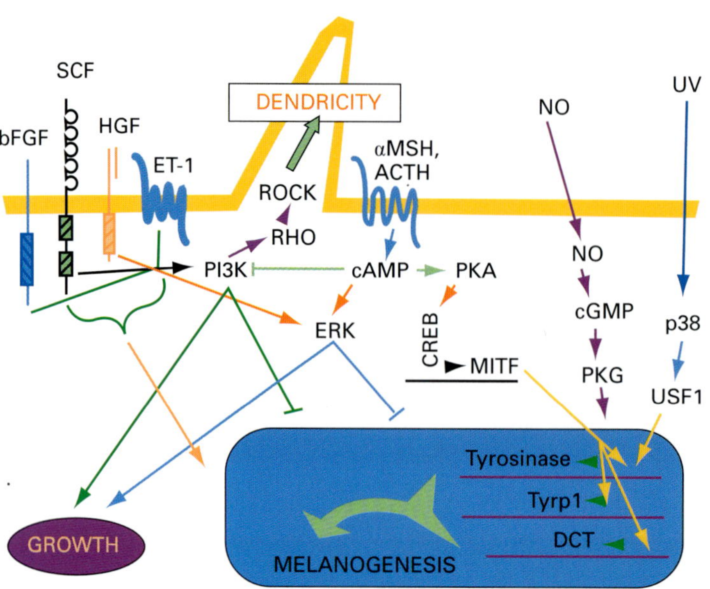

Figure 1.20

Summary of the molecular mechanisms involved in the regulation of melanocyte proliferation and differentiation.

References

1. Le Douarin N, *The Neural Crest*, Cambridge: Cambridge University Press (1982).
2. Hearing VJ, Tsukamoto K, Enzymatic control of pigmentation in mammals, *FASEB* J (1991) **5**:2902–9.
3. Thody AJ, Higgins EM, Wakamatsu K et al., Pheomelanin as well as eumelanin is present in human epidermis, *J Invest Dermatol* (1991) **97**:340–4.
4. Ortonne JP, Marks R, *Photodamaged Skin: Clinical Signs, Causes and Management,* London: Martin Dunitz (1991).
5. Quevedo WCJ, Fitzpatrick TB, Pathak MA, Jimbow K, *Sunlight and Man*, Tokyo: University of Tokyo Press (1974) 165–94.
6. Agin PP, Desrochers DL, Sayre RM, The relationship of immediate pigment darkening to minimal erythemal dose, skin type and eye color, *Photodermatol* (1985) **2**:288–94.
7. Jimbow K, Pathak MA, Fitzpatrick TB, Effect of ultraviolet on the distribution pattern of microfilaments and microtubules and on the nucleus in human melanocytes, *Yale J Biol Med* (1973) **46**:411–26.
8. Jimbow K, Fitzpatrick TB, Changes in distribution pattern of cytoplasmic filaments in human melanocytes during ultraviolet-mediated melanin pigmentation. The role of the 100-Angstrom filaments in the elongation of melanocytic dendrites and in the movement and transfer of melanosomes, *J Cell Biol* (1975) **65**:481–8.
9. Beitner H, Wennersten G, A qualitative and quantitative transmission electronmicroscopic study of the immediate pigment darkening reaction, *Photodermatol* (1985) **2**:273–8
10. Honigsmann H, Schuler G, Aberer W et al., Immediate pigment darkening phenomenon. A reevaluation of its mechanisms, *J Invest Dermatol* (1986) **87**:648–52.
11. Pathak MA, Stratton K, Free radicals in human skin before and after exposure to light, *Arch Biochem Biophys* (1968) **123**:468–76.
12. Sawamura D, Sato S, Kiuchi H et al., UVA induced darkening of lower epidermal cells as an in vitro system of immediate pigment darkening (IPD) and mechanisms of IPD, *J Dermatol* (1986) **13**:101–7.
13. Routaboul C, Denis A, Vinche A, Immediate pigment darkening: description, kinetic and biological function, *Eur J Dermatol* (1999) **9**:95–9.
14. Beitner H, The effect of high dose long-wave ultraviolet radiation (UVA) on epidermal melanocytes in

human skin: a transmission electron microscopic study, *Photoimmunol Photomed* (1986) **3**:133–9.
15. Fitzpatrick T, Ultraviolet induced pigmentary changes: benefits and hazards, *Curr Probl Dermatol* (1986) **15**:25–38.
16. Alaluf S, Heath A, Carter N et al., Variation in melanin content and composition in type V and VI photoexposed and photoprotected human skin: the dominant tole of DHI, *Pigment Cell Res* (2001) **14**:337–47.
17. Rosen CF, Seki Y, Farinelli W et al., A comparison of the melanocyte response to narrow band UVA and UVB exposure *in vivo*, *J Invest Dermatol* (1987) **88**:774–9.
18. Duval C, Régnier M, Schmidt R, Distinct melanogenic response of human melanocytes in mono-culture, in co-culture with keratinocytes and in reconstructed epidermis, to UV exposure, *Pigment Cell Res* (2001) **14**:348–55.
19. Imokawa G, Yada Y, Kimura M, Signalling mechanisms of endothelin-induced mitogenesis and melanogenesis in human melanocytes, *Biochem J* (1996) **314**(Pt 1):305–12.
20. Young AR, Potten CS, Nikaido O et al., Human melanocytes and keratinocytes exposed to UVB or UVA in vivo show comparable levels of thymine dimers, *J Invest Dermatol* (1998) **111**:936–40.
21. Gilchrest BA, Park HY, Eller MS, Yaar M, Mechanisms of ultraviolet light-induced pigmentation, *Photochem Photobiol* (1996) **93**:1–10.
22. Keong CH, Kurumaji Y, Nishioka K, A quantitative study of the interaction of ultraviolet A and ultraviolet B in producing delayed pigmentation, *Photodermatol Photoimmunol Photomed* (1990) **7**:237–42.
23. Porges SB, Kaidbey KH, Grove GL, Quantification of visible light-induced melanogenesis in human skin, *Photodermatology* (1988) **5**:197–200.
24. Breathnach AS, Nazzaro-Porro M, Passi S, Picardo M, Ultrastructure of melanocytes in chronically sun-exposed skin of elderly subjects, *Pigment Cell Res* (1991) **4**:71–9.
25. Breathnach AS, Melanocyte distribution in forearm epidermis of freckled human subjects, *J Invest Dermatol* (1957) 253–61.
26. Breathnach AS, Electron microscopy of melanocytes and melanosomes in freckled human epidermis, *J Invest Dermatol* (1963) 389–94.
27. Bastiaens M, Huurne J, Gruis N, The melanocortin-l-receptor gene is the major freckle gene, *Hum Mol Genet* (2001) **10**:1701–8.
28. Gabe C, Buttener P, Weib J, Associated factors in the prevalence of more than 50 common melanocytic naevi, atypical melanocytic naevi and actinic lentigines: multicenter case–control study of the central malignant melanoma registry of the German Dermatological Society, *J Invest Dermatol* (1994) **102**:700–5.
29. Nakagawa H, Rhodes AR, Momtaz TK, Fitzpatrick TB, Morphologic alterations of epidermal melanocytes and melanosomes in PUVA lentigines: a comparative ultrastructural investigation of lentigines induced by PUVA and sunlight, *J Invest Dermatol* (1984) **82**:101–7.
30. Kadono S, Manaka I, Kawashima M et al., The role of the epidermal endothelin cascade in the hyperpigmentation mechanism of lentigo senilis, *J Invest Dermatol* (2001) **116**:571–7.
31. Naganumaa M, Yagi E, Fukuda M, Delayed induction of pigmented spots on UVB-irradiated hairless mice, *J Dermatol Sci* (2001) **25**:29–35.
32. Salisbury JR, Williams H, du Vivier AW, Tanning-bed lentigines: ultrastructural and histopathologic features, *J Am Acad Dermatol* (1989) **21**(4 Pt 1): 689–93.
33. Rhodes AR, Harrist TJ, Momtaz TK, The PUVA-induced pigmented macule: a lentiginous proliferation of large, sometimes cytologically atypical, melanocytes, *J Am Acad Dermatol* (1983) **9**:47–58.
34. Roth DE, Hodge SJ, Callen JP, Possible ultraviolet A-induced lentigines: a side effect of chronic tanning salon usage, *J Am Acad Dermatol* (1989) **20**(5 Pt 2):950–4.
35. Kelly JW, Rivers JK, MacLennan R et al., Sunlight: a major factor associated with the development of melanocytic naevi in Australian schoolchildren, *J Am Acad Dermatol* (1994) **30**:40–8.
36. Harrison S, MacLennan R, Speare R, Wronski I, Sun exposure and melanocytic naevi in young Australian children, *Lancet* (1994) **344**:1529–32.
37. Menzies S, Khalil M, Crotty K, Bonin A, The augmentation of melanocytic naevi in guinea pigs by solar-simulated light: an animal model for human melanocytic naevi, *Cancer Res* (1998) **58**:5361–6.
38. Whiteman DC, Green AC, Melanoma and sun exposure: where are we now? *Int J Dermatol* (1999) **38**:481–9.
39. Setlow RB, Woodhead AD, Temporal changes in the incidence of malignant melanoma: explanation from action spectra, *Mutat Res* (1994) **307**:365–74.
40. Noonan FP, Recio JA, Takayama H et al., Neonatal sunburn and melanoma in mice, *Nature* (2001) **413**:271–2.

41. Gilchrest BA, Eller MS, Geller AC, Yaar M, The pathogenesis of melanoma induced by ultraviolet radiation, *N Engl J Med* (1999) **340**:1341–8.
42. Teraki E, Tajima S, Manaka I et al., Role of endothelin-1 in hyperpigmentation in seborrhoeic keratosis, *Br J Dermatol* (1996) **135**:918–23.
43. Lao LM, Kumakiri M, Kiyohara T et al., Subpopulations of melanocytes in pigmented basal cell carcinoma: a quantitative, ultrastructural investigation,) *J Cutan Pathol* (2001) **28**:34–43.
44. Lowe C, Goodman-Lowe G, Suntanning in hammerhead sharks, *Nature* (1996) **383**:677.
45. Friedmann PS, Wren F, Buffey J, Macneil S, Alpha-MSH causes a small rise in cAMP but has no effect on basal or ultraviolet-stimulated melanogenesis in human melanocytes, *Br J Dermatol* (1990) **123**:145–51.
46. Allan AE, Archambault M, Messana E, Gilchrest BA, Topically applied diacylglycerols increase pigmentation in guinea pig skin, *J Invest Dermatol* (1995) **105**:687–92.
47. Park HY, Perez JM, Laursen R et al., Protein kinase C-beta activates tyrosinase by phosphorylating serine residues in its cytoplasmic domain, *J Biol Chem* (1999) **274**:16470–8.
48. Bertolotto C, Bille K, Ortonne JP, Ballotti R, In B16 melanoma cells, the inhibition of melanogenesis by TPA results from PKC activation and diminution of microphthalmia binding to the M-box of the tyrosinase promoter, *Oncogene* (1998) **16**:1665–70.
49. Romero-Graillet C, Aberdam E, Biagoli N et al., Ultraviolet B radiation acts through the nitric oxide and cGMP signal transduction pathway to stimulate melanogenesis in human melanocytes, *J Biol Chem* (1996) **271**:28052–6.
50. Eller MS, Gilchrest BA, Tanning as part of the eukaryotic SOS response, *Pigment Cell Res* (2000) **13**(Suppl 8):94–7.
51. Romero-Graillet C, Aberdam E, Clement M et al., Nitric oxide produced by ultraviolet-irradiated keratinocytes stimulates melanogenesis, *J Clin Invest* (1997) **99**:635–42.
52. Gordon PR, Mansur CP, Gilchrest BA, Regulation of human melanocyte growth, dendricity, and melanization by keratinocyte derived factors, *J Invest Dermatol* (1989) **92**:565–72.
53. Abdel-Malek ZA, Swope VB, Amornsiripanitch N, Nordlund JJ, *In vitro* modulation of proliferation and melanization of S91 melanoma cells by prostaglandins, *Cancer Res* (1987) **47**:3141–6.
54. Hunt G, Todd C, Cresswell JE, Thody AJ, Alpha-melanocyte stimulating hormone and its analogue Nle4DPhe7 alpha-MSH affect morphology, tyrosinase activity and melanogenesis in cultured human melanocytes, *J Cell Sci* (1994) **107**(Pt 1): 205–11.
55. Hara M, Yaar M, Gilchrest BA, Endothelin-1 of keratinocyte origin is a mediator of melanocyte dendricity, *J Invest Dermatol* (1995) **105**:744–8.
56. Yohn JJ, Smith C, Stevens T et al., Autoregulation of endothelin-1 secretion by cultured human keratinocytes via the endothelin B receptor, *Biochim Biophys Acta* (1994) **1224**:454–8.

56a. Swope VB, Abdel-Malek Z, Sauder DN, Nordlund JT, A new role for epidermal cell-derived thymocyte activating factor IL-1 as an agonist for distinct epidermal cell function, *J Immunol* (1989) **142**:1943–9.

57. Kock A, Schwarz T, Micksche M, Luger TA, Cytokines and human malignant melanoma. Immuno- and growth-regulatory peptides in melanoma biology, *Cancer Treat Res* (1991) **54**:41–66.
58. Kameyama K, Tanaka S, Ishida Y, Hearing VJ, Interferons modulate the expression of hormone receptors on the surface of murine melanoma cells, *J Clin Invest* (1989) **83**:213–21.
59. Halaban R, Langdon R, Birchall N et al., Basic fibroblast growth factor from human keratinocytes is a natural mitogen for melanocytes, *J Cell Biol* (1988) **107**:1611–19.
60. Imokawa G, Kawai M, Mishima Y, Motegi I, Differential analysis of experimental hypermelanosis induced by UVB, PUVA, and allergic contact dermatitis using a brownish guinea pig model, *Arch Dermatol Res* (1986) **278**:352–62.
61. Jimbow K, Uesugi T, New melanogenesis and photobiological processes in activation and proliferation of precursor melanocytes after UV-exposure: ultrastructural differentiation of precursor melanocytes from Langerhans cells, *J Invest Dermatol* (1982) **78**:108–15.
62. Quevedo WC, Jr, Szabo G, Virks J, Sinesi SJ, Melanocyte populations in UV-irradiated human skin, *J Invest Dermatol* (1965) **45**:295–8.
63. Sato T, Kawada A, Uptake of tritiated thymidine by epidermal melanocytes of hairless mice during ultraviolet light radiation, *J Invest Dermatol* (1972) **58**:71–3.
64. Rosdahl IK, Szabo G, Mitotic activity of epidermal melanocytes in UV-irradiated mouse skin, *J Invest Dermatol* (1978) **70**:143–8.
65. Libow LF, Scheide S, DeLeo VA, Ultraviolet radiation acts as an independent mitogen for normal human melanocytes in culture, *Pigment Cell Res* (1988) **1**:397–401.

66. Imokawa G, Kobayashi T, Miyagishi M et al., The role of endothelin-1 in epidermal hyperpigmentation and signaling mechanisms of mitogenesis and melanogenesis, *Pigment Cell Res* (1997) **10**:218–28.
67. Hachiya A, Kobayashi A, Ohuchi A et al., The paracrine role of stem cell factor/c-kit signaling in the activation of human melanocytes in ultraviolet-B-induced pigmentation, *J Invest Dermatol* (2001) **116**:578–86.
68. Imokawa G, Kobayasi T, Miyagishi M, Intracellular signaling mechanisms leading to synergistic effects of endothelin-1 and stem cell factor on proliferation of cultured human melanocytes. Cross-talk via trans-activation of the tyrosine kinase c- kit receptor, *J Biol Chem* (2000) **275**:33321–8.
69. Halaban R, Langdon R, Birchall N et al., Paracrine stimulation of melanocytes by keratinocytes through basic fibroblast growth factor, *Ann NY Acad Sci* (1988) **548**:180–90.
70. Abdel-Malek Z, Swope VB, Suzuki I et al., Mitogenic and melanogenic stimulation of normal human melanocytes by melanotropic peptides, *Proc Natl Acad Sci USA* (1995) **92**:1789–93.
71. Medrano EE, Im S, Yang F, Abdel-Malek ZA, Ultraviolet B light induces G1 arrest in human melanocytes by prolonged inhibition of retinoblastoma protein phosphorylation associated with long-term expression of the p21Waf-1/SDI-1/Cip-1 protein, *Cancer Res* (1995) **55**:4047–52.
72. Quevedo WC, Szabo G, Virks J, Influence of age and UV on the populations of dopa-positive melanocytes in human skin, *J Invest Dermatol* (1969) **52**:287–90.
73. Snell RS, Bischitz PG, The melanocytes and melanin in human abdominal wall skin: a survey made at different ages in both sexes and during pregnancy, *J Anat* (1963) **97**:361–76.
74. Gilchrest BA, Blog FB, Szabo G, Effects of aging and chronic sun exposure on melanocytes in human skin, *J Invest Dermatol* (1979) **73**:141–3.
75. Grichnik JM, Ali WN, Burch JA et al., KIT expression reveals a population of precursor melanocytes in human skin, *J Invest Dermatol* (1996) **106**:967–71.
76. Kawaguchi Y, Mori N, Nakayama A, Kit(+) melanocytes seem to contribute to melanocyte proliferation after UV exposure as precursor cells, *J Invest Dermatol* (2001) **116**:920–5.
77. Swope VB, Medrano EE, Smalara D, Abdel-Malek ZA, Long-term proliferation of human melanocytes is supported by the physiologic mitogens alpha-melanotropin, endothelin-1, and basic fibroblast growth factor, *Exp Cell Res* (1995) **217**:453–9.
78. Suzuki E, Nagata D, Kakoki M et al., Molecular mechanisms of endothelin-1–induced cell-cycle progression: involvement of extracellular signal-regulated kinase, protein kinase C, and phosphatidylinositol 3-kinase at distinct points, *Circ Res* (1999) **84**:611–19.
79. Busca R, Bertolotto C, Abbe P et al., Inhibition of Rho is required for cAMP-induced melanoma cell differentiation, *Mol Biol Cell* (1998) **9**:1367–78.
80. Katoh H, Yasui H, Yamaguchi Y et al., Small GTPase RhoG is a key regulator for neurite outgrowth in PC12 cells, *Mol Cell Biol* (2000) **20**:7378–87.
81. Scott GA, Cassidy L, Rac1 mediates dendrite formation in response to melanocyte stimulating hormone and ultraviolet light in a murine melanoma model, *J Invest Dermatol* (1998) **111**:243–50.
82. Fritz G, Kaina B, RhoB encoding a UV-inducible Ras-related small GTP-binding protein is regulated by GTPases of the Rho family and independent of JNK, ERK, and p38 MAP kinase, *J Biol Chem* (1997) **272**:30637–44.
83. Raposo G, Tenza D, Murphy DM et al., Distinct protein sorting and localization to premelanosomes, melanosomes, and lysosomes in pigmented melanocytic cells, *J Cell Biol* (2001) **152**:809–24.
84. Ancans J, Hoogduijn MJ, Thody AJ, Melanosomal pH, pink locus protein and their roles in melanogenesis, *J Invest Dermatol* (2001) **117**:158–9.
85. Du J, Fisher DE, Identification of Aim-1 as the underwhite mouse mutant and its transcriptional regulation by MITF, *J Biol Chem* (2002) **277**:402–6.
86. Hara M, Yaar M, Byers HR et al., Kinesin participates in melanosomal movement along melanocyte dendrites, *J Invest Dermatol* (2000) **114**:438–43.
87. Byers HR, Yaar M, Eller MS et al., Role of cytoplasmic dynein in melanosome transport in human melanocytes, *J Invest Dermatol* (2000) **114**:990–7.
88. Virador VM, Muller J, Wu X et al., Influence of alpha-melanocyte-stimulating hormone and ultraviolet radiation on the transfer of melanosomes to keratinocytes, *FASEB J* (2002) **16**:105–7.
89. Galibert MD, Carreira S, Goding CR, The Usf-1 transcription factor is a novel target for the stress-responsive p38 kinase and mediates UV-induced tyrosinase expression, *EMBO J* (2001) **20**:5022–31.
90. Eisen T, Easty DJ, Bennett DC, Goding CR, The POU domain transcription factor Brn-2: elevated expression in malignant melanoma and regulation of melanocyte-specific gene expression, *Oncogene* (1995) **11**:2157–64.

91. Carreira S, Dexter TJ, Yavuzer U et al., Brachyury-related transcription factor Tbx2 and repression of the melanocyte-specific TRP-1 promoter, *Mol Cell Biol* (1998) **18**:5099–108.
92. Galibert MD, Yavuzer U, Dexter TJ, Goding CR, Pax3 and regulation of the melanocyte-specific tyrosinase-related protein-1 promoter, *J Biol Chem* (1999) **274**:26894–900.
93. Tassabehji M, Read AP, Newton VE et al., Waardenburg's syndrome patients have mutations in the human homologue of the Pax-3 paired box gene, *Nature* (1992) **355**:635–6.
94. Pingault V, Bondurand N, Kuhlbrodt K et al., SOX10 mutations in patients with Waardenburg–Hirschsprung disease, *Nat Genet* (1998) **18**:171–3.
95. Watanabe A, Takeda K, Ploplis B, Tachibana M, Epistatic relationship between Waardenburg syndrome genes MITF and PAX3, *Nat Genet* (1998) **18**:283–6.
96. Southard-Smith EM, Kos L, Pavan WJ, Sox10 mutation disrupts neural crest development in Dom Hirschsprung mouse model, *Nat Genet* (1998) **18**:60–4.
97. Jacquemin P, Lannoy VJ, O'Sullivan J et al., The transcription factor onecut-2 controls the microphthalmia-associated transcription factor gene, *Biochem Biophys Res Commun* (2001) **285**: 1200–5.

Section I

THE DEVELOPMENT OF THE MELANOCYTE

2

Influence of endothelin 3 on the development of pigment cells from the neural crest

Elisabeth Dupin and Nicole M. Le Douarin

Origin and migration of pigment cell precursors from the neural crest

In vertebrates, melanin-synthesizing pigment cells are responsible for coloration of the eye, hair and skin. Melanocytes derive from progenitors, the melanoblasts, that are unpigmented themselves but have the potential to produce melanin. Pigment cells have a double origin in the embryo. Those in the retinal pigmented epithelium are derived from the neural epithelium whereas the majority of melanocytes, which are found in epidermal and dermal layers of the skin and the choroid layer of the eye, are derived from the neural crest (NC).[1,2]

The NC forms on the mediodorsal aspect of the neural tube according to a cranio–caudal gradient. This ectodermal structure is transitory as NC cells undergo an epithelio–mesenchymal transition, become migratory and disperse along definite pathways throughout the developing embryo. The NC-derived cells settle in many embryonic locations and, in addition to melanocytes, yield multiple derivatives, including most of the neurons and all the glial cells in the ganglia of the peripheral nervous system, Schwann cells lining the peripheral nerves, and various glandular and endocrine cell types. Melanocytes are generated along almost the entire axis of the embryo whereas some other NC derivatives, such as the chromaffin cells of the adrenal medulla and the enteric nerve cells, are generated from very restricted regions of the neuroaxis. In addition to neural and pigment cells, the cephalic NC from the level of the diencephalon yields mesenchymal cell types forming the so-called mesectoderm, including the facial and head dermis and connective tissues, the smooth muscles of the walls of arterial trunks and most of the skull vault (i.e. parietal and frontal bones).[2,3]

Pioneer explantation experiments in chick embryos first demonstrated the NC origin of pigment cells and established the general timing of melanoblast invasion of the skin along the dorsoventral axis. However, at early stages, melanoblasts are unpigmented and cannot be recognized from the surrounding cells. This is why their migration pathways were largely unknown until cell markers were devised to follow melanocyte precursors. The temporal and spatial dispersion of melanoblasts was revealed thanks to the construction of quail-chick neural primordium chimera. The migration paths, final location and terminal differentiation of donor quail NC cells were thus followed when grafts of the whole neural primordium were carried out isochronically (donor and host embryos are at the same developmental stage) and isotopically (the level of the grafted segment corresponds to the level of the excised segment). At trunk level, NC cell migration proceeds mainly in two streams, one dorso-ventrally near the neural tube within the anterior part of the somite, and the other, medio-laterally between the superficial ectoderm and the somites (Fig. 2.1). The latter pathway is used by melanocyte precursors that invade the subectodermal mesenchyme during embryonic day 3 (E3) and E4 of chick development.[4,5] NC cells stay in the 'migration staging area' near the neural tube before entering the dorso-lateral pathway. Thus, pigment cell precursors migrate 1 day later than other NC derived-cells which follow the ventral path leading to form

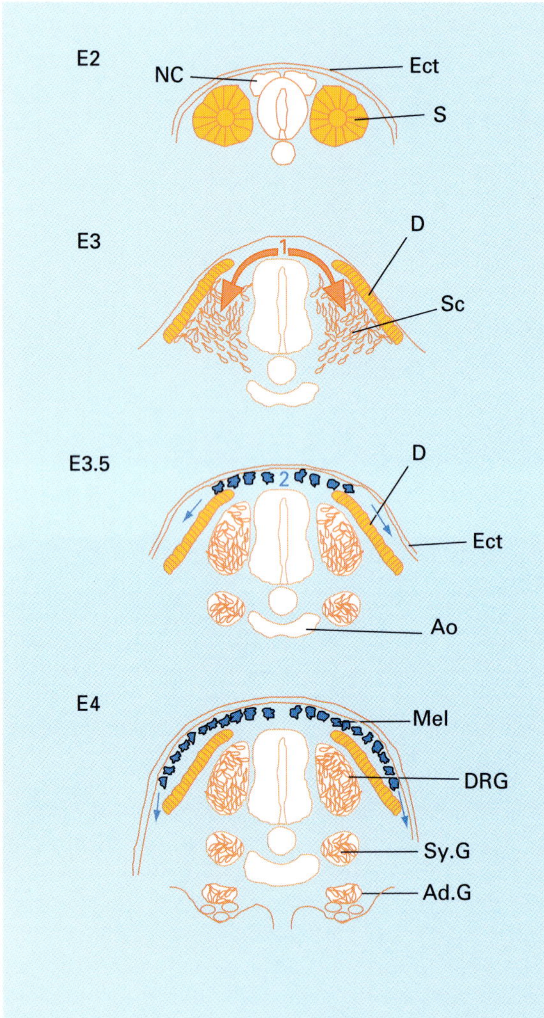

Figure 2.1

Migration of avian trunk neural crest (NC) cells between embryonic day 2 (E2) and E4. The first wave (1) of migratory cells (in red) migrate dorso-ventrally within the sclerotome (Sc) to populate the dorsal root (DRG), sympathetic (Sy.G) ganglia adrenal gland (ADG). Later, a second wave of NC cells (2) in blue start to migrate medio-laterally between superficial ectoderm (Ect) and dermomyotome (D) and will give rise to epidermal melanocytes (Mel).

the peripheral nervous system. As described in quail-chick neuroepithelium chimeras, prospective melanocytes migrate essentially through the mesenchyme. Then they massively invade the epidermis at E5–E6, a process that is completed around E7. The differentiation of epidermal melanin-synthesizing cells occurs at E9 after active cell proliferation in the feather germs.[1,2,5]

The segregation of the pigment cell lineage from pluripotent NC cells

The pluripotency of the NC cell population raised the question of how melanoblasts and neural precursors are segregated and specified. Do melanocytes derive from multipotent cells or is the melanocytic lineage segregated early from the other cell types derived from the NC? To address these questions, alternative approaches have consisted of examining, either *in vivo* or *in vitro*, the fate of isolated crest cells.

The first *in vitro* cloning analysis of quail trunk NC cells revealed a dual origin of pigment cells.[6] Colonies formed by NC cells plated at limiting dilution either contained only pigment cells or both pigmented and unpigmented cells, whereas a third type of colony was devoid of melanocytes. The finding that unpigmented cells within mixed NC colonies include neurons revealed the existence of common precursors for melanocytes and neural cells.[7,8] Therefore, in the early migratory trunk NC, pigment cell precursors comprise both already committed (unipotent) and pluripotent cells. The developmental potential of individual NC cells *in vitro* was further studied by using single-cell plating under microscopic control and culture on a feeder-layer of 3T3 fibroblasts.[9] The progeny of migratory NC cells isolated from the quail mesencephalon was analysed with a panel of lineage markers. These studies provided evidence for a large heterogeneity of the proliferation and differentiation potentials of individual crest cells. Most progenitors gave rise to two to five different cell types, with various combinations of phenotypes, whereas others generated only glial cells or neurons. In these experiments, pigment cells were generated from multipotent cells or from bipotent glial-melanocytic precursors (Fig. 2.2). Unpigmented melanoblasts were identified in multiphenotypic colonies from trunk and cephalic NC cells also by labelling with an early marker of avian melanocytes.[10] Furthermore, some clones contained all the main phenotypes derived from the cephalic NC including glial cells, adrenergic and

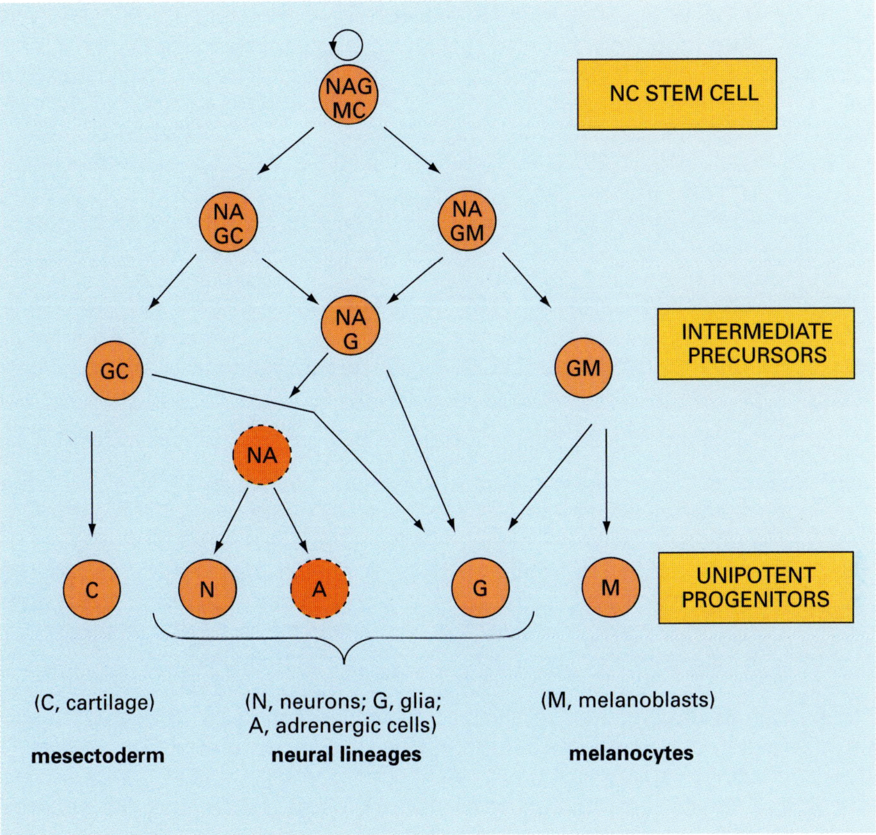

Figure 2.2

Model for the segregation of cell lineages derived from the cephalic neural crest (NC). Diagram illustrating the different progenitors from quail mesencephalic NC cells grown in clonal cultures. The presence of cartilage (C), neurons (N), glial cells (G), adrenergic cells (A) and melanocytes (M) was recorded in the colonies. Progenitors have been classified according to the number of these distinct phenotypes in their progeny. The results are consistent with the generation of unipotent progenitors from a totipotent stem cell through several intermediate oligopotent precursors. Filiations between precursors are only hypothetical.

non-adrenergic neurons, melanocytes and cartilage, a mesectodermal derivative. Such clones were therefore considered to derive from a totipotent NC precursor.[9–12] One can hypothesize that NC precursors are lineally related (Fig. 2.2), thus supporting the view that, as NC cells divide during migration, progressive restriction takes place in the developmental potentials of the cells generated from an initial pool of multipotent stem cells.

Pluripotency of NC cells was confirmed for mammalian cells by *in vitro* clonal analysis. Multipotent progenitors from the rat trunk NC give rise to neurons, glial cells and fibroblasts, and are able to self-maintain after serial propagation.[13] The development of pigment cells was not evaluated in this study. However, Ito et al.[14] have shown that NC cells isolated from mouse embryos at day 9.5 of gestation include common precursors for melanocytes and neurons.

Consistent with *in vitro* cell cultures, lineage studies in the avian embryo demonstrated that some individual premigratory and migratory NC cells are multipotent *in vivo*.[15,16] These studies investigated the fate of single precursor cells labelled by injection with fluorescent dye when still in the neural tube. The descendants of the labelled NC cells were found to populate distinct derivatives in many cases and could contain cell types as diverse as sensory neurons, adreno-medullary cells and presumptive pigment cells. In these experiments, the melanogenic fate of labelled cells was deduced from their localization in the skin but could not be ascertained due to dye dilution with cell divisions before the stage of melanogenesis. Other labelled cells populated only one NC derivative, suggesting an early specification of some precursors in the premigratory NC.

One way to investigate the timing of the restrictions of developmental options consists of challenging NC-derived cells with new environments. For example, the developmental capacities of cells en route or present in NC derivatives was investigated in single-cell cultures. These experiments consistently showed loss of differentiation options as development proceeded. However, they also revealed that pluripotent precursors still existed at advanced stages of migration, even in NC derivatives. Thus, NC cells in the epidermis, that are normally fated to become melanocytes, retain multiple developmental potentials. When isolated from the skin at early stages, these cells are able to give rise to neurons *in vitro*.[17] However, from E6 in quail epidermis, none of the crest-derived cells are still able to express non-melanogenic fate in the same culture conditions.

Taken together, these results show that NC cells are heterogeneous in their developmental potentialities, including multipotent stem-cell-like progenitors as well as already committed precursors. Therefore, appropriated signals from the environment are required to promote the final expression of the characteristic phenotypes adopted in each NC derivative. Knowing which factors influence the expression of developmental potentialities of NC cells locally and are responsible for final-fate decisions is of great importance for understanding the molecular mechanisms underlying NC multipotency.

The role of endothelin 3 in the onset and maintenance of the melanocyte phenotype

The characterization of environmental influences provided by embryonic structures, extracellular matrix molecules and/or growth factors, on the phenotypic choice of NC cells remains a major issue in understanding NC cell differentiation.[2,18] Mouse genetics proved to be very useful for knowledge about the factors that influence the migration, survival and differentiation of NC melanocytic precursors. Two well-known mouse-spotting mutants with clear defects in melanogenesis are *white dominant-spotting* (*w*) and *Steel* (*sl*). The *w* locus encodes the receptor tyrosine kinase c-kit, whereas the *sl* locus encodes its cognate ligand, steel factor (SLF).[19–22] *In vitro* studies of mouse and avian NC suggest that SLF promotes survival and moderate proliferation of melanocytes or their precursors.[23–25]

Recently, genetics and gene targeting in the mouse have led to the identification of endothelins (EDN) as crucial factors in the development of subsets of NC cell types. The endothelins 1, 2 and 3 (EDN1, EDN2 and EDN3) are a family of 21 aa peptides, endowed with vasoactive activity, which bind to heptahelical G-protein-coupled receptors of two types in mammals, endothelin receptor A and B (EDNRA and EDNRB). EDNRA displays a preferential affinity for EDN1, whereas EDNRB accepts all three peptides equally.[26]

The function of EDN3 and EDNRB in pigment cell development was discovered when knock-out mice were generated. The EDN3/EDNRB ligand/receptor plays a crucial role in the development of two NC-derived lineages: the melanocytes and the enteric nerve cells. Targeted mutation of the *EDNRB* gene in mice as well as the spontaneous piebald-lethal (s^l) mouse mutant are characterized by coat colour spots and megacolon. Similar defects result from targeted disruption or spontaneous mutation (lethal spotting, *ls*) of the *EDN3* gene.[27,28] Conditional mutation in the mouse revealed that the requirement for functional *EDNRB* corresponds to a restricted period of melanoblast early migration.[29]

The expression patterns of *EDNRB* and *EDN3* in the developing avian embryo suggested a role for these genes from the early stages of NC ontogenesis. *EDNRB* starts to be expressed by NC cells before they leave the neural primordium and may therefore be acting before cells enter the migration path to the skin. At a later stage, only cells that migrate dorso-ventrally and, later on, their neural derivatives, express *EDNRB*, whereas melanoblasts and melanocytes are *EDNRB*-negative.[30] A third type of endothelin receptor, referred to as EDNRB2 since it binds the three types of endothelins with equal affinity, has been cloned in the quail and is expressed by early melanoblasts as soon as they enter the medio-lateral migration pathway and, later on, by differentiated melanocytes.[31] *EDNRB2* is not present in crest cells migrating dorso-ventrally, thus *EDNRB2* and *EDNRB* display complementary expression patterns in avian NC cells and their derivatives. *EDN3* is expressed in the environment in which melanoblasts migrate, *i.e.* by the ectoderm from E3 and later by the epidermis.[32] These data therefore argue for a paracrine action exerted by EDN3, *via* EDNRB2, on NC cells during migration in the skin and melanogenic differentiation.

The effect of EDN3 was explored on quail NC cells cultured *in vitro*. Treatment with EDN3 caused a dose-dependent increase of cell proliferation and delayed the onset of melanogenesis. However, after 10 days of culture in the presence of EDN3, numerous melanocytes differentiated and distributed in a reproducible pattern of pigmented and unpigmented cells (Fig. 2.3).[33] The nature of the

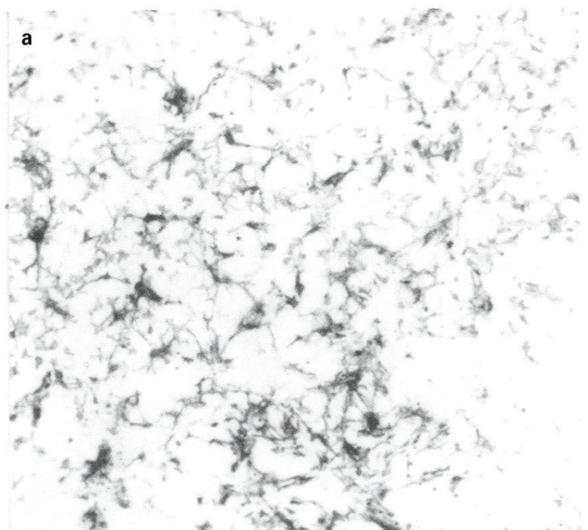

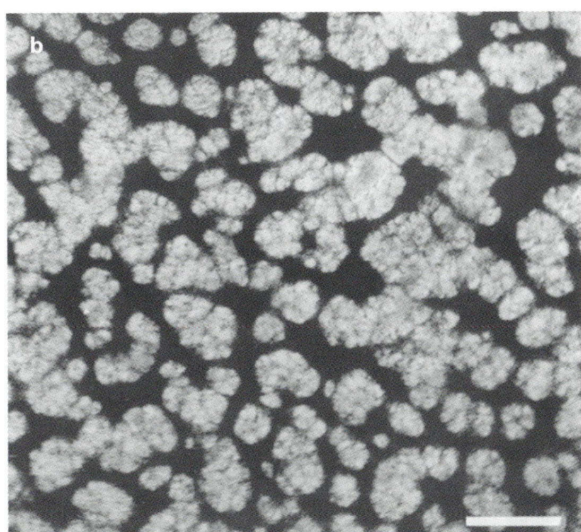

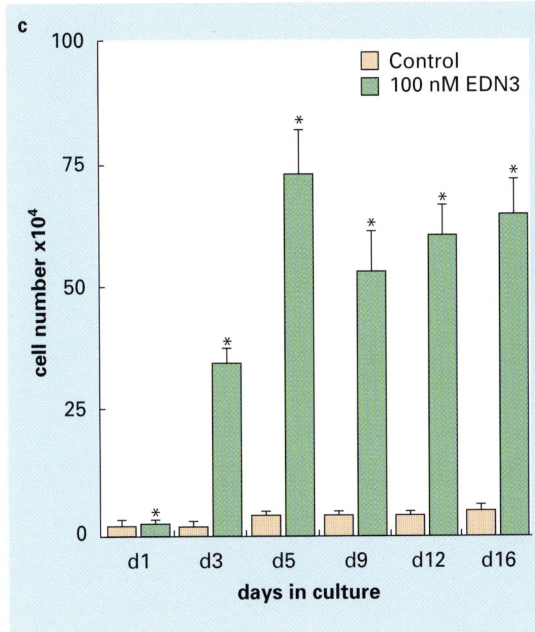

Figure 2.3

Effects of endothelin (EDN) 3 on melanogenesis and cell division by quail neural crest (NC) cells *in vitro*. (a, b) Effect of EDN3 on the pigmentation by trunk NC cells after 11 days in culture. In control medium (a), melanocytes remain dispersed whereas EDN3-treated cultures (b) show reproducible pattern of pigment cells and unpigmented pre-melanocytes. (c) Quantification of EDN3-induced changes of the total cell number at different time points. Cultures of quail trunk NC cells were analysed during a culture period of 16 days. Significant differences are indicated by a star at the top of columns. (From Lahav et al.[33]).

precursors that respond to EDN3 was investigated in NC clonal cultures. Among six different types of progenitors that were defined by cell phenotypes in the clones, EDN3 dramatically increased the survival of three types of clonogenic cells, those yielding both melanocytes and glial cells, and those generating melanocytes only and glial cells only. EDN3 also stimulated NC cell division, promoting a large increase of the total cell number in treated clones.[34] The action of EDN3 was stronger on melanogenic than on glial precursors, which explains that the most prominent effect of EDN3 is to expand pigment cells. It can therefore be concluded that prolonged exposure to EDN3 triggers a positive and selective effect on the survival and proliferation of melanogenic and glial progenitors.

These effects of EDN3 on trunk NC cells *in vitro* are mediated through EDNRB and EDNRB2. EDN3 increases the number of *EDNRB*-expressing cells only transiently, whereas it expands the population of *EDNRB2*-expressing melanocytic cells during the whole culture period. In culture conditions which promote melanogenesis, expression by crest cells of *EDNRB* declines to be replaced by

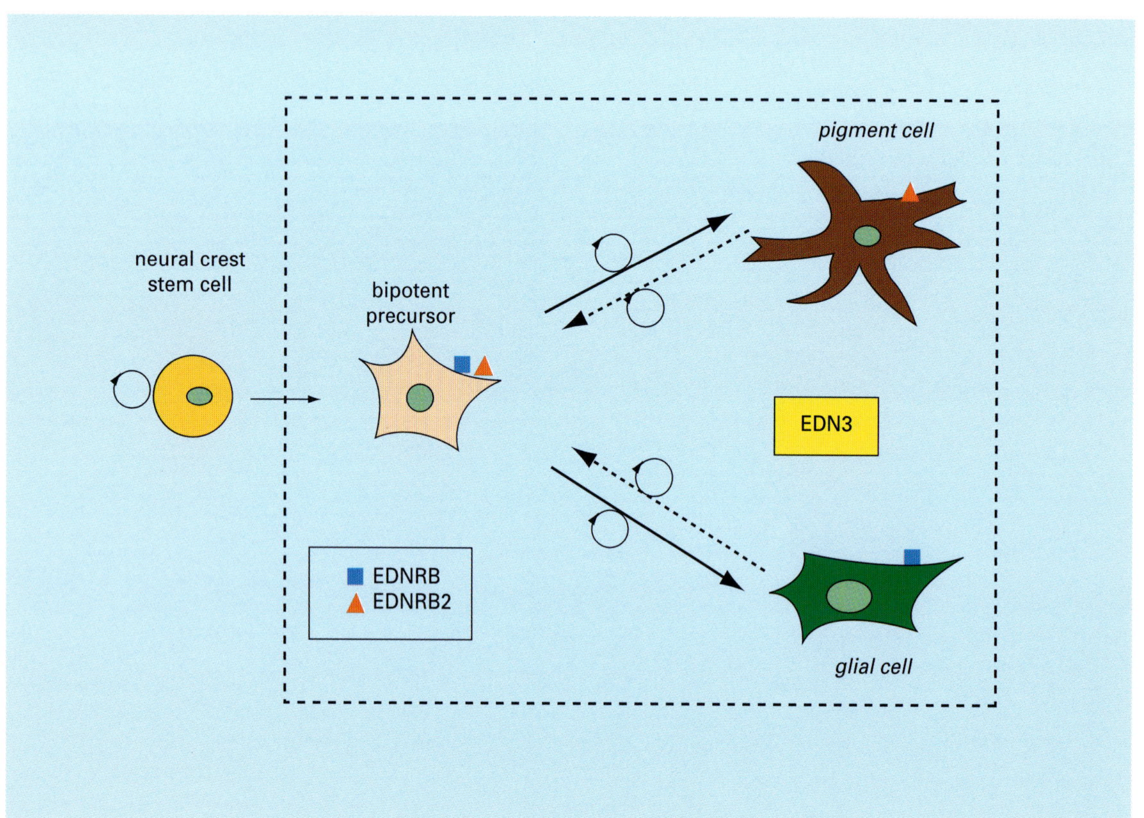

Figure 2.4

Summary of the action of endothelin (EDN) 3 on neural crest (NC) precursors and NC-derived cells. EDN3 favours the survival and proliferation of bipotent glial-melanocytic progenitors derived from NC stem cells in the early NC. Activation by EDN3 of the melanogenic differentiation program involves the induction of the EDN receptor EDNRB2 expression by developing melanoblasts, whereas differentiating glial cells continue to express EDNRB. Whether the bipotent cells are able to co-express both types of receptors remains to be ascertained. At later stages, differentiated pigment cells in the epidermis and glial cells in peripheral nerves are able to revert to the immature bipotent stage of their common NC ancestor under prolonged *in vitro* exposure to EDN3.

that of *EDNRB2*.[34] This is in agreement with the dynamic expression of *EDNRB* and *EDNRB2 in vivo*, which shows, at first, expression of *EDNRB* by virtually all premigratory and early migratory NC cells but, later, swiches off *EDNRB* and the onset of *EDNRB2* in cells which migrate medio-laterally to the skin. It is important to note that *EDNRB2*-positive NC cells remain in close contact with the superficial ectoderm that expresses *EDN3*. Therefore it is likely that, during avian skin development, EDN3 in the epidermis promotes the survival and proliferation of melanoblasts and melanocytes *via* activation of *EDNRB2*.

Since melanocytes continue to strongly express *EDNRB2* while differentiating in the epidermal environment which synthesizes EDN3 peptide, the question was raised as to whether this terminal differentiation within the epidermis could also be controlled by EDN3. To further investigate the role of EDN3 on the differentiation of NC derivatives, we have tested the effect of EDN3 on the behaviour of pigment cells isolated from the quail embryonic skin.

Clonal cultures of already pigmented melanocytes isolated from the epidermis show high proliferative activity in the presence of EDN3. Upon addition of 100 nmol/l EDN3, dividing pigment cells progressively lose melanogenic traits and, under prolonged treatment, generate a mixed progeny containing not only melanocytes but also cells expressing glial-specific proteins.[35] Therefore, epidermal pigment cells *in vitro* can be reversed to the bipotent stage of glial-melanocytic NC progenitor, which suggests that strong proliferative signals such as EDN3 are able to alter the stability of the pigment cell phenotype.

Interestingly, the bipotent glial-melanocytic NC stage can also be recapitulated by embryonic glial cells. Schwann cells purified from sciatic nerves and cultured individually, respond to EDN3/EDNRB signaling by yielding descendant colonies composed of both glial cells and melanocytes. The onset of melanocytic properties by dividing Schwann cells occurs progressively, by sequential induction of EDNRB2, early melanocyte antigens and, later on, melanin synthesis (Dupin et al., in preparation).

As summarized in Figure 2.4, these results show that the selection and expansion of melanogenic precursors depend on the local action of EDN3 on bipotent glial-melanocytic cells derived from NC stem cells. The immature bipotent stage of this common ancestor can be recapitulated *in vitro* by differentiated pigment and glial cells when they are submitted to high doses of EDN3. Reciprocal conversion between pigment and glial phenotypes *in vitro* thus provides evidence for the plasticity of NC cell fate and suggests that EDN3, due to its strong proliferative activity on NC precursors and NC-derived cells, could play a role in several pathologies *in vivo*, implicating both glia and melanocytes, such as neurofibromatosis and tumours of mixed origin.

Acknowledgements

This work was supported by the Centre National pour la Recherche Scientifique and Collège de France and by a grant from the Association pour la Recherche contre le Cancer (N° 5578).

References

1. Le Douarin N, *The Neural Crest*, Cambridge: Cambridge University Press (1982) 259.
2. Le Douarin NM, Kalcheim C, *The Neural Crest* (second edn), New York: Cambridge University Press, (1999) 445.
3. Couly GF, Coltey PM, Le Douarin NM, The triple origin of skull in higher vertebrates: a study in quail-chick chimeras, *Development* (1993) **117**:409–29.
4. Teillet MA, Le Douarin NM, La migration des cellules pigmentaires étudiée par la méthode des greffes hétérospécifiques de tube nerveux chez l'embryon d'oiseau, *C R Acad Sci, Série III, Paris* (1970) **270**:3095–8.
5. Teillet MA, Recherches sur le mode de migration et la différenciation des mélanoblastes cutanés chez l'embryon d'oiseau: etude expérimentale par la méthode des greffes hétérospécifiques entre embryons de Caille et de Poulet, *Annales d'Embryologie et de Morphogenèse* (1971) **4**:95–109.
6. Cohen AM, Konigsberg IR, A clonal approach to the problem of neural crest determination, *Dev Biol* (1975) **46**:262–80.
7. Sieber-Blum M, Cohen AM, Clonal analysis of quail neural crest cells: they are pluripotent and differentiate *in vitro* in the absence of noncrest cells, *Dev Biol* (1980) **80**:96–106.

8. Sieber-Blum M, Commitment of neural crest cells to the sensory neuron lineage, *Science* (1989) **243**: 1608–11.
9. Baroffio A, Dupin E, Le Douarin NM, Clone-forming ability and differentiation potential of migratory neural crest cells, *Proc Natl Acad Sci USA* (1988) **85**:5325–9.
10. Dupin E, Le Douarin NM, Retinoic acid promotes the differentiation of adrenergic cells and melanocytes in quail neural crest cultures, *Dev Biol* (1995) **168**:529–48.
11. Dupin E, Baroffio A, Dulac C et al., Schwann-cell differentiation in clonal cultures of the neural crest, as evidenced by the anti-Schwann cell myelin protein monoclonal antibody, *Proc Natl Acad Sci USA* (1990) **87**:1119–23.
12. Baroffio A, Dupin E, Le Douarin NM, Common precursors for neural and mesectodermal derivatives in the cephalic neural crest, *Development* (1991) **112**:301–5.
13. Stemple DL, Anderson DJ, Isolation of a stem cell for neurons and glia from the mammalian neural crest, *Cell* (1992) **71**:973–85.
14. Ito K, Morita T, Sieber-Blum M, *In vitro* clonal analysis of mouse neural crest development, *Dev Biol* (1993) **157**:517–25.
15. Bronner-Fraser M, Fraser SE, Cell lineage analysis reveals multipotency of some avian neural crest cells, *Nature* (1988) **335**:161–4.
16. Bronner-Fraser M, Fraser SE, Developmental potential of avian trunk neural crest cells *in situ, Neuron* (1989) **3**:755–66.
17. Richardson MK, Sieber-Blum M, Pluripotent neural crest cells in the developing skin of the quail embryo, *Dev Biol* (1993) **157**:348–58.
18. Anderson DJ, Cellular and molecular biology of neural crest cell lineage determination, *Trends Genet* (1997) **13**:276–80.
19. Reith AD, Bernstein A, Molecular biology of the *W* and *Stell* loci. In: *Genome Analysis. Vol. 3: Genes and Phenotypes*, New York: Cold Spring Harbor Laboratory Press (1991) 105–33.
20. Williams DE, de Vries P, Namen AE et al., The Steel factor, *Dev Biol* (1992) **151**:368–76.
21. Galli SJ, Zsebo KM, Geissler EN, The kit ligand, stem cell factor, *Adv Immunol* (1993) **55**:1–96.
22. Lecoin L, Lahav R, Dupin E, Le Douarin NM, Development of melanocytes from neural crest progenitors. In: CM Chuong, ed. *Molecular Basis of Epithelial Appendage Morphogenesis*, Georgetown, USA, RG Landes Company (1998) 131–54.
23. Murphy M, Reid K, Williams DE et al., Steel factor is required for maintenance, but not differentiation, of melanocyte precursors in the neural crest, *Dev Biol* (1992) **153**:396–401.
24. Lahav R, Lecoin L, Ziller C et al., Effect of the Steel gene product on melanogenesis in avian neural crest cell cultures, *Differentiation* (1994) **58**:133–9.
25. Reid K, Nishikawa SI, Bartlett PF, Murphy M, Steel factor directs melanocyte development *in vitro* through selective regulation of the number of c-kit(+) progenitors, *Dev Biol* (1995) **169**:568–79.
26. Sakurai T, Yanagisawa M, Masaki T, Molecular characterization of endothelin receptors. *Trends Pharmacol Sci* (1992) **13**:103–8.
27. Hosoda K, Hammer RE, Richardson JA et al., Targeted and natural (piebald-lethal) mutations of endothelin-B receptor gene produce megacolon associated with spotted coat color in mice, *Cell* (1994) **79**:1267–76.
28. Greenstein-Baynash A, Hosoda K, Giaid A et al., Interaction of endothelin-3 with endothelin-B receptor is essential for development of epidermal melanocytes and enteric neurons, *Cell* (1994) **79**:1277–85.
29. Shin MK, Levorse JM, Ingram RS, Tilghman SM, The temporal requirement for endothelin receptor-B signalling during neural crest development, *Nature* (1994) **402**:496–501.
30. Nataf V, Lecoin L, Eichmann A, Le Douarin NM, Endothelin-B receptor is expressed by neural crest cells in the avian embryo, *Proc Natl Acad Sci USA* (1996) **93**:9645–50.
31. Lecoin L, Sakurai T, Ngo MT et al., Cloning and characterization of a novel endothelin receptor subtype in the avian class, *Proc Natl Acad Sci USA* (1998) **95**:3024–9.
32. Nataf V, Amemiya A, Yanagisawa M, Le Douarin NM, The expression pattern of endothelin 3 in the avian embryo, *Mech Dev* (1998) **73**:217–20.
33. Lahav R, Ziller C, Dupin E, Le Douarin NM, Endothelin 3 promotes neural crest cell proliferation and mediates a vast increase in melanocyte number in culture, *Proc Natl Acad Sci USA* (1996) **93**:3892–7.
34. Lahav R, Dupin E, Lecoin L et al., Endothelin 3 selectively promotes survival and proliferation of neural crest-derived glial and melanocytic precursors *in vitro, Proc Natl Acad Sci USA* (1998) **95**: 14214–19.
35. Dupin E, Glavieux C, Vaigot P, Le Douarin NM, Endothelin 3 induces the reversion of melanocytes to glia through a neural crest-derived glial-melanocytic progenitor, *Proc Natl Acad Sci USA* (2000) **97**:7882–7.

3

The role of early melanoblast markers in the migration of neural crest cell derivatives

Patrick Pla, Alice Jouneau, Laure Lecoin, Hervé Kempf, Ahmed Mansouri and Lionel Larue

In the truncal part of vertebrate embroys, neural crest cells (NCC) migrate via two different pathways. One pathway lies between the neural tube and the somites and is known as the dorso-ventral pathway. The second lies between the somites and the ectoderm and is known as the dorso-lateral pathway. NCC follow the dorso-lateral pathway after proliferating in the migration staging area (MSA) located between the neural tube, the somite and the ectoderm. After completing their migration, NCC give rise to many different types of cell. In birds, the differentiation of NCC is a function of the rostro-caudal location of these cells. In the cephalic region, NCC give rise to chondrocytes, osteocytes, smooth muscle cells, connective tissue cells, neurons, Schwann cells (cranial sensory and ciliary ganglia) and melanocytes. In the vagal region, from somites 1 to 7, NCC give rise to smooth muscle cells, connective tissue cells, neurons, Schwann cells (cranial and spinal sensory ganglia, and enteric, sympathetic and parasympathetic ganglia) and melanocytes. In the truncal region, from somites 8 to 28, NCC give rise to neurons, Schwann cells (spinal sensory, sympathetic and parasympathetic ganglia), chromaffin cells in the adrenal medulla and melanocytes. Finally, in the lumbosacral region, from somites 28 onwards, NCC give rise to neurons, Schwann cells (spinal sensory, enteric, sympathetic and parasympathetic ganglia) and melanocytes (for review see reference 1). Here, we will concentrate on the migration of NCC at the truncal level.

The fundamental cellular mechanisms associated with the formation of NCC derivatives are delamination, determination, proliferation, migration, homing and differentiation. So far, 90 loci have been shown to be associated with the determination of mouse coat color. These loci are obviously associated with the melanocyte lineage. A large number of the genes associated with these loci or this lineage have been cloned, generally from mice in the first instance and then from birds. The patterns of expression of the genes encoding Kit, Mitf, Sox10, endothelin receptors (Ednr), Pax3 and β1-integrin are partially known. The results of these studies show that the fundamental cellular and molecular mechanisms underlying the formation of NCC derivatives have been well conserved throughout vertebrate evolution. Until recently, the classical approaches used for these species were different: grafting experiments and organ culture were routinely used for chicken, and mostly genetic techniques were used for mouse. In addition to the differences in the timing of development and the approach used, there are other differences between mammals and birds during the development of NCC derivatives. For instance, in birds, NCC delaminate from the dorsal part of the neural tube once it is closed. In mice, NCC start to delaminate before neural tube closure. The pattern of expression of certain genes may also differ slightly between mammals and birds at the temporal and spatial levels.

Skin melanoblasts cannot migrate in the dorso-lateral pathway

To investigate the function of the proteins involved in NCC migration, we searched for a cell line able to migrate in both the dorso-ventral and dorso-lateral pathways after grafting in chicken embryos at the level of the MSA. Cells were labeled with a fluorescent marker and grafted into early trunk NCC migratory pathways. The migratory behavior of the cells was assessed by fixing and labeling the host embroys 18 hours after grafting. The embryos were embedded in paraffin, sectioned, and observed under a fluorescent microscope. An initial screening of cell lines was previously initiated, but none of the cell lines tested had the desired characteristics.[2,3] We therefore extended this screen to novel cell lines after *in vitro* or *in ovo* grafting. All the cell lines tested were found to be migrating in the dorso-ventral pathway or not migrating at all; none were found to be migrating in the dorso-lateral pathway. We therefore grafted cells that originally migrated in the dorso-lateral pathway: cells of the melanocyte lineage. Cells of the melanocyte lineage may be classified according to age and location in the embryo during development: (i) the founder melanoblasts are limited in number, and are determined and directly derived from the NCC, (ii) the precursor melanoblasts are derived from the founder melanoblasts; they proliferate in the MSA prior to migration in the dorso-lateral pathway, (iii) the migrating melanoblasts are derived from the precursors; they proliferate, migrate, cross the basement membrane separating the dermis from the epidermis, and colonize the epidermis, (iv) the skin melanoblasts are derived from the migrating melanoblasts, and (v) the melanocytes are the ultimate stage of differentiation of this lineage in which melanin is produced. Melan-a and melb-a, a mouse melanocyte line and a mouse skin melanoblast line, respectively, were grafted into chicken embryos. Melb-a and melan-a cells migrated very efficiently in the dorso-ventral pathway but not in the dorso-lateral pathway (Fig. 3.1 and data not shown). These melanocyte and melanoblast cell lines were originally derived from the skin of a newborn mouse. They had, therefore, lost the ability to migrate in their original pathway, the dorso-lateral pathway. There are two possible non-mutually exclusive reasons for this: crucial proteins were down- or upregulated during the normal differentiation process and/or during the establishment of these cells in culture. In conclusion, these cells were not appropriate for our goal.

ES cells can migrate in both the dorso-lateral and dorso-ventral pathways

We decided to use a non-transformed cell line 'upstream' from the NCC. Embryonic stem (ES) cells are derived from the inner cell mass of the blastocyst and, in culture, the differentiation status of these cells is similar to that of cells of the epiblast. ES cells present numerous advantages, including the ability to differentiate, *in vivo* and *in vitro*, into melanocytes,[4,5] and the possibility of genetic manipulation. ES cells can be chemically labeled with CFSE or genetically marked with genes encoding LacZ or GFP. The migratory behavior of ES cells was assessed by fixing and labeling the host embryos at various times 18–96 hours after grafting, examining them either by means of paraffin sections, as described above, or directly by confocal scanning fluorescence microscopy (Fig. 3.2a–c). ES cells were detected in both pathways. Four types of embryo were distinguished: (i) ES cells maintained at the grafting site but no migration observed (no migration), (ii) migration of at least one cell in the dorso-ventral (DV) pathway (DV embryos), (iii) migration of at least one cell in the dorso-ventral and at least one cell in the dorso-lateral (DL) pathway (DV+DL embryos), and (iv) migration of at least one cell in the dorso-lateral pathway (DL embryos). The percentage of each type of embryo was then determined (Fig. 3.2d). For DL+DV embryos, we determined whether the majority of the cells migrated in one pathway or the other (Fig. 3.2e). Finally, the distance of migration and the mean number of migrating cells were determined. The mean number of wild-type migrating cells was seven. Molecular differentiation was detected by monitoring the expression of melanoblast markers, such as Mitf, in cells migrating in the dorso-lateral pathway, but the proliferation of ES cells was not observed in such an environment. Unfortunately,

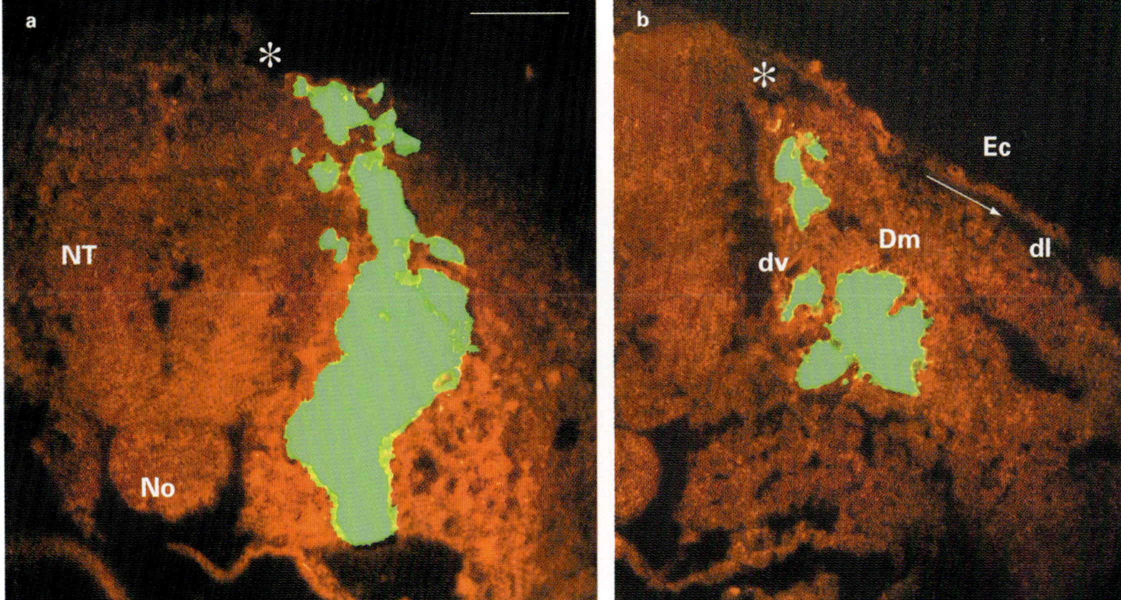

Figure 3.1

Skin melanoblast cells migrate in dorso-ventral pathway of neural crest cells when grafted into chicken embryo. Melanoblast cells were labeled with a green fluorescent marker (CFSE) before grafting. False colors are used to show the melanoblast cells. Embryos were fixed 18 hours after grafting, immunostained with an anti-laminin antibody that recognizes the basal lamina of embryo epithelia (red), embedded in paraffin, sectioned and viewed under a fluorescence microscope. Cells were grafted into embryos at the position of the asterisk (*) either *in vitro* (a) or *in ovo* (b). NT = neural tube; No = notochord; Ec = ectoderm; Dm = dermomyotome. Scale bar: 45 μm.

the lack of proliferation of ES cells in chicken embryos is a major limitation of this system, restricting our conclusions as to the migration process.

Murine ES cells are able to migrate simultaneously in the dorso-ventral and dorso-lateral pathways for at least 96 hours. This suggests that the required proteins are present in sufficient amounts in ES cells for these cells to mimic the migration of neural crest cells. We decided to assess the expression of various melanoblast markers by various techniques: RT-PCR, Northern and Western blot analyses, and binding of radiolabeled ligands. According to our expression criteria, ES cells produced the proteins β1-integrin (Itgb1), Kit and Pax3 but did not produce Mitf or endothelin receptors. We investigated the role of these proteins during neural crest cell migration by increasing or reducing expression of the corresponding genes in ES cells. Heterozygous and homozygous ES cells were produced by knocking out the *Kit*, *Itgb1* and *Pax3* genes, and hemizygous ES cells producing Mitf or various endothelin receptors were also produced. Hemizygous ES cells were produced by random integration of a ubiquitous expression vector containing the human CMV enhancer together with the chicken β-actin promoter.

Migration of ES cells lacking Itgb1

Cell motility is controlled by receptors that mediate cell-substrate adhesion. Integrins are the main family of extracellular matrix receptors.[6] As many as 11 integrin subunits associate with the β1-integrin subunit (Itgb1). *In vivo*, β1-integrin is expressed in migrating neural crest cells.[7,8] The pattern of expression of the *Itgb1* gene was studied in mice and birds, mainly in the neural tube and the dorso-ventral pathway. On the dorso-lateral pathway, only indirect information is available[2] and the results obtained are summarized in Figure 3.3a–c. It was shown that $\alpha_4\beta_1$ and $\alpha_5\beta_1$ were important for dorso-lateral migration.[2] ES cells produce the $\alpha_5\beta_1$, $\alpha_3\beta_1$, $\alpha_6\beta_1$ and $\alpha_v\beta_1$ integrin subunits.[9,10] We investigated further the role of β1-integrins in cell migration by grafting nullizygous (*Itgb1*$^-$/*Itgb1*$^-$) and

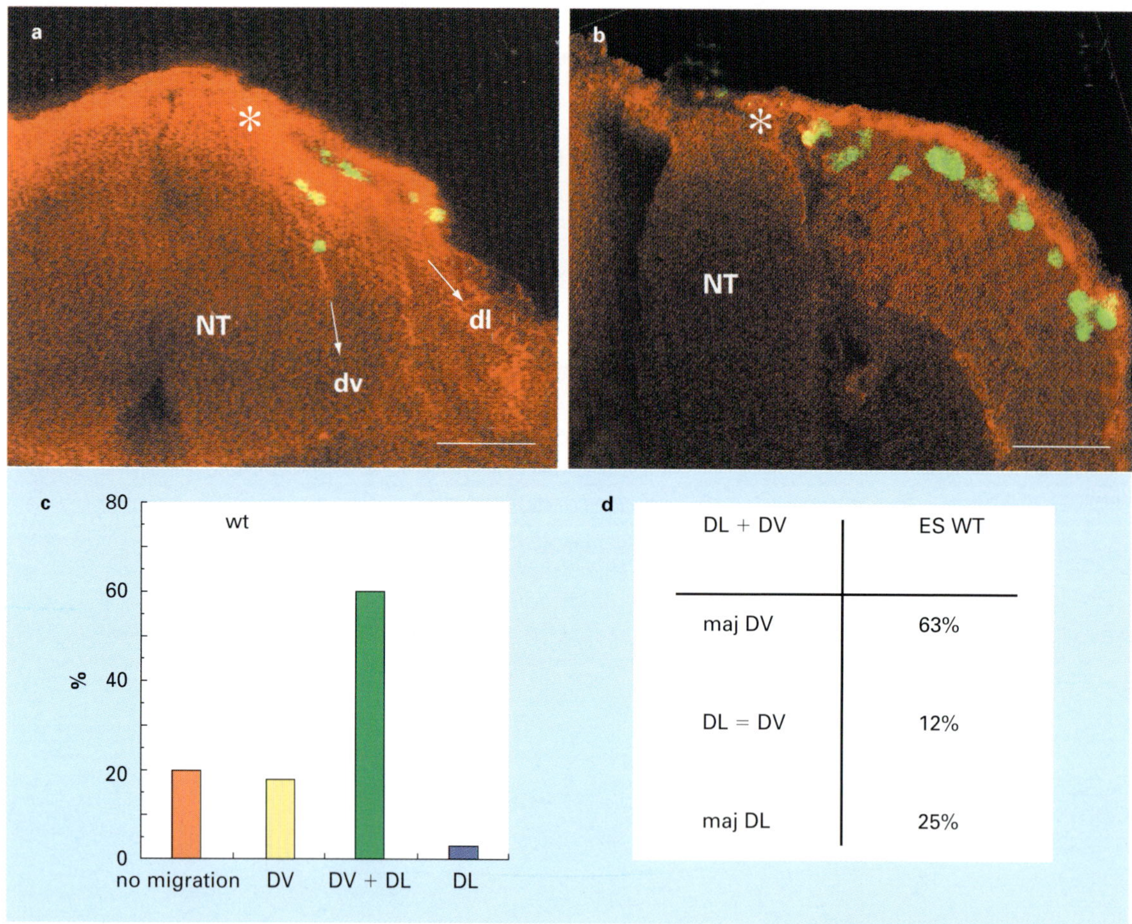

DL + DV	ES WT
maj DV	63%
DL = DV	12%
maj DL	25%

Figure 3.2

Murine ES cells migrate in the dorso-ventral (DV) and dorso-lateral (DL) pathways of neural crest cells when grafted into chicken embryo. (a,b) Cells were labeled with a green fluorescent marker (CFSE) before grafting at the position of the asterisk (*). Embryos were fixed 18 hours after grafting, immunostained with anti-laminin antibody that recognizes the basal lamina of embryo epithelia (red), and analyzed by optical scanning with a confocal scanning fluorescence microscope. (a) Example of a transverse section of DL+DV embryo: at least one cell migrated in each of the two pathways, with the majority of cells following the DL pathway: five cells in the DL pathway and three cells in the DV pathway. (b) One example of DL embryos. (c) The embryos were classified as follows: embryos with no migrating cells, embryos containing cells migrating in the DV pathway, embryos containing cells migrating in the DL+DV pathways and embryos containing cells migrating in the DL pathway. (d) Analysis of embryos containing cells migrating in the DL+DV pathways. For each embryo, the cells migrated preferentially in the DL or DV pathway (maj DL or maj DV, respectively) or migrated equally in both pathways (DL = DV). NT= neural tube. The arrows indicate the dorso-ventral (dv) or dorso-lateral (dl) pathway. Scale bars for a and b correspond to 30 and 20 μm, respectively.

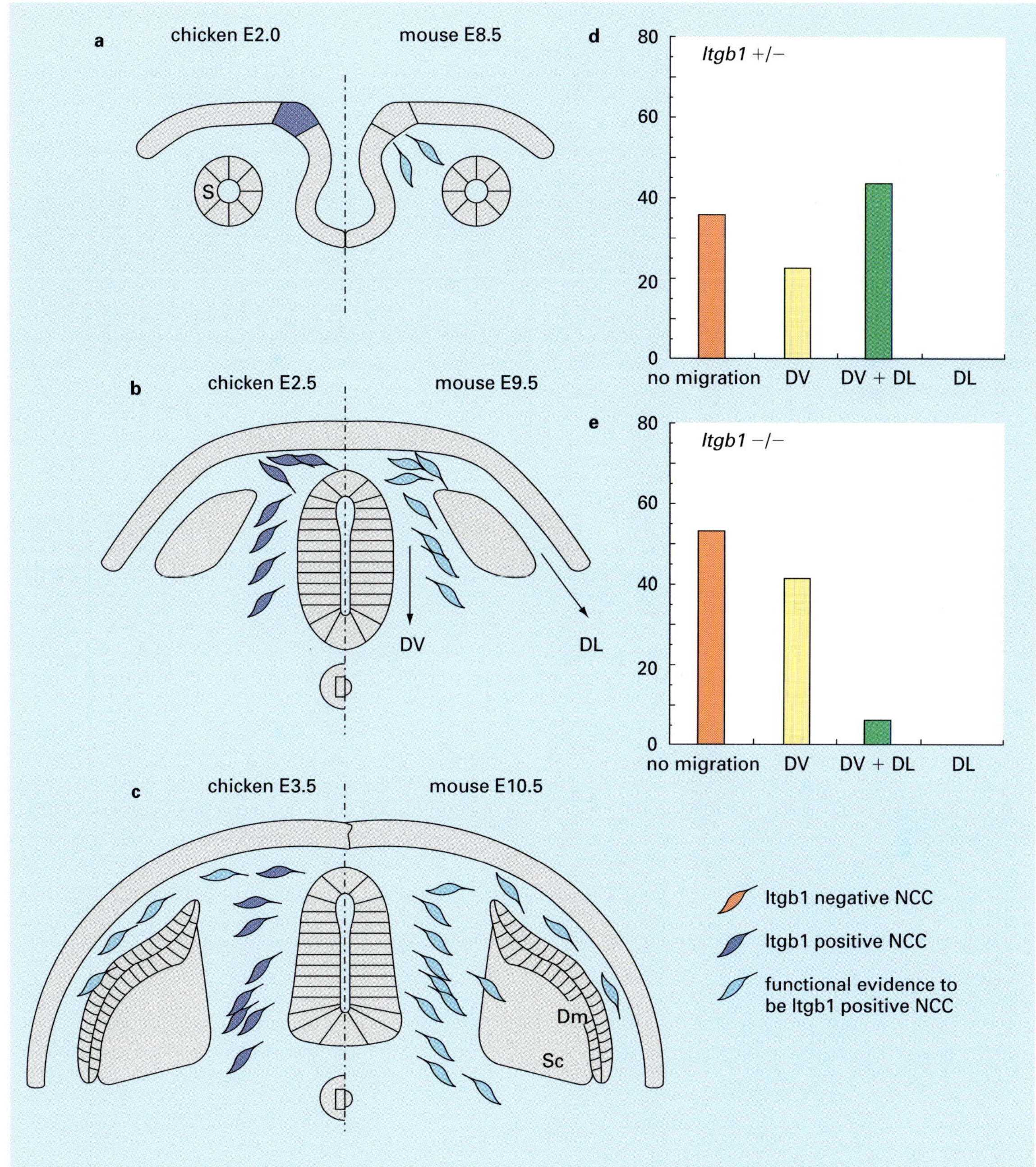

Figure 3.3

Itgb1 expression pattern and migration of *Itgb1−/−* ES cells in chicken embryo. (a–c) Schematic transverse section of chicken (left) and mouse (right) embryos at comparable periods of development from E2 to E3.5 and E8.5–E10.5, respectively. The expression pattern of Itgb1 in neural crest cells (NCC) is visualized according to a color code (pink: no expression, blue: expression, and light blue: functional evidence to be Itgb1-positive). The cells not derived from NCC cells are in gray. *Itgb1+/−* (d) and *Itgb1−/−* (e) ES cells were grafted into E2.5 chicken embryos, fixed, labeled and observed on E3.5.

heterozygous (*Itgb1*$^{+}$/*Itgb1*$^{-}$) ES cells into chicken embryos and assessing their ability to migrate in chicken neural crest cell pathways. The *Itgb1*$^{+}$/*Itgb1*$^{-}$ ES cells behaved similarly to the wild-type cells (Figs 3.2 and 3.3d). In contrast, the migration of *Itgb1*$^{-}$/*Itgb1*$^{-}$ ES cells in the dorso-lateral pathway was severely impaired. Indeed, only 6% of embryos grafted with nullizygous cells were classified as DL+DV, versus 43% for embryos grafted with heterozygous ES cells (Fig. 3.3d,e). However, $\beta 1^{-}/^{-}$ ES cells were still able to migrate ventrally *in vivo*, although less efficiently than heterozygous ES cells. First, 53% of embryos grafted with nullizygous ES cells contained non-migrating cells, versus 35% for embryos grafted with heterozygous cells. Second, although the number of grafted cells was similar, the mean number of migrating cells in embryos grafted with $\beta 1^{+}/^{-}$ ES cells was about eight, whereas that for embryos grafted with $\beta 1^{-}/^{-}$ ES cells was three.

The behavior of β1-integrin-deficient ES cells demonstrated the differential involvement of β1-integrins in dorso-ventral and dorso-lateral migration. Although their motility was reduced, *Itgb1*$^{-}$/*Itgb1*$^{-}$ ES cells were able to migrate in the dorso-ventral pathway, and this migration was qualitatively similar to that of β1-integrin-producing cells. In contrast, dorso-lateral migration was severely impaired. This is consistent with previous results for chimeras obtained from albino mouse blastocysts injected with *Itgb1*$^{-}$/*Itgb1*$^{-}$ ES cells. Some *Itgb1*$^{-}$/*Itgb1*$^{-}$ cells were found in ventral derivatives of neural crest cells, such as the peripheral nervous system and the adrenal medulla, but pigmented melanocytes derived from *Itgb1*$^{-}$/*Itgb1*$^{-}$ ES cells were not detected.[11,12] Thus, β1-integrin is required for the melanocyte lineage.

Migration of ES cells lacking Kit

Kit is a tyrosine-kinase receptor that interacts with stem cell factor (SCF), its ligand. Kit is expressed and has been shown to be important in hematopoietic and germ cells, as well as melanocytes.[13] The expression pattern of Kit has been determined in mice and birds and is summarized in Figure 3.4a–c. In mice, numerous Kit alleles have been identified, and analysis of these mutants suggested that this tyrosine-kinase receptor plays a role in the migration, survival and/or proliferation of pigment cell precursors throughout their development.[14,15] KIT mutations have been discovered in humans; these mutations lead to a syndrome known as piebaldism.[16,17] However, no direct role of the Kit receptor in early dorso-lateral migration has been clearly established. We investigated the role of Kit in cell migration further by generating nullizygous ($Kit^{W\text{-}lacZ/W\text{-}lacZ}$) and heterozygous ($Kit^{W\text{-}lacZ/+}$) ES cells, grafting them into chicken embryos and assessing migration in the chicken neural crest cell pathway.[11,18] Eighteen hours later, the migration of heterozygous and homozygous cells was assessed and embryos classified accordingly (Fig. 3.3c,d). No difference in migratory behavior was observed between $Kit^{W\text{-}lacZ/W\text{-}lacZ}$ and $Kit^{W\text{-}lacZ/+}$ ES cells. The number of migrating $Kit^{W\text{-}lacZ/W\text{-}lacZ}$ and $Kit^{W\text{-}lacZ/+}$ ES cells was similar to the number of migrating wild-type cells and no obvious cell proliferation was observed.

Mice have the same phenotype in the absence of SCF, the Kit ligand, as in the absence of Kit. SCF is not produced in ES cells, thereby eliminating the possibility of an autocrine loop. In the chicken embryo, dorso-lateral migration occurs 18 hours after ventral migration.[19] The onset of endogenous Steel expression in the ectoderm occurs at the same time as the dorso-lateral migration of endogenous crest cells.[20] However, it has been suggested that neural crest cells themselves may transiently express the *SCF* gene during their stay in the migration staging area.[21] Therefore, it is not clear whether SCF is available for ES cells at the start of migration. It is also unknown whether the chicken SCF induces an identical response following interaction with a mouse Kit receptor. In any case, the behavior of Kit-deficient cells suggests that Kit is not necessary for the migration of neural crest cell at this stage. Thus, ES cells may already possess the correct set of molecules, or at least an acceptable combination of proteins, required for migration in the dorso-ventral and dorso-lateral pathways.

Migration of ES cells lacking Pax3

Pax3 belongs to the family of paired-box-containing transcription factors. The expression pattern of *Pax3* has been studied in mice and birds,[22] and is summarized in Figure 3.5a–c. Mutations

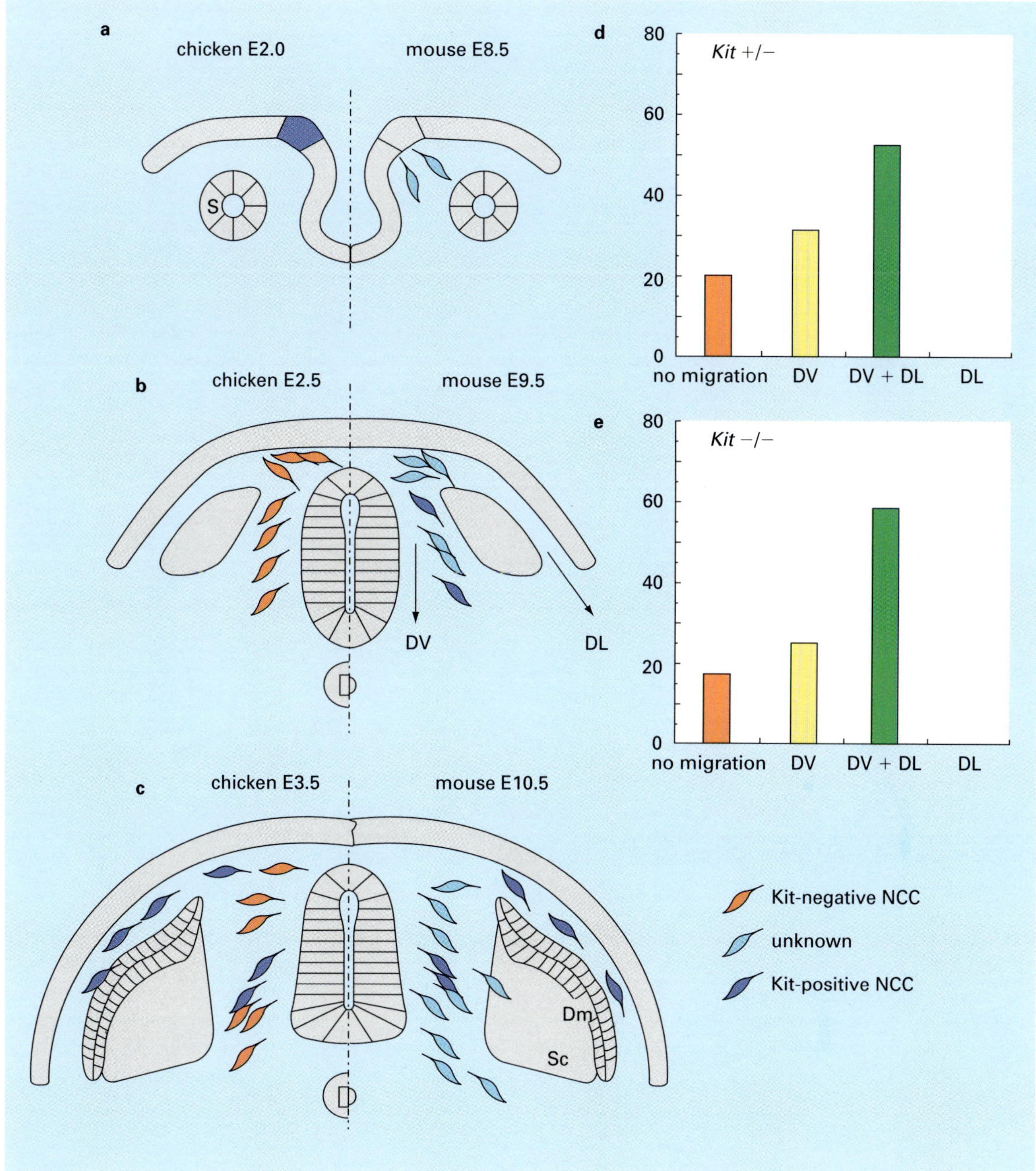

Figure 3.4

Kit expression pattern and migration of *Kit*$^{-}$/$^{-}$ ES cells in chicken embryo. (a–c) Schematic transverse sections of chicken (left) and mouse (right) embryos at comparable periods of development from E2 to E3.5 and E8.5–E10.5, respectively. The expression of *Kit* in neural crest cells (NCC) is visualized according to a color code (pink: no expression, blue: expression, and light blue: unknown). The cells not derived from NCC are in gray. *Kit*$^{W\text{-}lacZ/+}$ (d) and *Kit*$^{W\text{-}lacZ/W\text{-}lacZ}$ (e) ES cells were grafted into E2.5 chicken embryos, fixed, labeled and observed on E3.5.

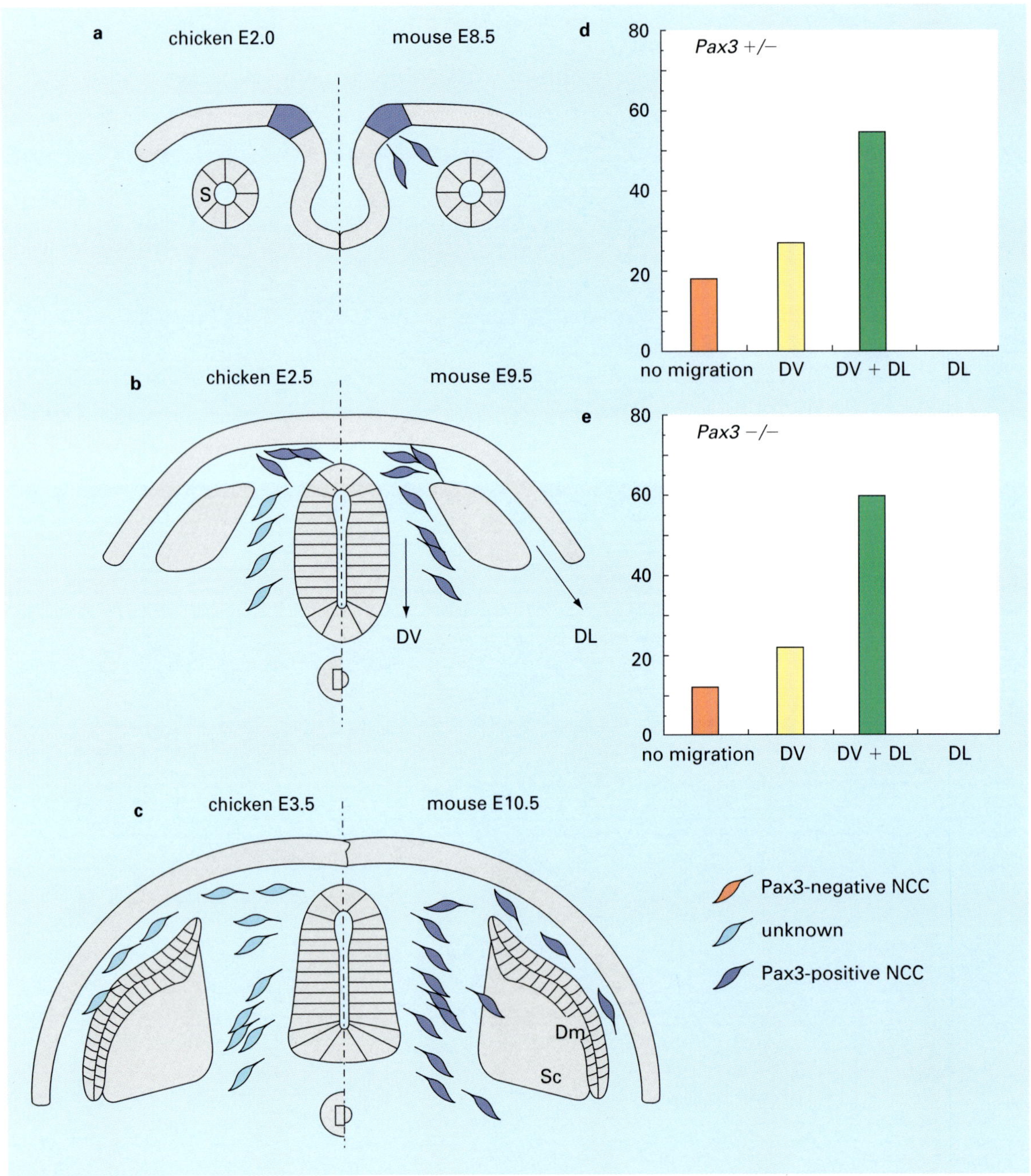

Figure 3.5

Pax3 expression pattern and migration of *Pax3* $^{-/-}$ ES cells in chicken embryo. (a–c) Schematic transverse sections of chicken (left) and mouse (right) embryos at comparable periods of development from E2 to E3.5 and E8.5–E10.5, respectively. The expression *Pax3* in neural crest cells (NCC) is visualized according to a color code (pink: no expression, blue: expression, and light blue: unknown). The cells not derived from NCC are in gray. *Pax3+/–* (d) and *Pax3–/–* (e) ES cells were grafted into E2.5 chicken embryos, fixed, labeled and observed on E3.5.

in the *Pax3* gene lead to developmental defects in mammals, known as Waardenburg syndrome types I and III in humans.[23,24] A classical mouse *Pax3* mutant, Splotch, lacks limb muscle, suffers from spina bifida and exencephalia, and displays defects in NCC derivatives.[25–27] The observed phenotypes involved similar defects, suggesting loss-of-function mutations leading to defects in cell proliferation and/or migration. The role of Pax3 in cell migration was investigated further by producing $Pax3^{LacZ/+}$ and $Pax3^{LacZ/LacZ}$ ES cells in which the bacterial β-galactosidase gene of *Escherichia coli* was inserted into the *Pax3* locus by homologous recombination.[28,29] The mice produced from $Pax3^{LacZ/+}$ ES cells had a phenotype identical to that of Splotch mice.[28] Homozygous $Pax3^{LacZ/LacZ}$ animals died on embryonic day 14 (E14) and displayed the same defects as Splotch mice.

The contribution of mutant neural crest cells to melanocyte formation has been analyzed by grafting $Pax3^{LacZ/+}$ and $Pax3^{LacZ/LacZ}$ ES cells into chick embryos. Heterozygous and homozygous ES cells were labeled with CFSE, grafted into chicken embryos and fixed. The proportions of embryos in which ES cells did not migrate, or migrated exclusively dorso-ventrally, were similar in embryos grafted with heterozygous and homozygous ES cells (Fig. 3.5d,e). In embryos in which ES cells migrated both dorso-laterally and dorso-ventrally, the number of cells following each pathway was determined. These embryos were classified according to whether the majority of cells followed the dorso-lateral (maj DL) or dorso-ventral (maj DV) pathway. In the absence of *Pax3*, the proportions of maj DL and maj DV embryos were equal, at 50%. In the presence of *Pax3*, wild-type or heterozygous cells, the proportion of maj DV embryos was 80%. This suggests that ES cells lacking *Pax3* have a stronger tendency to migrate dorso-laterally than ES cells with *Pax3*. Finally, the mean migration distance was similar for wild-type, heterozygous and homozygous *Pax3* ES cells. Moderate levels of β-galactosidase activity were detected by whole-mount LacZ-staining in homozygous and heterozygous ES cells containing *Pax3* during migration in chicken embryos. Staining of paraffin-embeded sections revealed that cells migrating dorso-laterally and dorso-ventrally expressed β-galactosidase. These results suggest that *Pax3* continues to be expressed in the migrating cells. $Pax3^{LacZ/LacZ}$ <-> $Pax3^{+/+}$ chimeric murine embryos were produced and analyzed. The analysis of several chimeras on E9 and E11 revealed that the neural crest cells of the rostral neural tube (hindbrain) seem to migrate more efficiently that those located caudally. In addition, more caudal neural crest cells were able to migrate and blue staining for β-galactosidase activity was detected in cells in dorsal root ganglia and spinal ganglia. The dorsal root ganglia of highly chimeric embryos were smaller at early stages of development but were later rescued by wild-type cells. Indeed, older embryos (E11.5) displayed normally formed spinal and dorsal root ganglia in all cases. Thus, *Pax3* does not display cell-autonomous action in neural crest cells, in contrast with other tissues.[29]

Migration of ES cells expressing EdnrB1 or EdnrB2

Endothelins (ET) and endothelin receptors (Ednr) were originally discovered in the vascular system.[30–32] These proteins were shown to be important in NCC development, because the classical coat color Piebald lethal (s^l) and lethal spotting (*ls*) mutants were found to be associated with mouse EdnrB1 and its ligand ET3, respectively. The loss of expression of the gene encoding this receptor or its ligand induces the formation of large white spots on the animal's coat, due to the lack of melanoblasts, and megacolon, due to the absence of enteric ganglia in the posterior part of the intestine.[33,34] In humans, similar phenotypes have been described in patients with Hirschprung disease or Waardenburg syndrome type IV.[35] It has recently been shown that these patients have mutations in either *Ednrb1*[36] or the *ET3* gene.[37] These results indicate that both these proteins are important in the migration of NCC derivatives in the dorso-lateral and dorso-ventral pathways at the vagal and truncal levels. EdnrA and ET1, members of the same receptor and ligand families, respectively, have been shown to be involved in the development from the NCC of specific derivatives, cardiac and cephalic derivatives in particular, but were not involved in the melanocyte lineage.[38] To date, no function in NCC development has been assigned to ET2.

Ednr is a protein of about 430 amino acids, belonging to the G-coupled-heptahelical transmembrane receptor family. In mice, only two receptors from this family have been isolated,

EdnrA and EdnrB1. To date, three receptors have been isolated from birds and frogs: EdnrA, EdnrB1 and EdnrB2 (or EdnrC for *Xenopus*).[39] The EdnrB1 of birds has been partially cloned, with the N-terminal part of the protein still missing. Structural similarity between the various Ednr has been studied.[39–41] Unanswered questions remain concerning the classification of EdnrB2, classified in the B or C class, depending on the author. The similarity between sequences differs according to the domain considered. To simplify a complex situation, the N-terminal part of EdnrB2 is most similar to that of EdnrB1, the core region is most similar to that of EdnrA, and the C-terminal region is most similar to that of EdnrC. Accordingly, at a very simple level, it might be expected that the binding of endothelins would be similar for EdnrB1 and EdnrB2, and that the associated signaling would be similar for EdnrC and EdnrB2.

The expression patterns of Ednrb1 and Ednrb2 in the truncal region have been investigated,[40,42] and are summarized in Figure 3.6. In birds, qEdnrB1 is

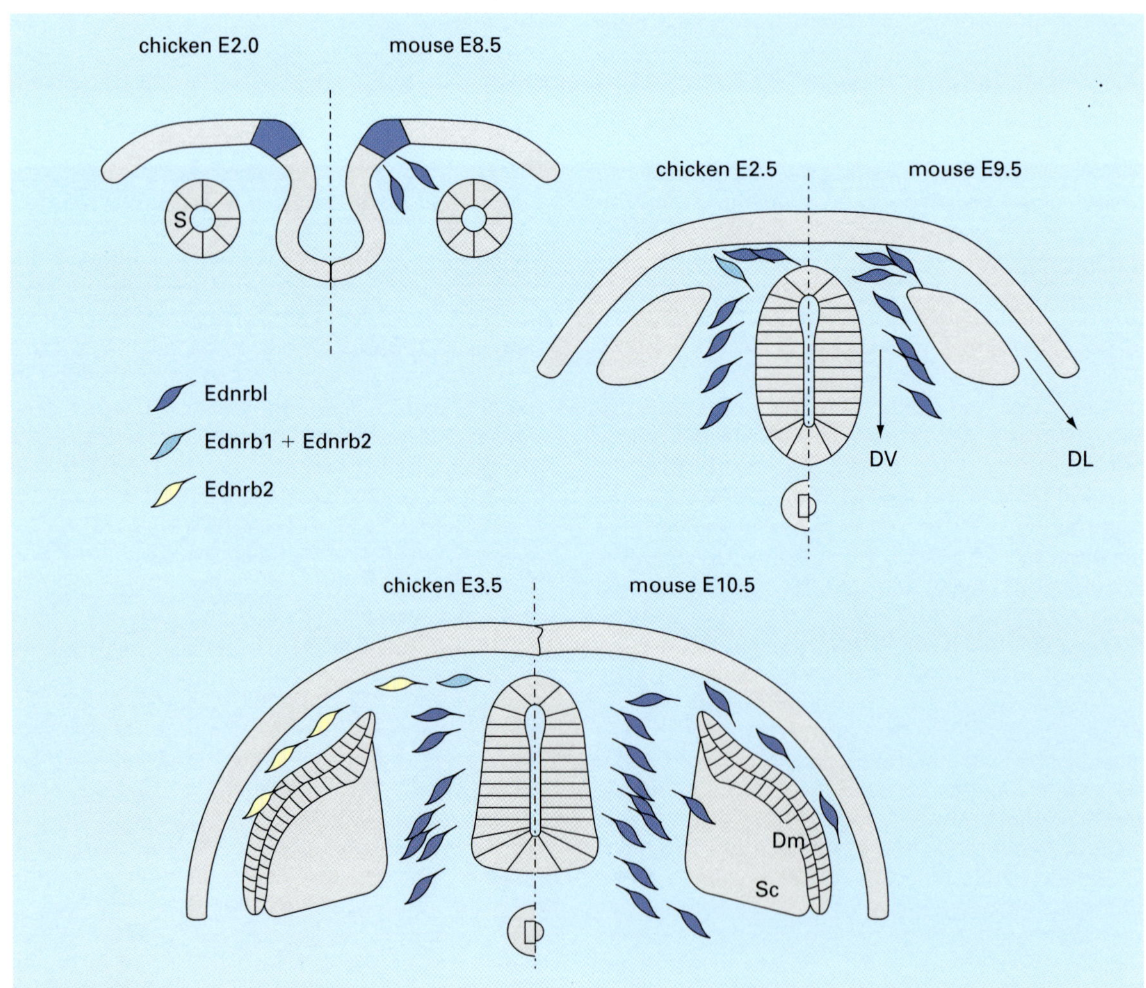

Figure 3.6

EdnrB1 and *EdnrB2* expression patterns. Schematic transverse sections of chicken (left) and mouse (right) embryos at comparable periods of development from E2 to E3.5 and E8.5–E10.5, respectively. The expression of *EdnrB1* (blue), *EdnrB2* (yellow) or both (green) is indicated. The cells not derived from NCC are in gray.

expressed from E2 onwards in the presumptive neural crest cells. Expression of qEdnrB1 is maintained in NCC derivatives following the dorsoventral pathway. On E3.5, cells following the dorso-lateral pathway express qEdnrB2, but no longer express qEdnrB1. *In vitro*, it has been shown that a very limited number of cells express qEdnrB1 and qEdnrB2 simultaneously. Such cells, expressing both qEdnrB1 and qEdnrB2, were not found *in vivo*, suggesting that they are not numerous if they are present at all. If such cells exist *in vivo*, they should be present, transiently, in the MSA. In mice, the situation is very simple: only one EdnrB has been cloned to date and mEdnrB1 is expressed in all NCC derivatives from E8.5 to E10.5 (Fig. 3.6).

ES cells do not produce significant amounts of Ednr. To evaluate the role of EdnrB in the migration of NCC, the full EdnrB cDNAs were introduced in a stable manner into ES cells. The mEdnrB1 or qEdnrB2 cDNAs were inserted, in the sense or antisense (as) direction, into an expression vector. ES cells were transfected with these expression vectors and selected on hygromycin for 12 days. Hemizygous (*qEdnrB2/–*, *mEdnrB1/–*, *asqEdnr B2/–* and *asmEdnrB1/–*) ES cells were produced. A minimum of 50 clones were picked and analyzed for each construct. Each clone was named according to the plasmid of origin. For instance, ES cell clones transfected with the vector containing the murine EdnrB1 cDNA were named mB1-i (i from 1 to 50). The expression of

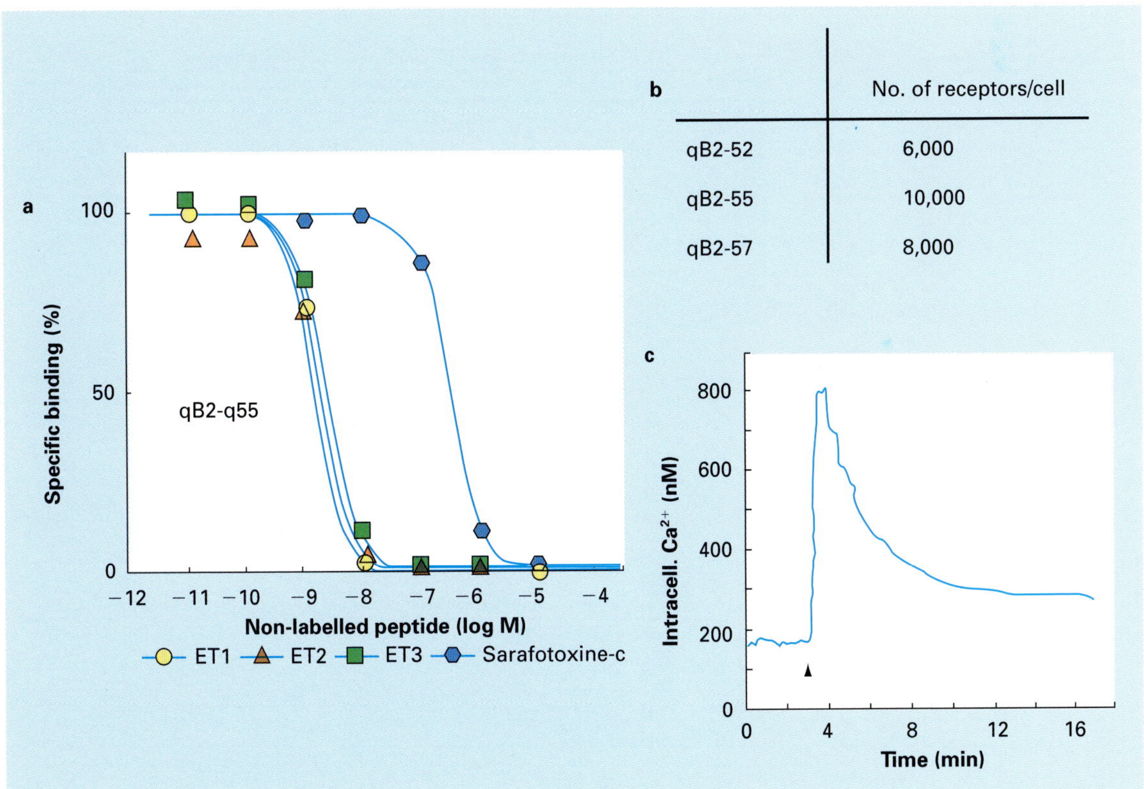

Figure 3.7

Evaluation of *EdnrB1* and *EdnrB2* expression using pharmacological criteria. (a) Competitive radio ligand-binding assay. Displacement of [^{125}I]ET1 to ES cells expressing qEdnrB2 (R1q55) by increasing concentrations of unlabeled endothelin-related peptides. (b) Estimated number of quail endothelin B2 receptors per cell, determined by Scatchard analysis of three different ES cells' clones expressing qEdnrB2. (c) Transient intracellular calcium influx in R1q55 ES cells after induction with 100 nM ET3.

these cDNA in the transfected ES cells was assessed by RT-PCR and Northern blot analysis (data not shown). To determine the number of receptors per cell and to check that mEdnrB1 or qEdnrB2 was effectively expressed at the membrane of these cells, classical pharmacological binding experiments were performed. [^{125}I]ET1 was used as a ligand and ET1, ET2, ET3 and sarafotoxin-C were used as competitors. Scatchard analysis showed that qB2-52, qB2-55 and qB2-57 possessed approximately 6000, 10,000 and 8000 receptors/cell, respectively (Fig. 3.7b). In this assay, we found that the apparent affinities of ET1, ET2 and ET3 for qEdnrB2 were similar, and that the apparent affinity of sarafotoxin-C for qEdnrB2 was no more than one-hundredeth that of its natural ligand, qEdnrB2 (Fig. 3.7a). Thus, the qEdnrB2 protein was effectively presented and properly processed at the membrane. Following induction by ligand binding, G-protein-coupled heptahelical transmembrane endothelin receptors are known to induce FAK and

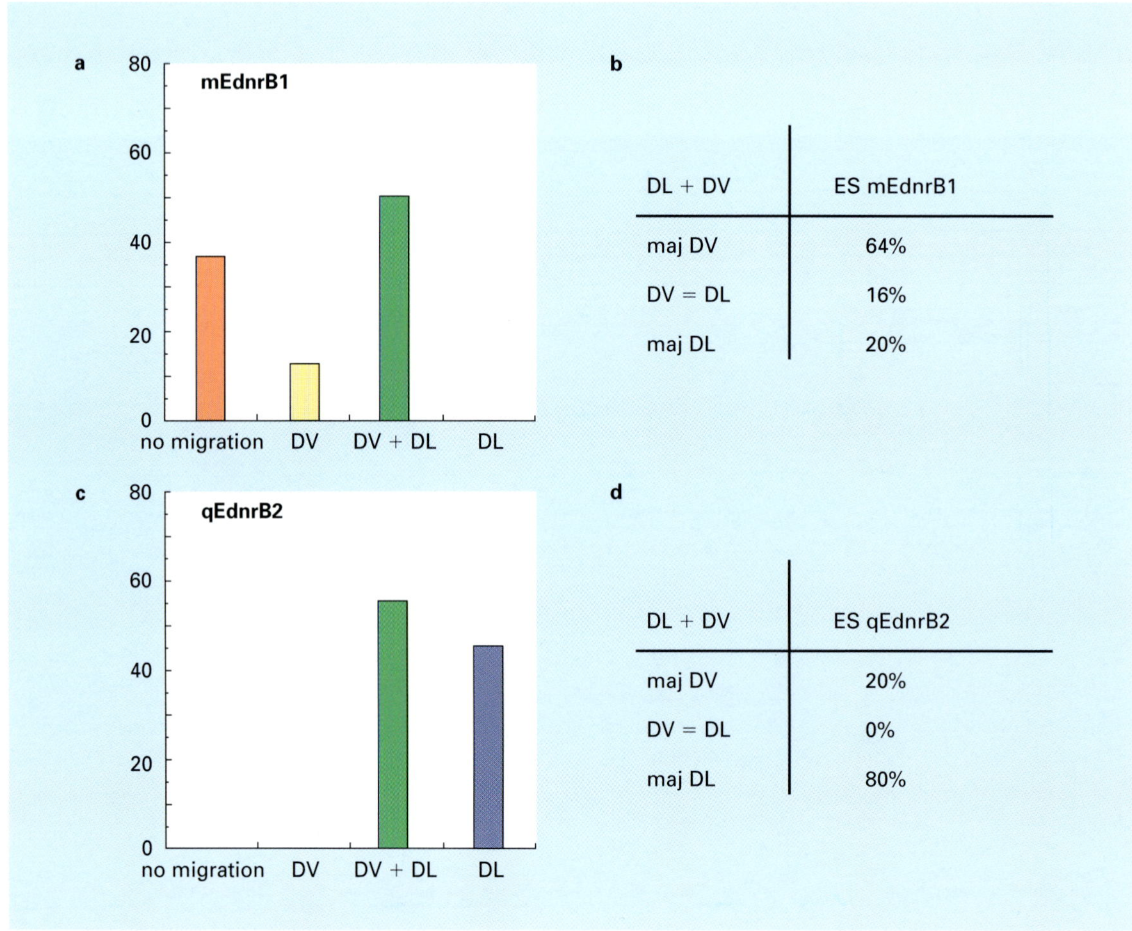

Figure 3.8

Migration of mEdnrB1 and qEdnrB2 ES cells in chicken embryo mEdnrB1 (a) and qEdnrB2 (c) ES cells were grafted into E2.5 chicken embryos, fixed, labeled and observed on E3.5. (b,d) Analysis of embryos containing cells migrating in the DL+DV pathways. For each embryo, the cells migrated preferentially in the DL or DV pathway (maj DL or maj DV, respectively), or equally in both pathways (DL = DV). In the presence of qEdnrB2, migration in the DL pathway is greatly stimulated.

phospholipase Cβ, and to stimulate calcium influx and to repress adenylate cyclase. We investigated whether this receptor was active in ES cells by performing a calcium transient assay (Fig. 3.7c and data not shown).

To investigate further the role of qEdnrB2 and mEdnrB1 in cell migration, these various ES cells were grafted into chicken embryos to test their ability to migrate in chicken neural crest cell pathways. We found that *mEdnrB1/–* and *asqEdnr B2/–* ES cells behaved similarly to wild-type cells (Figs 13.2, 3.8 and data not shown). In contrast, the migration of *qEdnrB2/–* ES cells in the dorso-lateral pathway was clearly stimulated. Indeed, 45% of the embryos grafted with *qEdnrB2/–* ES cells were dorso-lateral, versus 0–6% for embryos grafted with the various control ES cells (Fig. 3.8 and data not shown). The proportion of DL+DV cells was similar in the various cell lines (45–60%), but the large majority (80%) of *qEdnr B2/–* ES cells migrated in the dorso-lateral pathway, with only a small minority (20%) of control cells migrating in the dorso-ventral pathway. Thus, qEdnrB2 induced the dorso-lateral migration of ES cells grafted into chicken embryo, but mEdnrB1 did not seem to promote preferential migration one pathway or the other. There was, therefore, a good correlation between the pattern of expression and the migration of ES cells expressing *mEdnrB1* and *qEdnrB2*. To increase our understanding of the role of these receptors in the migration of NCC derivatives, the full-length *qEdnrB1* should be cloned, expressed in ES and grafted into chicken embryo.

After 18 hours, the mean number of migrating cells in embryos grafted with *qEdnrB2/–* ES cells was similar to wild-type ES cells, at about eight. However, cell proliferation is stimulated *in vitro* in the presence of endothelins and their receptors.[43] To follow the cells for 48 and 72 hours in the chicken embryo, the *lacZ* gene was introduced into the qB2-55 ES cells clone. The numbers of blue *lacZ*-expressing cells in embryos grafted with qB2-55 LacZ and LacZ ES cells were identical 48 and 72 hours after the graft (data not shown). This suggests that the presence of EdnrB2 in ES cells is not sufficient to induce ES cell proliferation *in ovo*.

In conclusion, this novel way of using wild-type and mutant ES cells has already proven to be useful, and further studies will provide new information about the roles of various proteins in NCC lineages. The experiments described here provide insight into the molecular mechanisms underlying the dorso-lateral migration of melanoblasts.

Acknowledgements

We would like to thank Catherine Chollet and Jeanine Marchetti for helping us in calcium influx experiments (U367 INSERM). This work was supported by a grant from Institut Curie and a grant from Fondation de France.

References

1. Le Douarin NM, Kalcheim C, *The Neural Crest* (Cambridge University Press: Cambridge, 1999) 445.
2. Beauvais A, Erickson CA, Goins T et al., Changes in the fibronectin-specific integrin expression pattern modify migratory behaviour in the embryonic environment, *J Cell Biol* (1995) **128:**699–713.
3. Erickson CA, Tosney KW, Weston JA, Analysis of migratory behavior of neural crest and fibroblastic cells in embryonic tissues, *Dev Biol* (1980) **77:**142–56.
4. Doetschman T, Eistetter H, Katz M et al., The *in vitro* development of blastocyst-derived embryonic stem cell lines: formation of visceral yolk sac, blood islands and myocardium, *J Emb Exp Morph* (1985) **87:**27–45.
5. Yamane T, Hayashi SI, Mizoguchi M et al., Derivation of melanocytes from embryonic stem cells in culture, *Dev Dyn* (1999) **216:**450–8.
6. Hynes RO, Integrins: versatility, modulation, and signaling in cell adhesion, *Cell* (1992) **68:**11–25.
7. Duband J-L, Rocher S, Chen W-T et al., Cell adhesion and migration in the early vertebrate embryo: Location and possible role of the putative fibronectin receptor complex, *J Cell Biol* (1986) **102:**160–78.
8. Krotoski DM, Domingo C, Bronner-Fraser M, Distribution of a putative cell surface receptor for fibronectin and laminin in the avian embryo, *J Cell Biol* (1986) **103:**1061–71.
9. Coppolino MG, Woodside MJ, Demaurex N et al., Calreticulin is essential for integrin-mediated calcium signalling and cell adhesion, *Nature* (1997) **386:**843–7.

10. Fässler R, Meyer M, Consequences of lack of β1 integrin gene expression in mice, *Genes Dev* (1995) **9**:1896–19.
11. Beauvais-Jouneau A, Pla P, Bernex F et al., A novel model to study the dorsolateral migration of melanoblasts, *Mech Dev* (1999) **89**:3–14.
12. Fässler R, Pfaff M, Murphy J et al., Lack of β1 integrin gene in embryonic stem cells affects morphology, adhesion, and migration but not integration into the inner cell mass of blastocysts, *J Cell Biol* (1995) **128**:979–88.
13. Ashman LK, The biology of stem cell factor and its receptor C-kit, *Int J Biochem Cell Biol* (1999) **31**:1037–51.
14. Cable J, Jackson IJ, Steel KP, Mutations at the W locus affect survival of neural crest-derived melanocytes in the mouse, *Mech Dev* (1995) **50**:139–50.
15. MacKenzie MA, Jordan SA, Budd PS et al., Activation of the receptor tyrosine kinase Kit is required for the proliferation of melanoblasts in the mouse embryo, *Dev Biol* (1997) **192**:99–107.
16. Spritz RA, Giebel LB, Holmes SA, Dominant negative and loss of function mutations of the c-kit (mast/stem cell growth factor receptor) proto-oncogene in human piebaldism, *Am J Hum Genet* (1992) **50**:261–9.
17. Spritz RA, Holmes SA, Ramesar R et al., Mutations of the KIT (mast/stem cell growth factor receptor) proto-oncogene account for a continuous range of phenotypes in human piebaldism, *Am J Hum Genet* (1992) **51**:1058–65.
18. Bernex F, De Sepulveda P, Kress C et al., Spatial and temporal patterns of c-kit-expressing cells in WlacZ/+ and WlacZ/WlacZ mouse embryos, *Development* (1996) **122**:3023–33.
19. Erickson CA, Duong TD, Tosney KW, Descriptive and experimental analysis of the dispersion of neural crest cells along the dorsolateral path and their entry into ectoderm in the chick embryo, *Dev Biol* (1992) **151**:251–72.
20. Lecoin L, Lahav R, Martin FH et al., Steel and C-Kit in the development of avian melanocytes: a study of normally pigmented birds and of the hyperpigmented mutant silky fowl, *Dev Dyn* (1995) **203**:106–18.
21. Guo CS, Wehrle-Haller B, Rossi J et al., Autocrine regulation of neural crest cell development by steel factor, *Dev Biol* (1997) **184**:61–9.
22. Goulding MD, Lumsden A, Gruss P, Signals from the notochord and floorplate regulate the region specific expression of two Pax genes in the developing spinal cord, *Development* (1993) **117**: 1001–16.
23. Tassabehji M, Read AP, Newton VE et al., Waardenburg's syndrome patients have mutations in the human homologue of the *Pax-3* paired box gene, *Nature* (1992) **355**:635–6.
24. Tassabehji M, Read AP, Newton VE et al., Mutations in the PAX3 gene causing Waardenburg syndrome type 1 and type 2, *Nat Genet* (1993) **3**:26–30.
25. Auerbach R, Analysis of the developmental effects of a lethal mutation in the house mouse, *J Exp Zool* (1954) **127**:305–29.
26. Franz T, Kothary R, Characterization of the neural crest defect in Splotch (Sp1H) mutant mice using a *lacZ* transgene, *Dev Brain Res* (1993) **72**:99–105.
27. Moase CE, Trasler DG, Spinal ganglia reduction in the splotch-delayed mouse neural tube defect mutant, *Teratology* (1989) **40**:67–75.
28. Mansouri A, Gruss P, Pax3 and Pax7 are expressed in commissural neurons and restrict ventral neuronal identity in the spinal cord, *Mech Dev* (1998) **78**:171–8.
29. Monsouri A, Pla P, Larue L et al., Pax 3 acts cell autonomously in the neural tube and somites by controlling cell surface properties, *Development* (2001) **128**:1995–2005.
30. Elshourbagy NA, Korman DR, Wu HL et al., Molecular characterization and regulation of the human endothelin receptors, *J Biol Chem* (1993) **268**:3873–9.
31. Lin HY, Kaji EH, Winkel GK et al., Cloning and functional expression of a vascular smooth muscle endothelin 1 receptor, *Proc Natl Acad Sci U S A* (1991) **88**:3185–9.
32. Yanagisawa M, Kurihara H, Kimura S et al., A novel potent vasoconstrictor peptide produced by vascular endothelial cells, *Nature* (1988) **332**:411–15.
33. Baynash A, Hosoda K, Giaid A et al., Interaction of endothelin-3 with endothelin-B receptor is essential for development of epidermal melanocytes and enteric neurons, *Cell* (1994) **79**:1277–85.
34. Hosoda K, Hammer RE, Richardson JA et al., Targeted and natural (piebald-lethal) mutations of endothelin-B receptor gene produce megacolon associated with spotted coat color in mice, *Cell* (1994) **79**:1267–76.
35. Spritz RA, Piebaldism, Waardenburg syndrome, and related genetic disorders —molecular and genetics aspects. In: Nordlund JJ, ed., *The Pigmentary System: Physiology and pathophysiology* (Oxford University Press: New York, NY, 1998) 207–15.

36. Puffenberger EG, Hosoda K, Washington SS et al., A missense mutation of the endothelin-B receptor gene in multigenic Hirschsprung's disease, *Cell* (1994) **79:**1257–66.
37. Edery P, Attie T, Amiel J et al., Mutation of the endothelin-3 gene in the Waardenburg–Hirschsprung disease (Shah–Waardenburg syndrome), *Nat Genet* (1996) **12:**442–4.
38. Clouthier DE, Hosoda K, Richardson JA et al., Cranial and cardiac neural crest defects in endothelin-A receptor-deficient mice, *Development* (1998) **125:**813–24.
39. Karne S, Jayawickreme CK, Lerner MR, Cloning and characterization of an endothelin-3 specific receptor (ETC receptor) from *Xenopus laevis* dermal melanophores, *J Biol Chem* (1993) **1268:**19126–33
40. Lecoin L, Sakurai T, Ngo MT et al., Cloning and characterization of a novel endothelin receptor subtype in the avian class, *PNAS* (1998) **95:**3024–9.
41. Parichy DM, Mellgren EM, Rawls JF et al., Mutational analysis of endothelin receptor b1 (rose) during neural crest and pigment pattern development in the zebrafish *Danio rerio*, *Dev Biol* (2000) **227:**294–306.
42. Nataf V, Lecoin L, Eichmann A et al., Endothelin-B receptor is expressed by neural crest cells in the avian embryo, *PNAS* (1996) **93:**9645–50.
43. Lahav R, Dupin E, Lecoin L et al., Endothelin 3 selectively promotes survival and proliferation of neural crest-derived glial and melanocytic precursors *in vitro*, *PNAS* (1998) **95:**14214–19.

4
The role of *microphthalmia* in pigment cell development

Heinz Arnheiter, Ling Hou, Minh-Thanh Nguyen, Atsuo Nakayama, Bénédicte Champagne, Jon H. Hallsson and Keren Bismuth

The *microphthalmia* locus and its alleles

Pigmentation is one of the most visible signs of variation among organisms and has intrigued scientists across many disciplines. Based on the analysis of a huge resource of pigment mutants in a variety of species, many of the genes affecting pigmentation have been identified in recent years. In the mouse alone, there are over 50 loci affecting coat color and their molecular analysis has already revealed a plethora of signaling pathways, transcription factors, pigment biosynthetic enzymes and motor proteins that act in concert to effect a pigment pattern.[1] Intriguingly, alterations in pigmentation are often part of syndromic disorders, either because the relevant pigment genes have pigment-independent roles in other organ systems[2] or because the pigment cells themselves have distinct roles besides providing color.[2,3] Hence, pigmentation cannot simply be viewed as an evolutionary adaptation for the purpose of display, camouflage, or light protection, but must be seen as an integrated part of an organism's physiology. The analysis of pigmentation genes is thus important far beyond the goal of understanding pigmentation.

Among the pigment loci that control pigment cell development (rather than pigment biosynthesis *per se*), *microphthalmia* is exceptional, since mutations at this locus affect both the neural-crest-derived melanocytes and the neuroepithelial-derived pigment cells of the retinal pigment epithelium (RPE) and the inner layer of the iris.[4–12] The locus is of interest because numerous independent alleles exist, from zebrafish[13] to humans,[14] that show a variety of genetic interactions, both between alleles as well as with alleles at other loci.[1,15] Many of these alleles have pleiotropic effects and in humans are associated with two forms of congenital deafness, Waardenburg syndrome IIa[14] and Tietz syndrome, which is characterized by profound deafness and uniform pigmentary dilution.[16] Mouse *microphthalmia* mutations—over 25 independent alleles have been described in this species—lead to varying degrees of loss of coat pigmentation, small, unpigmented or hypopigmented eyes, and an allele-dependent assortment of other symptoms, including deafness, mast cell deficiencies, and osteopetrosis (for a description of a selection of alleles, see Table 4.1). Homozygosity for phenotypically severe alleles, such as $Mitf^{mi}$ (*microphthalmia*), $Mitf^{mi-ew}$ (*mi-eyeless-white*), $Mitf^{Mi-wh}$ (*Mi-white*) or $Mitf^{vga-9}$ (a transgenic insertional allele), results in a cell-autonomous, early and complete abolishment of neural-crest-derived melanocyte development[10,11] and abnormalities in RPE development.[5–7,11,12,17–19] These phenotypes are thus distinct from albinism due to lack of pigment synthesis in otherwise unaltered pigment cells. Mice homozygous for the mildest allele, $Mitf^{mi-sp}$ (*mi-spotted*), however, appear entirely normal.[20,21] The presence of this allele leads to coat-color spotting only when it is combined with different *Mitf* alleles which, by themselves in heterozygous form, produce no phenotype (Fig. 4.1). Nevertheless, compound heterozygotes need not necessarily have more severe phenotypes than their homozygous parents. In mice in which the semi-dominant allele $Mitf^{Mi-wh}$ is combined with other *Mitf* alleles, there is a remarkable normalization of the small-eye phenotype, even though the

Table 4.1 Selected microphthalmia alleles in the mouse.

Allele	Mode of induction	Heterozygous phenotype	Homozygous phenotype	Mutation	Remarks	Refs.
Mitf^{mi}	spontaneous or X-irradiation?	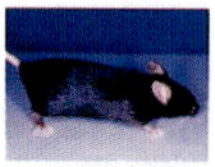	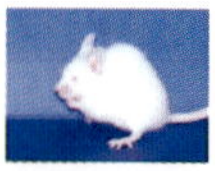	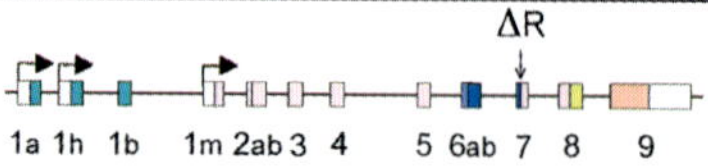 ΔR (1a 1h 1b 1m 2ab 3 4 5 6ab 7 8 9)	heterozygotes have belly spot, homozygotes have osteopetrosis	4-6, 9
Mitf$^{Mi\text{-}wh}$	spontaneous or X-irradiation?	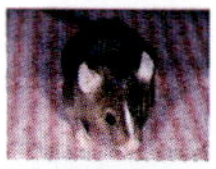	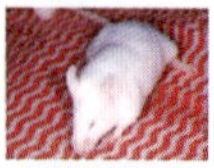	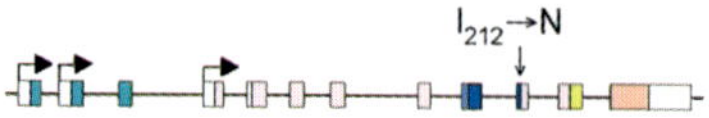 I_{212}→N	heterozygotes have belly spot and both heterozygotes and homozygotes are deaf but not osteopetrotic	6, 24
Mitf$^{mi\text{-}vit}$	spontaneous	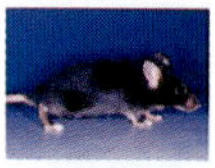	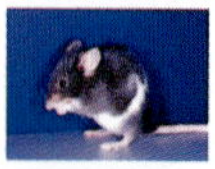	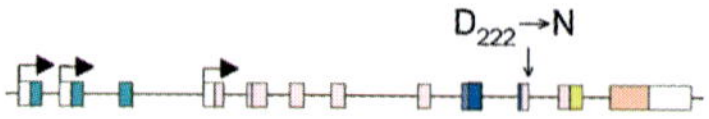 D_{222}→N	homozygotes show gradual depigmentation with age and early retinal degeneration	24, 62
Mitf$^{mi\text{-}ew}$	spontaneous	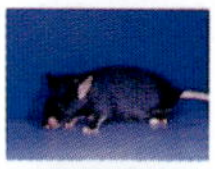	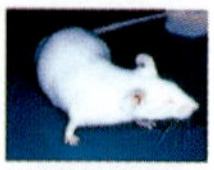	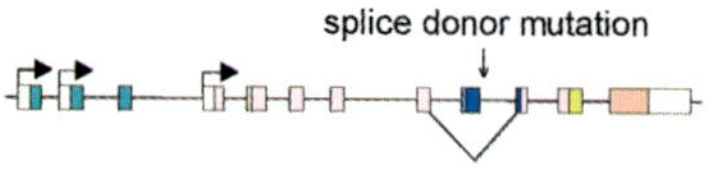 splice donor mutation		24, 26, 63
Mitf$^{mi\text{-}sp}$	spontaneous	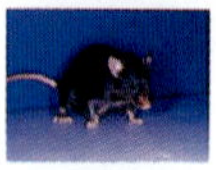	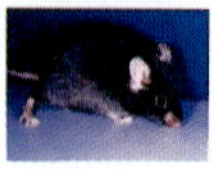	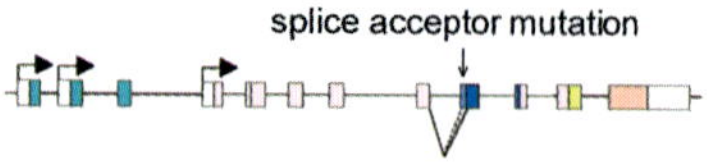 splice acceptor mutation	reduced tyrosinase activity in homozygotes	21, 24
Mitf$^{mi\text{-}bws}$	spontaneous	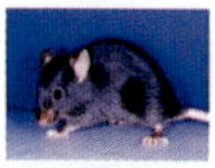	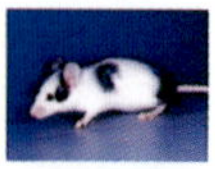	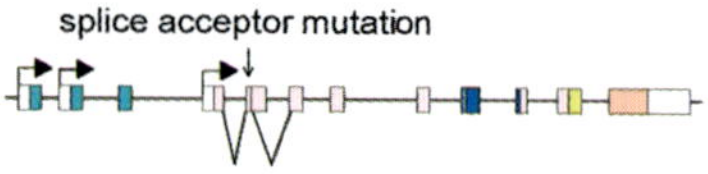 splice acceptor mutation		26, 64
Mitf$^{mi\text{-}rw}$	spontaneous	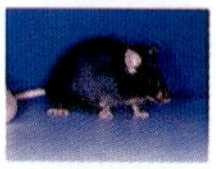	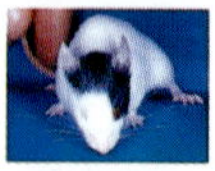	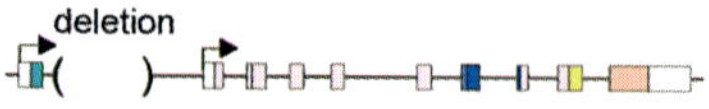 deletion		24, 65
Mitf$^{mi\text{-}bw}$	spontaneous	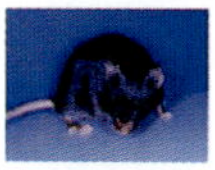	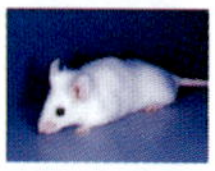	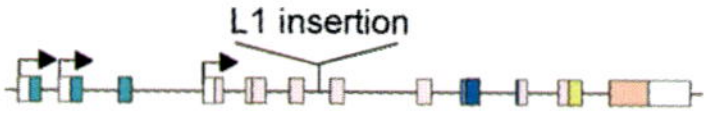 L1 insertion	homozygotes have normal black eyes	25
Mitf$^{vga\text{-}9}$	transgenic insertion	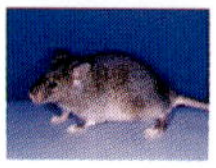	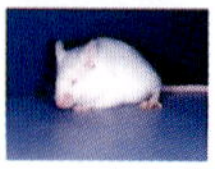	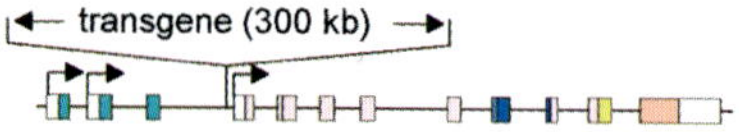 ← transgene (300 kb) →		8, 9

coat may remain entirely white.[17,22] Despite considerable insights into the function of the gene at *microphthalmia*, however, this phenomenon has still not been explained satisfactorily.

The *microphthalmia* gene and protein

The first identification of the *microphthalmia* gene, now termed *Mitf*, was provided by Hodgkinson and co-workers.[9] The gene encodes a transcription factor of the basic helix-loop-helix–leucine zipper (bHLH–LZ) class which, together with TFE3, TFEB and TFEC, belongs to the MITF-TFE subfamily of bHLH-Zip proteins. The four mammalian members of this subfamily share very similar bHLH and leucine zipper domains and, *in vitro*, form all possible combinations of homo- and heterodimers among each other but not with other bHLH and bHLH–LZ proteins.[9,23]

All currently known *microphthalmia* alleles have alterations in *Mitf* (Table 4.1, references 9, 24–26, and unpublished data). Based on this fact, it is now firmly established that *Mitf* is the sole gene affected by mutations at this locus. The gene, schematically depicted in Figure 4.2, resides on mouse chromosome 6 at 40 map units and is spread over at least 60 kbp. The human homolog lies on chromosome 3p at ~73 Mbp from the telomere. Messenger RNAs are initiated from at least three distinct promoters,[24,26] and the corresponding protein isoforms, here termed A-MITF, H-MITF, and M-MITF, differ in their amino termini but share exons 2–9. A-MITF was originally isolated as *Mitf-a* from a kidney cDNA library,[27] H-MITF was originally found in heart,[24]

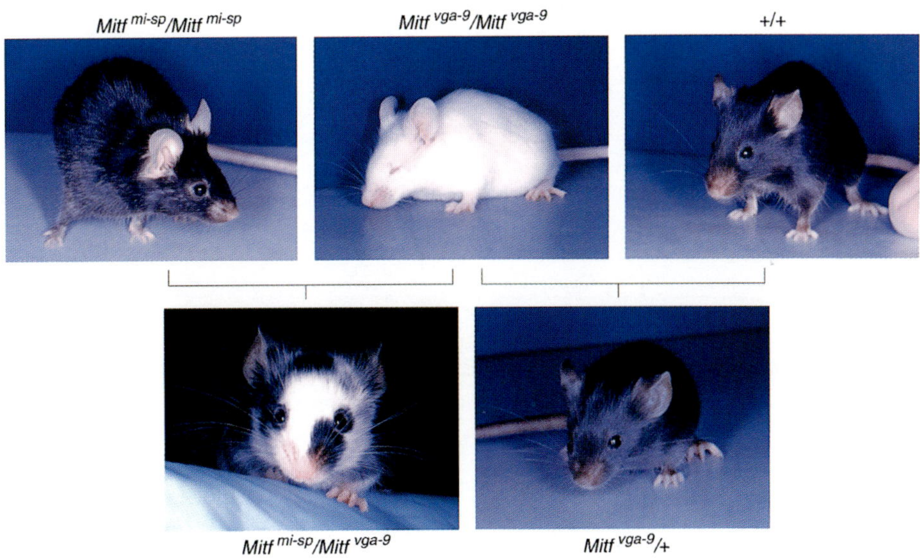

Figure 4.1

Mitf^{mi-sp} is a hypomorphic allele. The allele is characterized by its inability to generate the (+) isoforms of MITF but creates no visible phenotype, even when homozygous. When combined with other *Mitf* alleles, however, a spotting phenotype is revealed. The lower picture on the left shows a mouse in which *Mitf*$^{mi-sp}$ is combined with the transgenic insertional allele *Mitf*$^{vga-9}$ (*Mitf*$^{mi-sp}$/*Mitf*$^{vga-9}$). By comparison, a cross between a *Mitf*$^{vga-9}$/*Mitf*$^{vga-9}$ and a wild-type mouse produces offspring that show no white spotting (lower right, *Mitf*$^{vga-9}$/+).

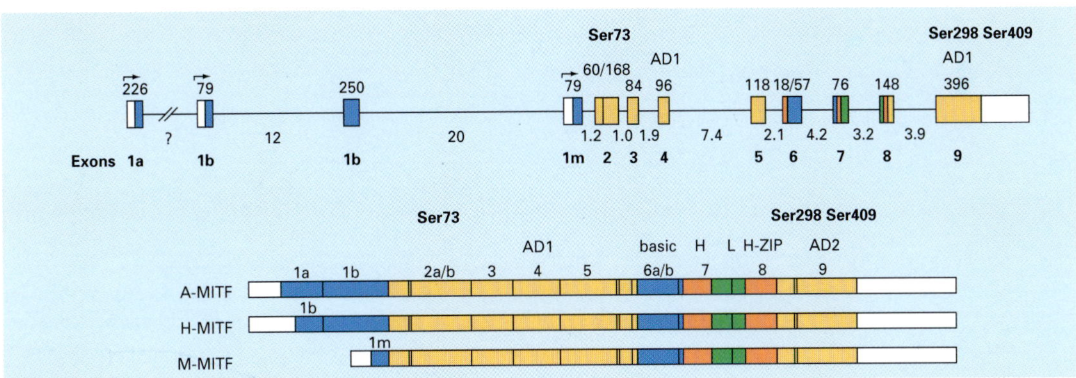

Figure 4.2

The mouse *Mitf* gene and its protein products. The upper part of the figure shows the genomic organization of the gene. The boxes represent exons, with the numbers written on top indicating the corresponding numbers of coding base pairs. The sizes of the corresponding introns (in kbp) are given below. Residues whose phosphorylation is involved in regulating MITF activity are in exon 2b (Ser.73) and exon 9 (Ser298, whose importance is inferred from a mutation in human *MITF*,[60] and Ser409). There is evidence for two activation domains, one encoded by exon 4 (AD1) and one by exon 9 (AD2). Three transcriptional start sites at exon 1a, 1h and 1m are indicated by arrows. The lower part of the figure shows the three major MITF isoforms, A-MITF, H-MITF, and M-MITF, which differ at their amino teminal ends but share the sequences encoded by exons 2–9. Alternative splicing generates additional isoforms which are not shown in the figure (for details see text).

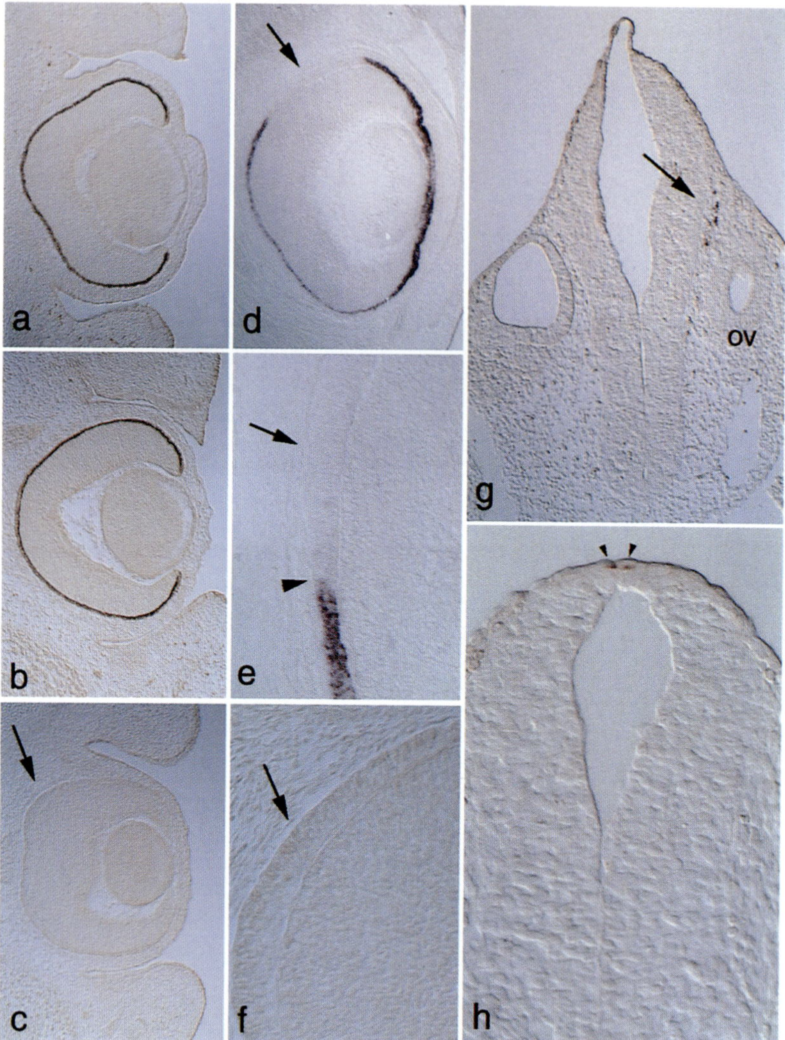

Figure 4.3

Expression of *Mitf* in eye and neural crest of wild-type and mutant embryos. (a–c, f) Cross sections through developing eyes of hamster embryos (E12.5). The sections were labeled by immunocytochemistry for MITF. (a) Wild type. Note pigmented RPE which, upon inspection at higher magnification,[30] shows nuclear MITF labeling and cytoplasmic pigment granules. (b) $Mitf^{Wh}/+$ embryo. RPE shows similar characteristics as wild type. (c) $Mitf^{Wh}/Mitf^{Wh}$ embryo. Note absence of pigmentation and absence of MITF labeling. Arrow points to a thickened part of the RPE. (f) A higher magnification of the thickened RPE shown in (c). (d, e) *In situ* hybridization of cross sections through developing eyes (E16.5) of $Mitf^{mi}/Mitf^{mi}$ embryos. These embryos express MITF mRNA (encoding non-functional protein) in RPE. Note interruption of labeling of the RPE (arrow). In addition to MITF mRNA, this part also downregulates other RPE markers and upregulates a number of retinal markers. The region will transdifferentiate into a second retina that will eventually degenerate. (e) A higher magnification of (d), where arrowhead points to the sharp transition between the transdifferentiating RPE and the abnormal, but not transdifferentiating, part of the RPE. For details, see reference 12. (g, h) *In situ* hybridization for MITF of E10.5 (29 pairs of somites) wild-type mouse embryos. (g) Otic vesicle area. Note positive cells on the ventromedial neural crest migration pathway in the vicinity of the caudal part of the otic vesicle (arrow). (h) *Mitf* expression in rare premigratory neural crest cells in the trunk area where the cells lie on top of the roof plate of the neural tube (arrowheads).

and M-MITF in melanocytes.[9] Additional transcriptional start sites, giving rise to B-MITF and C-MITF, have been described in humans.[28]

Cloning of cDNAs and RT-PCR reactions has identified a number of additional isoforms. Notably, the choice of an alternate splice acceptor in exon 6 leads to inclusion or exclusion of the sequence ACIFPT upstream of the basic domain, with the corresponding proteins usually referred to as the (+) and (−) isoforms of MITF.[9,23,24,26] Alternative splicing of this sequence is common to A-MITF, H-MITF and M-MITF.[26] The distinction between the (+) and (−) isoforms is functionally important, as the above-mentioned allele, $Mitf^{mi-sp}$, which behaves genetically as a hypomorphic allele for pigmentation (Fig. 4.1), cannot generate the (+) isoform.[24] It is unknown, however, whether the $Mitf^{mi-sp}$ phenotype is due to an overall reduction in the total amount of MITF protein or a lack of functions unique to the (+) isoform. *In vitro*, both isoforms bind DNA, though the (−) isoform does so with a modestly decreased affinity.[23] Interestingly, a similar alternate splice choice is seen upstream of the basic domain in the bHLH–LZ protein MAX, where the inclusion of nine residues appears to influence the affinity and kinetics of the interaction with DNA.[29]

In addition to the above-mentioned exon 6 splice choice, exon 2b is also subject to alternative splicing. The functional importance of this exon is evident in mice homozygous for $Mitf^{mi-bws}$ (*mi-black and white spotting*) (see Table 4.1) in which, due to a base substitution upstream of the splice acceptor for exon 2a, the balance of mRNA isoforms as tested in heart is shifted towards exclusion of exon 2b.[26] Interestingly, exon 2b contains a serine residue, which serves as an important target for MAP kinase-dependent phosphorylation in melanocytes (see below).

Mitf expression during development

Mitf expression patterns during development have been studied by standard non-radioactive *in situ* hybridization and immunocytochemical analyses.[10–12] The advantages of these techniques lie in the single-cell resolution and in the fact that they measure the presence of the actual players, mRNAs and proteins. Because of limited sensitivities, however, they fall short in the detection of low-level gene expression and, evidently, do not discriminate between bioactive and inactive proteins. Nonetheless, they provide important clues about the developmental roles of *Mitf*.

Expression in the developing eye

With *in situ* hybridization probes capable of detecting all isoforms of MITF mRNA, the first expression in the mouse is observed at the 22 somite stage in the budding optic vesicle.[12,18] This expression pattern, similarly seen at the protein level, encompasses areas of the neural ectoderm that give rise to the *Mitf*-negative future retina, as well as areas that give rise to the *Mitf*-positive future RPE.[12] The mechanisms that lead to the rapid and locally restricted downregulation of *Mitf* in the prospective retina involve signals from the overlaying surface ectoderm, notably fibroblast growth factors (FGF). This is based on the observation that experimental application of FGF1 or FGF2 leads to *Mitf* downregulation in the future RPE, and the subsequent development of an epithelium that, by the level of cell proliferation, gene expression and lack of pigmentation, resembles the prospective retina. Conversely, removal of the surface ectoderm, which leads to retention of *Mitf* expression in the prospective retina, induces this epithelium to differentiate into pigmented RPE, and re-addition of FGFs prevents this change of cell specification.[12] Thus, the downregulation of *Mitf* in the future neuroretina is crucial for the initial patterning of the optic neuroepithelium, but why *Mitf* is expressed at all in the future retina, albeit only transiently, is far from clear. In *Mitf* mutant embryos, the formation of an optic vesicle and cup, the spatially and temporally precise downregulation of *Mitf*, and the development of a retina are initially unchanged.[12] Only during later development does the mutant eye become abnormal, most likely following alterations in the RPE.

In fact, as shown in Figure 4.3 c,f for hamster embryos homozygous for the $Mitf^{Wh}$ (*anophthalmic white*) allele, which is characterized by a truncation of the MITF protein in the loop domain between helix 1 and helix 2,[30] the RPE still forms an epithelium but remains unpigmented and includes areas of excessive proliferation, particularly in the dorsal parts (arrow in Fig. 4.3 c,f). In mouse embryos homozygous for *Mitf*$^{mi-ew}$ or other alleles that express MITF mRNA but no functional protein, these hyperproliferating areas downregulate *Mitf* (arrows in Fig. 4.3d,e) and other genes normally expressed in RPE, upregulate genes normally expressed in retina, and eventually transdifferentiate into a stratified second retina.[12] This second retina is topologically inverted with respect to the first,[12,17,19] suggesting that retinal polarity does not simply follow a hypothetical anterior-to-posterior gradient of a polarity-inducing factor.

In conclusion, *Mitf* is an important regulator of early eye development during a period when critical cell fate decisions are made. Either due to the dysbalance between the increased growth rate of the RPE and the unchanged growth rate of the retina,[6] or other alterations in the physiology of the mutated RPE, the closing of the optic fissure is perturbed. Subsequently, the eye may not expand, perhaps because intraocular pressure may not build up properly[5,17] or because the secondary vitreous may not form correctly.[7]

Expression in the neural crest

The first *Mitf* expression in the neural crest is observed at the 25–26 somite stage in migratory cells in the head region and caudal to the otic vesicle (Fig. 4.3 g). Based on coexpression of markers such as *Dct* (dopachrome tautomerase, also known as tyrosinase-related protein 2) and *Kit* (a receptor tyrosine kinase), these *Mitf*-positive cells are operationally defined as melanoblasts.[11] In the mouse, melanoblasts usually migrate on a dorsolateral pathway underneath the surface ectoderm, but in the otic vesicle area, they also migrate ventro-medially (arrow in Fig. 4.3g) and eventually become incorporated into the stria vascularis of the inner ear. Here, they are involved in the regulation of the ionic composition of the endolymph, which controls the function of the auditory hair cells[31] (hence the deafness in *Mitf* mutant mice which lack strial melanocytes,[8] but whether deafness in human Waardenburg IIa and Tietz syndromes is due to melanocyte deficiencies has not yet been investigated in detail).

Soon after the first expression in the rostral area, neural crest cells become progressively *Mitf*-positive in an anterior-to-posterior sequence along the body axis.[11] Intriguingly, over the entire trunk area, there are initially (at embryonic day (E) 10.5) no more than approximately 10 premigratory *Mitf*-positive cells, which lie on top of the roof plate of the neural tube (arrowheads in Fig. 4.3h point to two of these cells that, by chance, were found in the same section). Soon thereafter, *Mitf*-positive melanoblasts are found on the dorso-lateral migration pathway and their numbers increase, either because of clonal expansion of the early precursors or because of *de novo* expression of *Mitf* in previously *Mitf*-negative cells. In *Mitf* mutant embryos, provided the mutations still allow for the expression of MITF mRNA, migratory *Mitf*-positive cells still appear, but their numbers do not increase appreciably above the initial number, and at E12.5 the cells become undetectable.[11] This observation argues against a process by which *Mitf*-positive cells are continuously recruited from *Mitf*-negative precursors, and suggests that, barring extensive melanoblast migration along the body axis, trunk melanocytes are largely derived from the small number of trunk precursor cells. This line of reasoning is consistent with the interpretation of the phenotypes of allophenic chimeras presented earlier,[32] and supports the view that melanoblast specification occurs before migration, *i.e.* before the cells reach their final destination. Outside the trunk area, however, *Mitf* is turned on only after the first melanoblast precursors have started to migrate, and so *Mitf* expression in these areas would not seem to reflect the initial number of precursors. The picture is further complicated by the fact that other areas of the crest, in particular the vagal crest, may give rise to *Mitf*-positive cells that are not melanocytic (see below).[11]

Expression and role of specific MITF isoforms

The question of which MITF isoform is expressed in any given cell type has not yet been addressed thoroughly. It appears that M-MITF is fairly specific to neural-crest-derived melanocytes.[27] Whether it plays a selective role in these cells can be addressed in mice carrying the allele *Mitf*$^{mi-bw}$ (*black-eyed white*) (Table 4.1). This allele is characterized by the insertion of an L1 transposable element in intron 3 of *Mitf* and appears to affect M-MITF expression but not A-MITF or H-MITF expression.[25] Mice homozygous for this allele are entirely white (or, depending on the background, may have just minor pigment spots) but have normal-sized and darkly pigmented eyes, suggesting that A-MITF and H-MITF, if at all expressed in neural-crest-derived melanoblasts, cannot rescue these cells effectively, and that M-MITF is not required for eye development and pigmentation of the RPE and inner layer of the iris.

Despite suggestions that it is specific to melanocytes, M-MITF has been amplified from mouse heart,[26] which is not considered to contain melanocytes but is, in part, made up of other neural crest derivatives. In fact, during development, *Mitf* expression can be found in individual cells around the dorsal aorta and the atrio-ventricular bulbar cushion,[11] sites known to be derived from the vagal neural crest. Perhaps M-MITF is not specific to neural-crest-derived melanoblasts but more generally to neural-crest-derived cells, albeit only a small subset of them.

Low-level *Mitf* expression is also found throughout the myocardium, but, based on Northern and PCR analyses, this expression likely corresponds to A-MITF and H-MITF.[9,24,26] Paradoxically, a tissue survey by Northern blots reveals the heart to be the major site of *Mitf* expression in the adult,[9] even though none of the *Mitf* alleles have so far been found to to cause heart defects, not even those that encode dominant-negative forms of MITF (unpublished observation). The intensity of the Northern signal in heart is based on the fact that virtually all myocardial cells, though each at a low level, contribute to the *Mitf* signal in heart mRNA, whereas, by comparison, the few melanocytes strongly positive for *Mitf* in skin, for instance, make little overall contribution to skin mRNA.

In contrast to M-MITF, A-MITF is more ubiquitously expressed and may be the major isoform expressed in the RPE.[27] By now, accustomed to the opportunities presented by a large allelic series, we are not surprised to also find an allele that may speak to the role of A-MITF. In fact, $Mitf^{mi-rw}$ (*mi-red-eyed white*) (Table 4.1) is characterized by a deletion of exons 1h and 1b and surrounding sequences, but leaves intact exons 1a and 1m and at least 6 kb of the corresponding M promoter region.[24,26] The mutant mouse has a characteristic black head spot (see Table 4.1) and may have a small black spot at its lower belly but otherwise is white and variably microphthalmic. If A-MITF is indeed the major isoform in the RPE, the *microphthalmia* phenotype can be explained by the absence of functional A-MITF protein, since, due to the deletion, no open reading frame can be maintained by skipping exons 1b and 1h. Nevertheless, H-MITF, and perhaps other isoforms, are also missing, and so the selective role of A-MITF for eye development must await further scrutiny. More difficult to explain, however, is the coat phenotype of these mice, whose black spots suggest the regional presence of fully functional M-MITF. Intriguingly, both pigmented and unpigmented skin of adult $Mitf^{mi-rw}$ mice show MITF mRNAs at high levels (higher than in wild-type skin), but these mRNAs have not been characterized in detail and it is not known whether they are translated into functional protein.[24]

The regulation of *Mitf* expression during development

Insights into the molecular mechanisms that regulate the onset of *Mitf* expression during development and its maintenance thereafter come from two approaches. The first involves *in vitro* tests of factors that recognize specific sequence motifs in the regulatory regions upstream of the respective transcriptional start sites, and the second the analysis of mutations in genes other than *Mitf* that may affect the development of pigment cells or other cells by regulating *Mitf*. Both approaches should eventually merge into a coherent picture of how the discrete *Mitf* isoforms are turned on and off in different cell types and at different time points.

Most of the analysis of the regulation of *Mitf* expression so far has concentrated on the M-MITF regulatory region, where an array of transcription factors have been found to bind (for a recent review, see reference 33). These include SOX10, PAX3, CREB, LEF1, and BRN2. Using the standard armamentarium of *in vitro* assays, such as transient transfection and mobility shift assays, the high mobility group protein SOX10, known for its capacity to bend DNA and, *in vitro,* activate a large variety of promoters, has been found to prominently stimulate human M-MITF transcription.[34–37] A less prominent activity is found for PAX3, whose binding site is juxtaposed to that of SOX10, and which may cooperate with SOX10 in regulating the promoter.[34,35,38] To date, coexpression of *Sox10* and *Mitf* in melanoblasts is indirectly inferred from the coexpression of *Sox10* and *Tyrp1* (tyrosinase-related protein 1) (unpublished observation) which itself is largely coexpressed with *Mitf*;[15] no evidence, however, is available for coexpression of *Mitf* with *Pax3*.

The *in vivo* importance of *Sox10* and *Pax3* is underscored by the fact that mutations in each of these two genes independently lead to pigment alterations. In fact, in humans, both genes have been implicated in Waardenburg-type pigmentary/deafness syndromes, *PAX3* in Waardenburg syndrome type I,[39] and *SOX10* in Waardenburg–Hirschsprung syndrome or Waardenburg syndrome type IV.[40] It is tempting to speculate, therefore, that the common denominator of the pigmentary defects in these syndromes is the lack of *Mitf*. There are, however, two problems with this sort of interpretation. First, since both *Sox10* and *Pax3* mutations inhibit neural crest development more generally than *Mitf* mutations, mutant neural crest cells may be lost before they are normally capable of turning on M-MITF. Second, both *Sox10* and *Pax3* have more expansive expression patterns than M-MITF, and yet M-MITF is activated only in a small subset of neural crest cells.

This latter problem has led to the notion that additional factors, in particular factors that are under cell-extrinsic signaling control, must be involved in *Mitf* regulation. In fact, the elevation of cAMP levels stimulates pigment gene expression in mature melanocytes and melanoma cells, and does so, indirectly, by stimulating transcription of *Mitf*.[41] Little information is available, however, on the role of cAMP on *Mitf* expression during melanoblast development. On the other hand, KIT signaling is clearly important for melanoblast development, as *Kit* mutations seem to interfere with the proliferation and survival of melanoblasts at similar time points as do *Mitf* mutations.[10] Nevertheless, while *in vivo* and under certain *in vitro* culture conditions, signaling through KIT may be involved in the maintenance of *Mitf* expression, it is clearly not involved in its onset.[10,15] Similarly, the other signaling pathway that is critical to melanoblast development, endothelin-3/endothelin-B receptor, is not required for the onset of *Mitf* expression (unpublished observation). In fact, these pathways, rather than regulating *Mitf* expression, may regulate MITF activity post-transcriptionally (see below).

Recent evidence suggests, however, that the Wnt signaling pathway may regulate M-MITF at the transcriptional level. This is inferred from several observations. First, the zebrafish Mitf promoter that is responsible for neural-crest-derived melanocyte expression (called the Mitf-a promoter) depends on functional binding sites for LEF1/TCF.[42] These are transcription factors whose activating transcriptional role depends on the association with β-catenin, which is stabilized by Wnt signaling. The pathway is conserved throughout evolution and LEF1/TCF binding sites are conserved in both the mouse and human M-MITF promoters.[43] Second, *in vitro*, zebrafish Mitf is downregulated by expression of dominant-negative TCF3.[42] Third, in *Wnt-1/Wnt-3a* double knockout mouse embryos, the number of *Dct*-positive melanoblasts is substantially reduced,[44] as it is in *Mitf* mutant embryos.[10,11] Fourth, in both zebrafish *in vivo*[42] and mouse neural crest cell cultures,[45] Wnt overexpression expands the pool of melanocytes. Activation by Wnt signaling alone, however, cannot be sufficient for M-MITF expression, as not all cells subject to Wnt signaling turn on M-MITF.

The above observations, in sum, have led to the proposal that the transcriptional activation of M-MITF is the result of a stochastic event that occurs only when a variety of transcription factors accumulate together in a cell, each by chance, to a level above a critical threshold.[33] 'Stochastic', however, is perhaps but a euphemism for acknowledging that we do not really understand the underlying mechanisms. Even less is known about the regulation of the other MITF promoters, except that distinct transcription factors must be involved, as the factors implicated in the regulation of M-MITF do not seem to play a role, for instance, in RPE development.

Regulation of *Mitf* target genes

As evident from the analysis of the various *Mitf* mutations, *Mitf* has a dual role, one in melanoblast proliferation and survival and one in differentiation or maintenance of the differentiated function. *Mitf* must thus affect target genes that control cell proliferation, as well as target genes that affect cell differentiation. Little is known about the first group of genes and whether the same or different sets of proliferation targets are accessed in RPE and in the neural crest whose cells, as mentioned above, differ dramatically in their proliferative response to *Mitf* mutations. In contrast, differentiation targets have been analyzed in some detail. Most of these studies, however, are confined to *in vitro* analyses of the respective promoter regions, and evidence for a direct regulation of the endogenous genes by *Mitf* is scarce at best.

The most detailed information is available for the *Dct*, *Tyrp1*, and *Tyr* (tyrosinase) genes which encode pigment enzymes, whose expression is largely restricted to melanocytes and whose regulatory regions share common *Mitf*-responsive E-box motifs.[27,46–51] As shown in Table 4.2, *Mitf*-responsive E-box motifs are also found in other genes expressed in melanocytes, as well as in genes considered *Mitf* targets in mast cells and osteoclasts. E-boxes, however, are frequent in promoter regions and are regulated by a wide variety of bHLH and bHLH–LZ proteins. To explain, then, why pigment genes are silent in non-pigment cells or *Mitf*-responsive osteoclast genes silent in melanoblasts, we have to invoke additional levels of regulation. Undoubtedly, the precise core sequence of an E-box, as well as its surrounding sequences, will influence DNA/protein interactions, and so will the type, isoform and nuclear concentration of the respective E-box binding proteins, their affinities for a given E-box motif, the regulation of their activities through post-translational modifications and interactions with other proteins, and the temporal hierarchy of events that render a given E-box motif competent to bind to and be regulated by a bHLH protein.

There is increasing evidence for regulation of the putative *Mitf* target genes at each of these levels. As shown in Table 4.2, genes expressed in melanocytes generally share the CATGTG core motif flanked by a 5′T/3′N or 5′N/3′A,[52] whereas genes expressed in osteoclasts and mast cells contain MITF-regulated E-boxes whose sequences are less constrained. There are, however, exceptions to this rule, notably the perfect 'melanocyte-type' E-box in the promoter of the osteoclast gene mTRAP, the E-boxes in the promoter of the quail pigment gene QNR-71, whose central dinucleotides differ from those in the CATGTG E box, or the E-box in the promoter of *Kit* which is thought to be regulated by *Mitf*[53] (although its MITF binding has not been a consistent finding[52]) and which is expressed in melanocytes and other cells as well. Nevertheless, it is conceivable that, in conjunction with distinct threshold requirements for *Mitf*, the different MITF isoforms in pigment cells (A-MITF in RPE and M-MITF in neural crest) preferentially regulate the constrained CATGTG motif, whereas isoforms in other cell types prefer different E-box motifs. This rationale would then predict that, at physiological levels, one MITF isoform may not fully replace the function of another, and different E-box binding proteins may not replace *Mitf*.

Although the pigment genes *Dct*, *Tyrp1* and *Tyr* are turned on in both RPE and neural crest melanoblasts, the temporal sequence of their expression and their sensitivity to *Mitf* mutations differ in the two cell types.[11] This, and other observations, argue for additional layers of control. *In vitro*, MITF has been found to interact with, and be regulated by, the transcriptional coactivators/-histone acetyl transferases CBP/P300,[54,55] whose availability for interaction with MITF may vary with the cell type, developmental time, or presence of competing factors. Also, the formal possibility exists that the formation of distinct heterodimers between MITF and the related TFE proteins may play a role. Although the *Tfe* genes do not seem to be expressed appreciably in melanoblasts during the relevant developmental periods,[11] in some cell types, such as osteoclasts, MITF/TFE3 heterodimers have indeed been observed.[56] Based on the analysis of knockout mutations in each of the three *Tfe* genes and the combination of these knockouts with different *Mitf* alleles, however, there is no evidence for an essential role for MITF/TFE heterodimers *in vivo* (Steingrimsson et al., in press).

Recent reports that, in melanocytes and melanoma lines, MITF is modified in both activity and stability by MAP-kinase-dependent phosphorylation through ERK2[57–59] and RSK,[59] and in activity by GSK3-mediated phosphorylation,[60] have added yet another layer of control. Although there is still little information about the role of these post-translational modifications during development, the analysis of some *Mitf* alleles *in vivo* and of cultured neural crest cells allow us a first glimpse into their importance. As mentioned, the allele $Mitf^{mi-bws}$ preferentially excludes exon 2b, which contains the serine residue (Ser73) that is phosphorylated by ERK2, and the homozygous mice are spotted. Nevertheless, whether this

Table 4.2 Core sequences and surrounding sequences of E-boxes reported to bind and respond to MITF *in vitro*. Group A shows E-boxes from the promoter regions of genes expressed in cells of the melanocyte lineage, and group B, E-boxes from the promoter regions of genes expressed in mast cells or osteoclasts. The E-box consensus is highlighted in blue, with central dinucleotides diverging from the 'melanocyte' E-box in light blue. Nucleotides conforming to the criteria in Aksan and Goding[52] are labeled in light gray.

	Gene	MITF responsive element	Reference
A	hTyr TDE	G A T **CATGTG** A T G	52
	mTyr TDE	A A T **CATGTG** A A G	
	qTyr TDE	G G T **CATGTG** A T G	
	tTyr TDE	G A T **CATGTG** A T G	
	hTyr M-box	A G T **CATGTG** C T T	
	mTyr M-box	A G T **CATGTG** C T T	
	qTyr M-box	A A T **CATGTG** C T A	
	tTyr M-box	G C T **CATGTG** A C A	
	hTyr InrE	A G A **CATGTG** A T A	
	mTyr InrE	A A A **CATGTG** A T A	
	qTyr InrE	C A A **CATGTG** A T A	
	tTyr InrE	G A A **CATGTG** A T A	
	hTYRP1 M-box	G G T **CATGTG** C T A	
	mTYRP1 M-box	A G T **CATGTG** C T G	66
	mTYRP1 M-box	A G T **CATGTG** C T G	67
	mTYRP1 E-box	A T A **CAAGTG** T G A	
	mTRP2 M-box	G G T **CATGTG** C T A	
	mTRP2 E-box	A C A **CATGTC** A G A	
	mTbx2	G G A **CATGTG** A G A	69
	hTRP-2 M-box	G G T **CATGTG** C T A	52
	hTRP2 E-box	G A G **CACATG** A G C	
	mMC1R motif 1	C A T **CATGTG** G C C	68
	mMC1R motif 2	T G G **CACATG** C C C	
	QNR-71 (-55--44)	C A T **CACATG** A T G	70
	QNR-71 (-109--98)	A A G **CACATG** A G C	
	mc-Kit	G A G **CACCTG** C C A	53

Table 4.2 contd

B									
mTRAP	G	G	T	**CATGTG**	A	G	N	71
mMCP-4	C	T	C	**CATGTG**	C	T	C	72
mp75 E-box (-146--135)	C	C	T	**CACTTG**	A	C	T	73
mp75 E-box (-24--13)	A	C	C	**CAGCTG**	C	T	C	
integrin α4	A	G	T	**CACTTG**	G	T	G	74
mMCP6-1				**CACATG**				75
mMCP6-2				**CATCTG**				
mMCP-2	C	C	C	**CACATG**	C	T	C	76
mMCP-9	A	C	C	**CATATG**	C	T	C	

phenotype is specifically due to loss of Ser73 or other parts or all of exon 2b requires further exploration. Furthermore, GSK3-mediated phosphorylation at Ser298, which enhances DNA binding of MITF, appears to be biologically important, as this residue is mutated in a family with Waardenburg syndrome IIa.[60] Yet another line of evidence comes from the analysis of embryos that are homozygous for a *Kit* null allele, marked by a knocked-in *LacZ* gene.[61] KIT is activated by KIT ligand and, acting through the RAS–RAF pathway, activates ERK2. Mutant embryos normally lose their melanoblasts around E12.5, but small numbers of the cells can be maintained in culture, provided they are given endothelin-3.[15] Moreover, these cells maintain *Mitf* expressions and the normal temporal sequence of expression of several pigment genes. Thus, *Dct* is turned on at day 1 of explantation, *Silver* at 4 days, and *Tyrp1* at 5 days, as observed in wild type. *Tyr,* whose expression should start at 6 days, however, is not turned on at all in mutant cultures and, hence, the cells remain unpigmented. Both *Tyr* expression and pigmentation can be rescued by exposure of the cells to hepatocyte growth factor, which signals through the tyrosine kinase receptor MET, or by elevating cAMP, which mimics part of the KIT signaling pathway. As discussed by Hou et al.,[15] these experiments have intriguing implications for the temporal and gene-specific regulation of *Mitf* target genes by extrinsic signals. During development, then, KIT signaling seems to have a dual role: one in promoting cell proliferation and survival, and the other in regulating cell differentiation. Interestingly, in melanoma cells, KIT is consistently downregulated, while other receptor tyrosine kinases are upregulated. In what way signaling through KIT and other receptor tyrosine kinases differs during melanocyte development and in mature melanocytes and melanomas remains a fascinating question.

Conclusions

Mutations at the *microphthalmia* locus have provided us with an extraordinary opportunity to gain insights into the mechanisms that control the birth, life and death of pigment cells in vertebrates. Thanks to the invaluable contributions by geneticists over six decades, we now have access to a large allelic series that has illuminated well-established textbook principles of genetics and added a few intriguing twists. *Microphthalmia* has taught us, once again, that widely expressed genes may have visible effects only in discrete locations, and that the action of a gene does not necessarily lie where the fattest Northern band is found in a tissue survey. It has also taught us that null mutations, still the standard in today's approach to gene function studies, often miss part of the picture. Without mutations generating dominant-negative proteins, for instance, we may still be ignorant about MITF's role in bone remodeling and would hardly know anything about its role in mast cells. *Microphthalmia* has also given us some living examples of intriguing allelic interactions that lead to exacerbation or complementation of phenotypes, and we predict that the continuing collection of *Mitf* alleles will give us many more such cases in the future. Further, it has shown us that, despite the sharing of the bulk of exons, *Mitf* in fact represents at least three transcription units, each with its preferred expression pattern and likely its distinct mutational consequences. This illustrates the futility of counting genes as single transcription units and then comparing their numbers between species without carefully analyzing the organization of each individual gene. Finally, *microphthalmia* has reminded us that mutations in animals are invaluable when it comes to analyzing human disorders, even if the genetics show species-specific differences, such as haploid insufficiency in humans and haploid sufficiency in mice.

As has been noted earlier, spontaneous mutations are experiments done by Nature and, thus, oblivious of the power, or the failure, of the human intellect. They are indisputable in fact, but challenging in the need for explanations. What, for instance, makes $Mitf^{mi-rw}$ mice have black spots on the head and belly but not the flanks, while the spots in $Mitf^{mi-bws}$ mice are more evenly distributed? Until recently, it was the analysis of random mutants that provided all the mechanistic insights, but now molecular biology and biochemistry have raced ahead and whetted our appetites for designer mutants. Thus, we now need to test the roles of each *Mitf* isoform independently, and to generate point mutations in the residues predicted to serve as targets for extracellular signaling. It will be fascinating to investigate whether it is by chance or for intrinsic mechanistic reasons, that Nature has not yet provided us with all the mutations that are required to explore these issues thoroughly.

Acknowledgements

We thank William J. Pavan and Colin Goding for helpful discussions, and Lynn D. Hudson for comments on the manuscript.

References

1. Mouse Genome Database (MGD), Mouse Genome Informatics Web Site, The Jackson Laboratory, Bar Harbor, Maine. World Wide Web (URL: http://www.informatics.jax.org/) (April, 2002).
2. King RA, Hearing VJ, Creel DJ et al., Albinism. In: Scriver CR et al., eds, *The Metabolic and Molecular Basis of Inherited Disease*, 8th edn (McGraw-Hill: New York, 2001) 5587–627.
3. Deol MS, The relationship between abnormalities of pigmentation and of the inner ear, *Proc R Soc Lond B Biol Sci* (1970) **175**:201–17.
4. Hertwig P, Neue Mutationen und Kopplungsgruppen bei der Hausmaus, *Z Indukt Abstammungs- u. Vererbungsl* (1942) **80**:220–46.
5. Müller G, Eine entwicklungsgeschichtliche Untersuchung über das erbliche Kolobom mit Mikrophthalmus bei der Hausmaus, *Z Mikrosk Anat Forsch* (1950) **56**:520–58.
6. Packer SO, The eye and skeletal effects of two mutant alleles at the microphthalmia locus of Mus musculus, *J Exp Zool* (1967) **165**:21–45.
7. Scholtz CL, Chan KK, Complicated colobomatous microphthalmia in the microphthalmic (mi/mi) mouse, *Development* (1987) **99**:501–8.
8. Tachibana M, Hara Y, Vyas D et al., Cochlear Disorder associated with melanocyte anomaly in mice with a transgenic insertional mutation, *Mol Cell Neurosci* (1992) **3**:433–45.
9. Hodgkinson CA, Moore KJ, Nakayama A et al., Mutations at the mouse microphthalmia locus are associated with defects in a gene encoding a novel basic-helix-loop-helix-zipper protein, *Cell* (1993) **74**:395–404.
10. Opdecamp K, Nakayama A, Nguyen MT et al., Melanocyte development in vivo and in neural crest cell cultures: crucial dependence on the Mitf basic-helix-loop-helix-zipper transcription factor, *Development* (1997) **124**:2377–86.
11. Nakayama A, Nguyen MT, Chen CC et al., Mutations in microphthalmia, the mouse homolog of the human deafness gene MITF, affect neuroepithelial and neural crest-derived melanocytes differently, *Mech Dev* (1998) **70**:155–66.
12. Nguyen M, Arnheiter H, Signaling and transcriptional regulation in early mammalian eye development: a link between FGF and MITF, *Development* (2000) **127**:3581–91.
13. Lister JA, Robertson CP, Lepage T et al., Nacre encodes a zebrafish microphthalmia-related protein that regulates neural-crest-derived pigment cell fate, *Development* (1999) **126**:3757–67.
14. Tassabehji M, Newton VE, Read AP, Waardenburg syndrome type 2 caused by mutations in the human microphthalmia (MITF) gene, *Nat Genet* (1994) **8**:251–5.
15. Hou L, Panthier JJ, Arnheiter H, Signaling and

transcriptional regulation in the neural crest-derived melanocyte lineage: interactions between KIT and MITF, *Development* (2000) **127**:5379–89.

16. Smith SD, Kelley PM, Kenyon JB et al., Tietz syndrome (hypopigmentation/deafness) caused by mutation of MITF, *J Med Genet* (2000) **37**:446–8.
17. Konyukhov B, Osipov VV, Interallelic complementation of microphthalmia and white genes in mice, *Genetika* (1968) **4**:65–76.
18. Bora N, Conway SJ, Liang H et al., Transient overexpression of the Microphthalmia gene in the eyes of Microphthalmia vitiligo mutant mice, *Dev Dyn* (1998) **213**:283–92.
19. Bumsted KM, Barnstable CJ, Dorsal retinal pigment epithelium differentiates as neural retina in the microphthalmia (mi/mi) mouse, *Invest Ophthalmol Vis Sci* (2000) **41**:903–8.
20. Wolfe HG, *Mouse News Lett* (1962) **26**:35.
21. Wolfe HG, Coleman DL, Mi-spotted: a mutation in the mouse, *Genet Res Camb* (1964) **5**:432–40.
22. Hollander WF, Complementary alleles at the *mi*-locus in the mouse, *Genetics* (1968) **60**:189.
23. Hemesath TJ, Steingrimsson E, McGill G et al., Microphthalmia, a critical factor in melanocyte development, defines a discrete transcription factor family, *Genes Dev* (1994) **8**:2770–80.
24. Steingrímsson E, Moore KJ, Lamoreux ML et al., Molecular basis of mouse microphthalmia (mi) mutations helps explain their developmental and phenotypic consequences, *Nat Genet* (1994) **8**:256–63.
25. Yajima I, Sato S, Kimura T et al., An L1 element intronic insertion in the black-eyed white (Mitf[mi-bw]) gene: the loss of a single Mitf isoform responsible for the pigmentary defect and inner ear deafness, *Hum Mol Genet* (1999) **8**:1431–41.
26. Hallsson JH, Favor J, Hodgkinson C et al., Genomic, transcriptional and mutational analysis of the mouse microphthalmia locus, *Genetics* (2000) **155**:291–300.
27. Amae S, Fuse N, Yasumoto K et al., Identification of a novel isoform of microphthalmia-associated transcription factor that is enriched in retinal pigment epithelium, *Biochem Biophys Res Commun* (1998) **247**:710–15.
28. Shibahara S, Yasumoto K, Amae S et al., Regulation of pigment cell-specific gene expression by MITF, *Pigment Cell Res* (2000) **13**:98–102.
29. Bousset K, Henriksson M, Luscher-Firzlaff JM, et al., Identification of casein kinase II phosphorylation sites in Max: effects on DNA-binding kinetics of Max homo- and Myc/Max heterodimers, *Oncogene* (1993) **8**:3211–20.
30. Hodgkinson CA, Nakayama A, Li H et al., Mutation at the anophthalmic white locus in Syrian hamsters: haploinsufficiency in the Mitf gene mimics human Waardenburg syndrome type 2, *Hum Mol Genet* (1998) **7**:703–8.
31. Steel KP, Kros CJ, A genetic approach to understanding auditory function, *Nat Genet* (2001, **27**: 136–7.
32. Mintz B, Gene control of mammalian pigmentary differentiation. I. Clonal origin of melanocytes, *Proc Natl Acad Sci U S A* (1967) **58**:344–51.
33. Goding C, Mitf from neural crest to melanoma: signal transduction and transcription in the melanocyte lineage, *Genes Dev* (2000) **14**:1712–28.
34. Potterf SB, Furumura M, Dunn KJ et al., Transcription factor hierarchy in Waardenburg Syndrome: regulation of MITF expression by SOX10 and PAX3, *Hum Genet* (2000) **107**:1–6.
35. Bondurand N, Pingault V, Goerich DE et al., Interaction among SOX10, PAX3 and MITF, three genes altered in Waardenburg syndrome, *Hum Mol Genet* (2000) **9**:1907–17.
36. Lee M, Goodall J, Verastegui C et al., Direct regulation of the Microphthalmia promoter by Sox10 links Waardenburg–Shah syndrome (WS4)-associated hypopigmentation and deafness to WS2, *J Biol Chem* (2000) **275**:37978–83.
37. Verastegui C, Bille K, Ortonne JP et al., Regulation of the microphthalmia-associated transcription factor gene by the Waardenburg syndrome type 4 gene, SOX10, *J Biol Chem* (2000) **275**:30757–60.
38. Watanabe A, Takeda K, Ploplis B et al., Epistatic relationship between Waardenburg syndrome genes MITF and PAX3, *Nat Genet* (1998) **18**:283–6.
39. Tassabehji M, Read AP, Newton VE et al., Mutations in the PAX3 gene causing Waardenburg syndrome type 1 and type 2, *Nat Genet* (1993) **3**:26–30.
40. Pingault V, Bondurand N, Kuhlbrodt K et al., SOX10 mutations in patients with Waardenburg–Hirschsprung disease, *Nat Genet* (1998) **18**:171–3.
41. Bertolotto C, Abbe P, Hemesath TJ et al., Microphthalmia gene product as a signal transducer in cAMP-induced differentiation of melanocytes, *J Cell Biol* (1998) **142**:827–35.
42. Dorsky RI, Raible DW, Moon RT, Direct regulation of nacre, a zebrafish MITF homolog required for pigment cell formation, by the Wnt pathway, *Genes Dev* (2000) **14**:158–62.
43. Takeda K, Yasumoto K, Takada R et al., Induction of melanocyte-specific microphthalmia-associated transcription factor by Wnt-3a, *J Biol Chem* (2000) **275**:14013–16.

44. Ikeya M, Lee SM, Johnson JE et al., Wnt signalling required for expansion of neural crest and CNS progenitors, *Nature* (1997) **389**:966–70.
45. Dunn KJ, Williams BO, Li Y et al., Neural crest-directed gene transfer demonstrates Wnt1 role in melanocyte expansion and differentiation during mouse development, *Proc Natl Acad Sci U S A* (2000) **97**:10050–5.
46. Bentley NJ, Eisen T, Goding CR, Melanocyte-specific expression of the human tyrosinase promoter: activation by the microphthalmia gene product and role of the initiator, *Mol Cell Biol* (1994) **14**:7996–8006.
47. Ganss R, Schutz G, Beermann F, The mouse tyrosinase gene. Promoter modulation by positive and negative regulatory elements, *J Biol Chem* (1994) **269**:29808–16.
48. Yasumoto K, Yokoyama K, Shibata K et al., Microphthalmia-associated transcription factor as a regulator for melanocyte-specific transcription of the human tyrosinase gene, *Mol Cell Biol* (1994) **14**:8058–70.
49. Yokoyama K, Yasumoto K, Suzuki H et al., Cloning of the human DOPAchrome tautomerase/tyrosinase-related protein 2 gene and identification of two regulatory regions required for its pigment cell-specific expression, *J Biol Chem* (1994) **269**:27080–7.
50. Yasumoto K, Yokoyama K, Takahashi K et al., Functional analysis of microphthalmia-associated transcription factor in pigment cell-specific transcription of the human tyrosinase family genes, *J Biol Chem* (1997) **272**:503–9.
51. Udono T, Yasumoto K, Takeda K et al., Structural organization of the human microphthalmia-associated transcription factor gene containing four alternative promoters, *Biochim Biophys Acta* (2000) **1491**:205–19.
52. Aksan I, Goding CR, Targeting the microphthalmia basic helix-loop-helix–leucine zipper transcription factor to a subset of E-box elements in vitro and in vivo, *Mol Cell Biol* (1998) **18**:6930–8.
53. Tsujimura T, Morii E, Nozaki M et al., Involvement of transcription factor encoded by the mi locus in the expression of c-kit receptor tyrosine kinase in cultured mast cells of mice, *Blood* (1996) **88**:1225–33.
54. Sato S, Roberts K, Gambino G et al., CBP/p300 as a co-factor for the Microphthalmia transcription factor, *Oncogene* (1997) **14**:3083–92.
55. Price ER, Ding HF, Badalian T et al., Lineage-specific signaling in melanocytes. C-kit stimulation recruits p300/CBP to microphthalmia, *J Biol Chem* (1998) **273**:17983–6.
56. Weilbaecher KN, Hershey CL, Takemoto CM et al., Age-resolving osteopetrosis: a rat model implicating microphthalmia and the related transcription factor TFE3, *J Exp Med* (1998) **187**:775–85.
57. Hemesath TJ, Price ER, Takemoto C et al., MAP kinase links the transcription factor Microphthalmia to c-Kit signalling in melanocytes, *Nature* (1998) **391**:298–301.
58. Xu W, Gong L, Haddad MM et al., Regulation of microphthalmia-associated transcription factor MITF protein levels by association with the ubiquitin-conjugating enzyme hUBC9, *Exp Cell Res* (2000) **255**:135–43.
59. Wu M, Hemesath TJ, Takemoto CM et al., c-Kit triggers dual phosphorylations, which couple activation and degradation of the essential melanocyte factor Mi, *Genes Dev* (2000) **14**:301–12.
60. Takeda K, Takemoto C, Kobayashi I et al., Ser298 of MITF, a mutation site in Waardenburg syndrome type 2, is a phosphorylation site with functional significance, *Hum Mol Genet* (2000) **9**:125–32.
61. Bernex F, De Sepulveda P, Kress C et al., Spatial and temporal patterns of c-kit-expressing cells in WlacZ/+ and WlacZ/WlacZ mouse embryos, *Development* (1996) **122**:3023–33.
62. Lamoreux ML, Boissy RE, Womack JE et al., The vit gene maps to the mi (microphthalmia) locus of the laboratory mouse, *J Hered* (1992) **83**:435–9.
63. Minor G, *Mouse News Lett* (1968) **38**:25.
64. Sweet HO, Recessive spotting mutation mapped to the Mitf-mi locus in chromosome 6, *Mouse Genome* (1996) **94**:145.
65. Southard JL, *Mouse News Lett* (1974) **51**:23.
66. Fang D, Setaluri V, Role of microphthalmia transcription factor in regulation of melanocyte differentiation marker TRP-1, *Biochem Biophys Res Commun* (1999) **256**:657–63.
67. Bertolotto C, Busca R, Abbe P et al., Different cis-acting elements are involved in the regulation of TRP1 and TRP2 promoter activities by cyclic AMP: pivotal role of M boxes (GTCATGTGCT) and of microphthalmia, *Mol Cell Biol* (1998) **18**:694–702.
68. Adachi S, Morii E, Kim D et al., Involvement of mi-transcription factor in expression of alpha-melanocyte-stimulating hormone receptor in cultured mast cells of mice, *J Immunol* (2000) **164**:855–60.
69. Carreira S, Liu B, Goding CR, The gene encoding the T-box factor Tbx2 is a target for the microphthalmia-associated transcription factor in melanocytes, *J Biol Chem* (2000) **275**:21920–7.
70. Turque N, Denhez F, Martin P et al., Characterization of a new melanocyte-specific gene (QNR-71)

expressed in v-myc-transformed quail neuroretina, *EMBO J* (1996) **15**:3338–50.

71. Luchin A, Purdom G, Murphy K et al., The microphthalmia transcription factor regulates expression of the tartrate-resistant acid phosphatase gene during terminal differentiation of osteoclasts, *J Bone Miner Res* (2000) **15**:451–60.
72. Jippo T, Morii E, Tsujino K et al., Involvement of transcription factor encoded by the mouse mi locus (MITF) in expression of p75 receptor of nerve growth factor in cultured mast cells of mice, *Blood* (1997) **90**:2601–8.
73. Jippo T, Lee YM, Katsu Y et al., Deficient transcription of mouse mast cell protease 4 gene in mutant mice of mi/mi genotype, *Blood* (1999) **93**:1942–50.
74. Kim DK, Morii E, Ogihara H et al., Impaired expression of integrin alpha-4 subunit in cultured mast cells derived from mutant mice of mi/mi genotype, *Blood* (1998) **92**:1973–80.
75. Morii E, Tsujimura T, Jippo T et al., Regulation of mouse mast cell protease 6 gene expression by transcription factor encoded by the mi locus, *Blood* (1996) **88**:2488–94.
76. Ge Y, Jippo T, Lee YM et al., Independent influence of strain difference and mi transcription factor on the expression of mouse mast cell, *Am J Pathol* (2001) **158**:281–92.

Section II

THE BIOCHEMISTRY OF MELANOGENESIS

5

The biochemistry of melanogenesis and its regulation by ultraviolet radiation

Taketsugu Tadokoro, Nobuhiko Kobayashi, Janusz Z. Beer, Barbara Z. Zmudzka, Kazumasa Wakamatsu, Sharon A. Miller, M. Lynn Lamoreux, Shosuke Ito and Vincent J. Hearing

Introduction

Melanin pigments, produced by melanocytes, give rise to virtually all color visible in the skin, hair and eyes of mammals.[1] Such pigments play a number of diverse and important roles, including thermoregulation in lower vertebrates, camouflage and sexual attraction in virtually all species, and photoprotection of the skin in higher mammals. Pigmentation patterns in the skin and hair are determined not only by the location of melanocytes in those tissues (as determined by the migration of melanoblasts during embryological development), but also by the type and number of melanins produced by functional melanocytes in a given location. Melanocytes must not only produce the melanin within membrane-bound organelles (termed melanosomes), but must then distribute those pigment granules to neighboring keratinocytes (which carry them to the surface of the skin or to the growing hair shaft). Thus, interactions between melanocytes and keratinocytes are critically important to the eventual color of tissue, and, of course, their final distribution plays a significant role in determining the photoprotective value of the pigment to the underlying cells. Factors that influence the eventual coloration of the skin and hair involve those acting within the melanocyte (*e.g.* the amount and type of melanins produced, the shape, size and number of melanosomes, and the transport of those melanosomes to the dendrites) and within the keratinocytes (*e.g.* the ability to ingest melanosomes, their packing individually or in complexes, their breakdown into smaller particles and their final distribution in the hair or at the surface of the skin).

The melanocyte:keratinocyte complex is a highly interactive milieu which responds quickly to a number of environmental stimuli, often in paracrine and/or autocrine manners.[2] Some of the major factors that influence melanocyte proliferation and differentiation include ultraviolet radiation (UV) (the focus of this meeting), melanocyte stimulating hormone (MSH), the antagonist agouti signal protein (ASP), endothelins (ET), steel factor, a variety of growth factors and cytokines, etc. It is known that UV can stimulate the production of ET1, the ET1 receptor (EDNRB), and POMC (the precursor of MSH) by keratinocytes, and those factors can then act as paracrine factors to stimulate melanocytes.[3–5] Melanocytes themselves respond to UV by increasing their expression of POMC and the MSH receptor (MC1R), the melanogenic enzymes tyrosinase and Tyrp1, protein kinase C, and other signaling factors. Those responses have been characterized in cell culture models, and need to be confirmed *in situ*, but it is clear that the responses of melanocytes and keratinocytes in the skin are quite complex, and may even vary significantly, depending on the type of UV used and the phototype of the skin irradiated.

Regardless of the mechanisms involved, the value of melanin to photoprotection of the skin is highly significant. In the United States, rates of basal and squamous cell carcinomas are 50 times higher in Caucasians than in African-Americans.[6] Although one might intuitively expect darker skin to have a higher incidence of melanoma (the transformed state of melanocytes), African-Americans actually have a 13-fold lower incidence of melanoma than do Caucasians. Whether the photoprotection afforded is due solely to the role of melanin as a sunscreen,[7] or whether other properties of melanins are involved, is an important question that remains to be resolved.

We have recently initiated a study aimed at characterizing the responses of melanocytes in the skin to UV and at measuring the efficacy of different types of melanins in photoprotection. Some preliminary considerations and findings of that study are included at the end of this chapter.

Biochemical determinants of melanin production

The complex nature of the regulation of mammalian pigmentation was understood many decades ago, based on the wide number of pigmentary genes that affected coat color in lower mammals, especially mice. The albino mouse has been maintained as an interesting curiosity for more than two millennia, and even 30 to 40 years ago, more than 60 discrete genetic loci had been identified that regulate pigmentation in mice. That number has recently grown to more than 90. Many of those genes specifically affect only melanocytes, but others affect other cell types as well. Some of them operate during embryologic development and migration, others are important to the survival and differentiation of melanoblasts to melanocytes, others are important to the specific production of melanin pigment within melanocytes, and yet others are involved in the mobilization of those granules to the dendrites of melanocytes and in their eventual distribution to neighboring keratinocytes.[8–10]

Of the more than 90 genes that are involved in regulating pigmentation, only five are specifically localized in melanosomes, the actual site of pigment formation, and play role(s) in the synthesis and deposition of melanin.[2,11,12] The first and most critical of those, known as tyrosinase, was identified biochemically almost 100 years ago as a polyphenol oxidase (Fig. 5.1); that enzyme was able to catalyze the rate-limiting step of hydroxylating the amino acid tyrosine to its dihydroxylated form, L-3,4-dihydroxyphenylalanine (DOPA). That reaction proceeds at negligible rates in the absence of that enzyme, and mutations in the gene-encoding tyrosinase (termed *Tyr*) were expected to be associated with albinism, a fact substantiated soon after *Tyr* was cloned. Although lower forms of tyrosinase have a relatively broad specificity towards hydroxylated (and in some cases even non-hydroxylated) phenols, as one moves up the evolutionary tree, the specificity of tyrosinase became more and more restrictive until, in higher mammals, the enzyme will essentially react only with tyrosine (and the dihydroxylated derivatives DOPA and 5,6-dihydroxyindole (DHI). Once DOPA is generated, it can be spontaneously further oxidized to DOPAquinone, which then cyclizes to produce an orange intermediate, known as DOPAchrome. DOPAchrome will spontaneously decarboxylate to give rise to DHI, which can then further oxidize to indole-5,6-quinone. It is the polymerization of these various quinone and indole–quinone intermediates that gives rise to the high molecular weight, insoluble and quite black pigment known as DHI eumelanin. For more than 80 years, this pathway (sometimes referred to as the Raper–Mason pathway) was accepted as the sole mechanism by which eumelanins were generated, and it was thought simply that the amount of melanin produced correlated directly with the amount of tyrosinase present.

But the rush to clone the gene encoding tyrosinase demonstrated very quickly that nature was not quite so simple. Initially, the cloned gene thought to be tyrosinase was actually mapped to the *brown* locus in mice, and turned out to be an enzyme closely related to tyrosinase; that enzyme is now termed tyrosinase-related protein 1 (Tyrp1). Soon thereafter, the *Tyr* gene was cloned and was mapped to the *albino* locus as expected, but along the way, a second tyrosinase-related enzyme, known as DOPAchrome tautomerase (Dct), was also cloned and was mapped to the *slaty* locus in mice. One might ask why we need other enzymes to regulate melanin production downstream of tyrosinase. There are various possible answers, among them a very attractive one related to the question of toxicity. When melanins and their precursors are generated in melanocytes, the reactions give rise to a number of various toxic by-products, including o-quinones, semiquinones, hydroxyl radicals and hydrogen peroxide. Non-melanocytic cells (*e.g.* fibroblasts) transfected with *Tyr* will make melanin, but those cells are

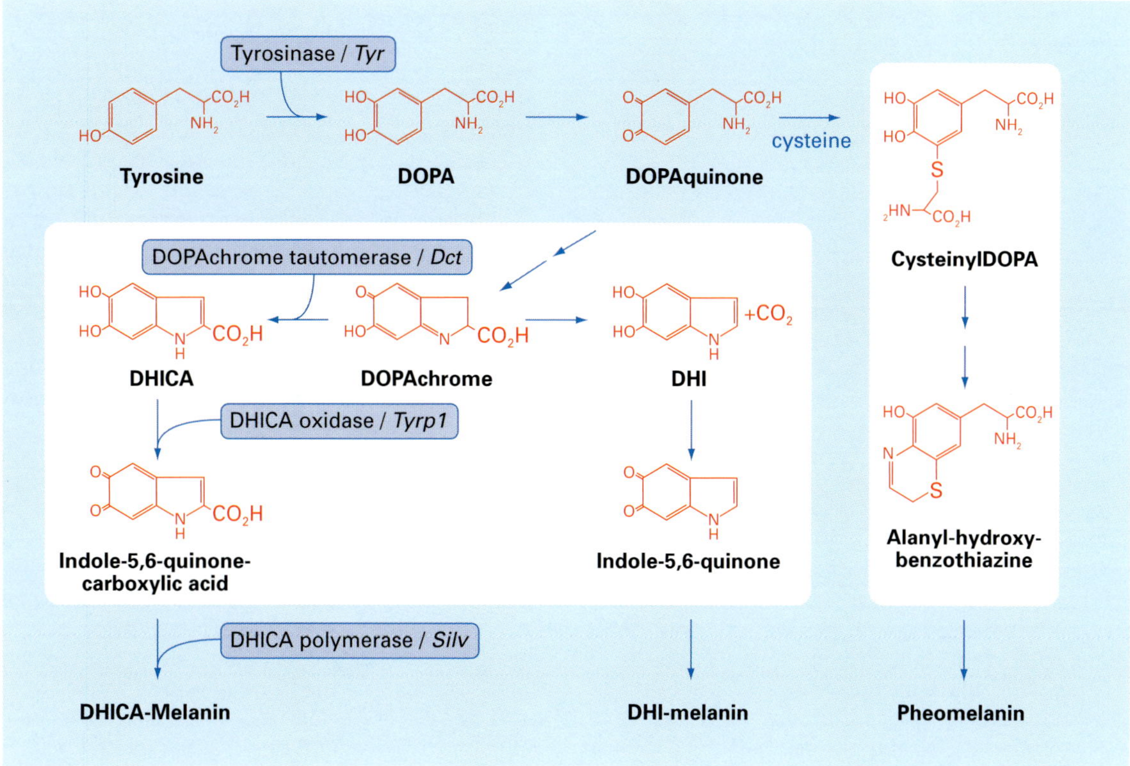

Figure 5.1

Schematic of the melanin biosynthetic pathway. The chemical reactions involved are summarized and the locations of action of the various melanogenic enzymes (tyrosinase, Tyrp1, Dct and Silv) are noted.

quickly killed if melanin production is significant, presumably due to their inability to handle the toxicity involved with that pathway.

So how do melanocytes deal with the cytotoxicity? One obvious answer is by sequestering the toxic intermediates within a membrane-bound organelle (the melanosome). In order to damage cytoplasmic components, those toxic compounds would have to pass through the melanosomal membrane. But more importantly, to damage the DNA in the nucleus, where more significant (and potentially heritable) damage could occur, they would have to penetrate the melanosomal membrane, avoid all the detoxifying systems in the cytoplasm (remember that as melanosomes produce pigment they are moving away from the nucleus towards the dendrites), and then pass through the nuclear membrane. So sequestering those toxic compounds within melanosomes is important in controlling the potential cytotoxicity associated with producing melanin. But an equally important approach is the presence of 'detoxifying' enzymes in the melanosome itself. We feel that Dct, and to some extent Tyrp1, fall into this category. Note the position of Dct in the melanogenic pathway (Fig. 5.1). Upon formation of DOPAchrome, if Dct is present, the DOPAchrome will be immediately converted to a carboxylated intermediate (DHICA) rather than spontaneously losing its carboxyl group, as occurs in the absence of Dct. Studies have shown that DHICA is significantly less toxic than DHI[13] and, initially, we felt that this was the importance of Dct. But recent studies have shown that, in reality, DOPAchrome is significantly more toxic than DHI or DHICA, and the importance of Dct may simply be to remove DOPAchrome from the milieu as quickly as possible.[14] In this regard, it should be noted that mutations of the gene encoding Dct typically result in the premature death of melanocytes, presumably through the increased cytotoxicity that results.

What about Tyrp1? Tyrp1 is downstream of Dct action, and is necessary because of the relative stability of DHICA. Tyrp1 is important in oxidizing DHICA, thus giving it a 'push' down the melanogenic pathway. As occurs for DHI, DHICA is oxidized to the indole–quinone form, which can then further oxidize and polymerize. Once that occurs, a chemically distinct type of melanin is produced, termed DHICA eumelanin (as distinct from the DHI eumelanin considered above). DHICA eumelanin is also dark, but has a brownish color rather than black, is poorly soluble, and is of an intermediate molecular weight. Chemical studies have found that in humans and other mammals, the majority of melanins produced in the skin and hair are actually combinations of DHICA and DHI eumelanins, with DHICA eumelanins generally occupying a significant portion of the total melanins present.[15,16]

A question that naturally arises is whether we have now identified all the enzymatic components involved in the melanogenic pathway. There is no final answer to that question at this time. Extensive studies to identify other members of the tyrosinase-related protein gene family have been negative. Certainly, a melanosomal matrix protein (known as Silv) plays a role in organizing the substructure of the melanosome and serves as a solid-phase matrix for the deposition of melanin on the internal fibrils, and some consider this a polymerase enzyme.[17] Mutations in the genes encoding Tyrp1 or Silv are often associated with the premature death of mutant melanocytes, and, although cytotoxicity might be anticipated as one possible mechanism resulting in such death, it is not really known at this point why or how that occurs. The final and fifth melanosomal protein is an enigma at this point; MART1 was initially identified as a melanoma antigen, but recent studies have shown that this protein is not only associated with the melanosome[18] but actually has the most similar profile to tyrosinase in its distribution.[19] Despite many attempts to define the role of MART1 as a structural or enzymatic component of the melanosome, there are simply no data at this point to provide a basis for predicting such a function.

Responses to the environment

How do melanocytes respond to their environment? The UV response, commonly known as the tanning response, is well known, although the mechanisms involved are just now being characterized. Most of what we know is based on responses of melanocytes to various factors in tissue culture, hardly the ideal model for determining what occurs *in situ*. Three-dimensional culture models of the skin are now evolving and should prove very useful for extending our knowledge of how melanocytes and keratinocytes respond to physiological stimuli, but ultimately this will have to be correlated with responses *in situ*. It is known that responses to UV closely mimic responses to MSH, and it may well be that melanocyte differentiation induced by UV is closely associated with increased expression of MC1R and thus a heightened sensitivity to MSH in the environment. Studies have shown that when MSH and UV stimulate melanocytes in culture, the expression of Dct, Tyrp1 and Silv are increased slightly (perhaps twofold) while expression of tyrosinase can be stimulated 10- to 20-fold or more.[20] Addition to ASP, an effective antagonist of MC1R, leads to a significant decrease in tyrosinase expression and activity (50–90%) but also leads to complete downregulation of expression of Dct, Tyrp1 and Silv.[21] So, it is clear that the major effects noted following the stimulation of melanocyte differentiation by MSH or by UV involve dramatic changes in tyrosinase activity, the rate-limiting factor in melanin production. Based on those studies, one might predict that levels of eumelanins would be increased in UV- or MSH-stimulated melanocytes, and that is, in fact, what happens.[21,22] Conversely, inhibition of melanogenesis by ASP leads to dramatic decreases in production of eumelanins, and eventually, as eumelanins are depleted in the melanocyte, the relatively constitutive levels of pheomelanin produced can be seen and the cells are considered to be pheomelanogenic.

The implications of such varying ratios of pheomelanin, DHICA-melanin and DHI-melanin on the functional properties are complicated. With respect to color (and thus effects on camouflage, etc.), it is clear that regulation of melanocyte function between pheomelanogenesis and eumelanogenesis is carried out at the level of the MC1R, even in humans. Upregulation of MC1R function results in dramatic increases in eumelanin production, while inhibition of MC1R function results in decreases of eumelanin function and, eventually, to visualization of the pheomelanin background. With respect to photoprotection from UV, *in situ* data are sorely lacking. Based on tissue culture and chemical analysis, the implication of producing pheomelanin or eumelanin has dramatic consequences for melanocytes (or melanin-containing keratinocytes) exposed to UV. DHI-melanins have the highest capacity for photoabsorption and have little or no phototoxicity (*i.e.* generation of toxic by-products when UV irradiated); but the cytotoxic implications of producing DHI-melanins are greater, as discussed above. At the other extreme, pheomelanins have little or no capacity to absorb UV, but have the advantage that they have little or no associated cytotoxicity either.[23] But studies have shown that irradiation of pheomelanins with UV actually gives rise to phototoxic by-products which may have deleterious effects on pheomelanin-containing cells.[24,25] It would seem that DHICA-melanins are the best compromise between a reasonable level of photoabsorptive properties, minimized cytotoxicity and no phototoxicity. Fortunately, this is the type of melanin that predominates in our skin and hair, with the exception of those with fair skin and red hair. Other chapters in this book deal with the consequences of that for skin cancer induction in those individuals.

Approaches to characterizing photoprotection *in situ*

Ultimately, we would like to understand the implications of producing various types of melanins in the skin on inherent photoprotection (which in turn may affect photosensitivity), and eventually we would like to design approaches to maximize that protective element. We have recently begun a collaboration amongst the co-authors of this article to measure the effects of UV on the skin *in situ*, and to elucidate the relative efficacies on photoprotection of producing different types of melanins. To this end, we have designed two different approaches based on considerations as noted below.

First, we have utilized mouse models to study the effect of producing different types of melanins on photosensitivity. This has been based on several key features: (a) although the majority of mouse skin is covered with hair, that on the ears and tail has a minimal amount of hair and the skin architecture is quite similar to that of human skin; (b) mice of different genotypes with varying amounts of melanogenic enzyme activities are available which can be used to compare different types of melanins in the skin; and (c) DNA damage-specific antibodies have been generated which allow us to directly measure DNA damage in UV-irradiated skin. The rationale behind our study considered the basic types of cell damage that follow UV irradiation. UV can directly damage biological membranes of keratinocytes, melanocytes and other types of cells in the skin. Although such damage generally leads to the death of the damaged cell, it has no long-range implications. In contrast, UV can also damage DNA, which if not appropriately repaired, may lead to mutations. If that mutation is in a key gene, for example p53 or another growth regulatory gene, malignant transformation can occur. This latter type of damage has lasting implications to the organism. There are several types of UV-induced DNA damage. We measured the most common, cyclobutane pyrimidine dimers (CPDs) and 6–4 photoproducts (64PPs). 64PPs are generally repaired relatively quickly, while the repair of CPDs takes longer. We confirmed this difference in the repair dynamics using antibodies to both types of DNA damage. Only results with the CPD antibodies are reported herein.

Fontana–Masson staining reveals the architecture of the skin in various coat color mutants (Fig. 5.2). In separate experiments, we have confirmed that the Fontana–Masson stain correlates well with eumelanin content but does not correlate with levels of pheomelanin. This can be seen clearly in Fig. 5.2, where eumelanins produced in the black, slaty and brown skins stain well, but pheomelanin in the recessive yellow and lethal yellow skin is not stained at all, nor, of course, is there any stain in the albino skin, which is devoid of all melanin. Chemical analysis of these skins (Table 5.1) reveals that there is no eumelanin or pheomelanin detected in albino skin, and that DHICA-eumelanin is formed predominantly in black skin and, to lesser extents, in brown and slaty skin, respectively. Eumelanins are detectable in the recessive yellow and lethal yellow skins, and increased amounts of pheomelanin are only

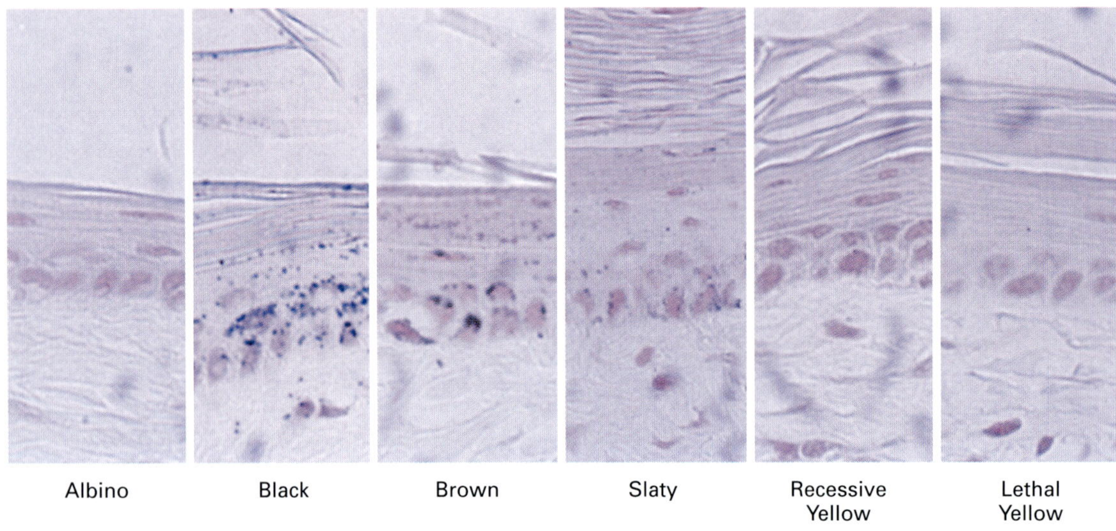

Figure 5.2

Architecture of mouse tail skins from various coat color mutants. Fontana–Masson staining is used to visualize the melanins in skin from the mouse mutants as noted.

found in the recessive yellow skin. When one then uses immunofluorescence to detect DNA damage (as CPDs) in those skin specimens, following their irradiation with UV, one can see that maximal protection (*i.e.* lowest UV sensitivity) is afforded in the black skin and that minimal protection (*i.e.* maximal damage) is seen in the albino skin. DNA damage in slaty and brown skin is higher than in black skin, but is significantly less than in the albino skin or in the pheomelanogenic skins. DNA damage in the recessive yellow skin was higher than in the black, brown and slaty skins, but was detectably less than in the albino skin. UV damage in the lethal yellow skin (which had significantly less eumelanin and pheomelanin than did all other types of skin, except albino) was at a level almost identical to the albino skin. These results show that pheomelanin affords little or no photoprotection, and that even a significant amount of eumelanin may be necessary to provide photoprotective benefit.

Assessing the situation in human skin is not nearly as simple, since humans are not as nicely inbred or genetically defined as are mice. Humans, however, can be grouped according to race, skin phototype, and experimentally-measured photosensitivity (usually expressed as minimal erythemal dose, MED). We have begun a large study aimed at examining subgroups of healthy human subjects of different phototypes, ranging from highly UV-sensitive to very UV-resistant, to explore relationships between DNA damage, melanin content and production, and the sensitivity of skin to UV radiation (photosensitivity). Several studies explored UV-induced DNA damage in human skin *in situ.* A paper reporting the most recent of such studies (on Caucasian skin) provides an overview.[26] In our study, the subjects are grouped according to their expected photosensitivity and racial/ethnic origin (African-American or Black; American-Indian or Alaska Native; Asian; Hispanic or Latino; Native Hawaiian or Pacific Islander; White). Their actual MED is determined using an FS lamp. The emission of this lamp contains approximately 60% UVA (315–400 nm) and 40% UVB (280–315 nm). The UVC component is removed by filtration through Kodacel. Finally, several 2×2-cm dorsal skin areas are exposed to 1 MED of the same UV radiation. The amount of UV radiation delivered to each experimental area is checked with a low-profile detector before and after exposure, and adjustments to the

Table 5.1 Chemical analysis and DNA damage in various types of mouse skin.

Genotype	*Mutant melanosomal Protein*	*Comment*	*DHICA-melanin (ng/mg skin)*	*DHI-melanin (ng/mg skin)*	*Pheomelanin (ng/mg skin)*	*Total melanin (ng/mg skin)*	*DNA damage (CPD)*
Albino	Tyrosinase	No melanin	0	0	0	0	25.0
Black	None	DHICA-rich	1206	594	7.8	1808	8.4
Brown	Tyrp1	DHICA-rich	507	144	16.0	667	10.4
Slaty	Dct	DHI-rich	249	1559	40.3	1848	10.3
Recessive yellow	MC1R	Pheomelanin-rich	67	455	53.8	576	20.1
Lethal yellow	ASP	Low melanin	291	38.4	3.6	333	24.5

Eumelanin and pheomelanin were determined as PTCA (n = 4–6) and AHP (n = 2) derivatives, as detailed in reference 28; values shown are the averages of determinations, corrected for recovery as detailed in reference 29. Background values obtained for albino skin were subtracted from all samples. Values for DHI-melanin were obtained by subtracting DHICA-melanin and pheomelanin values from total melanin values. DNA damage was measured by immunofluorescence of CPD damage, as detailed in reference 30; values shown represent the average of duplicate assays, and are caused by equivalent UV doses.

exposure time of each area are made. In this way, variations in the dose delivered to the individual 1 MED areas are minimal. The amount of radiation needed to produce 1 MED in the most resistant and most sensitive subjects varies by a factor of six (approximate range 150–1200 J/m^2). Shave biopsies are taken immediately prior to exposure, immediately following exposure (about 7 minutes), 1 day later and 7 days later. Those biopsies are examined immunohistochemically for UV damage, for melanin content, and for melanogenic enzyme expression using specific antibodies. Some preliminary findings of that study have provided a few surprises. For example, we have found that subjects vary widely in the amount of DNA damage they incur, and that this does not always correlate with the amount of pigment in the skin. The rate of DNA repair also differs widely from subject to subject, as does each patient's ability to repair DNA lesions back to baseline levels. It is known that other factors, *e.g.* thickness of stratum corneum, or modifications of molecular responses[27] may affect UV sensitivity. Even more surprisingly, we have found a wide variation in the response of various skins to produce melanin following UV irradiation. Some subjects respond in the classical, expected manner, in that there is an immediate increase in melanin content visible 1 day after irradiation and to a great extent 7 days after irradiation. But others actually decline in melanin content at 1 day, and occasionally decrease melanin content even further 1 week later. Again, this does not always correlate with constitutive skin pigmentation in a predictable manner. Even more surprising was the persistence of the pigmentation induced by UV; some subjects generated hyperpigmented skin in response to UV that was essentially back to constitutive levels within 2 weeks, whereas others maintained their pigmented tanning spots for months with little fading. The mechanisms behind all these variations in response are not known, and will provide a rich source for study in the coming years.

This study design allows us to assess the content of melanin in various skin types *in situ*, and to measure the efficacy of that pigment in preventing UV damage to DNA. Using specific antibodies, we can also quantify the proliferation of melanocytes and the expression of melanogenic enzymes in the skin following UV exposure. An example of our observations is shown in Fig. 5.3, where the expression of tyrosinase & Silv and of Dct & MART1 in human skin prior to UV exposure, 1 day later and 7 days later are shown. One can readily quantitate the number of antigen-positive melanocytes as well as the expression levels of the melanogenic proteins. Space does not allow a full consideration of the responses of the various types of melanocytes studied in different skin types or the melanocyte responses to produce melanin and the various melanosomal proteins. We will illustrate our findings with observations on three subjects representing different races (Table 5.2). Briefly, it can be seen that the relative numbers of melanocytes per

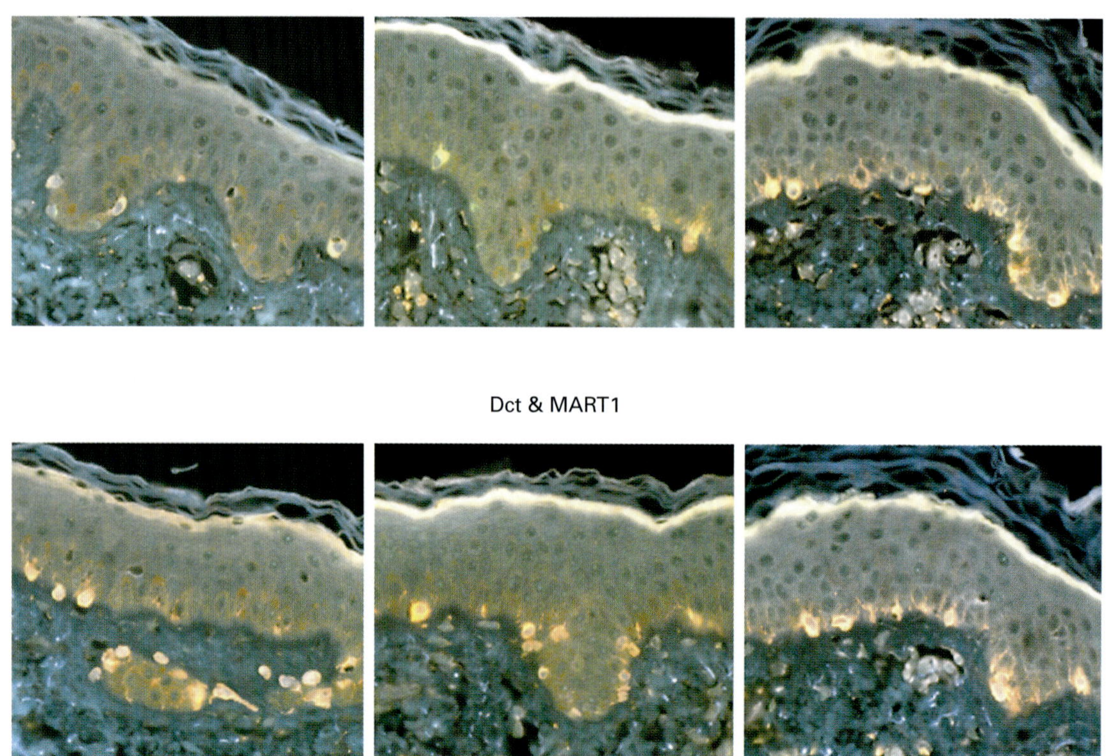

Figure 5.3

Immunohistochemical analysis of melanocyte number and melanosomal protein expression in African-American skin in response to UV radiation. From left to right, prior to UV, 1 day after UV and 7 days after UV. Top row was stained with antibodies recognizing tyrosinase (αPEP7h, green) and Silv (HMB45, red), while the bottom row was stained with antibodies recognizing TRP2 (αPEP8h, green) and MART1 (M2-9E3, red). Sections were examined by immunofluorescence microscopy and the merged red and green images are shown; colocalization of the two antigens is seen as yellow. Original magnification = 400X.

surface area of Asian and African-American skin was about twice that of the White skin prior to UV exposure, and that those numbers decreased by 10% or so 1 day later. One week later, these three subjects responded with increased numbers of melanocytes, ranging from 15 to 25%. Melanin content was more dramatically affected, ranging from a 10% increase in Asian skin 1 week after exposure, to an 85% increase in White skin and a 95% increase in African-American skin. Tyrosinase, Tyrp1 and Dct expression all increased significantly 1 week after UV radiation, some even as soon as 1 day after exposure. In sum, we found a wide variety of responses in these three subjects, and it will be important to collect data on a larger number of subjects to see how consistent these patterns are.

Conclusions

In conclusion, it is clear that melanin biosynthesis is regulated by a number of enzymatic and structural components of melanosomes which are

Table 5.2 Melanocyte proliferation and melanogenic enzyme expression following UV radiation *in situ*.

Race	*Time after UV*	*Melanocyte #*	*Melanin*	*Tyrosinase*	*Tyrp1*	*Dct*	*Silv*	*MART1*
White	Control	2.9 ± 0.3	3.82 ± 0.13	2.94 ± 0.18	3.56 ± 0.23	6.59 ± 0.50	4.36 ± 0.30	3.05 ± 0.58
	1 d later	2.6 ± 0.3	4.71 ± 0.30	5.73 ± 0.14	4.84 ± 0.22	10.25 ± 0.75	4.96 ± 0.21	2.51 ± 0.15
	7 d later	3.6 ± 0.3	7.14 ± 0.36	7.20 ± 0.25	7.95 ± 0.32	10.77 ± 0.54	6.77 ± 0.30	6.24 ± 0.65
Asian	Control	5.1 ± 0.4	8.89 ± 0.42	3.86 ± 0.60	5.14 ± 0.25	6.18 ± 0.39	4.35 ± 3.06	3.06 ± 0.12
	1 d later	4.3 ± 0.5	9.59 ± 0.48	3.82 ± 0.43	4.20 ± 0.21	7.41 ± 0.99	2.67 ± 2.72	2.21 ± 0.27
	7 d later	6.5 ± 0.7	9.80 ± 0.44	5.85 ± 0.29	6.68 ± 0.63	8.76 ± 1.33	4.12 ± 3.16	2.25 ± 0.25
African-American	Control	4.7 ± 0.4	8.82 ± 1.17	4.45 ± 0.11	5.38 ± 0.48	7.42 ± 0.21	4.29 ± 0.18	2.21 ± 0.74
	1 d later	4.2 ± 0.2	14.51 ± 0.71	7.36 ± 0.41	9.40 ± 0.47	12.67 ± 0.44	6.58 ± 0.23	2.26 ± 0.58
	7 d later	5.4 ± 0.3	17.04 ± 0.84	7.85 ± 0.41	10.67 ± 0.33	24.75 ± 1.56	10.05 ± 1.10	6.96 ± 0.89

Data are reported as the means ± SEM (n = 9). Melanocyte number is reported as the number of melanocytes counted in a single field at 400X; all other measurements reported for antibody staining are in arbitrary units of the integrated density of the stain noted.

modulated in response to various physiological agents, such as UV radiation. The type of melanin synthesized, the quantity of pigment produced and the properties of the melanosomes within which they are deposited, determine the visible color, the cytotoxicity and the photoprotective capacity. Melanin plays an obvious role in shielding nuclear DNA in the skin from UV damage, but the photoprotective value of melanin far exceeds its function as a sunscreen, and other properties of melanin, *e.g.* its antioxidant and radical scavenging properties, are also no doubt of great importance to the cells. Future study will be directed to further elucidating the mechanisms involved in melanocyte responses to UV radiation and in optimizing the photoprotective role of the pigment produced.

References

1. Nordlund JJ, Boissy RE, Hearing VJ et al., *The Pigmentary System: Physiology and Pathophysiology* (Oxford University Press: New York, 1998).
2. Hearing VJ, The melanosome: the perfect model for cellular responses to the environment, *Pigment Cell Res* (2000) **13**:23–34.
3. Suzuki I, Tada A, Ollmann M et al., Agouti signalling protein inhibits melanogenesis and the response of human melanocytes to α-melanotropin, *J Invest Dermatol* (1997) **108**:838–42.
4. Tada A, Suzuki I, Im S et al., Endothelin-1 is a paracrine growth factor that modulates melanogenesis of human melanocytes and participates in their responses to ultraviolet radiation, *Cell Growth Differ* (1998) **9**:575–84.
5. Abdel-Malek ZA, Scott MC, Suzuki I et al., The melanocortin-1 receptor is a key regulator of human cutaneous pigmentation, *Pigment Cell Res* (2000) **13** (Suppl 8):156–62.
6. Halder RM, Bridgeman-Shah S, Skin cancer in African-Americans, *Cancer* (1995) **75**:667–73.
7. Zeise L, Chedekel M, Fitzpatrick T, eds, *Melanin: Its Role in Human Photoprotection* (Valdenmar Publishing Company: Overland Park, 2001).
8. Spritz RA, Hearing VJ, Genetic disorders of pigmentation. In: Hirschhorn K, Harris H, eds, *Advances in Human Genetics* (Plenum Press: New York, 1994) 1–45.
9. King RA, Hearing VJ, Oetting WS, Abnormalities of pigmentation. In: Rimoin DL, Connor JM, Pyeritz RE, eds, *Emery and Rimoin's Principles and Practice of Medical Genetics* (Churchill Livingstone: New York, 1997) 1171–203.
10. King RA, Hearing VJ, Creel D et al., Albinism. In: Scriver CR, Beaudet AL, Sly WS et al., eds, *The Metabolic and Molecular Bases of Inherited Disease* (McGraw-Hill: New York, 2001) 5587–628.
11. Hearing VJ, The regulation of melanin production. In: Nordlund JJ, Boissy RE, Hearing VJ et al., eds, *The Pigmentary System: Physiology and Pathophysiology* (Oxford University Press: New York, 1998) 423–38.
12. Hearing VJ, Biochemical control of melanogenesis and melanosomal organization, *J Invest Dermatol Symp Proc* (1999) **4**:24–8.
13. Urabe K, Aroca P, Tsukamoto K et al., The inherent

cytotoxicity of melanogenic intermediates: a revision, *Biochim Biophys Acta* (1994) **1221**:272–8.
14. Matsunaga J, Riley PA, Solano F et al., *Biosynthesis of neuromelanin and melanin: the potential involvement of macrophage migration inhibitory factor and DOPAchrome tautomerase as rescue enzymes. Catecholamine Research: From Molecular Insights to Clinical Medicine* (Kluwer Academic/Plenum Publishing: New York, 2002) in press.
15. Ito S, Wakamatsu K, Ozeki H, Chemical analysis of melanins and its application to the study of the regulation of melanogenesis, *Pigment Cell Res* (2000) **13**:103–9.
16. Ozeki H, Wakamatsu K, Ito S et al., Chemical characterization of eumelanins with special emphasis on 5,6-dihydroxyindole-2-carboxylic acid content and molecular size, *Anal Biochem* (1997) **248**:149–57.
17. Chakraborty AK, Platt JT, Kim KK et al., Polymerization of 5,6-dihydroxyindole-2-carboxylic acid to melanin by the pMel17/silver locus protein, *Eur J Biochem* (1996) **232**:257–63.
18. Kawakami Y, Battles JK, Kobayashi T et al., Production of recombinant MART-1 proteins and specific antiMART-1 polyclonal and monoclonal antibodies: use in the characterization of the human melanoma antigen MART-1, *J Immunol Meth* (1997) **202**:13–25.
19. Kushimoto T, Basrur V, Matsunaga J et al., A new model for melanosome biogenesis based on the purification and mapping of early melanosomes, *Proc Natl Acad Sci U S A* (2001) **98**:10698–703.
20. Aroca P, Urabe K, Kobayashi T et al., Melanin biosynthesis patterns following hormonal stimulation, *J Biol Chem* (1993) **268**:25650–5.
21. Sakai C, Ollmann M, Kobayashi T et al., Modulation of murine melanocyte function *in vitro* by agouti signal protein, *EMBO J* (1997) **16**:3544–52.
22. Alaluf S, Heath A, Carter N et al., Variation in melanin content and composition in type V and VI photoexposed and photoprotected human skin: the dominant role of DHI, *Pigment Cell Res* (2001) **14**: 337–47.
23. Jimbow K, Reszka K, Schmitz S et al., Distribution of eu- and pheomelanins in human skin and melanocytic tumors, and their photoprotective vs. phototoxic properties. In: Zeise L, Chedekel MR, Fitzpatrick TB, eds, *Melanin: Its Role in Human Photoprotection* (Valdenmar Publishing Company: Overland Park, 1995) 155–76.
24. Hill HZ, Li W, Xin P et al., Melanin: a two edged sword? *Pigment Cell Res* (1997) **10**:158–61.
25. Hill HZ, Hill GJ, Cieszka K et al., Comparative action spectrum for ultraviolet light killing of mouse melanocytes from different genetic coat color backgrounds, *Photochem Photobiol* (1997) **65**:983–9.
26. Katiyar SK, Matsui MS, Mukhtar H, Kinetics of UV light-induced cyclobutane pyrimidine dimers in human skin in vivo: an immunohistochemical analysis of both epidermis and dermis, *Photochem Photobiol* (2000) **72**:788–93.
27. Cridland NA, Martin MC, Stevens K et al., Role of stress responses in human cell survival following exposure to ultraviolet C radiation, *Int J Rad Biol* (2001) **77**:365–74.
28. Ito S, Fujita K, Microanalysis of eumelanin and pheomelanin in hair and melanomas by chemical degradation and liquid chromatography, *Anal Biochem* (1985) **144**:527–36.
29. Ozeki H, Ito S, Wakamatsu K et al., Spectrophotometric characterization of eumelanin and pheomelanin in hair, *Pigment Cell Res* (1996) **9**:265–70.
30. Kobayashi N, Nakagawa A, Muramatsu T et al., Supranuclear melanin caps reduce ultraviolet induced DNA photoproducts in human epidermis, *J Invest Dermatol* (1998) **110**:806–10.

Section III

TRANSCRIPTIONAL CONTROL OF MELANOGENESIS

6 The regulation of the Microphthalmia transcription factor

David E. Fisher

Among the numerous coat color mutants which have been described in the mouse, a fascinating subgroup comprises the white-spotting mutants. These mutations cause loss of melanocytes, rather than loss of pigment, within viable melanocytes. A number of these white-spotting loci have been cloned. Prominent among these genes are the cytokine Steel factor, its receptor c-Kit, and the Microphthalmia transcription factor genes. The mechanistic understanding of how these factors impact on melanocyte numbers stands to produce substantial insights pertinent to neural crest development, normal pigmentation, abnormal pigmentation, and, possibly, even the biology of malignant melanoma.

The Microphthalmia transcription factor gene (MITF) was cloned by Arnheiter and colleagues.[1] The gene predicts a helix-loop-helix transcription factor with significant homology to c-Myc within its DNA binding motif. The structure of the MITF gene has been extensively analyzed by Shibahara and colleagues,[2,3] and consists of multiple promoters, each linked to unique initial exons tethered to a common downstream coding region. One of the promoters appears to produce a melanocyte-specific expression pattern[4] and has become the subject of considerable interest, as its regulation appears to be abnormal in several pigmentation/deafness conditions in humans. Mutations in MITF were recognized to occur in Waardenburg syndrome type IIA.[5] In addition, Waardenburg syndrome types I, III, and IV display considerable phenotypic overlap with type IIA, yet have distinguishing characteristics as well. The common phenotypic properties of all Waardenburg subtypes are the presence of a white forelock and variable degrees of deafness. These autosomal-dominant diseases represent a relatively common cause of inherited deafness in humans, and the mechanistic defect is thought to reside at the level of melanocyte loss either along the forehead midline or in the cochlea, where inner-ear melanocytes appear to play an essential role in normal hearing.

Mice with heterozygous mutations in MITF exhibit white spotting along the ventral midline (semi-dominant alleles) or no significant detectable phenotype (recessive alleles). In contrast, most homozygous mutant MITF alleles in the mouse exhibit complete absence of melanocytes, thereby producing entirely white animals. In addition, defects in the retinal pigment epithelium produce ocular developmental defects resulting in small eyes. Additional defects are seen in the mast cell and osteoclast cell lineages. The latter phenotypes are most apparent in mice harboring dominant-negative, rather than recessive, alleles of MITF, even in homozygous form.

Interestingly, although MITF is essential for melanocyte development and survival, the melanocyte-specific phenotypes of the different mutations of MITF in the mouse display variations which convey significant information about MITF's function. For example, one allele, $MITF^{vit}$, displays essentially normal pigmentation at birth which is followed by progressive loss of melanocytes over the ensuing 6–12 months. This vitiligo phenotype is caused by a mutation in the helix-loop-helix region of MITF, which modestly disrupts DNA-binding activity[6,7] and provides genetic evidence for a continued requirement for MITF protein in post-developmental phases of melanocyte survival or proliferation. In addition, it is interesting that most null alleles of MITF do not produce a bone/osteoclast phenotype in homozygously affected mice, whereas the homozygous alleles which encode dominant-negative mutants display significant osteopetrosis. These differing behaviors led to the proposal[7] that, within the osteoclast cell lineage, MITF exists together with other related factors, which may at least partially compensate for its loss in null mutants, but which may be dominantly suppressed by the osteopetrotic mutants of MITF.

MITF contains a gene structure in which its DNA-binding domain is located near the center and at least one strong transactivation domain is found near the N-terminus (Fig. 6.1). A second transactivation domain likely exists near the C-terminus in a proline-rich region. Electrophoretic mobility gel-shift assays have been used to demonstrate that MITF recognizes the E-box DNA sequence CACGTG.[7] MITF is also capable of recognizing the pyrimidine substitution, CACGTG. Based on sequence homologies within MITF's DNA-binding region, it was found that MITF could either homodimerize or heterodimerize with three related family members called TFE3, TFEB, and TFEC.[7] This distinct transcription factor family (referred to as MiT) was suggested to harbor overlapping DNA-binding and transcriptional functions. Genetic/phenotypic behavior suggests that MITF is likely to be the major member of this family, with functional importance in the melanocyte lineage, whereas other family members likely play important roles in the osteoclast lineage in addition to MITF (see below).

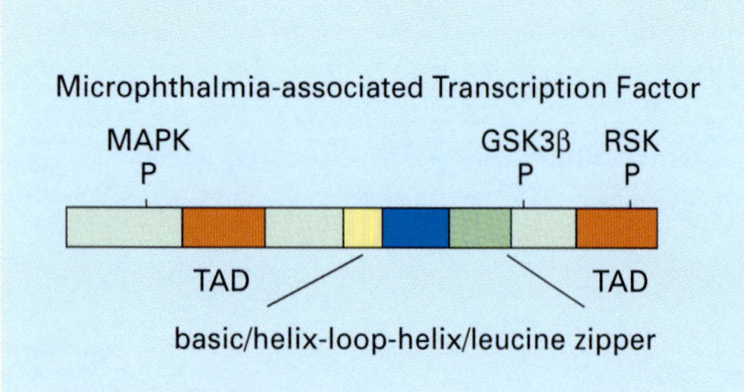

Figure 6.1

The MITF protein is characterized by a basic helix-loop-helix-leucine zipper DNA-binding and dimerization domain. This region bears considerable homology to the corresponding region in the c-Myc proto-oncogene family. Two transactivation domains likely mediate MITF's transcriptional activity, one located N-terminal to the DNA-binding region, the other located in a proline-rich region near the C-terminus. MITF has been found to undergo multiple phosphorylations, including those mediated by MAP kinase and RSK, which influence both transcriptional activity and degradation, and GSK3β, which influences DNA-binding activity.[25]

MITF as a transcriptional regulator of pigmentation

The identification of MITF as an E-box binding factor was accompanied by the observation that MITF could transcriptionally upregulate reporter constructs driven by the promoters for multiple pigmentation enzyme genes.[7–9] The identification of conserved E-box-like sequences in the tryosinase, TRP1, and TRP2 promoters suggested that MITF may be an important regulator of the pigmentation program in melanocytes through its recognition of these elements.

An important signaling pathway which regulates pigmentation is the pathway stimulated by melanocyte-stimulating hormone (MSH). Signaling studies indeed demonstrated that stimulation of melanocytes or melanoma cells with MSH produce significant upregulation of MITF expression.[10,11] This signaling pathway (Fig. 6.2) involves the MSH receptor (Mc1r) as well as a number of intermediates which are not entirely understood. Possible routes to nuclear targets include via protein kinase A or, alternatively, a Ras/Raf/MAPK/RSK pathway. Regardless, the CREB/ATF1 family of transcription factors is ultimately activated by phosphorylation and binds the MITF melanocyte-specific promoter at a cyclic AMP response element binding site. Stimulation of MSH thus results in transcriptional activation of the melanocyte-specific MITF promoter and a burst of MITF gene expression. It appears likely that downstream targets of MITF are subsequently upregulated in a manner which contributes to the pigmentation response initiated by MSH.

The MITF promoter, as mentioned above, has focused the attention of investigators examining the genetic relationships among Waardenburg syndrome subtypes in humans. The genetic causes of Waardenburg syndrome type I and certain cases of type IV are two other transcription factors, Pax3 and Sox10. The MITF melanocyte-specific promoter contains consensus DNA-binding sites for both of these factors, and their transcriptional activity on the MITF promoter[12–16] is likely to explain the phenotypic overlap among humans with mutations in these three transcription factor genes. In addition, the MITF promoter contains a consensus element for TCF/Lef, which has been shown to mediate Wnt signaling, an important pathway in melanocyte development.[17] The signaling pathways from Wnt or MSH to MITF, thus, are likely to play an important role in modulating the pigment response under a variety of physiologic conditions.

MITF is targeted by c-Kit

Given the striking phenotypic overlap of MITF loss, as well as c-Kit or Steel factor loss, in mutant mice, studies several years ago examined the possibility that these factors may lie within a common mechanistic pathway in melanocytes. It was discovered that Steel factor triggers Kit-dependent activation of MAP kinase, and MAP kinase, in turn, directly phosphorylates MITF at Ser 73[18] (see Fig. 6.3). Ser 73-phosphorylated MITF displays a mobility shift on gel electrophoresis. Transcriptional assays also suggested that MITF, when phosphorylated at Ser 73, recruits p300,[19] a transcriptional coactivator which results in transcriptional stimulation of MITF.[20]

Another consequence of MAP kinase activation by Steel/Kit is the activation of the RSK family of kinases (Fig. 6.3). Activation of RSK was seen to produce phosphorylation of MITF at Ser 409, near the C-terminus of MITF.[21] In addition, phosphorylations by both MAP kinase and RSK were seen to significantly alter MITF protein stability.[21] Phosphorylation was found to target MITF for ubiquitination and proteosome-dependent degradation.[22,23] These observations collectively suggest that the phosphorylated form of MITF is, simultaneously, a transcriptional activator and a short-lived species which is a target for rapid destruction in the melanocyte.

The observation that MITF plays an essential role in melanocyte survival, both during mouse development and in post natal life, suggested the possibility that MITF expression may also be important in human malignant melanoma. This possibility is of potential clinical importance because of several features of melanoma. Firstly,

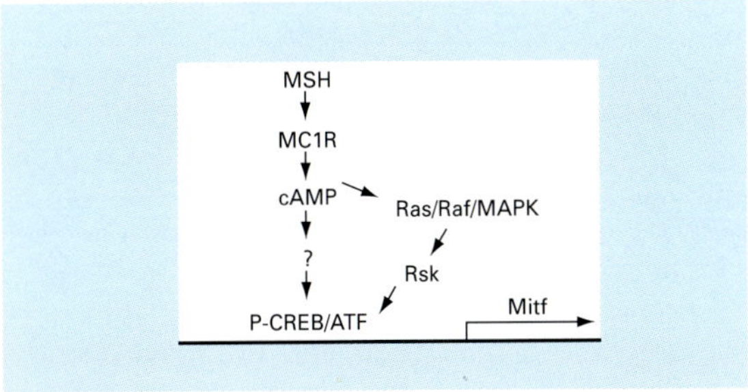

Figure 6.2

The melanocyte stimulating hormone (MSH) signaling pathway modulates MITF promoter activity in melanocytes. MSH binds and activates MC1R, a G-protein-coupled receptor, to upregulate cAMP. This leads to phosphorylation and activation of the CREB/ATF1 transcription factor family through intermediates which may include Rsk and possibly other paths as well. Activated CREB/ATF1 bind to a consensus cAMP response DNA sequence element within the melanocyte-specific MITF promoter, thereby triggering transcriptional upregulation of the MITF gene within melanocytes. This pathway may contribute to MSH's pigmentation phenotype, although the direct manner in which it does so remains to be determined.

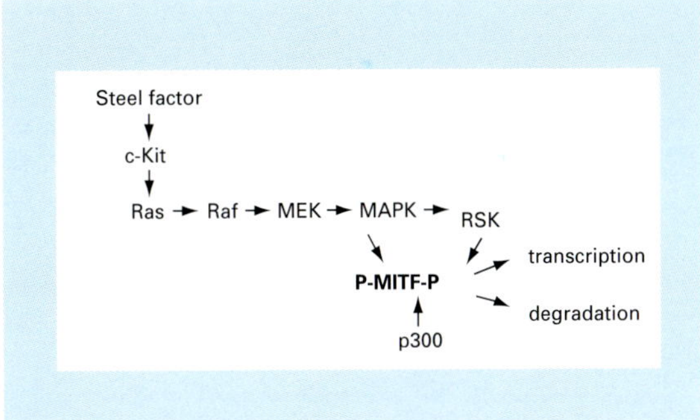

Figure 6.3

A biochemical pathway connects Steel/Kit signaling to MITF. The cytokine Steel factor activates its receptor, c-Kit, which, in turn, leads to MAP kinase activation. MAP kinase directly phosphorylates MITF at Ser 73, leading to recruitment of the transcriptional coactivator p300. MAP kinase also activates the RSK kinase family, members of which were also seen to directly phosphorylate MITF at Ser 409. A consequence of these two phosphorylations is the targeting of MITF for ubiquitination and proteosome-mediated degradation.

melanoma growth typically involves a vertical phase and, thus, is often associated with early metastasis. Metastatic melanoma is not infrequently the initial presentation of this cancer. Therefore, it is important to have histologic markers which help to identify the cell lineage of origin. In addition, it is not infrequently the case that melanomas are non-pigmented. A growth advantage of non-pigmented melanocytes and melanoma cells may provide a selection *in vivo* for this phenotype. In these tumors, it is particularly important to have histologic markers which help to identify the cell of origin.

For these reasons, a clinical correlative study was undertaken to examine the utility of MITF as a diagnostic marker in human malignant melanoma.[24] Seventy-six consecutive melanoma clinical specimens were analyzed (in collaboration with Drs Roy King and Martin Mihm). MITF expression was assessed by immunohistochemical staining using a monoclonal antibody. MITF was found to be expressed with a nuclear distribution in 100% of these tumors. In addition, 60 non-melanoma specimens were compared for MITF staining. MITF expression was absent in all but two of these tumors, the two positive lesions both being breast carcinomas. In addition, MITF was found to be expressed in epidermal melanocytes, as well as in a significant assortment of benign nevi.

Additional studies have examined the expression of MITF specifically in metastatic melanoma (in collaboration with Dr Scott Granter). These studies have revealed MITF expression to be positive in the vast majority of metastatic melanoma specimens as well. Another clinical use for MITF in melanoma diagnosis comes from cytologic specimens. Needle aspirates are obtained from draining lymph nodes in the region of a primary cutaneous melanoma in order to assess local disease spread. Although the cellular architecture is lost in such specimens, we found (in collaboration with Dr David Chhieng) that MITF was present and nuclear in 100% of 45 melanoma specimens diagnosed from these cytologic samples. In addition, the other melanoma markers, HMB45 as well as S100, were compared in side-by-side fashion. MITF was found to be more sensitive and more specific than either of the other two markers. Thus, MITF appears to be a sensitive and specific histologic marker for human melanoma.

MITF and osteoclast function

Several recent studies have been undertaken with MITF in the osteoclast lineage. Firstly, a striking similarity was noted between the c-Kit signaling pathway in melanocytes and the signaling pathway triggered by M-CSF in osteoclasts. The similarity is based on the mechanistic and biochemical similarity between the M-CSF receptor (c-Fms) and c-Kit. A series of biochemical analyses suggests that, in parallel to the Kit-MITF pathway outlined above in melanocytes, M-CSF triggers phosphorylation of MITF at Ser 73 within osteoclasts. Moreover, sequence comparisons revealed that the identical MAP kinase consensus sequence is conserved in the related transcription factor TFE3. Correspondingly, TFE3 was found to be similarly phosphorylated by M-CSF signaling within osteoclasts. These phosphorylations were also found to produce recruitment of the p300 coactivator. It therefore appears that similar signaling pathways exist within these two relatively unrelated cell types, stimulated by entirely different cytokines, but culminating in the nucleus at similar transcription factor targets. Within osteoclasts, the transcriptional profile of MITF and TFE3 target genes is likely to be distinct from the profile of melanocytes, and it remains to be seen how post-translational modifications of MITF and TFE3 might possibly alter such target genes.

One target gene of MITF has been recently identified within osteoclasts. This is a gene responsible for severe osteoclast dysfunction when it is mutated in humans. The gene encodes Cathepsin K, the factor responsible for the osteopetrosis syndrome called Pycnodysostosis. Cathepsin K is a secreted protease which functions to degrade the protein component of bone matrix. Although Cathepsin K deficiency does not produce a direct defect in bone mineral resorption, it nonetheless produces a significant degree of bone resorption defect due to the inability to degrade the protein component of bone. We observed that MITF and TFE3 both appear to target the Cathepsin K promoter. Three E-boxes were identified within the Cathepsin K promoter. These were shown to be bound by MITF, or transcriptionally activated in reporter assays by either MITF or TFE3 overexpression. In addition, overexpression of wild-type MITF was seen to significantly upregulate the endogenous Cathepsin K gene within primary human osteoclasts, whereas overexpression of mutant MITF failed to do so. Moreover, in reporter assays, it was found that the osteopetrotic mutants of MITF were capable of repressing Cathepsin K promoter activity as stimulated by either wild-type MITF or wild-type TFE3, but the non-osteopetrotic mutants of MITF did not interfere with the Cathepsin K promoter activity in these assays. Therefore, the transcriptional activities of both wild-type and dominant-negative MITF constructs/alleles suggest a phenotypic overlap with Cathepsin K deficiency and provide a mechanistic link between this transcription factor family and this essential secreted protease.

Future prospects

The importance of MITF in melanocyte biology, as well as in the biology of osteoclasts, has become increasingly clear as it has been recognized to play essential roles in multiple signaling pathways and as a downstream target gene of other transcription factors which are important to melanocyte development. The conserved expression of MITF in melanoma is also consistent with the possibility that it plays a functionally important role in this tumor, although that specific question still requires further analysis. One important direction for the continued study of MITF is a detailed and systematic survey of the transcriptional target genes which it regulates in the different cell types. It is possible that MITF regulates numerous genes involved in distinctive pathways, for example, pathways involving highly differentiated functions in melanocytes, such as pigmentation, or more global pathways, such as those involving cell cycle progression or survival. An important clinical problem relating to MITF is the deafness which occurs in humans carrying heterozygous deficiencies of the gene. It is likely that melanocyte survival in the inner ear is compromised by MITF haplo-insufficiency. It is also likely that MITF plays an essential role in the homeostasis of inner-ear biology. For example, it is likely that melanocytes play a role in modulating the ionic composition of the endolymph fluid which baths the inner-ear hair cells. How MITF deficiency may impact on such homeostasis remains to be seen, but could be of significant clinical importance, because a therapeutic intervention which focuses on MITF might significantly impact other etiologies of deafness due to factors which reside upstream of MITF (such as Sox 10 or Pax 3). Finally, the functional role of MITF in the biology of melanoma may be of significance if it were found that MITF plays a role in the survival or proliferation of the cell lineage. Such information would be of importance, not only in potentially identifying MITF as a therapeutic target, but also as a handle with which to identify additional genes of importance in regulating the survival or proliferation of pigment cells.

Acknowledgements

The author wishes to gratefully acknowledge the numerous colleagues and collaborators whose work has been cited in this manuscript. Collaborators include Drs C. Hodgekinson, E. Steingrimsson, N. Copeland, N. Jenkins, H. Arnheiter, M. Mihn, R. King, S. Granter, D. Chhieng, R. Ballotti, A. Tashjian, and numerous members of the author's laboratory over the years, including Drs T. Hemeseth, R. Price, K. Weilbaecher, M. Horstmann, C. Takemoto, H. Ding, M. Wu, W. Huber, G. McGill, G. Motychkova, and C. Hershey. Dr Fisher's laboratory is supported by a grant from the National Institutes of Health.

References

1. Hodgkinson CA, Moore KJ, Nakayama A et al., Mutations at the mouse microphthalmia locus are associated with defects in a gene encoding a novel basic-helix-loop-helix–zipper protein, *Cell* (1993) **74**:395–404.
2. Udono T, Yasumoto K, Takeda K et al., Structural organization of the human microphthalmia-associated transcription factor gene containing four alternative promoters, *Biochim Biophys Acta* (2000) **1491**:205–19.
3. Shibahara S, Yasumoto K, Amae S et al., Regulation of pigment cell-specific gene expression by MITF, *Pigment Cell Res* (2000) **13**:98–102.
4. Fuse N, Yasumoto K, Suzuki H et al., Identification of a melanocyte-type promoter of the

microphthalmia-associated transcription factor gene, *Biochem Biophys Res Commun* (1996) **219**:702–7.

5. Tassabehji M, Newton VE, Read AP, Waardenburg syndrome type 2 caused by mutations in the human microphthalmia (MITF) gene, *Nat Genet (*1994) **8**:251–5.
6. Steingrimsson E, Moore KJ, Lamoreux ML et al., Molecular basis of mouse microphthalmia (mi) mutations helps explain their developmental and phenotypic consequences, *Nat Genet* (1994) **8**:256–63.
7. Hemesath TJ, Steingrimsson E, McGill G et al., Microphthalmia, a critical factor in melanocyte development, defines a discrete transcription factor family, *Genes Dev* (1994) **8**:2770–80.
8. Yasumoto K, Yokoyama K, Shibata K et al., Microphthalmia-associated transcription factor as a regulator for melanocyte-specific transcription of the human tyrosinase gene, *Mol Cell Biol* (1994) **14**:8058–70.
9. Bentley NJ, Eisen T, Goding CR, Melanocyte-specific expression of the human tyrosinase promoter: activation by the microphthalmia gene product and role of the initiator, *Mol Cell Biol* (1994) **14**:7996–8006.
10. Bertolotto C, Abbe P, Hemesath TJ et al., Microphthalmia gene product as a signal transducer in cAMP-induced differentiation of melanocytes, *J Cell Biol* (1998) **142**:827–35.
11. Price ER, Horstmann MA, Wells AG et al., alpha-Melanocyte-stimulating hormone signaling regulates expression of microphthalmia, a gene deficient in Waardenburg syndrome, *J Biol Chem* (1998) **273**:33042–7.
12. Watanabe A, Takeda K, Ploplis B et al., Epistatic relationship between Waardenburg syndrome genes MITF and PAX3, *Nat Genet* (1998) **18**:283–6.
13. Bondurand N, Pingault V, Goerich DE et al., Interaction among SOX10, PAX3 and MITF, three genes altered in Waardenburg syndrome, *Hum Mol Genet* (2000) **9**:1907–17.
14. Lee M, Goodall J, Verastegui C et al., Direct regulation of the Microphthalmia promoter by Sox10 links Waardenburg–Shah syndrome (WS4)-associated hypopigmentation and deafness to WS2, *J Biol Chem* (2000) **275**:37978–83.
15. Potterf SB, Furumura M, Dunn KJ et al., Transcription factor hierarchy in Waardenburg syndrome: regulation of MITF expression by SOX10 and PAX3, *Hum Genet* (2000) **107**:1–6.
16. Verastegui C, Bille K, Ortonne JP et al., Regulation of the microphthalmia-associated transcription factor gene by the Waardenburg syndrome type 4 gene, SOX10, *J Biol Chem* (2000) **275**: 30757–60.
17. Takeda K, Yasumoto K, Takada R et al., Induction of melanocyte-specific microphthalmia-associated transcription factor by Wnt-3a, *J Biol Chem* (2000) **275**:14013–16.
18. Hemesath TJ, Price ER, Takemoto C et al., MAP kinase links the transcription factor Microphthalmia to c-Kit signalling in melanocytes, *Nature* (1998) **391**:298–301.
19. Price ER, Ding HF, Badalian T et al., Lineage-specific signaling in melanocytes. C-kit stimulation recruits p300/CBP to microphthalmia, *J Biol Chem* (1998) **273**:17983–6.
20. Sato S, Roberts K, Gambino G et al., CBP/p300 as a co-factor for the Microphthalmia transcription factor, *Oncogene* (1997) **14**:3083–92.
21. Wu M, Hemesath TJ, Takemoto CM et al., c-Kit triggers dual phosphorylations, which couple activation and degradation of the essential melanocyte factor Mi, *Genes Dev* (2000) **14**:301–12.
22. Wu M, Hemesath TJ, Takemoto CM et al., c-Kit triggers dual phosphorylations, which couple activation and degradation of the essential melanocyte factor Mi, *Genes Dev* (2000) **14**:301–12.
23. Xu W, Gong L, Haddad MM et al., Regulation of microphthalmia-associated transcription factor MITF protein levels by association with the ubiquitin-conjugating enzyme hUBC9, *Exp Cell Res* (2000) **255**:135–43.
24. King R, Weilbaecher KN, McGill G et al., Microphthalmia transcription factor. A sensitive and specific melanocyte marker for MelanomaDiagnosis, *Am J Pathol* (1999) **155**:731–8.
25. Takeda K, Takemoto C, Kobayashi I et al., Ser298 of MITF, a mutation site in Waardenburg syndrome type 2, is a phosphorylation site with functional significance, *Hum Mol Genet* (2000) **9**:125–32.

7

The regulation of the *tyrosinase*, *Tyrp-1* and *Tyrp-2* genes

Melanie Lee and Colin R. Goding

Melanocytes, the cells responsible for skin, hair and eye colour, arise from the mouse neural crest as non-pigmented melanoblast cells at embryonic day 10.5 (E10.5).[1] Following migration and proliferation during embryonic development, mature pigment-producing cells are found in the skin and hair follicles, as well as the inner ear, where they are required for hearing.[2,3] Melanocytes produce the pigment melanin in specialized organelles, termed melanosomes, in response to several environmental cues, including those promoting differentiation and those that arise in the epidermis in response to UV irradiation. Mutations in the genes that are specifically required for the development of the melanocyte lineage in the mouse, including commitment to the lineage, proliferation, migration, survival and differentiation, are often non-lethal and exhibit a coat-colour defect phenotype, allowing the identification of numerous loci implicated in the development of pigment cells (Mouse Genome Informatics: (http://www.informatics.jax.org/). A number of these genes have been cloned to date (http://www.cbc.umn.edu/ifpcs/micemut.htm),and encode proteins involved in the functioning of the melanosome, in addition to signaling molecules and transcription factors required for the development of the melanocytes. Here, we review the transcriptional regulation of three pigment cell-specific genes, *tyrosinase*, *Tyrp-1* and *Tyrp-2*. The *tyrosinase* gene product catalyses the key rate-limiting step in melanin biosynthesis, whilst the type of melanin produced is dependent upon the activity of the *tyrosinase*-related proteins, Tyrp-1 and Tyrp-2. Understanding the mechanisms involved in the regulation of the promoters of these genes should provide insight into how tissue-specific transcription may be achieved.

The *tyrosinase* gene

Tyrosinase maps to the albino locus in mouse, and mutations at this locus, affect *tyrosinase* activity and skin colour.[4] Genomic sequences for human[5,6] and mouse[7,8] *tyrosinase* have been isolated, and, in addition, partial *tyrosinase*-genomic sequences have been identified from chicken,[9] quail,[10] snapping turtle,[10] frog,[11] and ascidian.[12]

The 5′-regulatory regions of the human and mouse genes have since been studied extensively to determine how developmental and cell type-specific transcription of the *tyrosinase* gene is achieved (reviewed in reference 13).

Requirements for expression *in vivo* and identification of the *tyrosinase* enhancer

Initial investigations focused on the identification of the minimal promoter region required to direct melanocyte cell-specific expression of the *tyrosinase* gene in the mouse.[14,15] Analysis of a promoter–reporter construct deletion series revealed that 270 bp of the *tyrosinase* gene 5′-flanking sequence was sufficient to achieve melanoma cell-specific expression.[4] A *tyrosinase* minigene construct containing this 270 bp of 5′-regulatory sequence was introduced into the fertilized eggs of an albino mouse strain and found to direct specific expression of *tyrosinase* in both neural-crest-derived melanocytes and the optic-cup-derived retinal pigment epithelium, resulting in a mouse with pigmented skin and eyes.[15] During development, expression of the *tyrosinase* gene is first detected in the pigment epithelium of the retina at day 10.5 of gestation, whilst expression in the melanocytes of the hair follicle begins at day 16.5.[16] Further analysis of the transgenic mice harbouring the *tyrosinase* minigene demonstrated that expression from this construct mirrored that of the endogenous *tyrosinase* gene, indicating that the 270 bp 5′-flanking sequence is able to direct both temporal and cell type-specific expression of the *tyrosinase* gene during development.[14] However, although *tyrosinase* minigene constructs, containing between 270 bp and 5.5 kb of 5′-flanking sequence, were able to complement the albino phenotype, pigmentation levels were variable and rarely reached wild-type levels,[17] suggesting that additional remote regulatory region(s) may be present in the *tyrosinase* 5′-flanking region. Indeed, a 250 kb YAC construct covering the mouse *tyrosinase* gene was expressed in a copy-number-dependent, position-independent manner at levels comparable to the endogenous gene in transgenic mice.[18] As a consequence, the *tyrosinase* gene was postulated to contain, in addition to the proximal promoter, a region of DNA corresponding to elements described as locus control or matrix attachment regions, that permit the establishment of an open chromatin conformation and insulate a transgene from the influence of surrounding chromatin structure or regulatory regions.[19]

Consistent with the *tyrosinase* gene containing a potential enhancer element within the 155 kb 5′-flanking sequence of the *tyrosinase* gene that confers copy-number-dependent, position-independent expression from the 250 kb YAC construct,[18] a melanocyte cell-specific DNAase I hypersensitive region was identified −12 to −15 kb upstream of the transcription start site, indicating that factors binding to an element within this region may play a role in mediating cell-type-specific expression.[20,21] The potential regulatory importance of this region was supported by the previous observation that it lies within a 20 kb promoter fragment that is separated from the *tyrosinase* gene in melanocyte lines derived from homozygous *chinchilla-mottled* mice.[22] Further studies demonstrated that a 3.6 kb fragment of the *tyrosinase* promoter, encompassing the hypersensitive site and matrix attachment region, was able to direct expression of a *tyrosinase* transgene to levels comparable to the wild-type gene in mice. Transgene expression was confirmed to be position- and copy-number-independent.[20,21] Interestingly, transgene expression was restricted to the neural-crest-derived pigment cell lineages in one mouse strain background, indicating that, in this instance, a different enhancer region may be responsible for full *tyrosinase* gene expression in the retinal pigment epithelial cells arising from the optic cup.[21,22] Further analysis of the 3.6 kb fragment of the mouse *tyrosinase* gene regulatory sequences using promoter–reporter assays in a melanoma cell line, narrowed the enhancer region to 200 bp positioned −12.3 to −12.1 kb. A palindromic AP1 binding site within this 200 bp fragment was essential for promoter–reporter activation, and formed a melanoma cell-specific complex containing a fos protein family member in an electrophoretic mobility assay.[20] However, it is not yet clear whether this factor acts alone or in concert with other unidentified activities, or, indeed, whether it plays any role in the function of the enhancer *in vivo*. Nevertheless, there is no doubt that the enhancer region does play a key role in regulating *tyrosinase* expression as a type of locus control region[23] and analysis of the factors recognizing the enhancer should shed light on how it functions and whether it is responsive to specific environmental cues.

The proximal promoter region

Although the *tyrosinase* enhancer clearly plays a role in controlling *tyrosinase* expression, a major focus of attention has been the determination of the *cis*-regulatory elements within the 270 bp proximal promoter that are required for pigment cell-specific expression and the identification of their cognate transcription factors.

Analysis of the human *tyrosinase* gene proximal promoter region has identified several *cis*-regulatory elements and potential *trans*-acting factors. The region −300 to +80 contains sufficient information to direct melanoma cell-specific expression, although, as discussed below, expression is sub-optimal in the absence of an enhancer element located around 2.1 kb upstream.[24–26] Comparison of the mouse, human, quail and turtle proximal promoter regions revealed several conserved motifs, including an 11 bp motif, termed the M-box (AGTCATGTGCT), at position −104 to −99, and a related E-box (CATGTG) at position −12 to −7 of the human sequence,[25] predicted to bind members of the basic helix-loop-helix–leucine zipper (bHLH–LZ) family of transcription factors.

DNAase I footprinting analysis identified six protected regions (Fp1–Fp6) across the human *tyrosinase* proximal promoter (−300 to +80), although none of these footprints was cell-type-specific.[25] The importance of each of the protected regions for melanoma cell-specific *tyrosinase* gene expression was then assessed using a series of promoter–reporter deletion constructs.

Removal of Fp1 (−230 to −202), which was shown to bind to the ubiquitous transcription factor Oct-1, had little effect on promoter activity, indicating that this region does not play an important role in *tyrosinase* promoter function, at least in transfection assays. Region Fp2 (−185 to −179) contains a positive regulatory element, and region Fp3 (−145 to −119) contains a negative regulatory element. A single complex is formed in an electrophoretic mobility assay using oligonucleotides specific for either Fp2 or Fp3, but these complexes are not melanoma cell-specific and the protein(s) binding these elements have not been further characterized.[25]

Deletion of the proximal promoter to position −100 bp reduced expression to approximately 5% of the wild-type promoter, such that analysis of the requirement for regions Fp4–Fp6 was performed in the context of the full-length proximal promoter. Region Fp5 contains a functional Sp1 transcription factor binding site at −40 that is partially conserved and binds Sp1 in the mouse and quail promoters, but not that of the turtle.[25] Mutation of the Sp1 site in the context of the proximal promoter (−300 to +80) resulted in an eight-fold decrease in expression, confirming that Sp1 is likely to play a role in *tyrosinase* expression.[25] Although unlikely to mediate melanocyte-specific expression of the *tyrosinase* gene, the ubiquitously expressed factor Sp1 has been shown to facilitate the binding of the TFIID complex to the initiator element at a promoter lacking a TATA box,[27] and can also interact with, and is regulated by, the *retinoblastoma* gene product.[28,29] Therefore, a potential, but as yet unproven, mechanism by which Sp1 stimulates *tyrosinase* gene expression is by enhancing initiation at the non-canonical TATA box of the *tyrosinase* or by using Rb as a co-factor.

Mutation of the M-box located at −104 within Fp4, or bases within the putative initiator E-box and overlapping octamer element of Fp6, resulted in a 50-fold (Fp4) and 100-fold (Fp6) reduction in the activity of the *tyrosinase* promoter, respectively, highlighting an essential role for these regions for *tyrosinase* gene expression.[25] The M-box (also termed *tyrosinase* proximal promoter or TPE) and the initiator E-box bind the ubiquitous bHLH–LZ transcription factor, USF, as well as a tissue-restricted transcription factor, the microphthalmia-associated bHLH–LZ transcription factor, MITF, *in vitro*,[25,26,30] though it is important to note that which factor is detected in cell extracts using the electrophoretic mobility shift assay depends very much on the conditions used in the DNA-binding assay. The *tyrosinase* proximal promoter can be activated by Mitf in melanoma and non-melanocyte cell types,[25,26,30] and this is achieved predominantly through the initiator E-box, with the M-box being required for full activation.[25,26,30] Confirmation that Mitf indeed regulates *tyrosinase* expression comes both from the fact that a dominant-negative Mitf can repress the *tyrosinase* promoter in melanocyte cell lines,[31] as well as the fact that Mitf binding to the *tyrosinase* promoter can be detected using a chromatin immunoprecipitation assay[32]. The octamer motif overlapping the initiator E-box located within Fp6 can bind the POU domain ubiquitous transcription factor Oct1, as well as the related tissue-restricted POU domain protein, Brn-2,[33] that is expressed in melanoblasts, melanocytes and melanomas, and is, therefore, a potential regulator of *tyrosinase* expression during development.[33–35] Overexpression of Brn-2 in melanoma cells results in repression of the human *tyrosinase* proximal promoter −300 to +80,[33] most likely through competition for binding with Mitf at the overlapping initiator E-box within Fp6.[33] Consistent with this, a promoter–reporter construct, under the control of the *tyrosinase* E-box and octamer motif, is activated by Mitf in melanoma cells, and this activation is inhibited by co-transfection with a Brn-2 expression vector.[33] Therefore, an important aspect of regulation of the human *tyrosinase* promoter may involve changes in the ability of Brn-2 and Mitf to act at the initiator region. However, it is important to remember that the octamer motif found in the human promoter is absent from the mouse promoter and that, to date, there is no genetic evidence to support the observation that Brn-2 can regulate the human *tyrosinase* promoter or is required for regulation of melanocyte development.

The analysis of the human *tyrosinase* promoter focused primarily on those elements that were highly conserved between species, namely the M-box, initiator E-box and Sp1 binding site. Although these key elements are highly conserved between species, the characterization of the mouse *tyrosinase* promoter revealed a number of additional regulatory regions, and it is not yet clear how these relate to the elements described for the human promoter. Thus, experiments in which the expression of various deletion/point mutation promoter–reporter constructs were assessed in mouse melanoma cells and melanocytes revealed one negative regulatory region (−193 to −125 bp) and two positive regulatory elements (−245 to −230 bp and −104 to −93 bp),[17,36] the latter element corresponding to the conserved M-box. Intriguingly, transgenic mice expressing the 270 bp minigene construct with mutations in either or both of the two positive regulatory elements, did not reveal an essential role for these regions in pigment production.[36] However, interpreting the significance of these results is complicated by the fact that such a small region of the *tyrosinase* promoter is strongly subject to integration position-dependent effects.

Further analysis of the mouse *tyrosinase* promoter by *in vitro* DNAase I footprinting demonstrated that each of the functional regulatory elements is bound by proteins in extracts from both B16 and NIH-3T3 cells,[17] but does not contain a known transcription factor consensus binding site nor is it conserved within the promoters of other pigment cell-specific genes. Nevertheless, this region, as well as the mouse M-box, when multimerized upstream of a TK-CAT reporter construct, were able to direct transcription in B16 and NIH-3T3 cells,[17] consistent with their recognition by positive-acting transcription factors. In addition, the mouse initiator E-box was also demonstrated to be a target for transactivation by *Mitf*.[37]

The key role of E-box motifs, present within the M-box and at the initiator, in regulation of *tyrosinase* expression, was highlighted by the identification of a third CATGTG E-box motif located upstream from the proximal promoter. Expression studies demonstrated that the human *tyrosinase* gene promoter regions −209 to +56 and −616 to +56 were unable to efficiently direct melanoma cell-specific expression.[24] Further analysis led to the identification of an enhancer located in the region between −2.0 and −1.8 kb that conferred high-level pigment cell-specific expression of the human *tyrosinase* gene proximal promoter.[24] The 39 bp element of the human enhancer was further studied by DNAase I footprinting and found to be protected across a central 20 bp region by protein partially purified from human melanoma cells.[26] This region, termed the *tyrosinase* distal enhancer (TDE), confers pigment cell-type-specific expression of a heterologous reporter plasmid. An E-box motif was identified within this region, and mutation studies demonstrated that the integrity of this element is essential for enhancer activity. Like the other E-box motifs in the *tyrosinase* promoter, this element can bind both USF and Mitf and is regulated by Mitf.[26] The known elements regulating *tyrosinase*, expression as well as the *Tyrp-1* and *Tyrp-2* promoters are summarized in Fig. 7.1.

The results described above raise the question of how pigment cell-specific expression is achieved by the *tyrosinase* proximal promoter. Importantly, the key elements identified within the promoter may be recognized by factors present in non-expressing cell types and, to date, no element important for the activity of the proximal promoter has been described as binding proteins uniquely in melanocytes. One possibility is that tissue specificity is dictated by a combination of the spatial arrangement of the key elements along the promoter, which is remarkably conserved between species, acting in concert with a TATA region that may in itself act in a cell-type-specific fashion, as has been observed for the *Tyrp-1* promoter.[38]

The *Tyrp-1* gene

The mouse *tyrosinase*-related protein 1 (*Tyrp-1*) gene was originally identified as a cDNA encoding a protein that maps to the *brown* locus.[39] Rescue of the brown phenotype by a retrovirus carrying the mouse *Tyrp-1* in the immortal cell line melan-b, which is homozygous for the mutation at the brown locus gene, has been reported.[40] The human *Tyrp-1* gene including the 5′-regulatory sequences has also been isolated.[41]

Promoter–reporter construct analysis established that as little as 38 bp of the mouse *Tyrp-1* proximal promoter is sufficient to direct a low level of melanoma cell-specific expression.[42,43] A more rigorous investigation of the *Tyrp-1* promoter region was undertaken by introducing a series of deletions and point mutations into a *Tyrp-1* promoter–reporter construct and revealed several

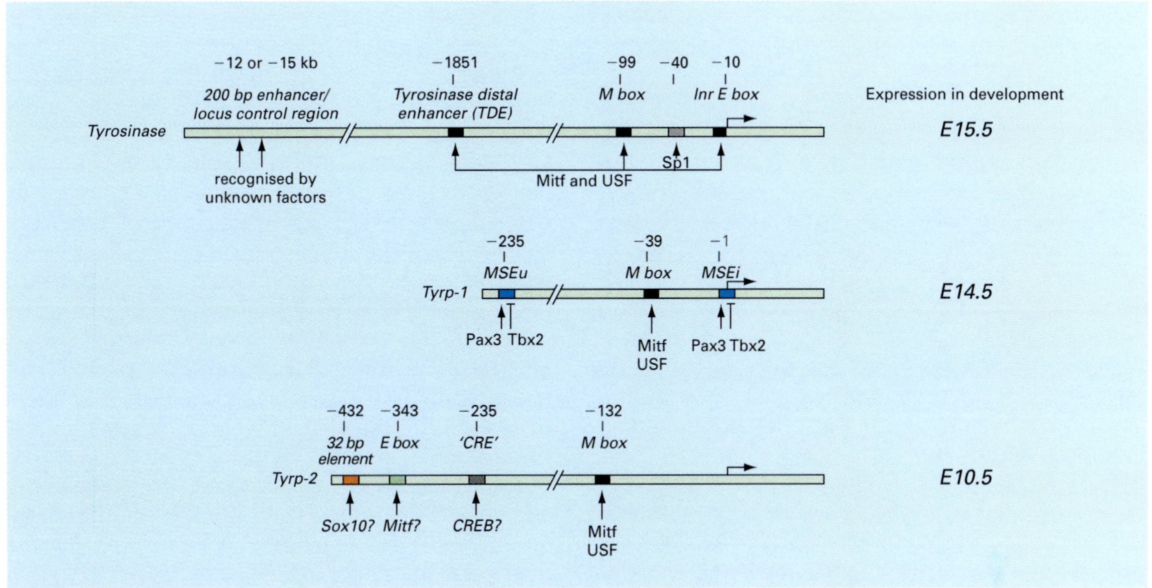

Figure 7.1

The *tyrosinase, Tyrp-1* and *Tyrp-2* promoters. Diagram indicating key elements and relative positions relative to the transcription start site of the *tyrosinase, Tyrp-1* and *Tyrp-2* promoters. Also indicated are the transcription factors likely to bind the key elements and the signals regulating their activity. Not shown are those elements for unidentified factors that have been shown to bind or those for which no defined function has been identified. E, Embryonic day.

interesting features, including a positive regulatory element between −332 and −319 and a negative regulatory element between −319 and −225.[38,43] It was postulated that pigment cell-specific gene expression might be attained by one or more pigment cell-specific transcription factors, acting through a common *cis*-regulatory element. Comparison of the mouse and human *tyrosinase* genes with the mouse *Tyrp-1* gene revealed that the only conserved region is the 11 bp M-box, located at position −44 to −34 in the *Tyrp-1* 5′-regulatory region.[43] Linker scanner mutations across the M-box, in the context of the proximal promoter (−322 to +114), confirmed that this element is essential for efficient expression of the *Tyrp-1* gene. The M-box is conserved in the human *Tyrp-1* promoter (position −48 to −38), and studies have shown that MITF activates the human *Tyrp-1* promoter through this element.[30] As discussed above for the *tyrosinase* gene, the core sequence of the M-box element contains a consensus binding site for members of the bHLH family of transcription factors can also bind to and be regulated by, both the 'melanocyte-specific' transcription factor Mitf[44,45] and the ubiquitous factor USF.[38,43] Consistent with this, the M-box can activate transcription from a heterologous promoter in a non-pigment cell fashion.[43] The lack of cell-type-specific binding to the M-box, together with the observation that a promoter–reporter construct under the control of multiple M-box elements is expressed equally well in melanocyte and non-melanocyte cell types, indicates that other elements contribute substantially to the pigment cell-specific expression of the *Tyrp-1* promoter.

In addition to the M-box, a strong positive regulatory element was identified between −332 and −319, with deletion or mutation of this region resulting in a 90% reduction in promoter activity. Closer inspection of this sequence revealed the presence of a non-consensus octamer motif. The most likely candidates for regulating the *Tyrp-1* promoter through this element are the ubiquitously expressed POU domain transcription factor, Oct-1, and the tissue-restricted Brn-2 transcription factor, suggesting that this element is also important for promoter activity, but is not primarily responsible for mediating melanocyte-specific expression of *Tyrp-1*.[43]

Given the failure to identify any elements capable of directing a uniquely pigment cell-specific expression pattern within the *Tyrp-1* promoter, attention turned more closely to the possibility that some control of cell-type-specific gene expression was mediated by the core promoter. Thus, a detailed analysis of the sequences −44 to +114 of the *Tyrp-1* promoter suggested that there is some cell-type specificity of the basal *Tyrp-1* promoter.[38] Analysis of a promoter–reporter construct, in which the region between −3 and +14 of the *Tyrp-1* gene was replaced with the corresponding sequences from the TK promoter, revealed the presence of a melanoma cell-specific negative regulatory element within the *Tyrp-1* initiator, and that the *Tyrp-1* TATA region also displayed an element of cell-type specificity. Significantly, the initiator region is bound *in vitro* by a 'melanocyte-specific' factor, originally termed MSF,[38] that was subsequently identified as the paired homeo domain transcription factor, Pax3,[46] which plays a critical role in melanocyte development by regulating *Mitf* expression.[47] Mutational analysis determined that the binding site for MSF/Pax3 within the initiator centres on a GTGTGA motif (−1 to +5), termed the melanocyte-specific initiator element (MSEi).[38,46] Inspection of the *Tyrp-1* proximal promoter identified a second binding site containing this motif, located between positions −256 and −232 (MSEu), that also binds MSF/Pax3 in a band shift.[38,46] The MSEu element lies within a previously identified negative regulatory region of the *Tyrp-1* promoter −319 to −225, consistent with mediation of melanocyte-specific repression.[43] However, further analysis of the MSEi and MSEu elements, by the introduction of point mutations within the context of the proximal *Tyrp-1* promoter, revealed that these regions are more complex, and actually contain overlapping positive and negative regulatory elements.[38] For example, the mutation of residues 3′ to the MSEi element did not influence MSF/Pax3 binding *in vitro*, but did relieve promoter repression *in vivo*, indicating that MSF/Pax3 is a positive, rather than negative, regulatory factor. Interestingly, mutation of MSEu and MSEi in combination, but not alone, in the context of the −334 to +114 construct, resulted in the de-repression of the *Tyrp-1* promoter in non-melanocyte cells.[38] This further supports the hypothesis that the repressor is not cell-type specific, and, therefore, expression of the *Tyrp-1* gene in melanocyte cells may result from the ability of the cell-type-specific MSF/Pax3 transcriptional activator to overcome the influence of the repressor. More recently, the MSEu and MSEi elements have been shown to be targets for the transcriptional repressor Tbx2,[48] a member of the T-box family of developmental regulators.[49,50] In other cell types, other members of the T-box family may play a role in preventing *Tyrp-1* expression.

Despite the fact that the *Tyrp-1* promoter, extending to around −330, is clearly cell-type specific in tissue culture cells, in transgenic animals up to 2.3 kb of upstream sequence is only active in the developing RPE, with no expression being observed in melanoblasts or melanocytes.[51,52] Presumably, additional elements, lying further upstream or downstream, are required for *Tyrp-1* expression, but their location has not been investigated.

The *Tyrp-2* (*DCT*) gene

The mouse *Tyrp-2* (*dopachrome tautomerase, DCT*) gene has been cloned and shown to be encoded at the *slaty* locus.[53] Expression of Tyrp-2 during development is first detected at around E10.5, and, in the adult, expression is observed in all neural-crest- and optic-cup-derived pigment cells.[54] The human *TYRP-2* gene has also been isolated and characterized to reveal several interesting features.[41,55–57] The transcription initiation start site predominantly utilized is located 427 bp from the translation start site, with a minor population of transcripts beginning at position −132. Analysis of promoter–reporter constructs demonstrated that 447 bp of the human *Tyrp-2* proximal promoter are sufficient to mediate melanocyte cell-specific expression. Further analysis revealed that two regions in combination are able to achieve this cell-type specificity.[57] These have been more clearly defined as the 32 bp element (located between −447 and −415) and the M-box (−138 to −128).[57] The ability of Mitf to activate the *Tyrp-2* promoter appears to be dependent on the cell type used, possibly reflecting a requirement for post-translational modifications of Mitf for efficient transactivation, as discussed later in this review, or, more likely, the fact that other elements contribute to cell-type-specific expression and that Mitf may not be competent to activate a promoter in the absence of a basal level of expression.[30,58] As might be expected from the results using the *tyrosinase* and *Tyrp-1* promoter, Mitf is able to bind to the M-box motif in a band shift assay, and also, weakly, to an E-box element identified between −341 and −346.[30,58] Experiments analysing the activation of a *Tyrp-2* promoter–reporter construct in response to an increase in cAMP levels revealed that the M- box is a more important regulatory element relative to the E-box, and also led to the identification of a potential CRE element located between −239 and −232.[58] The 32 bp element is not bound by Mitf in a band shift assay, despite possessing an E-box consensus sequence.[57] However, there is a consensus binding site for members of the Sox family of transcription factors within the 32 bp element, and it has recently been demonstrated that Sox10 transactivates the *Tyrp-2* promoter.[59] The *Tyrp-2* gene is expressed very early during melanogenesis, shortly after Sox10 is first detected in neural crest cells, consistent with a potential role for Sox10 in initiating *Tyrp-2* expression. However, further investigations are required to determine whether Sox10 is able to act directly upon the *Tyrp-2* promoter through the 32 bp element.

Regulation of transcription through the M-box and E-box elements

As discussed above, the only regulatory element conserved between the promoters of the mouse and human *tyrosinase*, *Tyrp-1* and *Tyrp-2* genes is the M-box that can be bound both by Mitf, the Mitf-related TFE3, TFEC and TFEB, and USF, comprised of homo- and heterodimers of the ubiquitous Usf1 and Usf2 transcription factors. Intriguingly, although the TFE family of proteins can heterodimerize with Mitf *in vitro*,[45] and activate transcription from *tyrosinase* or *Tyrp-1* reporters in transfection assays,[60] there is no evidence that these factors play any role in melanocyte development.[61] Moreover, although B16 melanoma cells clearly express both Mitf and TFE3, the two proteins do not co-immunoprecipitate, perhaps indicating that TFE3 may adopt a conformation incompatible with heterodimerization unless modified by phosphorylation in response to, as yet unidentified, signals.[60] Thus, regulation through the M-box and the tyrosinase initiator and enhancer E-box elements is most likely to occur via binding of USF and Mitf, both of which have been demonstrated to bind the *tyrosinase* promoter by chromatin immunoprecipitation assays,[32] and, as a consequence, be subject to signaling pathways that regulate the activity or abundance of these two key regulators.

Regulation of Mitf expression

Mitf is essential for development of the melanocyte lineage.[62,63] Mice with mutations at the *microphthalmia* locus exhibit a range of phenotypes, including loss of pigmentation, due to a lack of neural-crest-derived melanocytes[65,66] and small eyes, due to aberrant formation of the retinal pigment epithelium.[61] Mutations in the *MITF* gene in humans is associated with Waardenberg syndrome type II, a disease that is also characterized by pigmentary disorders and hearing loss.[67] Mitf expression is first detected in neural-crest-derived cells at day E10,[65] where its expression is under the control of several transcription factors, including Pax3, CREB, Sox10 and Lef1, that bind the melanocyte-specific Mitf-M promoter (reviewed in reference 68). Although the signaling pathways regulating Pax3 and Sox10 function are not known, the level of *Mitf* transcription is increased in response to Wnt signaling, through regulation of Lef1 (reviewed in reference 64) and, consistent with this, the Wnt pathway is essential for melanocyte development.[69,70] Regulation of factors, such as CREB, binding to the cAMP-response element, also play a major role in controlling Mitf expression. In this case, elevation of cAMP levels, for example by MSH signaling through the Mc1R, increases transcription from the *Mitf* promoter, resulting in a transient increase in Mitf protein levels, one consequence being increased transcription of *tyrosinase, Tyrp-1* and *Tyrp-2,* mediated though the M-box.[58,71–74]

While *Mitf* transcription is strongly regulated in response to cAMP and Wnt signaling, Mitf protein levels are also controlled by the MAP kinase signaling pathway, which lies downstream from receptor tyrosine kinases such as Kit. In this case, phosphorylation of Mitf by MAP kinase on Ser73 and by the MAP-kinase-activated kinase

RSK on Ser409, promote degradation of the Mitf protein via the ubiquitin-mediated targeting to the proteosome.[75,76]

In addition to regulation of the expression of *Mitf* RNA and Mitf protein, the ability of Mitf to activate transcription and, consequently, the regulation of the downstream target genes, such as *tyrosinase*, will also be affected by the interaction between Mitf and its cofactors. For example, the ability of Mitf to interact with the CBP/p300 transcription cofactor that binds the Mitf transcription activation domain[77] has been reported to be enhanced by phosphorylation on Ser73.[78] Moreover, experiments in which the adenovirus E1A protein, which can bind and sequester both p300/CBP and Rb -105/p107, was introduced into melan-a melanocytes resulted in transformation and dedifferentiation.[44] These effects were dependent upon the integrity of both the pRb and the p300/CBP interaction domains within E1A. *Mitf* RNA expression is downregulated in cells expressing E1A, most likely as a consequence of reduced CREB activity due to limitation of the p300/CBP cofactor, and the effects of E1A are reversed by overexpression of Mitf. Expression of E1A results in reduced levels of *tyrosinase* and *Tyrp-1*, and these repressive effects are mediated through the M-box element in the promoters of these genes. The low levels of *tyrosinase* and *Tyrp-1* expression result predominantly from reduced *Mitf* expression, but are, in part, due to impaired functioning of the residual Mitf.

Although much of the effect on E1A function may be a result of the sequestration of CBP/p300, Rb also appears to be involved. An interaction has also been demonstrated between Mitf and p105 Rb, both *in vitro*[38] and *in vivo* (Aksan et al., submitted) and, interestingly, co-immunoprecipitation experiments indicate that Mitf interacts specifically with the non-phosphorylated form of Rb (Aksan et al., submitted). Consistent with a role for Rb in regulation of Mitf transcriptional activity, the ability of Mitf to activate transcription of an M-box reporter construct in Rb-negative C33a cells is enhanced upon coexpression of either WT or non-phosphorylatable Rb (Aksan et al., submitted). Given the known regulation and roles of the Rb protein at both the G1-S transition of the cell cycle and during differentiation, the interaction of Mitf with non-phosphorylated Rb may potentially enhance the role of Mitf in regulating genes that are involved in specifying the melanocyte lineage.

Despite the clear demonstration that Mitf binds both p300/CBP and p105 Rb, to date, neither of these interactions has been demonstrated to influence the ability of Mitf to regulate transcription during development. Nevertheless, it seems likely that the interactions observed are relevant and that both CBP/p300 and Rb or Rb-related factors will play a key role in enabling Mitf to activate transcription of genes such as *tyrosinase* or *Tyrp-1*.

Requirements for Mitf DNA binding

Mitf has been shown to bind to the M-box and E-box elements within several pigment cell-specific promoters. However, the *tyrosinase*, *Tyrp-1* and *Tyrp-2* genes are dispensable for melanocyte development, and other Mitf target genes essential for specification of the melanocyte lineage remain to be identified. E-box motifs are found within the promoters of numerous genes, many of which are not regulated by Mitf, and there is often more than one bHLH–LZ family member expressed in any cell type. An important question is, therefore, how specificity in recruitment of bHLH–LZ family members to promoters is achieved. Insight into how Mitf is recruited to a subset of E-boxes has been gained from a detailed study of the requirements for Mitf binding. Whereas Mitf is recruited *in vitro* to all E-boxes comprising the sequence CACGTG that have been investigated,[45,79] E-boxes comprising the core sequence CATGTG exhibited differential abilities to bind Mitf. The results of *in vitro* and *in vivo* binding assays showed that Mitf will bind either TCATGTGN, NCATGTGA, or TCATGTGA, but not CATGTG E-boxes within any other context.[79] The significance of these observations becomes apparent when the Mitf-regulated E-box motifs of pigment cell-specific genes are inspected. The evolutionary conserved M-box motif of the *tyrosinase*, *Tyrp-1*, *Tyrp-2* and *QN71R* promoters, and also the *tyrosinase* TDE and initiator E-box, all contain a CATGTG E-box that possesses the flanking T residue.[79] More recently, two more Mitf target genes have been reported, the *Mcr1* and *Tbx2* promoters, and these also contain Mitf consensus sites that conform to this rule.[80,81] However, although these promoters bind Mitf *in vitro* and are activated by Mitf in transfection assays, it remains to be demonstrated that they are target genes of endogenous Mitf in cells or during development. As a result of exclusively possessing CATGTG E-boxes, melanocyte-specific promoters may avoid competition for binding between Mitf and other bHLH–LZ family members, particularly transcription factors that exclusively bind to CACGTG-type E-boxes. Moreover, the fact that only a subset of CATGTG motifs appears to bind Mitf has facilitated the identification of candidate Mitf target genes, for example, including the *p21* and *Bcl-2* promoters that both contain full consensus Mitf target elements (Goding et al., unpublished).

Regulation of *tyrosinase* in response to UV irradiation

In response to exposure to low levels of UV irradiation, epidermal melanocytes increase the production of melanin in melanosomes, which are then transferred to surrounding keratinocytes to protect from UV-induced DNA damage. This tanning response comprises both post-translational and transcriptional components.[82–86] Here we discuss only the regulation at the transcriptional level, and other aspects of the UV response will be reviewed by others.

Exposure of melanocyte and melanoma cell lines to UV irradiation results in the stimulation of transcription of the *tyrosinase* gene, as determined by semi-quantitative RT-PCR. A promoter–reporter construct, comprising the human *tyrosinase* proximal promoter, is also responsive to UV exposure.[32] The major regulatory elements of the *tyrosinase* gene are the M-box and the initiator E-box, that are target sites for Mitf. However, Mitf does not appear to be UV or stress regulated, indicating that an alternative transcription factor mediates the UV effect. The bHLH–LZ USF proteins are possible candidates, as Usf-1 is also able to bind to the *tyrosinase* M-box and E-box *in vitro*.[25,79] Chromatin immunoprecipitation assays demonstrated that both Usf-1 and Mitf are found at the *tyrosinase* promoter *in vivo* in untreated and UV-irradiated cells.[32] Although these results do not indicate which element is bound by Mitf and Usf-1, namely the M-box or the E-box, both proteins will be unable to bind to a single element simultaneously, and it is likely that occupancy at the promoter is a dynamic process. Expression of a dominant-negative non-DNA-binding Usf-1 protein resulted in the inhibition of the UV-induced activation of the *tyrosinase* promoter, strongly supporting a role for this factor in the UV response. Indeed, further investigations revealed that Usf-1 is phosphorylated in response to UV exposure or osmotic shock in both melanoma and non-melanocyte cells by a member of the p38 stress-responsive kinases, with phosphorylation appearing to enhance the ability of Usf-1 to activate transcription.

The conclusion principle here is that while Mitf, through binding to the M-box, may regulate basal level expression of the pigmentation genes and their activation in response to Wnt signaling or elevated cAMP levels, it is likely to be Usf-1 that is responsible for UV- or stress-mediated activation of the *tyrosinase* promoter.

Conclusions

The analysis of the *tyrosinase*, *Tyrp-1* and *Tyrp-2* promoters has led to the identification of several key elements required for their expression. This, in turn, has facilitated the identification of a number of sequence-specific transcription factors, including Mitf, USF, Pax3, Tbx2 and Sox10, that are clearly implicated in controlling expression of the pigmentation genes and mediating responsiveness to a variety of signaling pathways. Strikingly, however, despite the advances made, we still remain largely ignorant as to how the cell-type-specificity of expression is achieved. Moreover, it seems likely that additional, unidentified factors will also be involved in regulating the proximal *tyrosinase*, *Tyrp-1* and *Tyrp-2* promoters, and that additional enhancer elements required for *Tyrp-1* expression in melanoblasts have yet to be identified. The identification of these factors, as well as those mediating the activity of the tyrosinase enhancer, represents a major challenge and will lead, no doubt, not only to a greater understanding of the regulation of pigmentation genes, but also to key insights into controls operating during melanocyte development.

References

1. Mayer TC, The migratory pathway of neural crest cells into the skin of mouse embryos, *Dev Biol (*1973) **34**:39–46.
2. Steel KP, Barkway C, Another role for melanocytes: their importance for stria vascularis development in the mammalian inner ear, *Development* (1989) **107**:453–63.
3. Tachibana M, Sound needs sound melanocytes to be heard, *Pigment Cell Res* (1999) **12**:344–54.
4. Jackson IJ, Bennett DC, Identification of the albino mutation of mouse tyrosinase by analysis of an in vitro revertant, *Proc Natl Acad Sci U S A* (1990) **87**:7010–14.
5. Kikuchi H, Miura H, Yamamoto H et al., Characteristic sequences in the upstream region of the human tyrosinase gene, *Biochim Biophys Acta* (1989) **1009**:283–6.
6. Ponnazhagan S, Hou L, Kwon BS, Structural organization of the human tyrosinase gene and sequence analysis and characterization of its promoter region, *J Invest Dermatol* (1994) **102**:744–8.
7. Kwon BS, Haq AK, Wakulchik M et al., Isolation, chromosomal mapping, and expression of the mouse tyrosinase gene, *J Invest Dermatol* (1989) **93**:589–94.
8. Ruppert S, Muller G, Kwon B et al., Multiple transcripts of the mouse tyrosinase gene are generated by alternative splicing, *EMBO J* (1988) **7**:2715–22.
9. Ferguson CA, Kidson SH, Characteristic sequences in the promoter region of the chicken tyrosinase-encoding gene, *Gene* (1996) **169**:191–5.
10. Yamamoto H, Kudo T, Masuko N et al., Phylogeny of regulatory regions of vertebrate tyrosinase genes, *Pigment Cell Res* (1992) **5**:284–94.
11. Miura I, Okumoto H, Makino K et al., Analysis of the tyrosinase gene of the Japanese pond frog, Rana nigromaculata: cloning and nucleotide sequence of the genomic DNA containing the tyrosinase gene and its flanking regions, *Jpn J Genet* (1995) **70**:79–92.
12. Toyoda R, Sato S, Ikeo K et al., Pigment cell-specific expression of the tyrosinase gene in ascidians has a different regulatory mechanism from vertebrates, *Gene* (2000) **259**:159–70.
13. Ferguson CA, Kidson SH, The regulation of tyrosinase gene transcription, *Pigment Cell Res* (1997) **10**:127–38.
14. Beermann F, Schmid E, Schutz G, Expression of the mouse tyrosinase gene during embryonic development: recapitulation of the temporal regulation in transgenic mice, *Proc Natl Acad Sci U S A (*1992) **89**:2809–13.
15. Kluppel M, Beermann F, Ruppert S et al., The mouse tyrosinase promoter is sufficient for expression in melanocytes and in the pigmented epithelium of the retina, *Proc Natl Acad Sci U S A* (1991) **88**:3777–81.
16. Hou L, Panthier JJ, Arnheiter H, Signaling and transcriptional regulation in the neural crest-derived melanocyte lineage: interactions between KIT and MITF, *Development* (2000) **127**:5379–89.
17. Ganss R, Schutz G, Beermann F, The mouse tyrosinase gene. Promoter modulation by positive and negative regulatory elements, *J Biol Chem* (1994) **269**:29808–16.
18. Schedl A, Montoliu L, Kelsey G et al., A yeast artificial chromosome covering the tyrosinase gene confers copy number-dependent expression in transgenic mice, *Nature* (1993) **362**:258–61.
19. Grosveld F, van Assendelft G, Greaves D et al., Position-independent, high-level expression of the human ß-globin gene in transgenic mice, *Cell* (1987) **51**:975–85.
20. Ganss R, Montoliu L, Monaghan AP et al., A cell-specific enhancer far upstream of the mouse tyrosinase gene confers high level and copy number-related expression in transgenic mice, *EMBO J* (1994) **13**:3083–93.
21. Porter SD, Meyer CJ, A distal tyrosinase upstream element stimulates gene expression in neural crest-derived melanocytes of transgenic mice: position-independent and mosaic expression, *Development* (1994) **120**:2103–11.
22. Porter SD, Hu J, Gilks CB, Distal upstream tyrosinase S/MAR-containing sequence has regulatory properties specific to subsets of melanocytes, *Dev Genet* (1999) **25**:40–8.
23. Montoliu L, Umland T, Schütz G, A locus control region at −12 kb of the tyrosinase gene, *EMBO J* (1997) **15**:6026–34.
24. Shibata K, Muraosa Y, Tomita Y et al., Identification of a cis-acting element that enhances the pigment cell-specific expression of the human tyrosinase gene, *J Biol Chem* (1992) **267**:20584–8.
25. Bentley NJ, Eisen T, Goding CR, Melanocyte-specific expression of the human tyrosinase promoter: activation by the microphthalmia gene product and role of the initiator, *Mol Cell Biol* (1994) **14**:7996–8006.
26. Yasumoto K, Yokoyama K, Shibata K et al., Microphthalmia-associated transcription factor as a regulator for melanocyte-specific transcription of

the human tyrosinase gene, *Mol Cell Biol* (1994) **14**:8058–70.

27. Kaufman J, Smale ST, Direct recognition of initiator elements by a component of the transcription factor IID complex, *Genes Dev* (1994) **8**:821–9.
28. Chen LI, Nishinaka T, Kwan K et al., The retinoblastoma gene product RB stimulates Sp1-mediated transcription by liberating Sp1 from a negative regulator, *Mol Cell Biol* (1994) **14**:4380–9.
29. Kim SJ, Onwuta US, Lee YI et al., The retinoblastoma gene product regulates Sp1-mediated transcription, *Mol Cell Biol* (1992) **12**:2455–63.
30. Yasumoto K-I, Yokayama K, Takahashi K et al., Functional analysis of Microphthalmia-associated transcription factor in pigment cell-specific transcription of the human Tyrosinase family genes, *J Biol Chem* (1997) **272**:503–9.
31. Krylov D, Kasai K, Echlin DR et al., A general method to design dominant negatives to B-HLHZip proteins that abolish DNA binding, *Proc Natl Acad Sci U S A* (1997) **94**:12274–9.
32. Galibert M-D, Carreira S, Goding CR, The Usf-1 transcription factor is a novel target for the stress-responsive p38 kinase and mediates UV-induced tyrosinase expression, *Embo J* (2001) **20:**5022–31.
33. Eisen T, Easty DJ, Bennett DC et al., The POU domain transcription factor Brn-2: elevated expression in malignant melanoma and regulation of melanocyte-specific gene expression, *Oncogene* (1995) **11**:2157–64.
34. Thomson JA, Parsons PG, Sturm RA, In vivo and in vitro expression of octamer binding proteins in human melanoma metastases, brain tissue, and fibroblasts, *Pigment Cell Res* (1993) **6**:13–22.
35. Thomson JA, Murphy K, Baker E et al., The *brn-2* gene regulates the melanocytic phenotype and tumorigenic potential of human melanoma cells, *Oncogene* (1995) **11**:690–700.
36. Ganss R, Schmidt A, Schutz G et al., Analysis of the mouse tyrosinase promoter in vitro and in vivo, *Pigment Cell Res* (1994) **7**:275–8.
37. Yasumoto K-I, Mahalingam H, Suzuki H et al., Transcriptional regulation of the melanocyte-specific gnese by the human homolog of the mouse Microphthalmia protein, *J Biochem* (1995) **118**:874–81.
38. Yavuzer U, Goding CR, Melanocyte-specific gene expression: role of repression and identification of a melanocyte-specific factor, MSF, *Mol Cell Biol* (1994) **14**:3494–503.
39. Jackson IJ, A cDNA encoding tyrosinase-related protein maps to the brown locus in mouse, *Proc Natl Acad Sci U S A* (1988) **85**:4392–6.
40. Bennett DC, Huszar D, Laipis PJ et al., Phenotypic rescue of mutant brown melanocytes by a retrovirus carrying a wild-type tyrosinase-related protein gene, *Development* (1990) **110**:471–5.
41. Sturm RA, O'Sullivan BJ, Box NF et al., Chromosomal structure of the human TYRP1 and TYRP2 loci and comparison of the tyrosinase-related protein gene family, *Genomics* (1995) **29**:24–34.
42. Shibahara S, Taguchi H, Muller RM et al., Structural organization of the pigment cell-specific gene located at the brown locus in mouse. Its promoter activity and alternatively spliced transcript, *J Biol Chem* (1991) **266**:15895–901.
43. Lowings P, Yavuzer U, Goding CR, Positive and negative elements regulate a melanocyte-specific promoter, *Mol Cell Biol* (1992) **12**:3653–62.
44. Yavuzer U, Keenan E, Lowings P et al., The microphthalmia gene product interacts with the retinoblastoma protein in vitro and is a target for deregulation of melanocyte-specific transcription, *Oncogene* (1995) **10**:123–34.
45. Hemesath TJ, Steingrimsson E, McGill G et al., Microphthalmia, a critical factor in melanocyte development, defines a discrete transcription factor family, *Genes Dev* (1994) **8**:2770–80.
46. Galibert M-D, Yavuzer U, Dexter TJ et al., Pax3 and regulation of the melanocyte-specific TRP-1 promoter, *J Biol Chem* (1999) **274**:26894–900.
47. Watanabe A, Takeda K, Ploplis B et al., Epistatic relationship between Waardenburg syndrome genes MITF and PAX3, *Nat Genet (*1998) **18**:283–6.
48. Carreira S, Dexter TJ, Yavuzer U et al., Brachyury-related transcription factor Tbx2 and repression of the melanocyte-specific TRP-1 promoter, *Mol Cell Biol* (1998) **18**:5099–108.
49. Papaioannou VE, Silver LM, The T-box gene family, *BioEssays* (1998) **20**:9–19.
50. Smith J, T-box genes: what they do and how they do it, *Trends Genet* (1999) **15**:154–8.
51. Schmidt A, Tief K, Yavuzer U et al., Ectopic expression of RET results in microphthalmia and tumors in the retinal pigment epithelium, *Int J Cancer* (1999) **80**:600–5.
52. Raymond SM, Jackson IJ, The retinal pigment epithelium is required for development and maintenance of the mouse neural retina, *Curr Biol* (1995) **5**:1286–95.
53. Jackson IJ, Chambers DM, Tsukamoto K et al., A second tyrosinase-related protein, TRP-2, maps to and is mutated at the mouse *slaty* locus, *EMBO J* (1992) **11**:527–35.

54. Steel KP, Davidson DR, Jackson IJ, TRP-2/DT, a new early melanoblast marker, shows that steel growth factor (c-kit ligand) is a survival factor, *Development* (1992) **115**:1111–19.
55. Cassady JL, Sturm RA, Sequence of the human dopachrome tautomerase-encoding TRP-2 cDNA, *Gene* (1994) **143**:295–8.
56. Bouchard B, del Marmol V, Jackson IJ et al., Molecular characterisation of a human tyrosinase-related-protein-2 cDNA, *Eur J Biochem* (1994) **219**:127–34.
57. Yokoyama K, Yasumoto K, Suzuki H et al., Cloning of the human DOPAchrome tautomerase/tyrosinase-related protein 2 gene and identification of two regulatory regions required for its pigment cell-specific expression, *J Biol Chem* (1994) **269**:27080–7.
58. Bertolotto C, Busca R, Abbe P et al., Different cis-acting elements are involved in the regulation of TRP1 and TRP2 promoter activities by cyclin AMP: pivotal role of M boxes (GTCATGTGCT) and of Microphthalmia, *Mol Cell Biol* (1998) **18**:694–702.
59. Britsch S, Goerich DE, Riethmacher D et al., The transcription factor Sox10 is a key regulator of peripheral glial development, *Genes Dev* (2001) **15**:66–78.
60. Verastegui C, Bertolotto C, Bille K et al., TFE3, a transcription factor homologous to microphthalmia, is a potential transcriptional activator of tyrosinase and Tyrpl genes, *Mol Endocrinol* (2000) **14**:449–56.
61. Nakayama A, Nguyen MT, Chen CC et al., Mutations in microphthalmia, the mouse homolog of the human deafness gene MITF, affect neuroepithelial and neural crest-derived melanocytes differently, *Mech Dev* (1998) **70**:155–66.
62. Hodgkinson CA, Moore KJ, Nakayama A et al., Mutations at the mouse *microphthalmia* locus are associated with defects in a gene encoding a novel basic-helix-loop-helix-zipper protein, *Cell* (1993) **74**:395–404.
63. Hughes MJ, Lingrel JB, Krakowsky JM et al., A helix-loop-helix transcription factor-like gene is located at the *mi* locus, *J Biol Chem* (1993) **268**:20687–90.
64. Goding CR, Mitf from neural crest to melanoma: signal transduction and transcription in the melanocyte lineage, *Genes Dev* (2000) **14**:1712–28.
65. Opdecamp K, Nakayama A, Nguyen MT et al., Melanocyte development in vivo and in neural crest cell cultures: crucial dependence on the Mitf basic-helix-loop-helix-zipper transcription factor, *Development* (1997) **124**:2377–86.
66. Steingrimsson E, Moore KJ, Lamoreux ML et al., Molecular basis of mouse microphthalmia (mi) mutations helps explain their developmental and phenotypic consequences, *Nat Genet* (1994) **8**:256–63.
67. Tassabehji M, Newton VE, Read AP, Waardenburg syndrome type 2 caused by mutations in the human *microphthalmia* (*MITF*) gene, *Nat Genet* (1994) **8**:251–5.
68. Goding CR, Melanocyte development and malignant melanoma, *Forum (Genova)* (2000) **10**:176–87.
69. Dorsky RI, Moon RT, Raible DW, Control of neural crest cell fate by the Wnt signalling pathway, *Nature* (1998) **396**:370–3.
70. Ikeya M, Lee SMK, Johnson JE et al., Wnt signalling required for expansion of neural crest and CNS progenitors, *Nature* (1997) **289**:966–70.
71. Bertolotto C, Bille K, Ortonne J-P, Ballotti R, Regulation of tyrosinase gene expression by cAMP in B16 melanoma cells involves two CATGTG motifs surrounding the TATA box: implication of the microphthalmia gene product, *J Cell Sci* (1996) **134**:747–55.
72. Bertolotto C, Abbe P, Hemesath TJ et al., Microphthalmia gene product as a signal transducer in cAMP-induced differentiation of melanocytes, *J Cell Biol* (1998) **142**:827–35.
73. Aberdam E, Bertolotto C, Sviderskaya EV et al., Involvement of Microphthalmia in the inhibition of melanocyte lineage differentiation and of melanogenesis by agouti signal protein, *J Biol Chem* (1998) **273**:19560–5.
74. Price ER, Horstmann MA, Wells AG et al., α-Melanocyte-stimulating hormone signaling regulates expression of *microphthalmia*, a gene deficient in Waardenburg syndrome, *J Biol Chem* (1998) **273**: 33042–7.
75. Xu W, Gong L, Haddad MM et al., Regulation of microphthalmia-associated transcription factor MITF protein levels by association with the ubiquitin-conjugating enzyme hUBC9, *Exp Cell Res* (2000) **255**:135–43.
76. Wu M, Hemesath TJ, Takemoto CM et al., c-Kit triggers dual phosphorylations, which couple activation and degradation of the essential melanocyte factor Mi, *Genes Dev* (2000) **14**:301–12.
77. Sato S, Roberts K, Gambino G et al., CBP/p300 as a co-factor for the Microphthalmia transcription factor, *Oncogene* (1997) **14**:3083–92.
78. Price ER, Ding H-F, Badalian T et al., Lineage-specific signalling in melanocytes: c-Kit stimulation recruits p300/CBP to Microphthalmia, *J Biol Chem* (1998) **273**:17983–6.

79. Aksan I, Goding CR, Targeting the microphthalmia basic helix-loop-helix-leucine zipper transcription factor to a subset of E-box elements in vitro and in vivo, *Mol Cell Biol* (1998) **18**:6930–8.
80. Adachi S, Morii E, Kim D et al., Involvement of mi-transcription factor in expression of alpha-melanocyte-stimulating hormone receptor in cultured mast cells of mice, *J Immunol* (2000) **164**:855–60.
81. Carreira S, Liu B, Goding CR, The gene encoding the T-box transcription factor Tbx2 is a target for the microphthalmia-associated transcription factor in melanocytes, *J Biol Chem* (2000) **275**:21920–7.
82. Ota A, Park JS, Jimbow K, Functional regulation of tyrosinase and LAMP gene family of melanogenesis and cell death in immortal murine melanocytes after repeated exposure to ultraviolet B, *Br J Dermatol* (1998) **139(2)**:207–15.
83. Sturm RA, O'Sullivan BJ, Thomson JA et al., Expression studies of pigmentation and POU-domain genes in human melanoma cells, *Pigment Cell Res* (1994) **7**:235–420.
84. Hara H, Lee MH, Chen H et al., Role of gene expression and protein synthesis of tyrosinase, TRP-1, lamp-1, and CD63 in UVB-induced melanogenesis in human melanomas, *J Invest Dermatol* (1994) **102(4)**:495–500.
85. Imokawa G, Miyagishi M, Yada Y, Endothelin-1 as a new melanogen: coordinated expression of its gene and the tyrosinase gene in UVB-exposed human epidermis, *J Invest Dermatol* (1995) **105(1)**:32–7.
86. Imokawa G, Kobayashi T, Miyagishi M et al., The role of endothelin-1 in epidermal hyperpigmentation and signaling mechanisms of mitogenesis and melanogenesis, *Pigment Cell Res* (1997) **10(4)**: 218–28.

8
The molecular mechanisms of cAMP-induced melanogenesis

Corine Bertolotto

In humans, melanocytes originate from the neural crest, from which they migrate along the dorsolateral pathway, as melanoblast precursors, to reach the basal layer of the epidermis.[1] Subsequently, these cells differentiate to mature melanocytes possessing the specific enzymatic machinery responsible for melanin synthesis. Melanin synthesis takes place within specialized intracellular organelles termed melanosomes. Melanosomes are then transferred to surrounding keratinocytes to ensure a uniform skin colour and determine constitutive skin pigmentation ranging from black-brown to nearly white.[2] Three melanocyte-specific enzymes, tyrosinase, tyrosinase-related protein 1 (Tyrp1) and Tyrp2/DOPA chrome tautomerase (DCT), are involved in the enzymatic process that converts tyrosine to melanin pigments. Although these proteins have similar structures and features, they are expressed by different genes and possess distinct enzymatic activities. Tyrosinase, encoded by the *albino* locus of the mouse, is the rate-limiting enzyme in melanogenesis that catalyses the two initial steps of this process, hydroxylation of tyrosine to 3,4-dihydroxyphenylalanine (DOPA) and oxidation of DOPA to DOPA quinone.[3–5] Tyrosinase-related protein 1, which has been mapped in mouse to the *brown* locus, possesses, at least in mouse, a 5,6-dihydroxyindole-2-carboxylic acid (DHICA) oxidase activity[6] and Dct, encoded by the mouse *slaty* locus, is endowed with a DOPAchrome tautomerase activity.[7,8] Finally, the p protein, encoded by the *p* locus, also plays a key role in eumelanin synthesis but, to date, its function has not been well established. Recently, the p protein has been postulated to act as an ion exchanger and to maintain an acidic intramelanosomal pH, allowing tyrosinase to be active.[9] Two types of pigments are produced by melanocytes: eumelanins, which are black/brown pigments, and phaeomelanins, which are yellow/red. The constitutive skin pigmentation is physiologically increased by the ultraviolet (UV) radiation of the solar light and leads to skin darkening, also known as the tanning response. Skin darkening results from an increase in the number of melanocytes, in eumelanin synthesis and in the transfer of melanosomes to keratinocytes. Beyond its aesthetic and cultural role, the main function assigned to cutaneous pigmentation and melanin pigments is a photoprotective role against the carcinogenic effects of UV radiation. The ratio of eumelanins to phaeomelanins is variable, but the presence of eumelanins in epidermis has been correlated with improved skin protection against the UV-induced DNA damage that has been associated with the risk of skin cancer. Considering the key physiological role of melanin in photo-protection, a better understanding of the mechanisms involved in the control of the quantity and the quality of these pigments constitutes an issue of paramount importance.

Regulation of melanogenesis by melanotropic hormones and cAMP

Compelling evidence has demonstrated the involvement of the melanotropic hormones, adrenocorticotrophic hormone (ACTH) and alpha-melanocyte-stimulating hormone (αMSH), in the control of human pigmentation and, particularly, in eumelanin synthesis. The two melanotropic hormones, ACTH and αMSH, are locally produced in skin and derived from a common precursor, pro-opiomelanocortin (POMC). ACTH and αMSH act through binding to the melanocortin receptors type I (MC1R). In humans, mutations in POMC and MC1R are responsible for defects in eumelanin synthesis and lead to red-hair pigmentation.[10,11] In mouse, mutations at the *extension* locus, which renders the MC1R unable to bind αMSH, result in a yellow coat colour. Further, skin hyperpigmentation defects observed in patients suffering from Addison's disease or Cushing's syndrome have been explained by an ACTH overproduction.[12,13] An excessive production of αMSH, leading to skin hyperpigmentation, has also been reported.[14] Finally, administration of αMSH analogs ([norleucine-4, D-phenylalanine]- αMSH) increases skin pigmentation without sun exposure in human volunteers[15,16] and, *in vitro*, αMSH treatment increases melanin synthesis of cultured pigment cells. These data demonstrate that melanotropic hormones are essential regulators of cutaneous pigmentation. Binding of ACTH or αMSH to the Gαs-coupled MC1R leads to adenylate cyclase activation, elevation of intracellular cAMP, and activation of protein kinase A (PKA). PKA is then able to phosphorylate its substrates, among which the best characterized are CREB (cAMP-response element binding protein) and its co-activator CBP (CREB-binding protein) (Fig. 8.1). CREB proteins activate the expression of specific genes containing consensus CRE (cAMP-response element) sequences in their promoters (TGACCTCA).[17,18] Interestingly, patients with McCune–Albright syndrome display large hyperpigmented areas caused by an activating mutation in the Gαs protein that controls the cAMP level.[19,20] Mutations in the type Iα regulatory sub-unit of PKA, leading to a constitutive activation of PKA, have been detected in patients with Carney syndrome, characterized by spotty skin pigmentation.[21,22] Taken together, these observations clearly demonstrate the importance of the melanotropic hormones and the cAMP pathway in the regulation of human pigmentation.

Regulation of melanogenesis by the cAMP/PKA pathway

Upregulation of melanin synthesis by αMSH results from an increase in the tyrosinase activity that has been ascribed either to post-translational modifications of a pre-existing enzyme or to an increase in its expression. Until now, no clear evidence in favor of the first hypothesis has been reported. However, it has been demonstrated that the increased expression of tyrosinase by αMSH

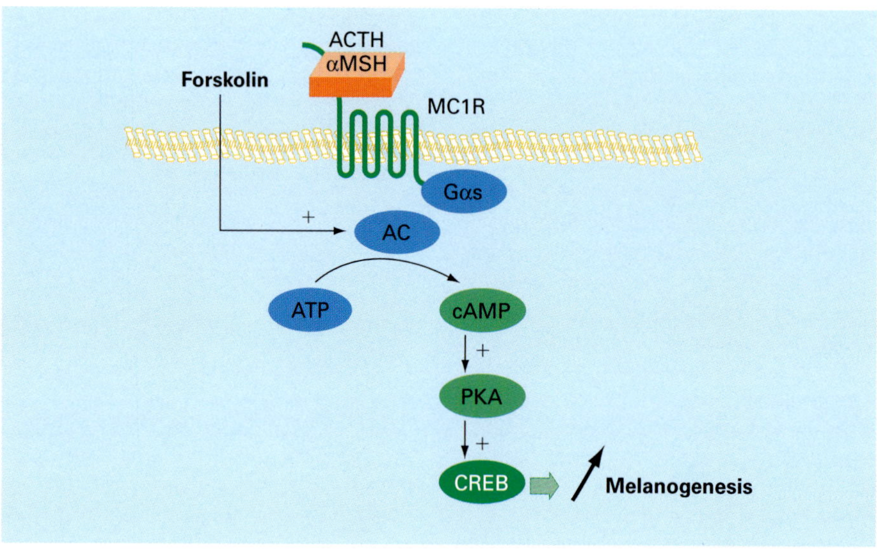

Figure 8.1

cAMP/PKA signaling pathway.

and cAMP involves a transcriptional mechanism. Indeed, αMSH, or pharmacological agents such as forskolin, IBMX or cholera toxin, that also elevate the intracellular cAMP content, potently stimulate the transcriptional activity of a 2.2 Kb fragment 5′ upstream of the transcriptional start site of the mouse *tyrosinase* gene[23] (Fig. 8.2). This 2.2 Kb promoter fragment has been previously shown to direct the melanocyte-specific expression of the enzyme in melanocyte.[24,25] Tyrosinase promoter activity is also increased by cAMP in the S91 mouse melanoma cells, in the G361 human melanoma cells and in normal human melanocytes.[23] Further, the human tyrosinase promoter is also responsive to cAMP, indicating the existence of common regulatory mechanisms between the two species. Stimulation of the tyrosinase promoter activity is also obtained by the overexpression of the catalytic subunit of PKA and PKI, the physiologic inhibitor of PKA, inhibit both the αMSH and PKA responses of the tyrosinase promoter.[26] Deletions and mutations in the tyrosinase promoter reveal that two regulatory elements, termed M-box (AGTCATGTGCT) and E-box (CATGTG), mediate its cAMP responsiveness.[23] Thus, αMSH, through PKA activation, stimulates tyrosinase expression by a transcriptional mechanism that involves M-box and E-box sequences. These sequences contain a CANNTG motif that is recognized by members of the basic helix-loop-helix (bHLH) transcription factor family. This transcription factor family includes ubiquitously-expressed proteins, such as myc, max,[27] upstream stimulatory factor, USF,[28] and tissue-specific expressed proteins such as myoD, myogenin,[29] and microphthalmia-associated transcription factor (MITF).[30,31] A few years ago, pigmentation disorders observed in microphthalmic mouse were associated with mutations of the b-HLH transcription factor encoded by the *microphthalmia* gene. These mice have small non-pigmented eyes, a lack of melanocytes in the skin and inner ear, a deficiency in mast cells, and osteopetrosis caused by osteoclast dysfunctions.[31–34] In humans, heterozygous mutations in MITF have been linked to abnormal pigmentation of the eyes, hair and skin, observed in patients with Waardenburg syndrome type IIa.[35–38] MITF is expressed as multiple isoforms, which contain different amino termini, termed MITF-M, MITF-A, MITF-H, and MITF-C.[39–41] MITF-M is specifically expressed in neural-crest-derived melanocytes while MITF-A is principally found in the pigmented epithelium of the retina. MITF-H, initially isolated from heart and MITF-C, present a wide distribution but their function has not

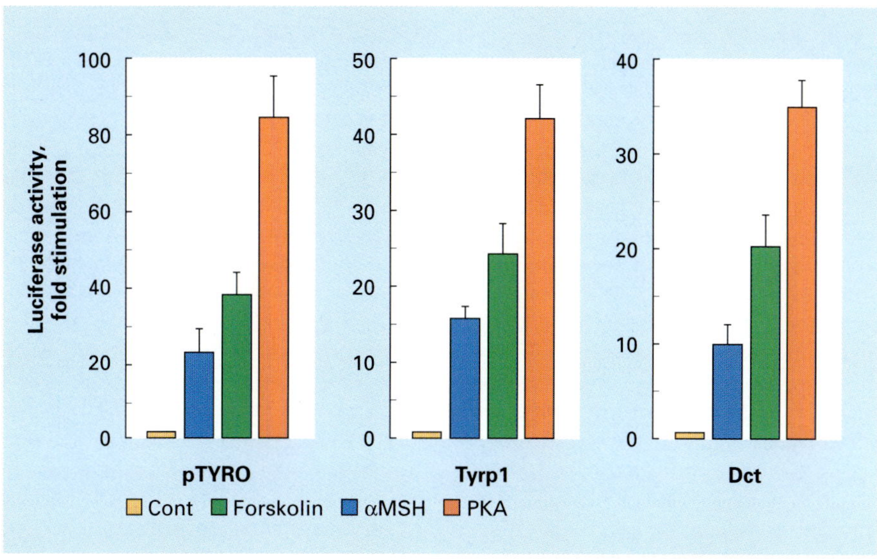

Figure 8.2

cAMP and PKA stimulate tyrosinase, tyrp1 and Dct promoter activities.

yet been determined. The fact that expression of the melanogenic enzymes is restricted to melanocytes suggests that their promoters contain regulatory elements responsible for their tissue-specific expression.[8,24,25] Interestingly, MITF recognizes the M-box sequence, and MITF binding to the M-box has been shown to play a key role in pigment cells' restricted expression of the melanogenic enzymes. In this context, it was tempting to propose that MITF could play a role in melanocyte differentiation and in mediating the cAMP effects on the tyrosinase promoter. Co-expression of MITF with the tyrosinase promoter, bearing either an intact or mutated M-box, reveals a total correlation between the cAMP sensitivity and MITF response.[23,26] These observations suggest that MITF is involved in the cAMP responsiveness of the tyrosinase promoter. However, a construction containing three M-boxes upstream a SV40 promoter does not respond to cAMP. Thus, it appears that the M-box needs additional elements to confer the cAMP responsiveness to the tyrosinase promoter.

It has been thought for many years that the regulation of melanin synthesis occurs at the level of tyrosinase, the rate-limiting enzyme in melanogenesis. However, Tyrp1 and Dct have been shown to play important roles in the switch from eumelanin to phaeomelanin. In 'lethal yellow' mouse, which exhibits a yellow coat colour, Tyrp1 and Dct expression is extinguished while tyrosinase is still expressed.[42–44] Additionally, transfection of fibroblasts with tyrosinase only allows phaeomelanin production,[45] while further overexpression of tyrosinase and Tyrp1 restores eumelanin synthesis.[46] This indicates that Tyrp1 and Dct also play a key role in eumelanin synthesis. cAMP-elevating agents also stimulate the transcriptional activities of Tyrp1 and Dct promoters (Fig. 8.2). Two regulatory elements, accountable for the cAMP responsiveness of the Tyrp1 promoter, were identified: the highly conserved M-box, and an E-box (CAAGTG), whose sequence differs from that of the tyrosinase promoter. Analysis of the Dct promoter indicated the involvement of another E-box (CACATG), a CRE-like motif and the M-box in its cAMP sensitivity. MITF also stimulates the transcriptional activity of the Tyrp1 and Dct promoters, and mutations of M-boxes in each promoter drastically abolished the response to MITF.[26] In conclusion, tyrosinase, Tyrp1 and Dct promoters share a common regulatory element, which is the M-box. However, the regulation by cAMP of each promoter can be acutely controlled through the involvement of other DNA sequences, such as E-box or CRE. This might allow a differential regulation of the enzyme expression, depending on the physiological context.

Nevertheless, MITF, through binding to the M-box, appears to play a key role in the regulation of melanogenic enzyme expression. This hypothesis has been confirmed by using dominant-negative forms of MITF, in which either the N-terminal transactivation domain is suppressed, or the arginine 215 in the DNA-binding domain of the basic region is deleted. As mentioned above, MITF is a bHLH protein that functions as a dimer. Both bHLH and trans-activation domains must be intact in each partnership to allow the transcription factor to be functional. Mutations affecting one of these MITF domains lead to the most severe phenotype in mice.[31] A dominant-negative form of MITF, in which the bHLH sequence is still present but the trans-activation domain is absent, is able to dimerize with wild-type protein. The resulting dimer can bind DNA but loses the ability to positively regulate its target genes because of the lack of the trans-activation domain in the mutant protein. In consequence, overexpression of this mutant has a strong inhibitory effect on the stimulation of the tyrosinase promoter by wild-type MITF. Additionally, this dominant-negative mutant of MITF completely blocks the cAMP sensibility of the tyrosinase promoter (Fig. 8.3).[47] Further, overexpression of the Mi-dn(R215del) preserves a transactivation domain intact and a dimerization activity, but fails to bind DNA. This dominant-negative MITF produces an inhibition of both basaly and αMSH-stimulated tyrosinase promoter activity.[48] Taken together, these results demonstrate that MITF is a key regulator of cAMP action.

Finally, it remained to elucidate how cAMP acts on MITF to regulate *tyrosinase* gene expression. It has been demonstrated that cAMP treatment of pigment cells stimulates MITF protein expression, reaching the maximum after 3–5 hours (Fig. 8.4).[47,48] As a consequence, MITF binding to the M-box of the melanogenic promoter is increased. Thus, increased melanogenesis could be explained by a two-step mechanism that requires, first, the accumulation of MITF, and then an increase in the melanogenic gene expression. Some have described MITF as a master gene of melanocyte differentiation, since enforced MITF

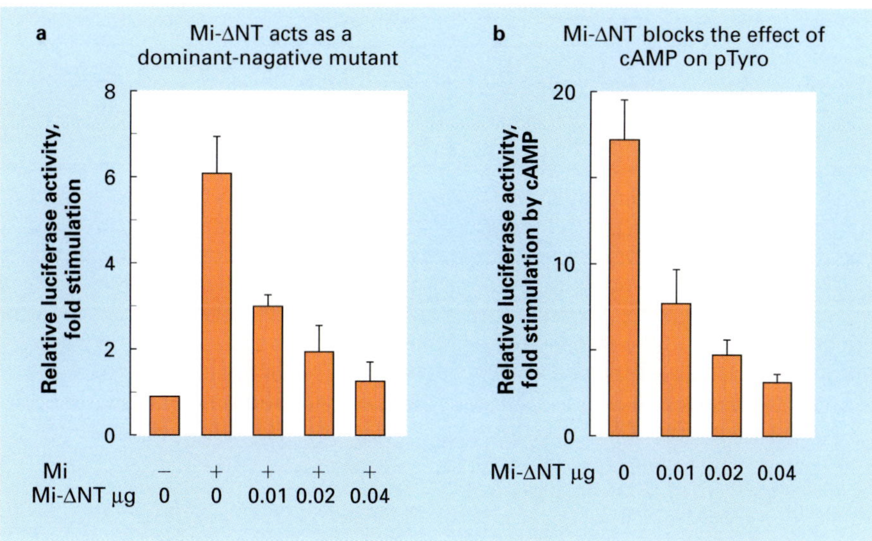

Figure 8.3

MITF plays a key role in the cAMP sensitivity of the tyrosinase promoter.[47]

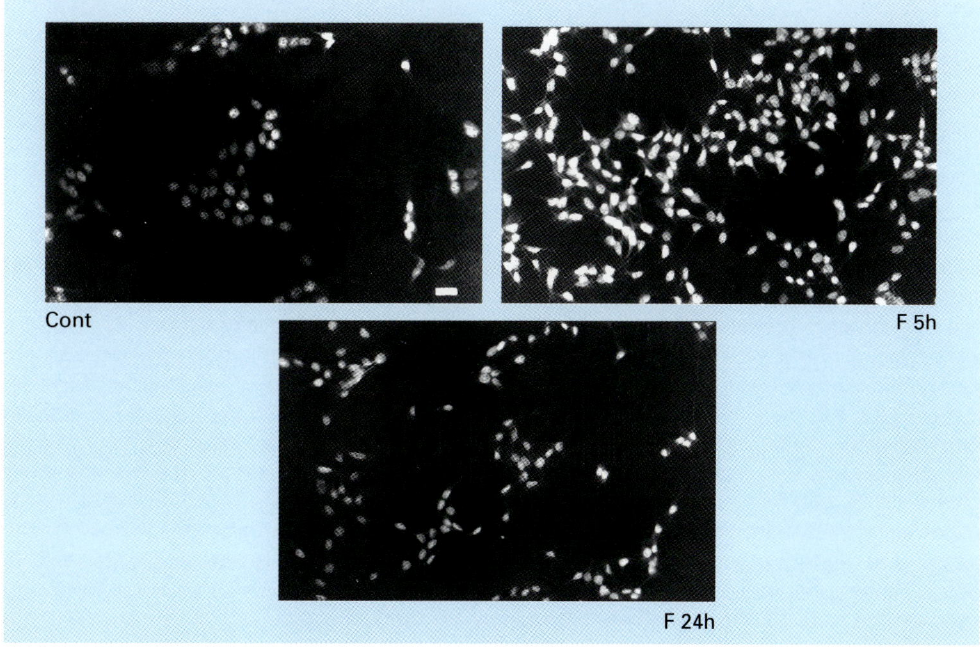

Figure 8.4

Forskolin increases MITF expression.[47]

expression in NIH3T3 cells confers to these cells characteristics of melanocytes.[49] Noteworthy, fibroblasts used in these experiments express Dct before transfection of MITF. Additionally, it has been recently demonstrated that the presence of MITF alone is not sufficient for tyrosinase expression in melanoblasts.[50] In other NIH3T3 cells, MITF is not able to stimulate the tyrosinase promoter activity and the tyrosinase promoter does not respond to cAMP. These observations suggest that MITF acts in concert with other melanocyte-specific transcription factors to fully transactivate the tyrosinase promoter and allow melanocyte differentiation. Further, the dissection of the cAMP signaling pathway has shown that cAMP regulates MITF expression by a transcriptional process that involves a CRE motif located in its promoter.[47,48] Mutations of the CRE site abolish the binding of the ubiquitously-expressed CREB transcription factor to the promoter, and block the cAMP sensitivity of the MITF promoter. Interestingly, in αMSH-treated cells, a slight increase in PP1α protein is observed. In the presence of cycloheximide, the decline of PP1α levels parallels the maintenance of phospho-CREB and sustained MITF mRNA expression, suggesting that PP1α may be involved in the regulation of MITF expression.[48] In NIH3T3 fibroblast cells, which contain a functional cAMP pathway, the cAMP elevating agent, forskolin, does not stimulate the MITF promoter activity.[47] Thus, it appears that the CRE in the microphthalmia promoter is turned off in fibroblasts while it is made functional in B16 cells, due to a cell-specific mechanism that remains to be elucidated. The fact that, in pigment cells, the cAMP response of the MITF promoter is not totally abolished when the CRE is mutated supports this former hypothesis. Identification of such a transcription factor would be of great interest to improve our knowledge of the regulation of melanogenesis by cAMP. Two other transcription factors, Pax3 and Sox10, expressed in melanocytes, have recently been involved in the regulation of the MITF promoter.[51–55] Mutations of Pax3 are associated with Waardenburg syndrome types I and III, and mutations in Sox10 have been detected in patients manifesting Waardenburg syndrome type IV, all of which are characterized by hypopigmentary troubles. The lack of cAMP sensitivity of the MITF promoter in NIH3T3 cells could be easily explained by the absence of such transcription factors. The roles of SOX10 and PAX3 in the cAMP responsiveness of the MITF promoter remain to be demonstrated.

In summary, αMSH, through PKA regulation, phosphorylates and activates CREB, which is bound to the CRE in the MITF promoter. In turn, MITF promoter activity is stimulated and MITF expression elevated. This results in an increased binding of MITF to the M-box of the tyrosinase promoter and an increased tyrosinase level, which leads to stimulation of melanogenesis. Taken together, these observations demonstrate that MITF action is of paramount importance in αMSH-induced melanogenesis and in the control of melanocyte differentiation (Fig. 8.5).

Regulation of melanogenesis by the cAMP/MAP kinase pathway

PKA is the major intracellular target of cAMP. However, cAMP also regulates several other signaling pathways in pigment cells. First, elevation of intracellular cAMP content results in activation of the MAP kinase. Interestingly, activation of the MAP kinase leads to inhibition of melanogenesis. Dominant-negative mutants of the MAP kinase pathway stimulate both basal and cAMP-induced tyrosinase promoter activity, and inhibition of MAP kinase by a pharmacological inhibitor increases tyrosinase expression.[56,57] Noteworthy, stimulation of the c-kit tyrosine kinase receptor by its ligand Steel factor also activates MAP kinase and leads to phosphorylation of MITF on Ser73 and Ser409.[58,59] Phosphorylation at these two sites has been shown to induce MITF degradation.[59,60] Thus, the inhibition of the MAP kinases is expected to increase MITF expression through stabilization of the protein. Recently, we have observed that inhibition of the MAP kinase pathway increases the MITF level. However, this effect is not mediated entirely by a stabilization of MITF, since we also observed, under these conditions, a stimulation of the transcriptional activity of the MITF promoter (Bertolotto C, unpublished work).

These compelling observations suggest that activation of the MAP kinase pathway inhibits melanogenesis. Activation of the MAP kinase by cAMP would be part of a of retro-control mecha-

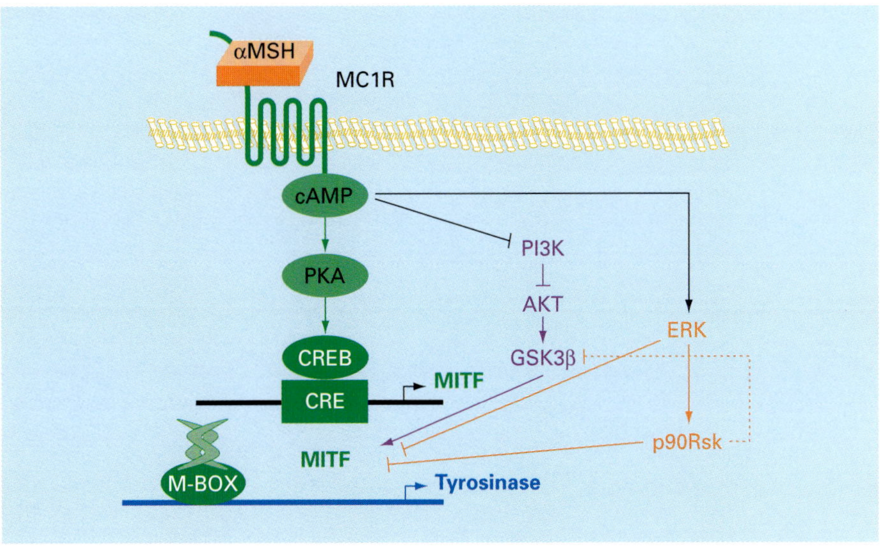

Figure 8.5

Molecular mechanisms of melanogenesis regulation by cAMP.

nism that prevents overproduction of melanin that could be toxic for melanocytes.

Regulation of melanogenesis by the cAMP/PI3 kinase pathway

Finally, cAMP elevation inhibits PI3 kinase activity. A specific inhibitor of the PI3K pathway mimics the cAMP effect on melanocyte differentiation and increases tyrosinase expression.[61] Additionally, cAMP leads to inhibition of the PI3K target, protein kinase B (PKB), also called AKT, resulting in the activation of the glycogen synthase kinase 3β (GSK3β) (Bertolotto C, unpublished work).[62] Further, expression of a dominant-negative mutant of AKT stimulates pigment synthesis.[63] Interestingly, mutation of Ser298 in MITF has been found in patients with Waardenburg syndrome type II. It has been shown that phosphorylation of this serine by GSK3β, *in vivo* and *in vitro*, promotes MITF DNA binding to the tyrosinase promoter.[64] Additionally, GSK3β is inhibited by the p90 ribosomal S6 kinase (Rsk), a downstream target of MAP kinase, pointing out a connection between the PI3K and MAP kinase pathways, which are both negative regulators of melanogenesis. Recently, we have shown that the PI3K/AKT inhibitor, Ly 294002, stimulates the transcriptional activity of the tyrosinase, Tyrp1 and Dct promoters. We also observed that Ly 294002 increases MITF protein level without affecting gene transcription, indicating that the PI3K/AKT pathway may regulate, in addition to the activity of MITF, its stability (Bertolotto C, unpublished work).

In conclusion, elevation of intracellular cAMP by αMSH leads to the activation of a complex network of signaling pathways that finally ends in melanocyte differentiation and upregulation of melanogenesis. Interestingly, all these pathways converge to MITF, strengthening the crucial role of this transcription factor in the regulation of melanogenesis (Fig. 8.5).

References

1. Le Douarin N, *The Neural Crest* (Cambridge University Press: Cambridge, UK, 1982).
2. Ortonne JP, The effects of ultraviolet exposure on skin melanin pigmentation, *J Int Med Res* (1990) **18**:8C–17C.
3. Hearing VJ, Jimenez M, Analysis of mammalian

pigmentation at the molecular level, *Pigment Cell Res* (1989) **2**:75–85.

4. Hearing VJ, Tsukamoto K, Enzymatic control of pigmentation in mammals, *FASEB J* (1991) **5**:2902–9.
5. Prota G, Some new aspects of eumelanin chemistry. In: Bagnara JT, ed, *Progress in Clinical and Biological Research. Advance in Pigment Cell Research* (AR Liss, Inc: New York, 1988) 101–24.
6. Kobayashi T, Urabe K, Winder A et al., Tyrosinase related protein 1 (TRP1) functions as a DHICA oxidase in melanin biosynthesis, *EMBO J* (1994) **13**:5818–25.
7. Kameyama K, Takemura T, Hamada Y et al., Pigment production in murine melanoma cells is regulated by tyrosinase, tyrosinase-related protein1 (TRP-1), DOPAchrome tautomerase (TRP2) and a melanogenic inhibitor, *J Invest Dermatol* (1993) **100**: 126–31.
8. Yokoyama K, Yasumoto KI, Suzuki H et al., Cloning of the human DOPAchrome tautomerase/tyrosinase-related protein 2 gene and identification of two regulatory regions required for its pigment cell-specific expression, *J Biol Chem* (1994) **269**: 27080–7.
9. Puri N, Gardner JM, Brillant MH, Aberrant pH of melanosomes in Pink-eyed dilution mutant melanocytes, *J Invest Dermatol* (2000) **115**:607–13.
10. Krude H, Biebermann H, Luck W et al., Severe early-onset obesity, adrenal insufficiency and red hair pigmentation caused by POMC mutations in humans, *Nat Genet* (1998) **19**:155–6.
11. Valverde P, Healy E, Jackson I et al., Variants of the melanocyte-stimulating hormone receptor gene are associated with red hair and fair skin in humans, *Nat Genet* (1995) **11**:328–30.
12. Lamerson CL, Nordlund JJ, Pigmentary changes in Addison's disease with adrenal insufficiency. In: Nordlund JJ, Boissy RE, Hearing VJ et al., eds, *The Pigmentary System: Physiology and Pathophysiology* (Oxford University Press: Oxford, 1998) **120**:1695–708.
13. Sowers JR, Lippman HR, Cushing's syndrome due to ectopic ACTH production: cutaneous manifestations, *Cutis* (1985) **36**:351–2, 354.
14. Pears JS, Jung RT, Bartlett W et al., A case of skin hyperpigmentation due to alpha-MSH hypersecretion, *Br J Dermatol* (1992) **126**:286–9.
15. Lerner AB, McGuire JS, Effect of alpha- and beta-melanocyte stimulating hormone on the skin colour of the man, *Nature* (1961) **189**:176–9.
16. Levine N, Sheftel SN, Eytan T et al., Induction of skin tanning by subcutaneous administration of a potent synthetic melanotropin, *JAMA* (1991) **226**: 2730–6.
17. Arias J, Alberts AS, Brindle P et al., Activation of cAMP and mitogen responsive genes relies on a common nuclear factor, *Nature* (1994) **370**:226–9.
18. Lalli E, Sassone-Corsi P, Signal transduction and gene regulation: the nuclear response to cAMP, *J Biol Chem* (1994) **269**:17359–62.
19. Schwindinger WF, Francomano CA, Levine MA, Identification of a mutation in the gene encoding the alpha subunit of the stimulatory G protein of adenylyl cyclase in McCune–Albright syndrome, *Proc Natl Acad Sci U S A* (1992) **89**:5152–6.
20. Weinstein LS, Shenker A, Gejman PV et al., Activating mutations of the stimulatory G protein in the McCune–Albright syndrome [see comments], *N Engl J Med* (1991) **325**:1688–95.
21. Casey M, Vaughan CJ, He J et al., Mutations in the protein kinase A R1alpha regulatory subunit cause familial cardiac myxomas and Carney complex, *J Clin Invest* (2000) **106**:R31–8.
22. Kirschner LS, Carney JA, Pack SD et al., Mutations of the gene encoding the protein kinase A type I-alpha regulatory subunit in patients with the Carney complex, *Nat Genet* (2000) **26**:89–92.
23. Bertolotto C, Bille K, Ortonne JP et al., Regulation of tyrosinase gene expression by cAMP in B16 melanoma cells involves two CATGTG motifs surrounding the TATA box: implication of the microphthalmia gene product, *J Cell Biol* (1996) **134**:747–55.
24. Ganss R, Schutz G, Beermann F, The mouse tyrosinase gene, *J Biol Chem* (1994) **269**:29808–16.
25. Lowings P, Yavuzer U, Goding R, Positive and negative elements regulate a melanocyte-specific promoter, *Mol Cell Biol* (1992) **12**:3653–62.
26. Bertolotto C, Bùsca R, Abbe P et al., Different cis-acting elements are involved in the regulation of TRP1 and TRP2 promoter activities by cyclic AMP: Pivotal role of boxes (GTCATGTGCT) and of microphthalmia, *Mol Cell Biol* (1998) **18**:694–702.
27. Blackwood EM, Eisenman RN, Max: a helix-loop-helix zipper protein that forms a sequence-specific DNA-binding complex with Myc, *Science* (1991) **251**:1211–17.
28. Gregor PD, Sawadogo M, Roeder RG, The adenovirus major late transcription factor USF is a member of the helix loop helix group of regulatory proteins and binds to DNA as a dimmer, *Genes Dev* (1990) **4**:1730–40.
29. Edmondson DG, Olson EN, Helix-loop-helix protein as regulators of muscle-specific transcription, *J Biol Chem* (1993) **268**:755–8.

30. Hemesath TJ, Steingrímsson E, McGill G et al., Microphthalmia, a critical factor in melanocyte development, defines a discrete transcription factor family, *Genes Dev* (1994) **8**:2770–80.
31. Steingrímsson E, Moore KJ, Lamoreux ML et al., Molecular basis of mouse microphthalmia (mi) mutations helps explain their developmental and phenotypic consequences, *Nat Genet* (1994) **8**:256–63.
32. Hodgkinson CA, Moore KJ, Nakayama A et al., Mutations at the mouse microphthalmia locus are associated with defects in a gene encoding a novel basic-helix-loop-helix–zipper protein, *Cell* (1993) **4**:395–404.
33. Hughes MJ, Lingrel JB, Krakowski JM et al., A helix-loop-helix transcription factor-like gene is located at the *mi* locus, *J Biol Chem* (1993) **268**: 20687–90.
34. Silvers WK, The coat color of mice. In: Springer-Verlag N-Y, ed, *A Model for Mammalian Gene Action and Interaction* (Springer-Verlag: Berlin, 1979).
35. Hughes AE, Newton VE, Liu XZ et al., A gene for Waardenburg syndrome type 2 maps close to the human homologue of the microphthalmia gene at chromosome 3p12–p14.1, *Nat Genet* (1994) **7**: 509–13.
36. Tachibana M, Evidence to suggest that expression of MITF induces melanocyte differentiation and haploinsufficiency of MITF causes Waardenburg syndrome type 2A, *Pigment Cell Res* (1997) **10**: 25–33.
37. Tassabehji M, Newton VE, Read AP, Waardenburg syndrome type 2 caused by mutations in the human microphthalmia (MITF), *Nat Genet* (1994) **8**:251–5.
38. Waardenburg PJ, A new syndrome combining developmental anomalies of eyelids, eyebrows and nose root with pigmentary defects of the iris and head hair and with congenital deafness, *Am J Hum Genet* (1951) **3**:195–253.
39. Fuse N, Yasumoto K, Takeda K et al., Molecular cloning of cDNA encoding a novel microphthalmia-associated transcription factor isoform with a distinct amino-terminus, *J Biochem* (1999) **126**: 1043–51.
40. Udono T, Yasumoto K, Takeda K et al., Structural organization of the human microphthalmia-associated transcription factor gene containing four alternative promoters, *Biochem Biophys Acta* (2000) **1491**: 205–19.
41. Yasumoto KI, Amae S, Udono T et al., Big gene linked to small eyes: many promoters make light work, *Pigment Cell Res* (1998) **11**:329–36.
42. Furumura M, Sakai C, Abdel-Malek Z et al., The interaction of agouti signal protein and melanocyte stimulating hormone to regulate melanin formation in mammals, *Pigment Cell Res* (1996) **9**:191–203.
43. Graham A, Wakamatsu K, Hunt G et al., Agouti protein inhibits the production of eumelanin and phaeomelanin in the presence and absence of alpha-melanocyte-stimulating hormone, *Pigment Cell Res* (1997) **10**:298–303.
44. Kobayashi T, Viera WD, Potterf B et al., Modulation of melanogenic protein expression during the switch from eu- to pheomelanogenesis, *J Cell Sci* (1995) **108**:2301–9.
45. Winder A, Wittbjer A, Odh G et al., Fibroblasts expressing mouse c locus tyrosinase produce an authentic enzyme and synthesize phaeomelanin, *J Cell Sci* (1993) **104**:467–75.
46. Winder A, Odh G, Rosengren E et al., Fibroblasts co-expressing tyrosinase and the b-protein synthesize both eumelanin and phaeomelanin, *Biochem Biophys Acta* (1995) **1268**:300–10.
47. Bertolotto C, Abbe P, Hemesath TJ et al., Microphthalmia gene product as signal transducer in cAMP-induced differentiation of melanocytes, *J Cell Biol* (1998) **142**:827–35.
48. Price ER, Horstmann MA, Wells AG et al., Melanocyte-stimulating hormone signaling regulates expression of *microphthalmia*, a gene deficient in Waardenburg Syndrome, *J Biol Chem* (1998) **273**:33042–7.
49. Tachibana M, Takeda K, Nobukini Y et al., Ectopic expression of MITF, a gene for Waardenburg syndrome type 2, converts fibroblasts to cells with melanocyte characteristics, *Nat Genet* (1996) **14**:50–4.
50. Hou L, Panthier JJ, Arnheiter H, Signaling and transcriptional regulation in the neural crest-derived melanocyte lineage: interactions between KIT and MITF, *Development* (2000) **127**: 5379–89.
51. Bondurand N, Pingault V, Goerich DE et al., Interaction among SOX10, PAX3, and MITF, three genes altered in Waardenburg syndrome, *Hum Mol Genet* (2000) **9**:1907–17.
52. Lee M, Goodall J, Verastegui C et al., Direct regulation of the microphthalmia promoter by sox 10 links Waardenburg–Shah syndrome (WS4)-associated hypopigmentation and deafness to WS2, *J Biol Chem* (2000) **275**: 37978–83.
53. Potterf SB, Furumura M, Dunn KJ et al., Transcription factor hierarchy in Waardenburg syndrome: regulation of MITF expression by SOX10 and PAX3, *Hum Genet* (2000) **107**:1–6.

54. Verastegui C, Bille K, Ortonne JP et al., Regulation of the microphthalmia-associated transcription factor gene by the Waardenburg syndrome type 4 gene, SOX10, *J Biol Chem* (2001) **275**: 30757–60.
55. Watanabe A, Takeda K, Ploplis B et al., Epistatic relationship between Waardenburg syndrome genes MITF and PAX3, *Nat Genet* (1998) **18**:283–6.
56. Englaro W, Rezzonico R, Durand-Clément M et al., Mitogen-activated protein kinase pathway and AP-1 are activated during cAMP-induced melanogenesis in B-16 melanoma cells, *J Biol Chem* (1995) **270**: 24315–20.
57. Englaro W, Bertolotto C, Buscà R et al., Inhibition of the mitogen-activated protein kinase pathway triggers B16 melanoma cell differentiation, *J Biol Chem* (1998) **273**:9966–70.
58. Hemesath TJ, Price ER, Takemoto C et al., MAPK links microphthalmia to c-kit signaling in melanocytes, *Nature* (1998) **391**:298–301.
59. Wu M, Hemesath TJ, Takemoto C et al., c-Kit triggers dual phosphorylations, which couple activation and degradation of the essential melanocyte factor mi, *Genes Dev* (2000) **14**:301–12.
60. Xu W, Gong L, Haddad MM et al., Regulation of microphthalmia-associated transcription factor MITF protein levels by association with the human ubiquitin-conjugating enzyme hUCB9, *Pigment Cell Res* (1999) **7**:31.
61. Buscà R, Bertolotto C, Ortonne JP, Inhibition of the phosphatidylinositol 3-kinase/p70S6-kinase pathway induces B16 melanoma cell differentiation, *J Biol Chem* (1996) **271**:1–7.
62. Kim S, Jee K, Kim D et al., Cyclic AMP inhibits Akt activity by blocking the membrane localization of PDK1, *J Biol Chem* (2001) **272**:12864–70.
63. Oka M, Nagai H, Ando H et al., Regulation of melanogenesis through phosphatidyl 3-kinase–AKT pathway in human G361 melanoma cells, *J Invest Dermatol* (2000) **115**:699–703.
64. Takeda K, Takemoto C, Kobayashi I et al., Ser 298 of MITF, a mutation in Waardenburg syndrome type 2, is a phosphorylation site with functional significance, *Hum Mol Genet* (2000) **9**:125–32.

9
The role of Wnt signaling in melanogenesis

Shigeki Shibahara

Introduction

Wnt proteins are cysteine-rich glycoproteins, comprising a group of secretory signaling molecules.[1–3] Wnt proteins regulate diverse developmental processes, such as patterning of the body axis and cell proliferation in certain adult tissues. The binding of Wnt to its receptor, Frizzled, leads to inactivation of glycogen synthase kinase-3β (GSK3β), followed by the accumulation of β-catenin. β-Catenin then activates the target genes through the interaction with a member of LEF-1/TCF transcription factors, containing a high-mobility-group (HMG) domain. Thus, β-catenin plays a critical role in Wnt signaling and its degradation is regulated by phosphorylation. The β-catenin destruction machinery includes GSK3β, a tumor-supressor protein APC, Axin, and Dishevelled. APC is inactivated in most colorectal cancers, resulting in activation of the Wnt pathway. A large number of Wnt molecules and their receptors have been identified to date, but only one LEF-1 and three TCFs are known as nuclear mediators of Wnt signalling in mammals.

Microphthalmia-associated transcription factor (Mitf), encoded by the mouse *Mitf* locus, plays a critical role in the differentiation of melanocytes that originate from the neural crest and of retinal pigment epithelium (RPE) derived from the optic cup of the brain. Mitf contains a basic helix-loop-helix and leucine zipper (bHLH–LZ) structure,[4,5] which permits Mitf to form homodimers or heterodimers and to bind to the E-box motif (CANNTG).[6] Heterozygous mutations in the *MITF* gene, the human counterpart of the *Mitf* gene, are associated with dominantly inherited auditory-pigmentary syndromes, which are characterized by sensorineural hearing loss and abnormal pigmentation of the hair and skin.[7–9] To date, there are at least five MITF isoforms with distinct N-termini, MITF-M, -H, -A, -B, and -C.[10–12] These isoforms share the entire downstream region, including the transcriptional activation domain and the bHLH–LZ domain (Fig. 9.1). Among these isoforms, MITF-M is exclusively expressed in melanocytes and melanoma cells, whereas other isoforms are expressed in various tissues and cultured cell lines.[10,11,13]

MITF-M as a target of Wnt signaling

Essential requirement of Mitf-M for melanocyte development was verified by the analysis of a recessive *Mitf* mutant, black-eyed white, $Mitf^{mi\text{-}bw}$.[14] This mutant mouse is characterized by the completely white coat color, deafness, and normally-pigmented RPE without any ocular abnormalities. The molecular lesion of $Mitf^{mi\text{-}bw}$ mice is the insertion of an L1 retrotransposable element in the *Mitf* gene, leading to complete repression of Mitf-M mRNA expression and certain reduction of Mitf-A and Mitf-H mRNA expression (Fig. 9.1). Thus, the $Mitf^{mi\text{-}bw}$ mutant may mimic the Mitf-M-deficient mice. These results indicate that MITF-M/Mitf-M is a key regulator of the melanocyte development but is dispensable for RPE development.

In zebrafish embryos, Wnt signaling directly activates *nacre*, a zebrafish *MITF* homolog, which is required for the formation of neural-crest-derived pigment cells.[15] Injection of β-catenin mRNA into zebrafish embryo increases the population of pigment cells of neural crest origin.[16] Moreover, targeted disruption of the *Wnt-1* and *Wnt-3* genes in the mouse causes

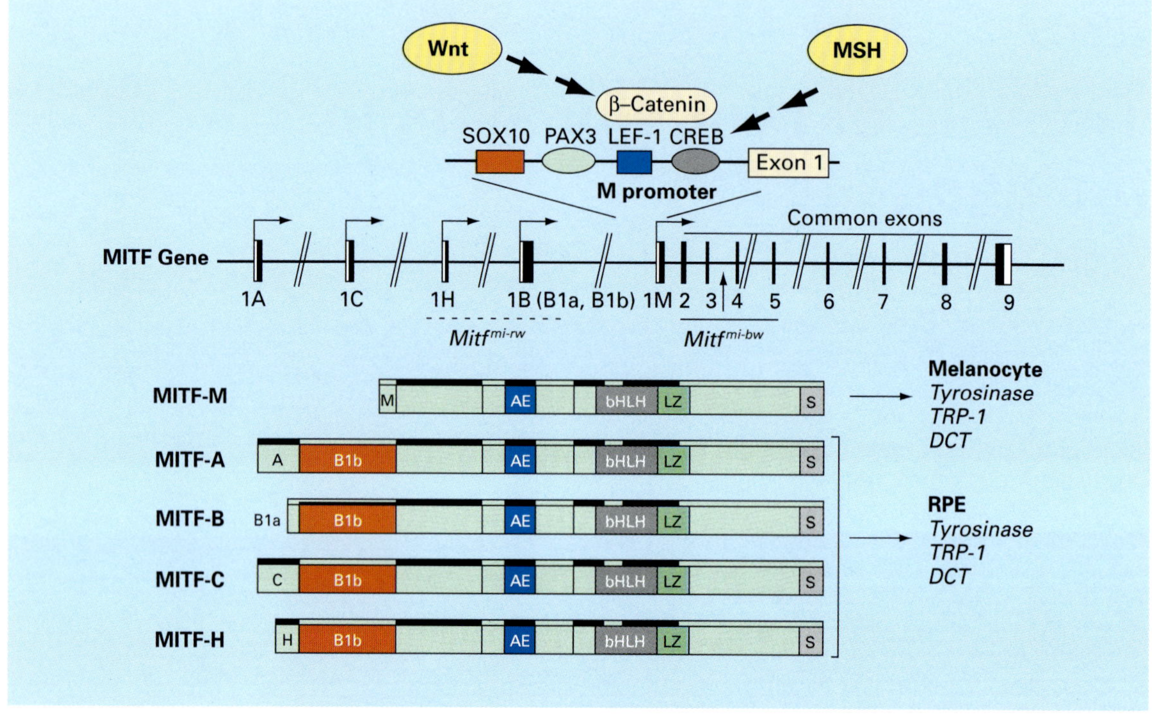

Figure 9.1

Multiple MITF isoforms encoded by the single *MITF* gene. Shown are the schematic representation of the MITF gene and five MITF isoforms. Also shown are extracellular signaling molecules, Wnt and MSH. The M promoter region is highlighted to show multiple *cis*-acting elements, which are bound by the indicated transcription factors. The direction of transcription is from left to right, indicated by arrows. The 5′- and 3′-untranslated exons are indicated by open boxes, and the protein-coding exons are indicated by closed boxes. All MITF isoforms differ at their N-termini but share the entire carboxyl-portion, encoded by common exons (exons 2–9). Domain B1a and domain B1b of MITF-B are encoded by exon 1B. Domains A, C, and H are encoded by exon 1A, putative exon 1C, and exon 1H, respectively. Note that exon 1C remains to be determined. The 3′-portion of exon 1B (exon B1b) is used as a second exon for generation of MITF-A, MITF-C, and MITF-H mRNAs. The transcriptional activation domain (AE), the bHLH–LZ structure, and the serine-rich region (S) are indicated. Also indicated are the equivalent positions of the deletion identified in red-eyed white *Mitf*$^{mi\text{-}rw}$ mice[42] and the insertion seen in black-eyed white *Mitf*$^{mi\text{-}bw}$ mice.[14]

deficiency of neural crest derivatives,[17] indicating that Wnt-1 and Wnt-3a are required for the expansion of neural crest precursors and determining the fates of neural crest cells. Direct gene transfer of Wnt-1 or β-catenin to mouse neural crest cells results in melanocyte expansion and differentiation.[18] Exogenously-added Wnt-3a protein to cultured murine melanocytes increased the expression of endogenous Mitf-M mRNA and transactivated the melanocyte-specific M promoter of the *MITF* gene through the LEF-1 site.[19] It was suggested that Wnt-3a signaling recruits β-catenin and LEF-1 to the M promoter, leading to the increased transcription from the M promoter. These results indicate a direct link between Wnt signaling and Mitf-M/MITF-M expression.

In addition to the LEF-1 site, the M promoter contains the separate *cis*-acting elements which are recognized by CREB,[20,21] PAX3,[22] and SOX10,[23–26] respectively (Fig. 9.1). CREB is functionally activated by MSH signalling, suggesting an important role of MITF-M in suntanning.[27] PAX3 is a transcription factor with a paired-homeodomain, and is responsible for

Waardenburg syndrome (WS) types I and III.[28] SOX10 is a new member of the SOX family transcription factors, with a high-mobility group box as a DNA-binding motif.[29] SOX10 is defective in some cases of Shah–Waardenburg syndrome, also known as Waardenburg–Hirschsprung disease, or WS4, which is characterized by aganglionic megacolon, sensorineural deafness, and pigmentation abnormalities.[30] Thus, SOX10 is responsible for differentiation of the melanocytes and intestinal ganglia cells. This notion is confirmed by the phenotypic consequences of Sox10 null (-/-) mice.[31] The Sox10 (-/-) mice showed no gross morphological abnormalities at birth, but were unable to breathe because lung alveoli did not expand. Taken together, these results indicate that multiple transcription factors are involved in the regulation of transcription from the M promoter.

Regulation of the DCT expression by MITF-M

Both melanocytes and RPE share the unique property of melanin production and express the three melanogenesis enzymes: tyrosinase, and tyrosinase-related protein 1 (TRP-1) and TRP-2, also called DOPAchrome tautomerase (DCT).[32] Tyrosinase is a rate-limiting enzyme in melanin biosynthesis, and both TRP-1 and DCT are the enzymes which determine the quality of melanin. These enzymes share about 40% amino acid identity, constituting the tyrosinase family. Among these melanogenic enzymes, DCT is characterized by its expression in migrating melanoblasts, as well as in the telencephalon of mouse embryos, where the *tyrosinase* and *TRP-1* genes are not normally expressed.[33] Moreover, DCT mRNA is abundantly expressed in a glioblastoma multiforme, the most malignant brain tumor, comprising undifferentiated cells,[34] and in retinoblastomas, which may be derived from an embryonic retinoblast.[35] Taken together, these results suggest that the *DCT* gene is expressed in some primitive cell types derived from the neural ectoderm.

Expression of *DCT* is almost entirely absent from neural crest cells in *nacre* (-/-) zebrafish embryos, and, conversely, misexpression of *nacre*-induced ectopic expression of DCT in wild-type and mutant embryos.[36] These results suggest that the *DCT* gene is a downstream target of Mitf. In mice, DCT mRNA expression becomes detectable in retina on embryonic day 9.5, before primitive retinal cells are commited to becoming RPE, and in migrating melanocytes at embryonic day 10.[33] The onset of Mitf expression is detectable in neural crest cells by embryonic day 9.5.[37] Thus, the *DCT* gene has been established as an early melanoblast marker and is likely to be regulated by Mitf-M in melanoblasts.

MITF-M and other MITF isoforms transactivated the *tyrosinase* and *TRP-1* gene promoters through the *cis*-acting DNA elements containing a CATGTG motif, such as M-box, but not the *DCT* gene promoter in cultured human melanoma cells,[38–40] as judged by transient coexpression assays. The *DCT* gene promoter was transactivated by MITF-M in B16 mouse melanoma cells,[20] and by MITF-M or other MITF isoforms in a human RPE cell line.[12] These results suggest that the transcriptional activation function of MITF may be differentially modulated by the abundance of other transcription factors in a given cell type.

Wnt signaling in RPE

A recessive *Mitf* mutant, red-eyed white, *Mitf*$^{mi\text{-}rw}$, exhibits small red eyes and white coat with some pigmented spots around the head and/or tail.[41] Its molecular defect is a deletion of the genomic DNA segment containing exons 1H and exon 1B (Fig. 9.1).[42] Thus, *Mitf*$^{mi\text{-}rw}$ mice completely lack Mitf-H and Mitf-B but may express aberrant Mitf-A, lacking domain B1b, encoded by the 3′-portion of exon 1B. However, deletion of exon B1b results in a frame shift in such aberrant mRNA species. It is, therefore, conceivable that the phenotype of *Mitf*$^{mi\text{-}rw}$ mice represents the loss of function of all Mitf isoforms containing domain B1b. Mitf isoforms with extended N-termini are, therefore, responsible for differentiation of RPE and development of normal eye.

The tumor-supressor protein, APC, is a critical component of the β-catenin destruction machinery, and is inactivated in most colorectal cancers. APC mutation is frequently associated with congenital hypertrophy of RPE.[43] In fact, the retinal lesions are present at birth and do not change with age, suggesting that Wnt signaling may be involved in RPE development. Congenital hypertrophy of RPE is composed of enlarged RPE and degenerated photoreceptors, and is reminiscent of the RPE abnormalities seen in some Mitf mutant mice.

In fetal RPE, Mitf isoforms, such as MITF-A/Mitf-A, are predominantly expressed.[10,11,44] Domain A of MITF-A shares 37% amino acid identity with the N-terminus of TFE3.[45,46] Moreover, three consecutive portions, covering the entire domain A, are aligned to cytoplasmic retinoic-acid-binding protein.[47] Interestingly, the portion of domain A that shows greater similarity to cytoplasmic retinoic-acid-binding protein, is less conserved in TFE3. In this context, abnormalities in retinoid metabolism are seen in a recessive *Mitf* mutant, *Mitf^{vitiligo}* (*Mitf^{vit}*).[48,49] The molecular lesion of *Mitf-M^{vit}* is the Asp222Asn substitution in helix 1 of the bHLH–LZ domain.[41] Thus, all MITF isoforms of the *Mitf^{vit}* mouse carry this Asp222Asn substitution. The *Mitf-M^{vit}* protein binds *in vitro* to DNA as either a homodimer or a heterodimer.[6] The homozygous *Mitf^{vit}* mice appear normal when young, with uniformly lighter color, but show age-dependent melanocyte loss and retinal degeneration.[48,49] In *Mitf^{vit}* mice, the earliest abnormality, detected by embryonic day 12, is multilayered RPE with hyper- and hypopigmented patches, but photoreceptor cells normally differentiate and begin to degenerate after postnatal day 30.[50] This slowly progressing retinal degeneration suggests a role of Mitf isoforms in the postnatal maintenance of retinal function. In fact, the RPE of postnatal *Mitf^{vit}* mice has been shown to decrease phagocytosis of rod outer segments[51] and to possess increased proliferation potential.[52] It is noteworthy that DCT is expressed in Y79 retinoblastoma cells and excised retinoblastomas.[35] Retinoblastoma is the most common primary intraocular tumor of childhood and represents the prototype of hereditary cancers in humans. DCT expression is upregulated by retinoic acid in Y79 retinoblastoma cells,[35] whereas the DCT expression is rather reduced by retinoic acid in melanoma cells.[35,53] The mechanism for the retinoic-acid-mediated induction of DCT mRNA remains to be investigated. Thus, the DCT gene will provide us with a good system for studying the network of transcription factors which are involved in retinoid metabolism and Wnt signalling.

References

1. Cadigan KM, Nusse R, Wnt signaling: a common theme in animal development, *Genes Dev* (1997) **11**:3286–305.
2. Eastman Q, Grosschedl R, Regulation of LEF-1/TCF transcription factors by Wnt and other signals, *Curr Opin Cell Biol* (1999) **11**:233–40.
3. Barker N, Morin PJ, Clevers H, The yin-yang of TCF/β-catenin signaling, *Adv Cancer Res* (2000) **77**:1–24.
4. Hodgkinson CA, Moore KJ, Nakayama A et al., Mutations at the mouse microphthalmia locus are associated with defects in a gene encoding a novel basic helix-loop-helix–zipper protein, *Cell* (1993) **74**:395–404.
5. Hughes MJ, Lingrel JB, Krakowsky JM et al., A helix-loop-helix transcription factor-like gene is located at the mi locus, *J Biol Chem* (1993) **268**: 20687–90.
6. Hemesath TJ, Steingrímsson E, McGill G et al., Microphthalmia, a critical factor in melanocyte development, defines a discrete transcription factor family, *Genes Dev* (1994) **8**:2770–80.
7. Tassabehji M, Newton VE, Read AP, Waardenburg syndrome type 2 caused by mutations in the human microphthalmia (*MITF*) gene, *Nat Genet* (1994) **8**:251–5.
8. Nobukuni Y, Watanabe A, Takeda K et al., Analyses of loss-of-function mutations of the *MITF* gene suggest that haploinsufficiency is a cause of Waardenburg syndrome type 2A, *Am J Hum Genet* (1996) **59**:76–83.
9. Amiel J, Watkin PM, Tassabehji M et al., Mutation of the MITF gene in albinism-deafness syndrome (Tietz syndrome), *Clin Dysmorphol* (1998) **7**:17–20.
10. Amae S, Fuse N, Yasumoto K et al., Identification of a novel isoform of microphthalmia-associated transcription factor that is enriched in retinal pigment epithelium, *Biochem Biophys Res Commun* (1998) **247**:710–15.
11. Fuse N, Yasumoto K, Takeda K et al., Molecular cloning of cDNA encoding a novel microphthalmia-associated transcription factor isoform with a distinct amino-terminus, *J Biochem (Tokyo)* (1999) **126**:1043–51.
12. Udono T, Yasumoto K, Takeda K et al., Structural organization of the human microphthalmia-associated transcription factor gene containing four alternative promoters, *Biochim Biophys Acta* (2000) **1491**:205–19.

13. Fuse N, Yasumoto K, Suzuki H et al., Identification of a melanocyte-type promoter of the microphthalmia-associated transcription factor gene, *Biochem Biophys Res Commun* (1996) **219**:702–7.
14. Yajima I, Sato S, Kimura T et al., An L1 element intronic insertion in the black-eyed white (*Mitf*$^{mi\text{-}bw}$) gene: the loss of a single Mitf isoform responsible for the pigmentary defect and inner ear deafness, *Hum Mol Genet* (1999) **8**:1431–41.
15. Dorsky RI, Raible DW, Moon RT, Direct regulation of *nacre*, a zebrafish *MITF* homolog required for pigment cell formation, by the Wnt pathway, *Genes Dev* (2000) **14**:158–62.
16. Dorsky RI, Moon RT, Raible DW, Control of neural crest cell fate by the Wnt signalling pathway, *Nature* (1998) **396**:370–3.
17. Ikeya M, Lee SM, Johnson JE et al., Wnt signalling required for expansion of neural crest and CNS progenitors, *Nature* (1997) **389**:966–70.
18. Dunn KJ, Williams BO, Li Y et al., Neural crest-directed gene transfer demonstrates Wnt1 role in melanocyte expansion and differentiation during mouse development, *Proc Natl Acad Sci U S A* (2000) **97**:10050–5.
19. Takeda K, Yasumoto K, Takada R et al., Induction of melanocyte-specific microphthalmia-associated transcription factor by Wnt-3a, *J Biol Chem* (2000) **275**:14013–16.
20. Bertolotto C, Buscà R, Abbe P et al., Different *cis*-acting elements are involved in the regulation of TRP1 and TRP2 promoter activities by cyclic AMP: Pivotal role of M boxes (GTCATGTGCT) and of microphthalmia, *Mol Cell Biol* (1998) **18**:694–702.
21. Price ER, Ding H-F, Badalian T et al., Lineage-specific signaling in melanocytes, *J Biol Chem* (1998) **273**:17983–6.
22. Watanabe A, Takeda K, Ploplis B et al., Epistatic relationship between Waardenburg syndrome gene MITF and PAX3, *Nat Genet* (1998) **18**:283–6.
23. Potterf SB, Furumura M, Dunn KJ et al., Transcription factor hierarchy in Waardenburg syndrome: regulation of MITF expression by SOX10 and PAX3, *Hum Genet* (2000) **107**:1–6.
24. Bondurand N, Pingault V, Goerich DE et al., Interaction among SOX10, PAX3 and MITF, three genes altered in Waardenburg syndrome, *Hum Mol Genet* (2000) **9**:1907–17.
25. Verastegui C, Bille K, Ortonne JP et al., Regulation of the microphthalmia-associated transcription factor gene by the Waardenburg syndrome type 4 gene, SOX10, *J Biol Chem* (2000) **275**: 30757–60.
26. Lee M, Goodall J, Verastegui C et al., Direct regulation of the Microphthalmia promoter by Sox10 links Waardenburg–Shah syndrome (WS4)-associated hypopigmentation and deafness to WS2, *J Biol Chem* (2000) **275**:37978–83.
27. Buscà R, Ballotti R, Cyclic AMP a key messenger in the regulation of skin pigmentation, *Pigment Cell Res* (2000) **13**:60–9.
28. Tassabehji M, Newton VE, Liu X-Z et al., The mutational spectrum in Waardenburg syndrome, *Hum Mol Genet* (1995) **4**:2131–7.
29. Pusch C, Hustert E, Pfeifer D et al., The SOX10/Sox10 gene from human and mouse: sequence, expression, and transactivation by the encoded HMG domain transcription factor, *Hum Genet* (1998) **103**:115–23.
30. Pingault V, Bondurand N, Kuhlbrodt K et al., SOX10 mutations in patients with Waardenburg–Hirschsprung disease, *Nat Genet* (1998) **18**:171–3.
31. Britsch S, Goerich DE, Riethmacher D et al., The transcription factor Sox10 is a key regulator of peripheral glial development, *Genes Dev* (2001)**15**: 66–78.
32. Shibahara S, Yasumoto K, Takahashi K, Genetic regulation of the pigment cell. In: Nordlund JJ, Boissy RE, Hearing VJ et al., eds, *The Pigmentary System. Physiology and Pathophysiology* (Oxford University Press: New York, 1998) 251–73.
33. Steel KP, Davidson DR, Jackson IJ, TRP-2/DT, a new early melanoblast marker, shows that steel growth factor (c-kit ligand) is a survival factor, *Development* (1992) **115**:1111–19.
34. Suzuki H, Takahashi K, Yasumoto K et al., Role of neurofibromin in modulation of expression of the tyrosinase-related protein 2 gene, *J Biochem (Tokyo)* (1998) **124**:992–8.
35. Udono T, Takahashi K, Yasumoto K et al., Expression of tyrosinase-related protein 2/DOPAchrome tautomerase in the retinoblastoma, *Exp Eye Res* (2001) **72**: 225–34.
36. Lister JA, Robertson CP, Lepage T et al., *nacre* Encodes a zebrafish microphthalmia-related protein that regulates neural-crest-derived pigment cell fate, *Development* (1999) **126**:3757–67.
37. Nakayama A, Nguyen MT, Chen CC et al., Mutations in *microphthalmia*, the mouse homolog of the human deafness gene *MITF*, affect neuroepithelial and neural crest-derived melanocytes differently, *Mech Dev* (1998) **70**:155–66.
38. Yasumoto K, Yokoyama K, Shibata K et al., Microphthalmia-associated transcription factor as a regulator for melanocyte-specific transcription of the human tyrosinase gene, *Mol Cell Biol* (1994) **14**:8058–70.

39. Yasumoto K, Yokoyama K, Takahashi K et al., Functional analysis of microphthalmia-associated transcription factor in pigment cell-specific transcription of the human tyrosinase family genes, *J Biol Chem* (1997) **272**:503–9.
40. Shibahara S, Yasumoto K, Amae S et al., Regulation of pigment cell-specific gene expression by MITF, *Pigment Cell Res* (2000) **13** (Suppl 8):98–102.
41. Steingrímsson E, Moore KJ, Lamoreux ML et al., Molecular basis of mouse microphthalmia (mi) mutations helps explain their developmental and phenotypic consequences, *Nat Genet* (1994) **8**:256–63.
42. Hallsson JH, Favor J, Hodgkinson C et al., Genomic, transcriptional and mutational analysis of the mouse microphthalmia locus, *Genetics* (2000) **155**:291–300.
43. Olschwang S, Tiret A, Laurent-Puig P et al., Restriction of ocular fundus lesions to a specific subgroup of APC mutations in adenomatous polyposis coli patients, *Cell* (1993) **75**:959–68.
44. Mochii M, Mazaki Y, Mizuno N et al., Role of Mitf in differentiation and transdifferentiation of chicken pigmented epithelial cell, *Dev Biol* (1998) **193**:47–62.
45. Yasumoto K, Amae S, Udono T et al., A big gene linked to small eyes encodes multiple Mitf isoforms: Many promoters make light work, *Pigment Cell Res* (1998) **11**:329–36.
46. Rehli M, Elzen ND, Cassady AI et al., Cloning and characterization of the murine genes for bHLH–ZIP transcription factors TFEC and TFEB reveal a common gene organization for all MiT subfamily members, *Genomics* (1999) **56**:111–20.
47. Shibahara S, Takeda K, Yasumoto K et al., Microphthalmia-associated transcription factor (MITF): Multiplicity in structure, function and regulation, *J Invest Dermatol Symp Proc* (2002) **6**:99–104.
48. Lerner AB, Shiohara T, Boissy RE et al., A mouse model for vitiligo, *J Invest Dermatol* (1986) **87**:299–304.
49. Smith SB, Duncan T, Kutty G et al., Increase in retinyl palmitate concentration in eyes and livers and the concentration of interphotoreceptor retinoid-binding protein in eyes of vitiligo mutant mice, *Biochem J* (1994) **300**:63–8.
50. Smith SB, Cope BK, McCoy JR et al., Reduction of phagosomes in the vitiligo (C57BL/6–mi^{vit}/mi^{vit}) mouse model of retinal degeneration, *Invest Ophthalmol Vis Sci* (1994) **35**:3625–32.
51. Sidman RL, Kosaras B, Tang M, Pigment epithelial and retinal phenotypes in the Vitiligo, mi^{vit}, mutant mouse, *Invest Ophthalmol Vis Sci* (1996) **37**:1097–115.
52. Tang M, Ruiz M, Kosaras B et al., Increased cell genesis in retinal pigment epithelium of perinatal Vitiligo mutant mice, *Invest Ophthalmol Vis Sci* (1996) **37**:1116–24.
53. Orlow SJ, Zhou BK, Chakraborty AK et al., High-molecular-weight forms of tyrosinase and the tyrosinase-related proteins: evidence for a melanogenic complex, *J Invest Dermatol* (1994) **103**:196–201.

Section IV

CELL SIGNALLING OF MELANOGENESIS

10 The role of the stress-activated protein kinases in UV-induced signaling pathways

Karen Yeow, Candice Cabane and Benoît Dérijard

Introduction

Mitogen-activated protein kinases (MAPK) are among the most widely represented signaling pathways in eucaryotes. They have been found in all eucaryotic cells in which they have been studied, from yeast to mammals. Most cells display several MAPK pathways, allowing the transduction of a whole set of stimuli, thereby permitting a co-ordinate response. In mammalian cells, three major groups of MAP kinases (or MAPK) have been identified: the ERK (extra cellular regulated kinase), the JNK (c-Jun N-terminal kinase) and the p38 MAPK.

Initially identified in 1991,[1] the MAPK ERK1 and ERK2 play a crucial role in the transmission of mitogenic signals from the membrane to the nucleus.[2] They are involved in a wide array of cellular processes[3] and are activated by threonine and tyrosine phosphorylation[4] in response to various extra cellular stimuli.[1,5] Phosphorylation of MAPK is mediated by a dual specificity protein kinase termed MAP kinase kinase (MAPKK). Finally, the MAPKK is itself activated through the phosphorylation of two serine threonine residues by an upstream MAP kinase kinase kinase (MAPKKK).[6] Thus, the MAPK signaling cascade represents the archetypal mechanism by which signals received at the cell surface, via the activation of specific receptors, may propagate in the cell and lead to a modification of cell functions (Fig. 10.1).

Several transduction pathways involving MAPK have already been described in yeast.[7] Nonetheless, until 1994, only one such pathway had been identified in mammals.[6] Since then, it has been shown that, in addition to the pathway leading to MAPK activation, at least two new MAPK pathways co-existed. These pathways, the JNK and p38 pathways, were termed stress-activated MAPK pathways with respect to their common stress-signal activators (Fig. 10.1).

The identification of the various members of the stress-activated MAPK signal transduction pathway is now virtually complete.[8–10] Begun in 1994 by the isolation of JNK1/SAPKα,[11,12] it was then followed by the cloning of its upstream activators. Like the other known MAPK, whose stimulation leads to the modification of gene transcription via specific activation of transcription factors, JNK1 was shown to be rapidly and highly activated by ultraviolet (UV) light, to bind to the N-terminal transactivation domain of c-Jun and to phosphorylate the latter on Ser63 and Ser73. Like UV, although to a lesser extent, Ha-Ras, EGF and phorbol esters also activate JNK.[11] Its apparent molecular weight (46 kDa) and biochemical properties correlated with the uncloned, but previously characterized, JNK-46 c-Jun N-terminal kinase.[13] In a similar manner to ERK1 and ERK2, two conserved Thr and Tyr residues of JNK have to be phosphorylated in order for this kinase to be activated.[11]

Finally it was shown that, besides c-Jun, JNK phosphorylates other transcription factors such as ATF2 (activating transcription factor-2),[14] and, more recently, Elk-1.[15] JNK seems, therefore, to play a crucial role in the transcriptional responses triggered by the transcription factors c-Jun, ATF2 and Elk-1.

In 1994, the field of MAPK research broadened, in addition to the cloning and biochemical characterization of JNK1, by the isolation of p38 MAPK.[16] Gram-negative bacteria LPS (lipopolysaccharide) triggers the potent and rapid stimulus involved in

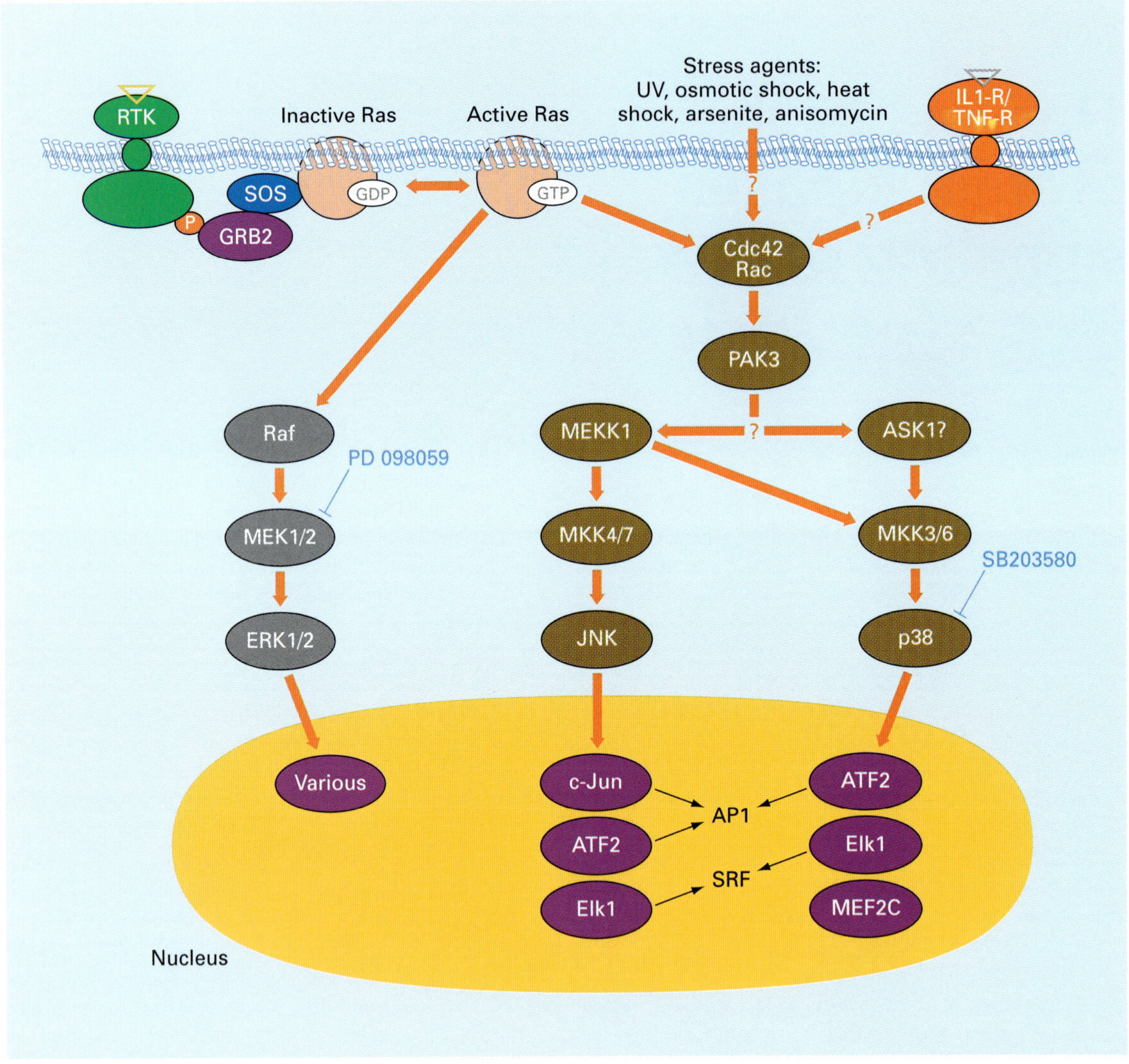

Figure 10.1

The three MAPK cascades, ERKs, JNK and p38 pathways, are shown with their upstream effectors, agonists and triggering agents. PD 098059 and SB203580 are inhibitors of the ERK activator MEK1 and of the p38 MAPK, respectively.

the mammalian cellular response to sepsis. LPS stimulation of mammalian cells was known to activate kinases and finally lead to an increase in specific gene expression. The p38 protein kinase, which was phosphorylated on Thr and Tyr residues in response to LPS activation, was purified using an anti-phosphotyrosine antibody[16] and its cDNA was thereby isolated. As was the case for JNK1, p38 displayed strong homologies with the *S. cerevisiae Hog1* gene product, especially within the activation site.[16,17] Hog1 is involved in yeast osmotic shock resistance by the stimulation of intracellular glycerol production. JNK1 and p38 both complement a yeast Δ*Hog1* knockout[16,17] and are activated by osmotic shock in mammalian cells.[18]

Similarly, p38 shares several substrates with JNK, such as ATF2[19,20] and Elk-1.[20] In addition, p38 also phosphorylates MEF-2C,[21] which, in turn, induces the transcriptional activation of c-Jun.[21]

Altogether, these observations strongly suggested that the pathways leading to JNK and p38 activation were identical, and would only diverge at the critical level of the MAPK (Fig. 10.1). Only the cloning of the activator of these two new MAPK, the MAPKK, would enable the distinction between these two pathways. Using degenerate PCR, cDNAs encoding two new MAPKK, termed MKK3 and MKK4, were isolated from a human fetal brain library (Fig. 10.1).[22] These MAPKK are phosphorylated on Ser and Thr residues within the activation domain (sub-domain VIII).[22] In a similar manner, the MAPKK MEK1 and MEK2 are phosphorylated on Ser. Both MKK3 and MKK4 are activated by the signals stimulating JNK1 and p38 (UV, IL-1, TNF, anisomycin). MKK3 phosphorylates p38 MAPK specifically on the activation domain Thr and Tyr residues, *in vitro* and *in vivo*. However, JNK1 is only phosphorylated by MKK4, both in *vitro* and *in vivo*.[22] In part, these results were confirmed with the rat homologues of MKK4 and JNK1, called SEK and SAPK, respectively.[23] Later, MKK6, another MAPKK closely related to MKK3, was shown to be an exclusive activator of p38[20] and MKK7, a JNK-specific activator.[24–26] No phosphorylation of ERK was observed with any of the SAPK activators (Fig. 10.1).

At the upstream level, MEKK1 (MAPK or ERK kinase kinase 1) was identified as being one of the MAPKKK upstream of JNK1.[27] From this point, a large group of JNK[8] and p38[28] MAPKKK had been characterized. Several putative elements had been suspected to lie upstream of the JNK and p38 core pathways. It was subsequently shown that the small Rho family of GTPases, Cdc42 and Rac1,[29–32] as well as their targets of the PAK (p21-activated kinase) family,[29,32,33] were among the factors upstream of JNK and p38. Similarly, some members of the wide heterotrimeric G-protein family were shown to link seven transmembrane receptors to the stress kinases core module (Fig. 10.1).[34]

In a given cell type, there are at least three highly homologous but distinct kinase signaling pathways with each of ERK, JNK and p38 as the ternary member of the cascade. Each cascade, when specifically activated by stimuli such as growth factors, inflammatory cytokines or stress agonists, modifies gene transcription and, thus, may lead to the control of various cell functions and, ultimately, to cell division or differentiation. ERK, JNK and p38 have specific activators ($MEK_{1,2}$, $MEK_{4,7}$, $MEK_{3,6}$, respectively), allowing for the specific manipulation of one or more of these pathways by the ectopic expression of members of the signaling cascade in either a positive or negative manner (expression of constitutive active or inactive mutants). Similarly, several inhibitors, among which PD0980 and SB203580 are the most widely used to block MEK1 and p38, respectively, have been developed.[35] These inhibitors, together with the constitutive active or inactive mutants of the kinases, are very useful and extensively employed to characterize MAPK functions.

Despite the tremendous amount of data accumulated on these pathways within a few years, it is quite surprising that the agonist that was so widely used to characterize the first stress kinase, ultraviolet radiation (UV),[13] has received such little attention from scientists in terms of physiological response. Indeed, the skin and the eyes being the only naturally UV-exposed tissue has certainly limited these investigations. Nevertheless, global environmental changes, such as ozone layer depletion, should make the issue of UV-radiation impact on skin of increasing concern to the scientific community. The purpose of this review is to gather the data obtained on the effects of UV radiation on stress-activated protein kinases on skin, using the overall data on the consequences of UV-induced stress kinase activation as a paradigm.

Physical considerations

Wavelength

Most biochemistry and cell biology laboratories are equipped with UVC lamps, to visualize DNA or as germicidal radiation in cell culture hoods. For this very simple reason, UVC (100–280 nm) has been primarily used to activate stress kinases. Nevertheless, these UV wavelengths are the least represented on the earth's surface. However, contrary to common thought, UVC is not completely blocked by the atmosphere (besides at high elevations, where they are normally less filtered) and their levels have increased in the past few years due to the depletion of stratospheric ozone.

A recent study on human T Lymphoma Molt4 cells has shown that ERKs were activated by 320–360 nm light within 1 minute of irradiation[36] (Fig. 10.2). p38 was also activated within 1 minute, but in response to a shorter wavelength (270–280 nm). In contrast, in this study, JNK was activated 10 minutes after irradiation with UV light at a narrow peak of 280 nm (Fig. 10.2). Although it appears to be the only one of that kind, and apparently rigorous, this study was limited to a particular cell type (not naturally exposed to UV light) and cannot account for MAPK UV activation in all cell types. Indeed, skin cells may have developed specialized features to adapt to prolonged UV irradiation. As far as skin cells are concerned, MAPK have been shown to be activated by all three UV types in several reports.[11,37–40] As discussed later, UV-induced MAPK activation is likely to be triggered by receptor clustering, which provides a possible explanation for cell-type-specific responses to UV.

Doses

Although UVC is the most widely used to activate MAPK in most cell types, it is the least used in skin cells because it is considered to be absorbed by the upper atmosphere. Nevertheless, doses of 60–80 J/m^2 of UVC are able to activate both ERK and JNK in JB6 cells,[39] as well as in keratinocytes.[41] More recently, p38 was shown to be activated by UVC doses of 60 J/m^2 in JB6 cells.[42] Despite the filtering action exerted by the upper atmosphere, such doses of UVC are close to what can be received after a 2-hour walk at an elevation of 2000 m on a sunny day.[43]

UVB is known to be responsible for most of the damaging effects of UV light,[44] although UVA is more penetrant on human skin.[45] Doses of UVB as low as 150–200 J/m^2 have been successfully used to activate all three MAPK in human cultured keratinocytes,[40,46–48] although much higher doses are commonly used.[37,39,40] On human skin, a dose of 2 MED (minimal erythema dose) of UVB is enough to trigger the activation of ERK, JNK and p38.[40,50]

Finally, UVA doses of 3000 J/m^2 can also activate all three MAPK in human keratinocytes.[40]

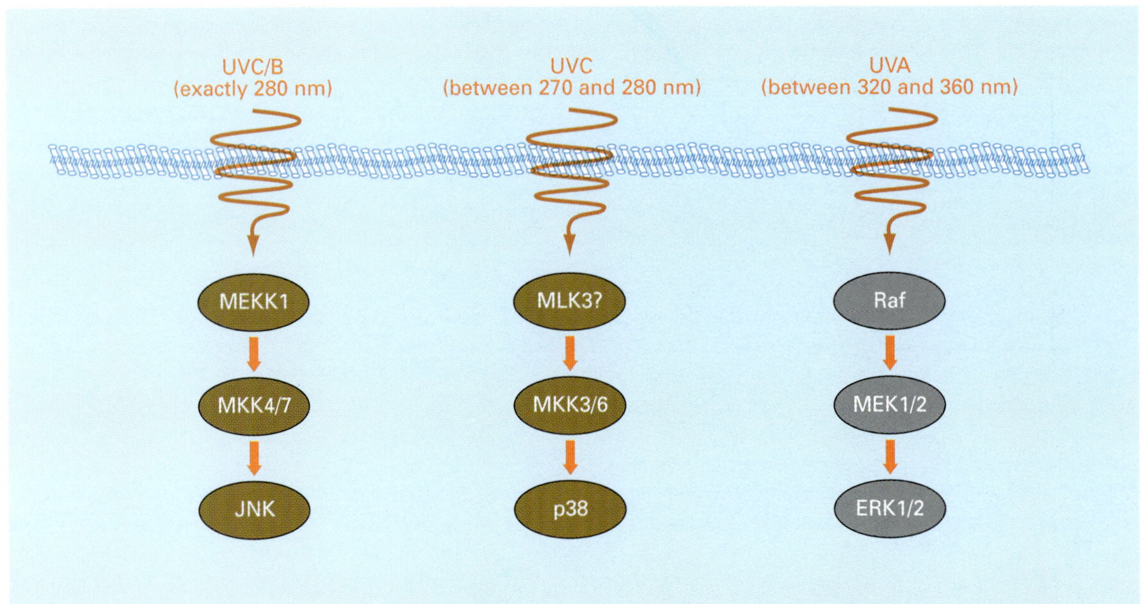

Figure 10.2

A study done on Molt4 cells (human T-lymphoma cultured cells) describes JNK as being activated by 280 nm UV light, p38 by 270–280 nm UVC and ERK by 320–360 nm UVA.

Mechanisms triggering UV-activation of the stress kinases

Receptor clustering

Receptor clustering is the most commonly accepted hypothesis to explain the UV radiation-mediated MAPK activation.[51,52] Since receptor distribution can vary tremendously from one cell type to another, UV-induced MAPK activation triggered by receptor clustering can vary accordingly between cell types. Thus, the process of receptor clustering in response to UV provides a plausible explanation for the cell-type-specific responses to UV irradiation. This ligand-independent activation leads to the phosphorylation of both ERK and JNK/p38 MAPK, respectively, through the clustering of RTKs (receptor tyrosine kinases), such as growth factor[53] and cytokine receptors.[54,55] Activation of these receptors independently of their ligands is likely to be due to dimerization or oligomerization of the receptors, thereby allowing auto- or transphosphorylation of their intracellular tails (Fig. 10.3a). Hence, the PTPs (protein tyrosine phosphatases) that rapidly dephosphorylate and, therefore, inactivate RTKs, are sensitive to UV-induced oxidation.[51]

DNA damage

DNA damage was first considered to be the main mechanism triggering the sequence of events leading to UV-induced activation of gene transcription, known as the mammalian UV response.[56] However, the rapid UV activation of RTKs,[57] as well as the possibility to activate MAPK in enucleated cells,[58] suggests that DNA damage is not always required to elicit the UV response.

One of the major arguments in favour of DNA damage as being an early event triggering stress kinase signaling lies in the observation that Cockayne's syndrome DNA-repair-deficient cells display poor JNK activation.[59] In addition, it is well documented that Cockayne's syndrome and Xeroderma pigmentosum cells show a significant UV susceptibility.[60]

Among the UV-induced proteins involved in DNA damage recognition, DDPK (DNA-dependent protein kinase) and ATM (ataxia telangiectasia mutated) have been shown to interact with and activate c-Abl, a proto-oncogene known to be an upstream activator of both JNK and p38.[61,62] These observations are the only biochemically relevant data linking UV-induced DNA damage to the stress kinase signaling pathways (Fig. 10.3b). This aspect of UV-induced DNA damage and its connections with signaling pathways was reviewed by D. Watters.[63]

Ribotoxic stress

Although recently described, and with a limited number of published observations, ribotoxic stress (Fig. 10.3c) represents an attractive hypothesis to explain UV-induced stress kinase activation.[64,65] Ribotoxic stress was first described through the effects of anisomycin, a protein synthesis inhibitor, both on the activation of SAPK and on the inhibition of the eukaryotic peptidyl transferase reaction. Despite the fact that anisomycin can potently activate SAPK at doses that are sub-inhibitory for protein synthesis,[66,67] these authors have shown that active ribosomes are required at the moment of anisomycin exposure. This is also the case when the ribotoxic stressor is UVC.[65] In addition, other ribotoxic stressors that interfere with the 28S rRNA anisomycin binding site can also activate the SAPK. However, the steps linking 28S rRNA damage, or the inhibition of the peptidyl transferase reaction, to the activation of stress kinases still need to be characterized.

Although ribotoxic stress has not yet been shown in skin cells, it represents an attractive alternative to receptor clustering or DNA damage.

The three mechanisms described above are obviously not exhaustive, and it is very likely that, depending on the cell type, there should be a prevalence of one over the others, since, for example, RTK distribution or the translating potential varies greatly from one cell type to another.

Stress-kinase-mediated activation of AP-1 and other transcription factors

The substrates of stress-activated MAP kinases reflect the important role played by these proteins in inflammatory signaling. In response to UV,

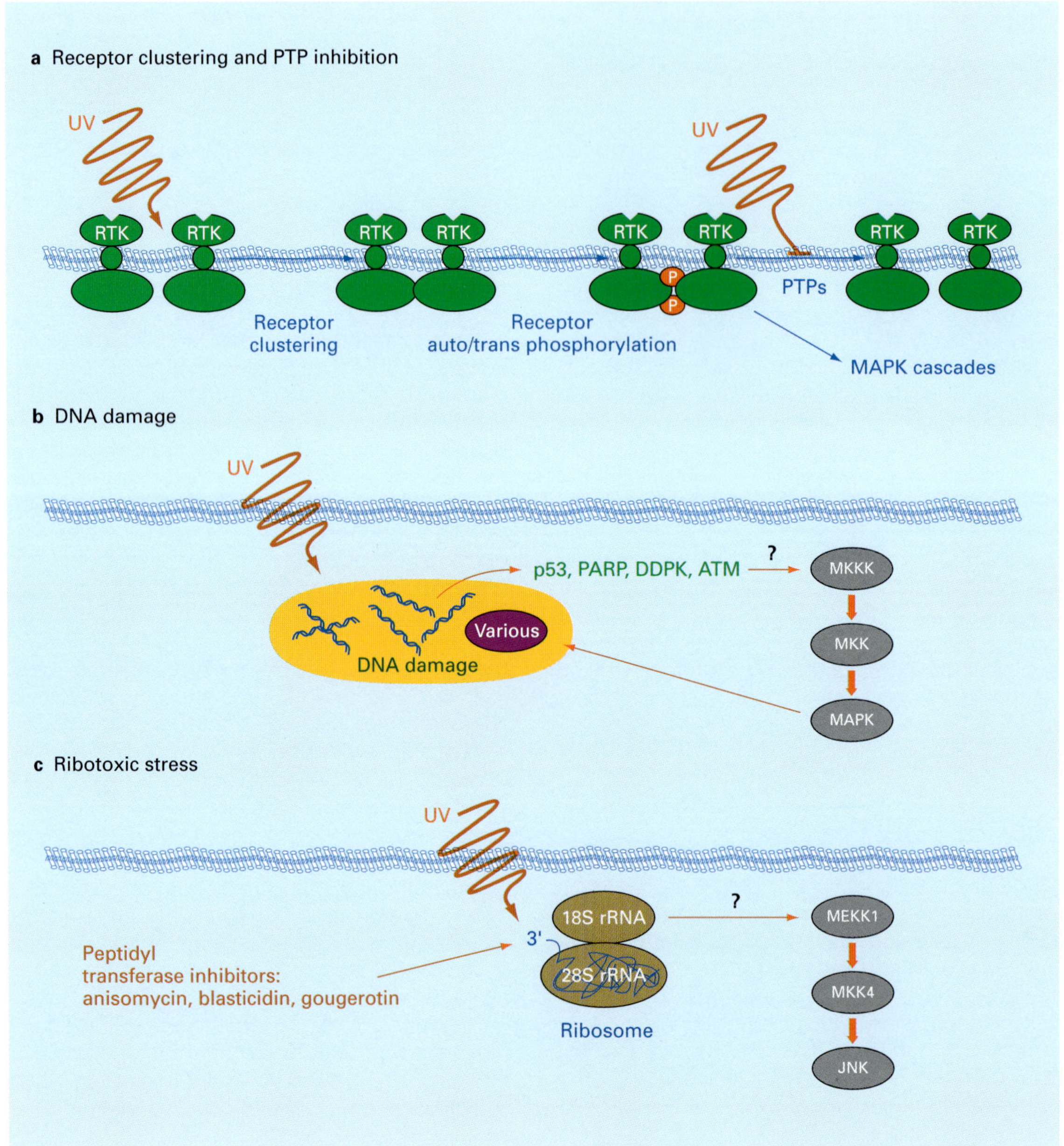

Figure 10.3

How does UV activate the MAP kinase cascades? (a) Ligand-independant receptor clustering leads to receptor autophosphorylation. (b) UV-induced DNA damage induces the expression of several DNA repair proteins that would activate the MAPK pathways through as yet unknown intermediates. (c) UV causes specific damage to the 3'end of 28S rRNA that leads to JNK activation. PTPs: protein tyrosine phosphatases. PARP: poly-ADP ribose polymerase. DDPK: DNA-dependent protein kinase. ATM: ataxia telangiectasia mutated.

mammalian cells display the activation of key transcription factors, such as AP1, p53,[68] GADD45,[69,70] p21,[71,72] NFκB[58,60] and c-Jun.[73,74] Changes in the expression and activities of these transcription factors affect the cell cycle,[75] as well as the cellular machinery for DNA repair.[76,77] The signaling pathways that are upregulated in response to UV in keratinocytes are summarized in Figure 10.4. This section will discuss some of the work on the involvement of these transcription factors in UV-induced carcinogenesis, with emphasis on the role of the AP-1 and ATF2 transcription factors.

The JNK and p38 kinases are the main stress-activated kinases involved in the activation of the AP-1 transcription factor. AP-1 is one of the main transcription factors known to be involved in the onset of carcinogenesis. This transcription factor is a heterodimer consisting of Fos and Jun proteins, either Jun-Jun homodimers or Fos-Jun heterodimers. There are three Jun isoforms (c-Jun, Jun B, and Jun D), and four Fos isoforms (c-Fos, Fos B, Fra-1 and Fra-2). AP-1 typically consists of c-Jun and Jun D, along with members of the *fos* and ATF2 family of transcription factors. AP-1 activation involves either phosphorylation or dephosphorylation of its molecular components.[9] The activation of transcription factors which, in turn, induce expression of c-Jun or c-Fos, can also result in AP-1 activation. Phosphorylation of the transactivating (NH_2 terminal) domains of c-Jun or ATF2 enhances their ability to activate transcription.[9] *In vivo*, the activation of the JNK kinase signaling pathway results in the phosphorylation of Ser63 and Ser73 of the c-Jun transactivating domain. Similarly, the JNK kinases can also phosphorylate the transactivating domains of Jun D and ATF2.

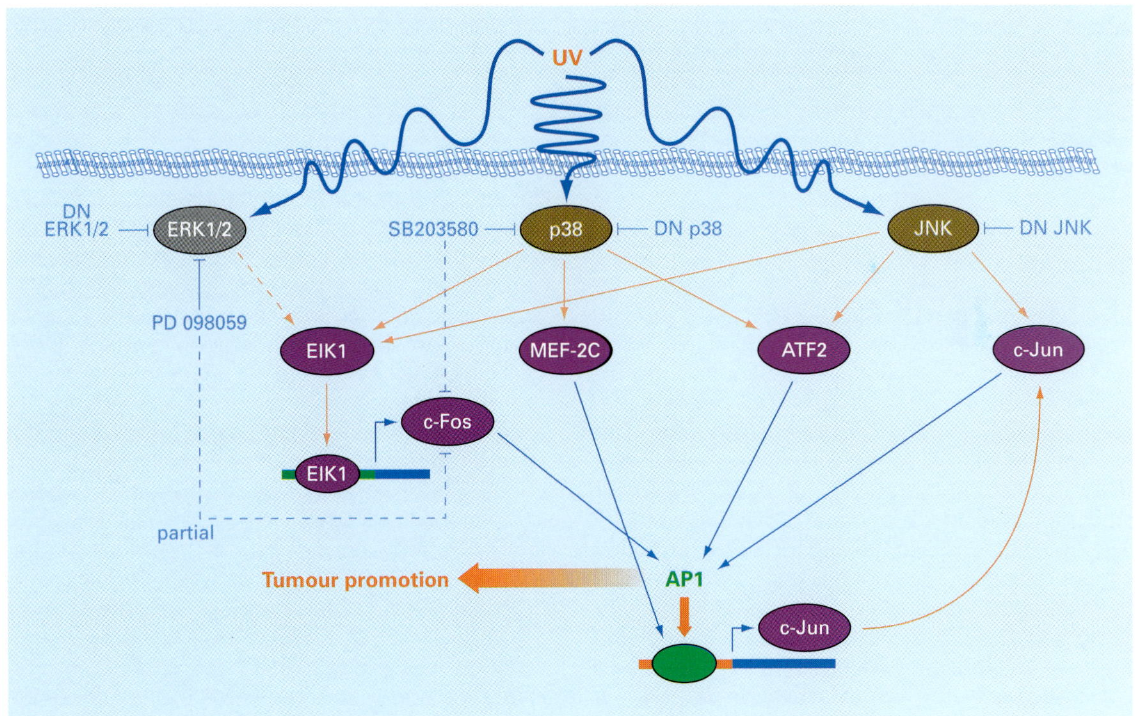

Figure 10.4

MAP kinase UV-induced AP1 activation in keratinocytes. The three MAPKs, ERKs, JNK and p38, lead to the transcriptional activation of c-Fos through Elk1 phosphorylation. Both JNK and p38 activate ATF-2 by direct phosphorylation, whereas c-Jun is only activated by JNK. MEF-2C, an activator of c-Jun transcription, is only activated by p38. All four events, therefore, lead to a massive activation of AP1 which, in turn, activates c-Jun transcription and induces tumour promotion.

The JNK and p38 kinases can also contribute to AP-1 activation by stimulating transcription of the genes encoding AP-1 components, such as c-Fos (Fig. 10.4). Transcription of the human *c-Fos* gene is exerted via the serum response element (SRE), located within the promoter region of the *c-Fos* gene,[78] as well as a cyclic AMP response element (CRE).[79] The SRE can be recognized by the serum response factor (SRF)-ternary complex factor (TCF), also known as Elk-1.[78] Activation of TCF via phosphorylation, in turn, triggers *c-Fos* gene transcription.[80] It has been shown that all three MAP kinase pathways are capable of phosphorylating (and thereby activating) TCF (Fig. 10.4), including the JNK and p38 pathways.[20] Indeed, the activation of p38 is thought to be required for UVB-induced *c-Fos* gene expression[81] and AP1 activation in human keratinocytes.[82]

An important role for JNK appears to be the regulation of the transcriptional activity of AP1, specifically in response to stress- and cytokine-induced stimuli (reviewed in reference 83). Phosphorylation of residues Ser63 and Ser73 in the activation domain of c-Jun by JNK results in increased transcription activity.[84] JNK can also phosphorylate several of the AP1 proteins, including Jun D.[83]

Role of AP1 in onset of photoaging and skin cancer

AP-1 is a multifunctional transcription factor known to play important roles in cell proliferation, differentiation, apoptosis, and transformation. The involvement of the AP-1 transcription factor has been invoked in the onset of many types of cancers, including UV-induced carcinogenesis.[85,86] Carcinogenesis is a multistep process, involving tumour initiation, promotion and progression.[87] The rate-limiting steps in tumorigenesis are thought to occur during the tumour promotion and progression stages, requiring chronic exposure to a tumour promoter.[87] Transactivation of AP-1 is thought to be important for progression through these stages of tumorigenesis.[88]

Elevated AP1 DNA binding and transactivation activity is characteristic of highly malignant spindle cell carcinoma cell lines.[89] In JB6 cells, AP-1 activation is required in tumour-promoter-induced transformation.[90] In this case, ERK activity is thought to be necessary for this activation of AP-1.[39] The transforming effects of mutant Ras proteins are thought to require AP1 activity: these oncoproteins have been shown to upregulate AP1 activity at the transcriptional and post-translational levels.[91] Analysis of the dimerization partners of Jun in tumour cells indicate a strong correlation between the activation of these proteins and malignant transformation. The Fra proteins, which can activate and phosphorylate AP1, are also activated in dividing keratinocytes, as well as in transformed cells.[89] In squamous cell carcinoma cells, the phosphorylated levels of c-Jun are present at high levels, and AP1 activity was found to be elevated in these cells.[89] In contrast, transgenic mice expressing a mutant form of c-Jun under the control of the human keratin-14 promoter are protected against skin tumour promotion.[92] Thus, the expression of high levels of AP1 correlates well with tumorigenesis in the skin, whereas abolishing AP1 activity appears to have a protective effect against tumorigenesis.

AP-1 regulates the transcription of many genes, some of which mediate neoplastic transformation.[93,94] UV-induced activation of AP1 causes an enhanced transcription of metalloproteinase genes, which leads to the degradation of collagen and elastin.[50,55,95] The upregulation of matrix metalloproteinases is one of the major causes of photoageing and various skin cancers.[50,55] Indeed, exposure of human skin to UVB irradiation causes a significant loss of procollagen synthesis, and this inhibition is dependent on c-Jun.[96] Although the AP1 transcription factor is involved in the onset of tumorigenesis, it also plays a role in regulating the transcription of other epithelial-specific genes. Other genes whose expression is altered in response to UVB in keratinocytes include ICAM-1[97] and keratins.[98] The promoters of keratins K5 and K14 (which are molecular markers of mitotically active keratinocytes) are able to interact with AP1.[99] In addition, AP1-dependent transcription is important for expression of the involucrin gene, an early keratinocyte differentiation marker.[100] Clearly, this transcription factor is involved in the upregulation of many genes involved in tumorigenesis and differentiation of the skin. Further research will be necessary in order to identify and isolate the subset of AP-1-responsive genes involved in the onset of skin cancer.

UV, stress kinases and apoptosis in skin

Role of the stress kinases in radiation resistance

One of the characteristics of malignant melanoma is its insensitivity to radiotherapy. The ability of many types of tumours to resist apoptosis is demonstrated by the presence of altered apoptosis signaling responses, including suppression of the death receptor or increased expression of apoptosis-inhibitory proteins.[101,102] In late-stage melanomas, many growth factors, cytokines, and their receptors, are overexpressed, which may contribute to tumour progression and apoptosis resistance.[103] The cell death or survival factors are regulated by the stress kinases and their respective downstream transcription factors, such as ATF2.[104]

ATF2 is known to be phosphorylated upon treatment of cells with various stress stimuli, thereby regulating the expression of its target genes, such as c-Jun. The stress kinases contribute to the regulation of ATF2 activation and stability, thereby playing an important role in the acquisition of apoptosis resistance.[105] However, ATF2 can directly affect radiation-induced apoptosis by upregulating TNFα expression.[104] In late-stage melanoma cells, TNFα functions as a survival factor.[104] ATF2-derived peptides have been used successfully in sensitizing late-stage human melanoma cell lines to UV-induced apoptosis, theoretically by out-competing endogenous ATF2 expression (Fig. 10.5).[105] This method of inhibiting endogenous ATF2 function may impede its downstream effects on TNFα, thereby increasing tumour cell apoptosis in the absence of this survival factor (Fig. 10.5).

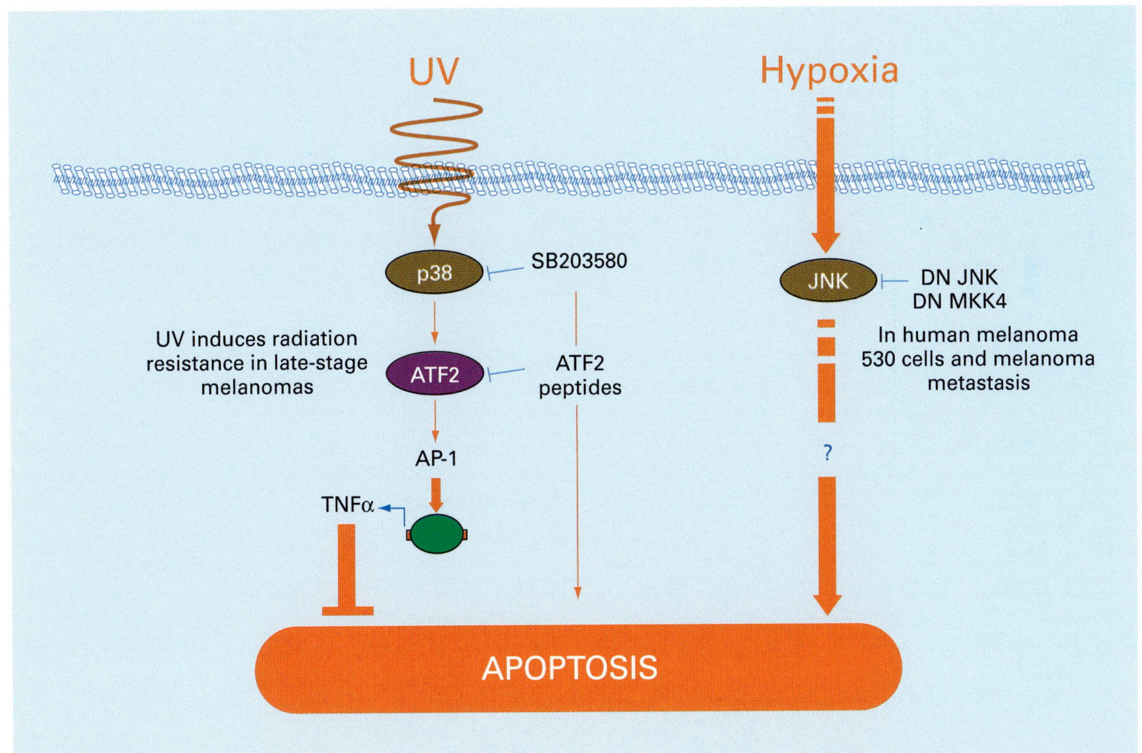

Figure 10.5

Stress-kinase- and UV-induced apoptosis in melanomas.

In addition to their effects on ATF2, the stress kinases also affect apoptosis via the Fas ligand. Through its action on an NFκB/Sp1 site on the Fas promoter, p38 downregulates the expression of this apoptotic-promoting ligand in late-stage melanoma cells.[104] Deletion or mutation of this region negates this effect, as does inhibition of p38 activity. It is thought that this effect of p38 on the Fas promoter directly involves the inhibition of IκB activity, via inhibition of the phosphorylation of the IκBα subunit.[104]

Finally, a recent study described data not directly involving UV-induced JNK activation but which rather concerned hypoxia-induced JNK activation in melanoma cells as well as metastasis (Fig. 10.5).[106] The study shows that the hypoxia-induced MAPK activation is specific to JNK, independent of Fas/Fas ligand expression, and is involved in hypoxia-mediated tumour cell apoptosis. Since it seems accepted that hypoxia selects for the most aggressive tumour via hypoxia-induced apoptosis,[107] the authors suggest that interfering with the JNK signaling pathway might be of therapeutical interest in melanomas.

Stress-kinase-induced activation of p53 and cytochrome *c* release

Skin overexposure to solar UV light leads to keratinocyte apoptosis. This enables the organism to rid itself of potentially malignant cells produced by DNA damage. This protective mechanism uses several pathways, some of which directly involve the stress-activated kinases.[108] The main UV-induced proteins triggering apoptosis via the stress kinases are p53 and cytochrome *c*. A brief overview of the situation in various cell types will be presented first, and the specific situation in skin cells will be discussed further.

The product of the p53 tumour suppressor gene is a transcription factor with a short half-life which plays a key role in DNA repair, apoptosis and cell cycle regulation.[109,110] p53 is expressed at basal levels in normal growth conditions but it is accumulated and post-translationally modified, and subsequently activated in response to stress and DNA damage.[109,110] The activation of p53 leads to cell-cycle arrest, thereby allowing the cell to monitor the extent of DNA damage and either initiate DNA repair or trigger programmed cell death, according to the DNA damage level. Several studies recently suggested that the regulation of p53 transcriptional activity is dependent on phosphorylation (Fig. 10.6), mainly by the stress kinases.[111–118] In addition, p53 activity is directly linked to its stability regulated by Mdm2,[119] JNK[120] and p38[121,122] in a phosphorylation-dependent manner. The relevance of the phosphorylation of all these sites on p53 still remains controversial and will have to be clarified further.[123]

As far as skin cells are concerned,[124] studies on the role of UV-induced stress kinase activation of p53 are surprisingly limited (Fig. 10.7). Indeed, only one study mentions the phosphorylation of p53 by p38 on Ser15 in response to UVB radiation in JB6 epidermal cells.[122] This phosphorylation stabilizes p53 by preventing its interaction with its negative regulator Mdm2. In fact, both ERK2 and p38 were shown to be responsible for Ser15 phosphorylation and to co-immunoprecipitate with p53. This was demonstrated using both dominant-negative forms of ERK2 and p38, as well as specific inhibitors. The role of JNK in this process was excluded using a recombinant active form of the kinase.[122]

Cytochrome *c* release from mitochondria upon UV irradiation has been shown to trigger the caspase 3 pathway (Fig. 10.6), leading to cell death.[125,126] This pathway was therefore examined in murine embryonic fibroblasts derived from JNK1 and -2 knockout mice.[127] It turns out that fibroblasts lacking both JNK1 and -2 activity are unable to activate caspase 3 (Fig. 10.6), and that these cells are thereby protected against UV-induced apoptosis.[127] Several intermediates potentially linking UV-induced JNK activation to cytochrome *c* release are suspected, and are represented in Figure 10.6. The Bcl2 protein, which exerts its antiapoptotic effects by preventing the release of cytochrome *c* from the mitochondria, is phosphorylated, and thereby inactivated, through the JNK pathway.[128] Another candidate might be the proapoptotic Bcl2 family member Bid, which, when proteolytically activated, can translocate to the mitochondria and trigger cytochrome *c* release.[127,129] In addition, Bid cleavage was also shown to be induced by the p38 pathway in response to oxidative stress.[130]

In human keratinocyte HaCat cells (Fig. 10.7), two studies have recently shown the UVB-induced activation of caspase 3[48] and Bid cleavage,[47] as well as mitochondrial cytochrome *c* release.[47] Although they need to be further confirmed by additional

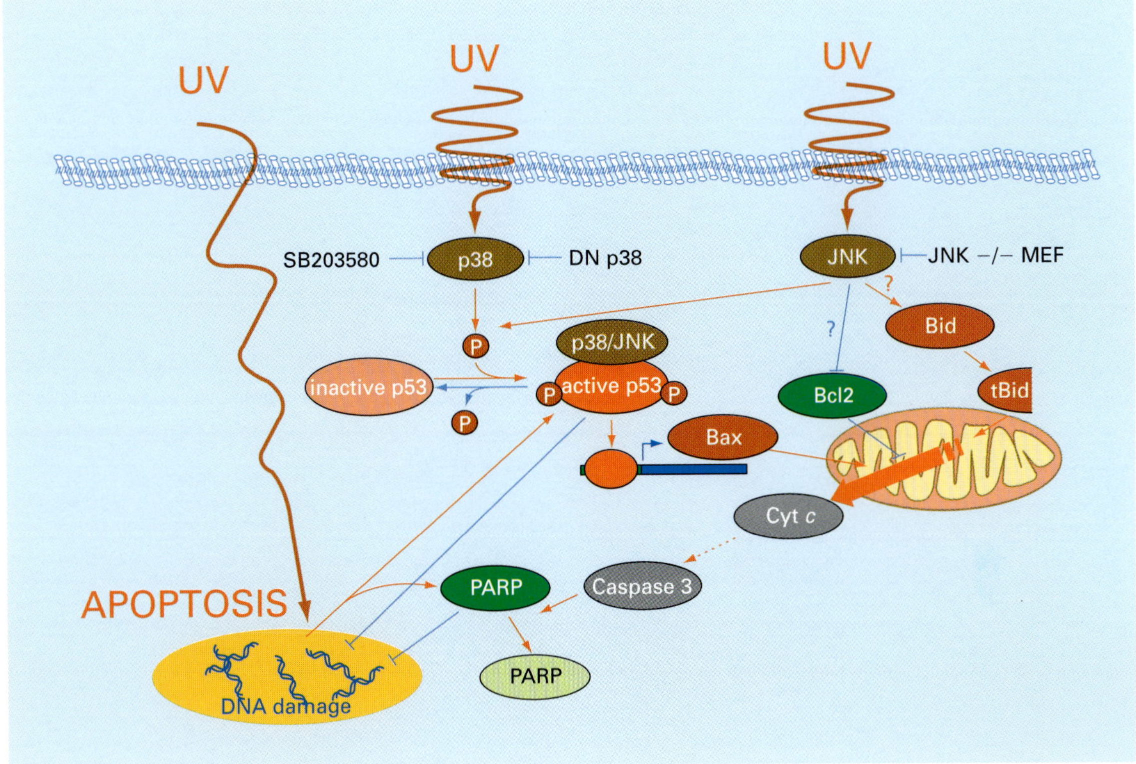

Figure 10.6

Stress-kinase- and UV-induced apoptosis. The main UV- and stress-kinase-induced apoptotic pathways encountered in various tissues, including skin, are depicted. Refer to text for details.

studies, these results provide new insight into the mechanisms triggering UVB-induced apoptosis in keratinocytes and have identified the p38 pathway as being a major pathway mediating mitochondrial cytochrome *c* release, which significantly contributes to the programmed cell death process.

Perspectives and conclusions

In light of the important roles played by the stress kinases in response to cellular-damaging agents, including UV light, it is surprising that they have received such little attention in the field of skin cell biology. Given that the skin is one of the largest organs in the human body, and the increasing levels of UV penetrating the Earth's atmosphere, it is crucial that the molecular events triggered in response to UV exposure in human skin be clarified. To date, much attention has been focused on the role of the AP-1 transcription factor in the onset of skin carcinogenesis. However, little is known regarding the involvement of other transcription factors, such as p53. Although much work has been done on the role of UV in p53 activation in non-skin cell types, surprisingly little is known on how UV modulates p53 function in the skin itself. Another major response to UV is the induction of apoptosis. In light of the critical role played by the stress kinases in apoptosis induction, an important area of research will be to characterize how these signaling pathways contribute towards apoptosis induction, and, thus, what role they play in the development of apoptosis resistance in skin cancers. It is well known that the stress kinase signaling pathway plays an important role in cell differentiation (such as in

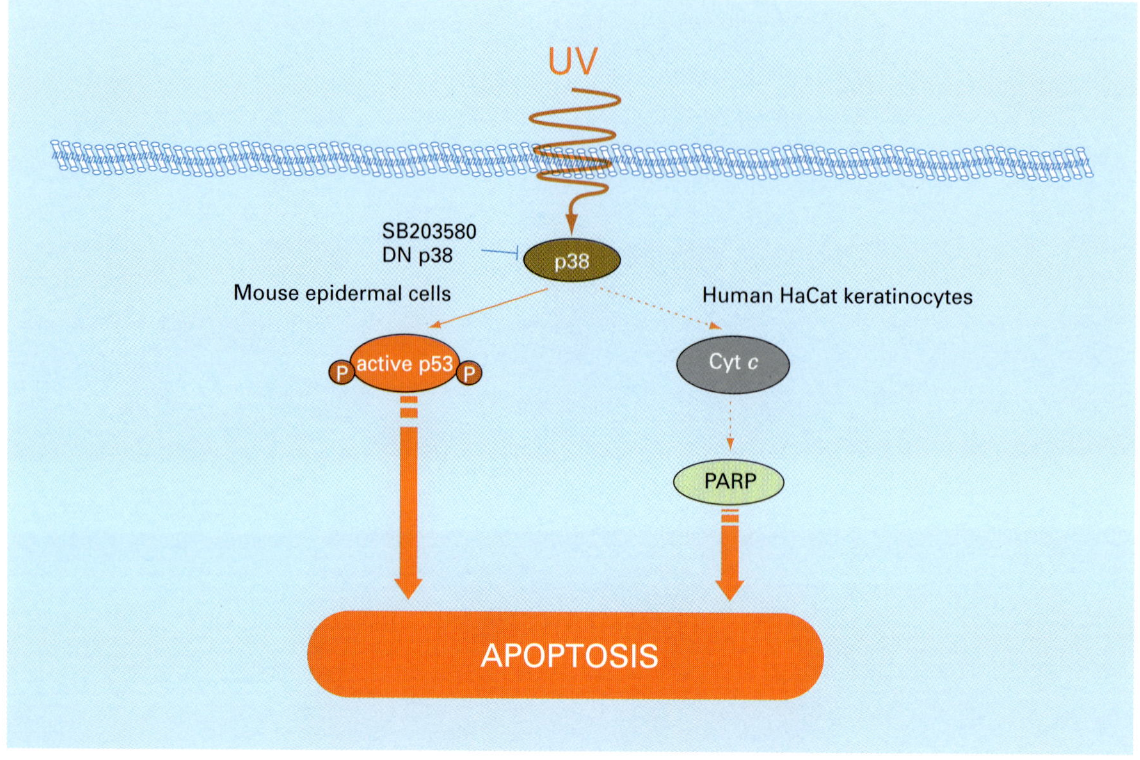

Figure 10.7

UV-induced p38-mediated apoptosis in keratinocytes.

muscle and neuronal cells), and there is evidence that this holds true for skin cells as well.[131] The identification of differentiation-specific targets of the stress kinase pathways in skin will be of great value in understanding how this process is dysregulated during cancer progression. Much work remains to be done in order to understand how the stress kinases are involved in the complex series of events that occurs between sun exposure and the onset of skin cancer.

References

1. Sturgill TW, Wu J, Recent progress in characterization of protein kinase cascades for phosphorylation of ribosomal protein S6, *Biochim Biophys Acta* (1991) **1092**:350–7.
2. L'Allemain G, Deciphering the MAP kinase pathway, *Prog Growth Factor Res* (1994) **5**:291–334.
3. Davis RJ, Transcriptional regulation by MAP kinases, *Mol Reprod Dev* (1995) **42**:459–67.
4. Ahn NG, Seger R, Krebs EG, The mitogen-activated protein kinase activator, *Curr Opin Cell Biol* (1992) **4**:992–9.
5. Cobb MH, Robbins DJ, Boulton TG, ERKs, extracellular signal-regulated MAP-2 kinases, *Curr Opin Cell Biol* (1991) **3**:1025–32.
6. Marshall CJ, MAP kinase kinase kinase, MAP kinase kinase and MAP kinase, *Curr Opin Genet Dev* (1994) **4**:82–9.
7. Davis RJ, MAPKs: new JNK expands the group, *Trends Biochem Sci* (1994) **19**:470–3.
8. Davis RJ, Signal transduction by the JNK group of MAP kinases, *Cell* (2000) **103**:239–52.
9. Kyriakis JM, Avruch J, Mammalian mitogen-activated protein kinase signal transduction pathways activated by stress and inflammation, *Physiol Rev* (2001) **81**:807–69.
10. Chang L, Karin M, Mammalian MAP kinase signalling cascades, *Nature* (2001) **410**:37–40.

11. Dérijard B, Hibi M, Wu IH et al., JNK1: a protein kinase stimulated by UV light and Ha-Ras that binds and phosphorylates the c-Jun activation domain, *Cell* (1994) **76**:1025–37.
12. Kyriakis JM, Banerjee P, Nikolakaki E et al., The stress-activated protein kinase subfamily of c-Jun kinases, *Nature* (1994) **369**:156–60.
13. Hibi M, Lin A, Smeal T et al., Identification of an oncoprotein- and UV-responsive protein kinase that binds and potentiates the c-Jun activation domain, *Genes Dev* (1993) **7**:2135–48.
14. Gupta S, Campbell D, Derijard B et al., Transcription factor ATF2 regulation by the JNK signal transduction pathway, *Science* (1995) **267**:389–93.
15. Whitmarsh AJ, Shore P, Sharrocks AD et al., Integration of MAP kinase signal transduction pathways at the serum response element, *Science* (1995) **269**:403–7.
16. Han J, Lee JD, Bibbs L et al., A MAP kinase targeted by endotoxin and hyperosmolarity in mammalian cells, *Science* (1994) **265**:808–11.
17. Dérijard B, Galcheva GZ, Wu IH et al., An osmosensing signal transduction pathway in mammalian cells, *Science* (1994) **265**:806–8.
18. Raingeaud J, Gupta S, Rogers JS et al., Pro-inflammatory cytokines and environmental stress cause p38 mitogen-activated protein kinase activation by dual phosphorylation on tyrosine and threonine, *J Biol Chem* (1995) **270**:7420–6.
19. Stein B, Brady H, Yang MX et al., Cloning and characterization of MEK6, a novel member of the mitogen-activated protein kinase kinase cascade, *J Biol Chem* (1996) **271**:11427–33.
20. Raingeaud J, Whitmarsh AJ, Barrett T et al., MKK3- and MKK6-regulated gene expression is mediated by the p38 mitogen-activated protein kinase signal transduction pathway, *Mol Cell Biol* (1996) **16**:1247–55.
21. Han J, Jiang Y, Li Z et al., Activation of the transcription factor MEF2C by the MAP kinase p38 in inflammation, *Nature* (1997) **386**:296–9.
22. Dérijard B, Raingeaud J, Barrett T et al., Independent human MAP-kinase signal transduction pathways defined by MEK and MKK isoforms, *Science* (1995) **267**:682–5.
23. Yan M, Dai T, Deak JC et al., Activation of stress-activated protein kinase by MEKK1 phosphorylation of its activator SEK1, *Nature* (1994) **372**:798–800.
24. Moriguchi T, Toyoshima F, Masuyama N et al., A novel SAPK/JNK kinase, MKK7, stimulated by TNFalpha and cellular stresses, *EMBO J* (1997) **16**:7045–53.
25. Yao Z, Diener K, Wang XS et al., Activation of stress-activated protein kinases/c-Jun N-terminal protein kinases (SAPKs/JNKs) by a novel mitogen-activated protein kinase kinase, *J Biol Chem* (1997) **272**:32378–83.
26. Tournier C, Whitmarsh AJ, Cavanagh J et al., Mitogen-activated protein kinase kinase 7 is an activator of the c-Jun NH2–terminal kinase, *Proc Natl Acad Sci U S A* (1997) **94**:7337–42.
27. Minden A, Lin A, McMahon M et al., Differential activation of ERK and JNK mitogen-activated protein kinases by Raf-1 and MEKK, *Science* (1994) **266**:1719–23.
28. Ono K, Han J, The p38 signal transduction pathway: activation and function, *Cell Signal* (2000) **12**:1–13.
29. Dérijard B, Bagrodia S, Davis RJ et al., Cdc42 and PAK-mediated signaling leads to Jun kinase and p38 mitogen-activated protein kinase activation, *J Biol Chem* (1995) **270**:27995–8.
30. Coso OA, Chiariello M, Yu JC et al., The small GTP-binding proteins Rac1 and Cdc42 regulate the activity of the JNK/SAPK signaling pathway, *Cell* (1995) **81**:1137–46.
31. Minden A, Lin A, Claret FX et al., Selective activation of the JNK signaling cascade and c-Jun transcriptional activity by the small GTPases Rac and Cdc42Hs, *Cell* (1995) **81**:1147–57.
32. Zhang S, Han J, Sells MA et al., Rho family GTPases regulate p38 mitogen-activated protein kinase through the downstream mediator Pak1, *J Biol Chem* (1995) **270**:23934–6.
33. Clerk A, Sugden PH, Activation of p21-activated protein kinase alpha (alpha PAK) by hyperosmotic shock in neonatal ventricular myocytes, *FEBS Lett* (1997) **403**:23–5.
34. Hamm HE, The many faces of G protein signaling, *J Biol Chem* (1998) **273**:669–72.
35. Davies SP, Reddy H, Caivano M et al., Specificity and mechanism of action of some commonly used protein kinase inhibitors, *Biochem J* (2000) **351**:95–105.
36. Kabuyama Y, Homma MK, Sekimata M et al., Wavelength-specific activation of MAP kinase family proteins by monochromatic UV irradiation, *Photochem Photobiol* (2001) **73**:147–52.
37. Englaro W, Derijard B, Ortonne JP et al., Solar ultraviolet light activates extracellular signal-regulated kinases and the ternary complex factor in human normal keratinocytes, *Oncogene* (1998) **16**:661–4.
38. Klotz LO, Pellieux C, Briviba K et al., Mitogen-activated protein kinase (p38-, JNK-, ERK-) activation pattern induced by extracellular and intracellular

singlet oxygen and UVA, *Eur J Biochem* (1999) **260**:917–22.

39. Huang C, Ma WY, Dong Z, The extracellular-signal-regulated protein kinases (Erks) are required for UV-induced AP-1 activation in JB6 cells, *Oncogene* (1999) **18**:2828–35.
40. Peus D, Meves A, Pott M et al., Vitamin E analog modulates UVB-induced signaling pathway activation and enhances cell survival, *Free Radic Biol Med* (2001) **30**:425–32.
41. Dhanwada KR, Dickens M, Neades R et al., Differential effects of UV-B and UV-C components of solar radiation on MAP kinase signal transduction pathways in epidermal keratinocytes, *Oncogene* (1995) **11**:1947–53.
42. Huang C, Ma WY, Maxiner A et al., p38 kinase mediates UV-induced phosphorylation of p53 protein at serine 389, *J Biol Chem* (1999) **274**:12229–35.
43. Holbrook NJ, Liu Y, Fornace AJ Jr, Signaling events controlling the molecular response to genotoxic stress, *Exs* (1996) **77**:273–88.
44. Shea CR, Parrish JA, *Nonionizing Radiations and the Skin* (Oxford University Press: Oxford 1991).
45. Lavker RM, Veres DA, Irwin CJ et al., Quantitative assessment of cumulative damage from repetitive exposures to suberythemogenic doses of UVA in human skin, *Photochem Photobiol* (1995) **62**: 348–52.
46. Pfundt R, van Vlijmen-Willems I, Bergers M et al., In situ demonstration of phosphorylated c-jun and p38 MAP kinase in epidermal keratinocytes following ultraviolet B irradiation of human skin, *J Pathol* (2001) **193**:248–55.
47. Assefa Z, Vantieghem A, Garmyn M et al., p38 mitogen-activated protein kinase regulates a novel, caspase-independent pathway for the mitochondrial cytochrome c release in ultraviolet B radiation-induced apoptosis, *J Biol Chem* (2000) **275**: 21416–21.
48. Shimizu H, Banno Y, Sumi N et al., Activation of p38 mitogen-activated protein kinase and caspases in UVB-induced apoptosis of human keratinocyte HaCaT cells, *J Invest Dermatol* (1999) **112**:769–74.
49. Nakamura S, Takahashi H, Kinouchi M et al., Differential phosphorylation of mitogen-activated protein kinase families by epidermal growth factor and ultraviolet B irradiation in SV40-transformed human keratinocytes, *J Dermatol Sci* (2001) **25**:139–49.
50. Fisher GJ, Talwar HS, Lin J et al., Retinoic acid inhibits induction of c-Jun protein by ultraviolet radiation that occurs subsequent to activation of mitogen-activated protein kinase pathways in human skin in vivo, *J Clin Invest* (1998) **101**: 1432–40.
51. Herrlich P, Bohmer FD, Redox regulation of signal transduction in mammalian cells, *Biochem Pharmacol* (2000) **59**:35–41.
52. Tyrrell RM, Activation of mammalian gene expression by the UV component of sunlight—from models to reality, *Bioessays* (1996) **18**:139–48.
53. Warmuth I, Harth Y, Matsui MS et al., Ultraviolet radiation induces phosphorylation of the epidermal growth factor receptor, *Cancer Res* (1994) **54**:374–6.
54. Rosette C, Karin M, Ultraviolet light and osmotic stress: activation of the JNK cascade through multiple growth factor and cytokine receptors, *Science* (1996) **274**:1194–7.
55. Fisher GJ, Datta SC, Talwar HS et al., Molecular basis of sun-induced premature skin ageing and retinoid antagonism, *Nature* (1996) **379**:335–9.
56. Sachsenmaier C, Radler-Pohl A, Zinck R et al., Involvement of growth factor receptors in the mammalian UVC response, *Cell* (1994) **78**:963–72.
57. Devary Y, Gottlieb RA, Smeal T et al., The mammalian ultraviolet response is triggered by activation of Src tyrosine kinases, *Cell* (1992) **71**:1081–91.
58. Devary Y, Rosette C, DiDonato JA et al., NF-kappa B activation by ultraviolet light not dependent on a nuclear signal, *Science* (1993) **261**:1442–5.
59. Dhar V, Adler V, Lehmann A et al., Impaired jun-NH2-terminal kinase activation by ultraviolet irradiation in fibroblasts of patients with Cockayne syndrome complementation group B, *Cell Growth Differ* (1996) **7**:841–6.
60. Stein B, Rahmsdorf HJ, Steffen A et al., UV-induced DNA damage is an intermediate step in UV-induced expression of human immunodeficiency virus type 1, collagenase, c-fos, and metallothionein, *Mol Cell Biol* (1989) **9**:5169–81.
61. Kharbanda S, Yuan ZM, Weichselbaum R et al., Determination of cell fate by c-Abl activation in the response to DNA damage, *Oncogene* (1998) **17**:3309–18.
62. Wang X, McGowan CH, Zhao M et al., Involvement of the MKK6-p38gamma cascade in gamma-radiation-induced cell cycle arrest, *Mol Cell Biol* (2000) **20**:4543–52.
63. Watters D, Molecular mechanisms of ionizing radiation-induced apoptosis, *Immunol Cell Biol* (1999) **77**:263–71.
64. Iordanov MS, Pribnow D, Magun JL et al., Ribotoxic stress response: activation of the stress-activated protein kinase JNK1 by inhibitors of the peptidyl

transferase reaction and by sequence-specific RNA damage to the alpha-sarcin/ricin loop in the 28S rRNA, *Mol Cell Biol* (1997) **17**:3373–81.

65. Iordanov MS, Pribnow D, Magun JL et al., Ultraviolet radiation triggers the ribotoxic stress response in mammalian cells, *J Biol Chem* (1998) **273**: 15794–803.
66. Cano E, Doza YN, Ben LR et al., Identification of anisomycin-activated kinases p45 and p55 in murine cells as MAPKAP kinase-2, *Oncogene* (1996) **12**:805–12.
67. Cano E, Hazzalin CA, Mahadevan LC, Anisomycin-activated protein kinases p45 and p55 but not mitogen-activated protein kinases ERK-1 and -2 are implicated in the induction of c-fos and c-jun, *Mol Cell Biol* (1994) **14**:7352–62.
68. Kastan MB, Onyekwere O, Sidransky D et al., Participation of p53 protein in the cellular response to DNA damage, *Cancer Res* (1991) **51**:6304–11.
69. Fornace AJ, Jr, Mammalian genes induced by radiation; activation of genes associated with growth control, *Annu Rev Genet* (1992) **26**:507–26.
70. Smith ML, Chen IT, Zhan Q et al., Interaction of the p53-regulated protein Gadd45 with proliferating cell nuclear antigen, *Science* (1994) **266**:1376–80.
71. el-Deiry WS, Tokino T, Velculescu VE et al., WAF1, a potential mediator of p53 tumor suppression, *Cell* (1993) **75**:817–25.
72. Di Leonardo A, Linke SP, Clarkin K et al., DNA damage triggers a prolonged p53-dependent G1 arrest and long-term induction of Cip1 in normal human fibroblasts, *Genes Dev* (1994) **8**:2540–51.
73. Herrlich P, Rahmsdorf HJ, Transcriptional and post-transcriptional responses to DNA-damaging agents, *Curr Opin Cell Biol* (1994) **6**:425–31.
74. Radler-Pohl A, Sachsenmaier C, Gebel S et al., UV-induced activation of AP-1 involves obligatory extranuclear steps including Raf-1 kinase, *EMBO J* (1993) **12**:1005–12.
75. Liu M, Pelling JC, UV-B/A irradiation of mouse keratinocytes results in p53-mediated WAF1/CIP1 expression, *Oncogene* (1995) **10**:1955–60.
76. Li R, Waga S, Hannon GJ et al., Differential effects by the p21 CDK inhibitor on PCNA-dependent DNA replication and repair, *Nature* (1994) **371**:534–7.
77. Waga S, Hannon GJ, Beach D et al., The p21 inhibitor of cyclin-dependent kinases controls DNA replication by interaction with PCNA, *Nature* (1994) **369**:574–8.
78. Janknecht R, Regulation of the c-fos promoter, *Immunobiology* (1995) **193**:137–42.
79. Ginty DD, Bonni A, Greenberg ME, Nerve growth factor activates a Ras-dependent protein kinase that stimulates c-fos transcription via phosphorylation of CREB, *Cell* (1994) **77**:713–25.
80. Janknecht R, Cahill MA, Nordheim A, Signal integration at the c-fos promoter, *Carcinogenesis* (1995) **16**:443–50.
81. Chen W, Bowden GT, Activation of p38 MAP kinase and ERK are required for ultraviolet-B induced c-fos gene expression in human keratinocytes, *Oncogene* (1999) **18**:7469–76.
82. Chen W, Bowden GT, Role of p38 mitogen-activated protein kinases in ultraviolet-B irradiation-induced activator protein 1 activation in human keratinocytes, *Mol Carcinog* (2000) **28**:196–202.
83. Ip YT, Davis RJ, Signal transduction by the c-Jun N-terminal kinase (JNK)—from inflammation to development, *Curr Opin Cell Biol* (1998) **10**:205–19.
84. Pulverer BJ, Kyriakis JM, Avruch J et al., Phosphorylation of c-jun mediated by MAP kinases, *Nature* (1991) **353**:670–4.
85. Barthelman M, Chen W, Gensler HL et al., Inhibitory effects of perillyl alcohol on UVB-induced murine skin cancer and AP-1 transactivation, *Cancer Res* (1998) **58**:711–16.
86. Huang C, Ma W, Bowden GT et al., Ultraviolet B-induced activated protein-1 activation does not require epidermal growth factor receptor but is blocked by a dominant negative PKClambda/iota, *J Biol Chem* (1996) **271**:31262–8.
87. Brown K, Balmain A, Transgenic mice and squamous multistage skin carcinogenesis, *Cancer Metastasis Rev* (1995) **14**:113–24.
88. Li JJ, Rhim JS, Schlegel R et al., Expression of dominant negative Jun inhibits elevated AP-1 and NF-kappaB transactivation and suppresses anchorage independent growth of HPV immortalized human keratinocytes, *Oncogene* (1998) **16**:2711–21.
89. Zoumpourlis V, Papassava P, Linardopoulos S et al., High levels of phosphorylated c-Jun, Fra-1, Fra-2 and ATF-2 proteins correlate with malignant phenotypes in the multistage mouse skin carcinogenesis model, *Oncogene* (2000) **19**:4011–21.
90. Li JJ, Dong Z, Dawson MI et al., Inhibition of tumor promoter-induced transformation by retinoids that transrepress AP-1 without transactivating retinoic acid response element, *Cancer Res* (1996) **56**:483–9.
91. Derijard B, Hibi M, Wu IH et al., JNK1: a protein kinase stimulated by UV light and Ha-Ras that binds and phosphorylates the c-Jun activation domain, *Cell* (1994a) **76**:1025–37.

92. Young MR, Li JJ, Rincon M et al., Transgenic mice demonstrate AP-1 (activator protein-1) transactivation is required for tumor promotion, *Proc Natl Acad Sci U S A* (1999) **96**:9827–32.
93. Su Z, Shi Y, Fisher PB, Cooperation between AP1 and PEA3 sites within the progression elevated gene-3 (PEG-3) promoter regulate basal and differential expression of PEG-3 during progression of the oncogenic phenotype in transformed rat embryo cells, *Oncogene* (2000) **19**:3411–21.
94. Matrisian LM, Matrix metalloproteinase gene expression, *Ann N Y Acad Sci* (1994) **732**:42–50.
95. Brenneisen P, Wenk J, Klotz LO et al., Central role of ferrous/ferric iron in the ultraviolet B irradiation-mediated signaling pathway leading to increased interstitial collagenase (matrix-degrading metalloprotease (MMP)-1) and stromelysin-1 (MMP-3) mRNA levels in cultured human dermal fibroblasts, *J Biol Chem* (1998) **273**:5279–87.
96. Fisher GJ, Datta S, Wang Z et al., c-Jun-dependent inhibition of cutaneous procollagen transcription following ultraviolet irradiation is reversed by all-trans retinoic acid, *J Clin Invest* (2000) **106**:663–70.
97. Krutmann J, Bohnert E, Jung EG, Evidence that DNA damage is a mediate in ultraviolet B radiation-induced inhibition of human gene expression: ultraviolet B radiation effects on intercellular adhesion molecule-1 (ICAM-1) expression, *J Invest Dermatol* (1994) **102**:428–32.
98. Bayerl C, Taake S, Moll I et al., Characterization of sunburn cells after exposure to ultraviolet light, *Photodermatol Photoimmunol Photomed* (1995) **11**:149–54.
99. Sinha S, Degenstein L, Copenhaver C et al., Defining the regulatory factors required for epidermal gene expression. *Mol Cell Biol* (2000) **20**:2543–55.
100. Hanley K, Ng DC, He SS et al., Oxysterols induce differentiation in human keratinocytes and increase Ap-1-dependent involucrin transcription, *J Invest Dermatol* (2000) **114**:545–53.
101. Deveraux QL, Stennicke HR, Salvesen GS et al., Endogenous inhibitors of caspases, *J Clin Immunol* (1999) **19**:388–98.
102. Deveraux QL, Reed JC, IAP family proteins—suppressors of apoptosis, *Genes Dev* (1999) **13**: 239–52.
103. Moretti S, Pinzi C, Spallanzani A et al., Immunohistochemical evidence of cytokine networks during progression of human melanocytic lesions, *Int J Cancer* (1999) **84**:160–8.
104. Ivanov VN, Ronai Z, p38 protects human melanoma cells from UV-induced apoptosis through down-regulation of NF-kappaB activity and Fas expression, *Oncogene* (2000) **19**:3003–12.
105. Bhoumik A, Ivanov V, Ronai Z, Activating transcription factor 2-derived peptides alter resistance of human tumor cell lines to ultraviolet irradiation and chemical treatment, *Clin Cancer Res* (2001) **7**: 331–42.
106. Kunz M, Ibrahim S, Koczan D et al., Activation of c-Jun NH2-terminal kinase/stress-activated protein kinase (JNK/SAPK) is critical for hypoxia-induced apoptosis of human malignant melanoma, *Cell Growth Differ* (2001) **12**:137–45.
107. Graeber TG, Osmanian C, Jacks T et al., Hypoxia-mediated selection of cells with diminished apoptotic potential in solid tumours, *Nature* (1996) **379**: 88–91.
108. Kulms D, Schwarz T, Molecular mechanisms of UV-induced apoptosis, *Photodermatol Photoimmunol Photomed* (2000) **16**:195–201.
109. Oren M, Regulation of the p53 tumor suppressor protein, *J Biol Chem* (1999) **274**:36031–4.
110. Prives C, Hall PA, The p53 pathway, *J Pathol* (1999) **187**:112–26.
111. Ashcroft M, Taya Y, Vousden KH, Stress signals utilize multiple pathways to stabilize p53, *Mol Cell Biol* (2000) **20**:3224–33.
112. Buschmann T, Potapova O, Bar-Shira A et al., Jun NH2–terminal kinase phosphorylation of p53 on Thr-81 is important for p53 stabilization and transcriptional activities in response to stress, *Mol Cell Biol* (2001) **21**:2743–54.
113. Giaccia AJ, Kastan MB, The complexity of p53 modulation: emerging patterns from divergent signals, *Genes Dev* (1998) **12**:2973–83.
114. Fuchs SY, Fried VA, Ronai Z, Stress-activated kinases regulate protein stability, *Oncogene* (1998) **17**:1483–90.
115. Meek DW, Multisite phosphorylation and the integration of stress signals at p53, *Cell Signal* (1998) **10**:159–66.
116. Sanchez-Prieto R, Rojas JM, Taya Y et al., A role for the p38 mitogen-acitvated protein kinase pathway in the transcriptional activation of p53 on genotoxic stress by chemotherapeutic agents, *Cancer Res* (2000) **60**:2464–72.
117. Wang J, Friedman E, Downregulation of p53 by sustained JNK activation during apoptosis, *Mol Carcinog* (2000) **29**(3):179–88.

118. Takekawa M, Adachi M, Nakahata A et al., p53-inducible wip1 phosphatase mediates a negative feedback regulation of p38 MAPK-p53 signaling in response to UV radiation, *EMBO J* (2000) **19**: 6517–26.
119. Haupt Y, Maya R, Kazaz A et al., Mdm2 promotes the rapid degradation of p53, *Nature* (1997) **387**: 296–9.
120. Fuchs SY, Adler V, Buschmann T et al., JNK targets p53 ubiquitination and degradation in nonstressed cells, *Genes Dev* (1998) **12**:2658–63.
121. Bulavin DV, Saito S, Hollander MC et al., Phosphorylation of human p53 by p38 kinase coordinates N-terminal phosphorylation and apoptosis in response to UV radiation, *EMBO J* (1999) **18**: 6845–54.
122. She QB, Chen N, Dong Z, ERKs and p38 kinase phosphorylate p53 protein at serine 15 in response to UV radiation, *J Biol Chem* (2000) **275**: 20444–9.
123. Blattner C, Tobiasch E, Litfen M et al., DNA damage induced p53 stabilization: no indication for an involvement of p53 phosphorylation, *Oncogene* (1999) **18**:1723–32.
124. Dore JF, Pedeux R, Boniol M et al., Intermediate-effect biomarkers in prevention of skin cancer, *IARC Sci Publ* (2001) **154**:81–91.
125. Yoshida H, Kong YY, Yoshida R et al., Apaf1 is required for mitochondrial pathways of apoptosis and brain development, *Cell* (1998) **94**:739–50.
126. Hakem R, Hakem A, Duncan GS et al., Differential requirement for caspase 9 in apoptotic pathways in vivo, *Cell* (1998) **94**:339–52.
127. Tournier C, Hess P, Yang DD et al., Requirement of JNK for stress-induced activation of the cytochrome c-mediated death pathway, *Science* (2000) **288**:870–4.
128. Yamamoto K, Ichijo H, Korsmeyer SJ, BCL-2 is phosphorylated and inactivated by an ASK1/Jun N-terminal protein kinase pathway normally activated at G(2)/M, *Mol Cell Biol* (1999) **19**:8469–78.
129. Bossy-Wetzel E, Newmeyer DD, Green DR, Mitochondrial cytochrome c release in apoptosis occurs upstream of DEVD-specific caspase activation and independently of mitochondrial transmembrane depolarization, *EMBO J* (1998) **17**:37–49.
130. Zhuang S, Demirs JT, Kochevar IE, p38 mitogen-activated protein kinase mediates bid cleavage, mitochondrial dysfunction, and caspase-3 activation during apoptosis induced by singlet oxygen but not by hydrogen peroxide, *J Biol Chem* (2000) **275**:25939–48.
131. Sayama K, Hanakawa Y, Shirakata Y et al., Apoptosis signal-regulating kinase 1 (ASK1) is an intracellular inducer of keratinocyte differentiation, *J Biol Chem* (2001) **276**:999–1004.

11

The effect of ultraviolet light on the production and processing of proopiomelanocortin in the skin

Thomas A. Luger, Thomas Brzoska, Markus Böhm, Meinhard Schiller,

Tanja Fisbeck and Thomas Scholzen

Introduction

One of the most important environmental factors responsible for skin cancer, premature aging and immunosuppression, is ultraviolet (UV) light.[1] Exposure to UV irradiation has been demonstrated to modify cellular immune responses, such as contact hypersensitivity (CHS), and to induce allergen-specific tolerance.[2] The immunosuppressive effects of UV light are mainly mediated by the short wavelength range (UVB 290–320 nm), which is mostly absorbed within the epidermis. Among UV-induced effects, such as DNA damage and keratinocyte apoptosis, the UV-mediated upregulation of proinflammatory cytokines, such as interleukin (IL)-1, IL-6, tumor necrosis factor (TNF)-α, as well as other mediators, appears to be a crucial event responsible for the immunomodulating activity of UV light.[3,4] On the other hand, treatment of keratinocytes with UV is well known to result in an increased production of immunosuppressing cytokines, such as IL-1 receptor antagonist (IL-1RA), transforming growth factor β (TGFβ) and IL-10.[2] In animal models, application of these cytokines has been shown to result in UV-like immunosuppression, and treatment with antibodies or antagonists directed against IL-10 was found to prevent UV-mediated immunosuppression.[5–7] Thus, suppressor cytokines released upon UV irradiation appear to function as crucial mediators of UV-induced immunosuppression.

Recently, epidermal cells have been shown to produce neuropeptides, such as substance P (SP), calcitonin gene-related peptide (CGRP), and proopiomelanocortin (POMC)-derived peptides—for example, the melanocortin α melanocyte-stimulating hormone (αMSH).[8] Among these neuropeptides, αMSH, in addition to its known pigment-inducing capacity, has a strong anti-inflammatory, as well as immunomodulating, potential.[9,10] Under normal conditions, POMC-derived peptides are detectable only in minimal amounts in epidermal cells. However, proinflammatory cytokines, such as IL-1, bacterial endotoxin and environmental factors, such as UV light, are potent inducers of POMC expression and αMSH release.[3] Therefore, this paper will briefly review the current knowledge on the UV-mediated induction of αMSH, as well as its potential role in skin inflammation.

Proopiomelanocortin (POMC)-derived neuropeptides

POMC-derived peptides are generated in a complex way involving transcriptional, translational and post-translational events, which ultimately result in the production of multifunctional peptides from a single, biologically inactive precursor protein (POMC). ACTH, β-endorphin and melanocortins, such as αMSH, are the best characterized and most widely studied products of POMC processing.[11] Melanocortins have a wide range of functional properties, which includes neuroendocrine, thermoregulatory, cognitive, behavioral, cardiovascular, pigmentary, lipolytic, antiinflammatory and immunomodulatory activities.[12]

Melanocortin production is controlled by the activity of tissue-specific prohormone convertases

(PC1, PC2), which determine the spectrum of POMC products actually generated by a given cell population. These enzymes belong to the subtilisin family of serine proteinases, and show homologies to the yeast protease kex2 and to furin, a product of the protooncogene fes/fps, suggesting that evolutionarily highly-conserved principles of propeptide cleavage are utilized to generate these neuropeptides.[13,14] In addition, ACTH may be cleaved into αMSH by the activity of neutral endopeptidase 24.11 (NEP), which is present on the surface of peripheral blood mononuclear cells (PBMC).[15]

The control of POMC transcription itself is not fully understood, and central, as well as peripheral, sites of POMC expression may differ in this respect.[16] Hypothalamus-derived corticotropin-releasing hormone (CRH, CRF) is a major regulator of pituitary POMC transcription. CRH stimulates POMC transcription in the anterior and neuro-intermediate lobes of the pituitary gland, but suppresses it in the pars intermedia, while glucocorticoids inhibit it.[16,17] Interestingly, both CRH and CRH receptors have already been detected in most extrapituitary sites of POMC expression, including the skin.[18] Thus, immunocompetent cells, as well as epidermal cells, can generate CRH, suggesting that CRH also plays a role in the control of extrapituitary POMC transcription.[17]

POMC-derived peptides exert their functional activities via melanocortin receptors, a group of heterodimeric guanine-nucleotide-binding protein-coupled receptors which are characterized by seven transmembrane domains. So far, five different melanocortin receptors have been cloned (MC1-R to MC5-R). The MC1-R is coded for by a gene locus that is crucially involved in determining mouse coat color (*extension* locus), while *agouti*, another key coat-color-determining gene locus, codes for a protein that operates as a high-affinity antagonist of both the MC1-R and the MC4-R.[17–19] While the exact ligand specificity and affinity of all known MC-R is not yet fully understood, convincing evidence supports that MC1-R has equally high affinities for αMSH and ACTH, that MC2-R specifically binds ACTH and that MC3-R specifically recognizes a heptapeptide core shared by ACTH and the melanotropins. MC4-R is considered specific for α-, β- and γMSH, while MC5-R binds ACTH and the melanotropins.[17,19] Depending on the cells studied, αMSH either up- or downregulates expression of its receptor, and there is evidence for a cooperation between distinct MC-R.[19]

Tissue expression of MC-R is thought to be quite selective. For example, MC1-R was primarily found to be expressed by melanocytes, but, recently, it was also detected on several cells within the skin, as well as cells of the hematopoietic system.[3] MC2-R is expressed by the adrenal cortex and some hematopoietic cells, MC3-R in placenta and gastrointestinal mucosa, and MC3-R as well as MC4-R in selected regions of the central nervous system. MC5-R showed the widest distribution, being found in skin, adrenal cortex, gonads, skeletal muscle and lymphoid tissues. In fact, MC1-R and MC5-R may be responsible for the majority of melanocortin effects on peripheral tissues.[17,19]

Effect of UV irradiation on the production of melanocortins and melanocortin receptors in keratinocytes

Human keratinocytes, including normal cells as well as several transformed keratinocyte cell lines (KB, A431, HaCaT), have been shown to express POMC mRNA and to release POMC-peptides such as αMSH, ACTH and α-endorphin.[20,21] Unstimulated human keratinocytes and transformed keratinocyte cell lines expressed only low levels of POMC mRNA, and did not release significant amounts of αMSH. Upon stimulation with LPS, tumor promoters or the proinflammatory cytokine IL-1, a significantly enhanced POMC peptide production was observed at both the transcriptional and translational levels.[2] Similarly, UV irradiation of keratinocytes in culture was found to be a potent inducer of POMC mRNA expression and of the release of αMSH, as well as ACTH.[22,23] Both short wavelength UVB (290–300 nm) and long wavelength UVA1 (340–400 nm) upregulated POMC synthesis in keratinocytes. Using semi-quantitative RT-PCR, it was demonstrated that POMC mRNA upregulation following UVB irradiation is time- and dose-dependent, with a maximum induction 10 and 24 hours after 10 J/m^2 UVA1 or 25 mJ/cm^2 UVB.[24] Maximum release of αMSH occurred 48–72 hours after UVB irradiation of keratinocytes in culture.[21]

For the post-translational generation of POMC-peptides, specific prohormone convertases (PC1 and PC2) are required. Whereas cleavage by PC1 gives rise to β-endorphin and ACTH, PC2 generates αMSH.[13] Among other epidermal cells, keratinocytes have recently been detected to produce both PC1 and PC2, as well as the PC2-specific binding protein, 7B2, which is required for the activation of pro-PC2 into PC2.[14] UVB irradiation also turned out to significantly upregulate the expression of both PC1 and PC2, as well as 7B2, in normal as well as transformed keratinocytes. Time and dose kinetics were similar when compared to those of POMC.[25,26] These findings indicate that UVB, in addition to upregulating POMC expression, also induces the generation of prohormone convertases in the skin required for the generation of POMC-peptides, such as αMSH and ACTH.

Most interestingly, the time after UVB irradiation of keratinocytes required for maximum POMC expression and αMSH release differs significantly from that needed for the optimal generation of proinflammatory cytokines. In contrast to UV-induced POMC mRNA expression, which peaks 10–24 hours post-UV, the expression of mRNA specific for IL-1, IL-6 or TNFα is generally already upregulated within 1–2 hours after UVB exposure, and, at 12 hours post-UV-irradiation, serum levels of circulating cytokines have been detected.[2] Moreover, proinflammatory cytokines, such as IL-1, turned out to be potent inducers of POMC mRNA expression and αMSH release by keratinocytes.[21] In the presence of IL-1RA, UVB was not able to upregulate POMC mRNA expression and αMSH release, suggesting that UVB indirectly via IL-1 upregulates αMSH production.[27] On the other hand, αMSH has been shown to antagonize particular proinflammatory activities of IL-1, such as fever, thymocyte proliferation and chemokine production, possibly by inhibiting the binding of IL-1β to the IL-1 receptor type 1.[2] These findings suggest that αMSH, released at later times after UV irradiation, is responsible for the downregulation of inflammatory responses preventing the host from deleterious consequences of an overshoot in the inflammatory response.

The relevance of these *in vitro* findings is further supported by studies demonstrating that irradiation of the skin in humans resulted in the induction of POMC expression and αMSH release. Accordingly, increased levels of circulating αMSH have been found in humans following UV irradiation. Moreover, following UV irradiation with a solar simulator (2MED) suction blister fluid obtained from UV-treated skin contained significantly increased levels of αMSH. In the same experiment, using mRNA from blister roofs and RT-PCR, the expression POMC mRNA was significantly upregulated following UV treatment.[28,29] In addition to POMC, the expression of both PC1 and PC2, as well as MC1-R, was also increased in epidermal cells derived from the suction blister roofs (Brzoska et al., unpublished observation). These data indicate that UV treatment generates increased amounts of melanocortins, as well as melanocortin receptors in the skin, which may contribute to UV-mediated effects, such as inflammation, pigmentation and keratinocyte proliferation.

αMSH as a mediator of immunity and inflammation

Several studies have focused on the recently-discovered functions of αMSH in inflammation and immunity. Accordingly, it has been detected that αMSH, especially its C-terminal region, has antipyretic and anti-inflammatory properties, in part by antagonizing the activities of selected proinflammatory cytokines.[3,10] Accordingly, there is evidence that αMSH functions as an antagonist of IL-1, as it inhibited the ability of IL-1 to augment the proliferation of murine thymocytes *in vitro*.[3] Since αMSH blocks binding of IL-1β to the IL-1 receptor type I, this peptide may serve as a functional antagonist of IL-1.[30,31] This is further supported by the observation that the pyrogenic activity of IL-1 was counteracted by αMSH and that systemic αMSH administration inhibited the capacity of IL-1β to enhance plasma levels of corticosterone.[32,33]

The role of αMSH to modulate the function of antigen-presenting cells (APC) is of particular importance, and has therefore been addressed by several investigations. Studies analyzing the expression of MC-R on monocytes provided clear evidence that peripheral blood-derived monocytes, after treatment with LPS which is well known to induce monocyte differentiation into macrophages, expressed significant amounts of MC-1R mRNA and protein.[34] In addition, monocytic cell lines (THP1, U937), as well as dendritic cells generated from peripheral blood-derived monocytes upon culture with IL-4, GM-CSF and monocyte-conditioned medium (MCM), were also found to express increased levels of MC-1R.[35,36] These data indicate that MC-1R expression is upregulated, irrespective of whether differentiation occurs into macrophages or dendritic cells.

There is evidence, from several studies, that αMSH regulates the migration and other functions of monocytes, possibly by modulating the secretion of chemokines such as IL-8 and Gro-α.[37] In addition, the production of proinflammatory nitric oxide and neopterin by macrophages was inhibited by αMSH.[38] Moreover, αMSH has been demonstrated to upregulate mRNA expression and release of IL-10 in monocytes in a dose-dependent manner.[39] On the other hand, the synthesis and release of proinflammatory cytokines, such as IL-1, IL-6 and TNFα, was downregulated by αMSH.[40] αMSH also turned out to be a potent inhibitor of IL-1-mediated effects, such as thymocyte proliferation and fever induction.[41] In addition to regulating cytokine production, there is evidence that αMSH downregulates the expression of MHC class I molecules on monocytes, and significantly suppresses the expression of accessory molecules, such as CD86 and CD40, on monocytes and dendritic cells.[34,36] Since αMSH blocks accessory signals and additionally induces suppressor factors such as IL-10, it may be one of the signals required for the downregulation of an immune response and possibly the induction of tolerance. This was further supported by recent experiments demonstrating that treatment of haptenized immature dendritic cells with αMSH resulted in the generation of CTLA$^+$-4 T-suppressor lymphocytes which, upon i.v. injection into naive mice, were able to induce hapten-specific tolerance.[42]

The molecular mechanisms underlying αMSH-mediated effects are not yet completely understood. The activation of the transcription factor NFκB appears to be a crucial event in immune and inflammatory responses. NFκB is activated by proinflammatory cytokines, such as IL-1 and TNFα, as well as endotoxin and other stimuli.[43] It controls the expression of many genes involved in inflammation, including cytokines, MHC class I, adhesion molecules or nitric oxide synthetase. Upon treatment with αMSH, the TNFα, IL-1-, LPS- and ceramide-mediated activation of NFκB was significantly suppressed in a dose- and time-dependent manner.[31,44] Moreover, the TNFα-mediated degradation of the inhibitory subunit IκBα and the nuclear translocation of the p65 subunit of NFκB was inhibited. The αMSH-mediated inhibition of NFκB activation appears to be dependent on cAMP. Suppression of NFκB activation was not cell specific, and could be observed in monocytes, monocytic cell lines (U937), keratinocytes and endothelial cells.[31,44,45] These data suggest that αMSH exerts its anti-inflammatory and immunomodulating effects by generally inhibiting NFκB activation.

In vivo, using a murine model of contact hypersensitivity (CHS), it has been demonstrated that systemic, as well as topical, application of αMSH blocks the elicitation as well as the sensitization phase of CHS and is capable of inducing hapten-specific tolerance.[46] Systemic αMSH did not affect the development of an experimental irritant dermatitis, and the tolerance induction by αMSH could be blocked by s.c. administration of an IL-10 antibody at the site of sensitization.[46] Interestingly, αMSH selectively induced the production of IL-10 by human peripheral blood monocytes *in vitro*, and a single, systemic application of αMSH suffices to induce a long-lasting elevation of IL-10 serum levels in mice.[3,39] *In vitro*, αMSH, however, was not able to affect the production of IL-10 by T-lymphocytes.[39] There is also evidence that αMSH inhibited the synthesis of IFNγ by T-lymphocytes and the production of IL-12 by monocytes (Becher et al., unpublished observation).[47,48] Like IL-10, αMSH may also be one of the signals which downregulate MHC class I expression.[49] Mitogen or endotoxin treatment upregulated MC1-R expression on human monocytes *in vitro*, while TNFα stimulated αMSH production by macrophages *in vitro*.[35] This suggests that proinflammatory stimuli increase the sensitivity of monocytes/macrophages to stimulation by αMSH and increase production of this immunosuppressive neuropeptide.

The main immunomodulatory function of αMSH is, apparently, to serve as a major negative-feedback signal to control and antagonize inflammatory immune responses. The elevated αMSH serum levels described in many chronic inflammatory diseases, like rheumatoid arthritis, viral and parasitic diseases, atopic eczema and psoriasis, may well reflect such a counter-regulatory task of αMSH for keeping proinflammatory immune responses in check.[10–17] However, clinical observations, like the positive correlation of high αMSH levels with an increased survival time of AIDS patients, question whether this fully reflects the spectrum of immunomodulatory properties of αMSH *in vivo*.[50]

Recent *in vitro* studies suggest that αMSH can also modulate the IL-4- or anti-CD40-driven IgE synthesis and release by B-cells. Accordingly, pharmacological doses of αMSH strongly inhibited induced IgE synthesis.[51] However, this activity of αMSH appears to require the presence of monocytes. This may be relevant to the pathobiology of atopy and allergic diseases, and is in line with indications that αMSH is a mast cell secretagogue, since it was shown to enhance the release of histamine by a human skin mast cells line *in vitro*.[52] Indeed, the function of αMSH as a mediator of allergic diseases has recently been supported in a murine model of allergy and asthma induced by sensitization to ovalbumin (OVA). In contrast to control animals, the levels of αMSH in the bronchoalveolar lavage fluids (BALF) were significantly downregulated during acute airway inflammation. On the other hand, treatment of mice with αMSH prior to sensitization or challenge with OVA significantly reduced the frequency of eosinophils and IL-5 levels in BALF, but increased IL-10 levels.[53] This further supports the notion that αMSH may play an important role as one of the mediators involved in the control of immune and inflammatory reactions in allergic diseases, such as asthma and atopic eczema.

There is evidence that αMSH also stimulates the cytokine production of normal melanocytes *in vitro*, which could be relevant in the context of the regulatory, non-pigmentary roles proposed for epidermal melanocytes.[17] Most notably, αMSH was found to be a potent, and apparently selective, stimulus for chemokine secretion by endothelial cells and fibroblasts, since it increased IL-8 secretion of human dermal microvascular endothelial cells as well as fibroblasts *in vitro*.[54,55] Although αMSH upregulates chemokine production, it has also been demonstrated to inhibit IL-8-mediated chemotaxis of neutrophils.[40] By this property, αMSH which, by inducing IL-8, is involved in the upregulation of adhesion molecule expression on endothelial cells and, by inhibiting the motility of neutrophils, may contribute to the accumulation of inflammatory cells at the site of inflammation.

Endothelial cells play a crucial role in inflammation and immune reactions. The multiple steps of recruitment and transmigration of inflammatory leukocytes to the vascular wall require the co-ordinated temporal and spatial expression and presentation of cellular adhesion molecules, such as E-selectin, L-selectin, vascular adhesion molecule-1 (VCAM-1), intercellular adhesion molecue-1 (ICAM-1), and β2 integrins on both endothelial cells and leukocytes.[56] The expression of these molecules can be induced by stimulation with UV light, tumor promoters, IL-1, TNFα and neuropeptides.[57,58] Recent investigations focused on the capacity of αMSH to modulate biologic functions of human dermal microvascular endothelial cells and their capacity to express melanocortin receptors. Accordingly, HDMEC constitutively expressed only low amounts of MC-1R, which were significantly upregulated upon stimulation with IL-1.[54] After binding to MC-1R in a dose-dependent manner, αMSH was capable of downregulating the LPS-induced expression of ICAM-1, VCAM and E-selectin.[45] Using *in vitro* adhesion assays, αMSH significantly suppressed the LPS-mediated adhesion of T- or B-lymphoblastoid cell lines to an HDMEC monolayer.[9,45] As in monocytes, the signaling pathway involved in the regulation of adhesion molecule expression appears to involve NFκB, since αMSH was capable of inhibiting the LPS- or IL-1-mediated activation of NFκB in HDMEC.[45] The *in vivo* effect of αMSH on vascular endothelial cells was investigated using a mouse model of leucocytoclastic vasculitis, the local Shwartzman reaction.[59] In this model, local subcutaneous injection of low-dose LPS (preparatory phase) is followed by systemic application of LPS after 24 hours (challenge). When mice were injected i.v. with αMSH prior to the preparatory phase, a marked reduction of vascular hemorrhage in the challenge phase was observed. This inhibition was also associated with a significantly diminished expression of E-selectin and VCAM-1, as determined by immunohistochemistry.[59] These findings suggest that αMSH, by modulating the expression of different cellular adhesion molecules, may prevent adhesion of inflammatory cells to the vascular wall that may, in turn, significantly contribute to the downregulation of an inflammatory response.

Conclusions

The production of the POMC-derived peptide, αMSH, in the skin is upregulated following injurious stimuli, such as UV irradiation, and appears to be a crucial mediator regulating post-injurious inflammation and immunomodulation. Accordingly, UV-induced epidermal-cell-derived αMSH is, apparently, one of the mediators responsible for the UV-mediated immunosuppression, as well as tolerance induction. The immunomodulating effects of αMSH are mainly exerted via interaction with the MC-1R, which is expressed on monocytes, macrophages and dendritic cells, whereas the anti-inflammatory function of αMSH can be explained by the capacity of αMSH to downregulate the expression of adhesion molecules on dermal microvascular endothelial cells. Proinflammatory signals, such as IL-1, TNFα or LPS, appear to be required to induce MC-1R expression on inflammatory cells and endothelial cells since, under normal conditions without pro-inflammatory stimuli, MC-1R is barely detectable on these cells. Inflammation constitutes a prerequisite for αMSH in order to exert its anti-inflammatory and immunomodulating activities. Therefore, the melanocortins may belong to the essential pathways that have evolved to check the persistent inflammatory reaction and to prevent uncontrolled and chronic inflammation.

Acknowledgements

This work was supported by grants from the Deutsche Forschungsgemeinschaft SFB 293 B7 and SCH 629 1-1 and the Centre de Recherche et Investigations Epidermiques et Sensorielles (CERIES), Paris.

References

1. Beissert S, Granstein RD, UV-induced cutaneous photobiology, *Crit Rev Biochem Mol Biol* (1996) **31**:381–404.
2. Luger TA, Schwarz T, Effects of UV-light on cytokines and neuroendocrine hormones. In: Krutmann J, Elmets C, eds, *Photoimmunology* (Blackwell: Oxford, 1995) 55–76.
3. Luger TA, Scholzen T, Grabbe S, The role of α-melanocyte stimulating hormone in cutaneous biology, *J Invest Dermatol Symp Proc* (1997) **2**:87–93.
4. Beissert S, Schwarz T, Mechanisms invoved in ultraviolet light-induced immunosuppression, *J Invest Dermatol Symp Proc* (1999) **4**:61–64.
5. Beissert S, Hosoi J, Kühn R et al., Impaired immunosuppressive response to ultraviolet radiation in interleukin-10-deficient mice, *J Invest Dermatol* (1996) **107**:553–7.
6. Lee HS, Kooshesh F, Sauder DN et al., Modulation of TGF-beta 1 production from human keratinocytes by UVB, *Exp Dermatol* (1997) **6**:105–10.
7. Shreedhar V, Giese T, Sung VW et al., A cytokine cascade including prostaglandin E2, IL-4, and IL-10 is responsible for UV-induced systemic immune suppression, *J Immunol Meth* (1998) **160**:3783–9.
8. Scholzen T, Armstrong CA, Bunnett NW et al., Neuropeptides in the skin: interactions between the neuroendocrine and the skin immune systems, *Exp Dermatol* (1998) **7**:81–96.
9. Luger TA, Kalden D, Scholzen TE et al., alpha-melanocyte-stimulating hormone as a mediator of tolerance induction, *Pathobiology* (1999) **67**: 318–21.
10. Lipton JM, Catania A, Antiinflammatory actions of the neuroimmunomodulator α-MSH, *Immunol Today* (1997) **18**:140–5.
11. Eberle AN, *The Melanotropins* (Karger: Basel, 1988).
12. Luger TA, Scholzen T, Brzoska T et al., Cutaneous immunomodulation and coordination of skin stress responses by alpha-melanocyte-stimulating hormone, *Ann N Y Acad Sci* (1998) **840**:381–94.
13. Seidah NG, Benjannet S, Hamelin J et al., The subtilisin/kexin family of precursor convertases. Emphasis on PC1, PC2/7B2, POMC and the novel enzyme SKI-1, *Ann N Y Acad Sci* (1999) **885**:57–74.
14. Seidah NG, Day R, Marcinkiewicz M et al., Precursor convertases: an evolutionary ancient, cell-specific, combinatorial mechanism yielding diverse bioactive peptides and proteins, *Ann N Y Acad Sci* (1998) **839**:9–24.
15. Deschodt Lanckman M, Vanneste Y, Loir B et al., Degradation of alpha-melanocyte stimulating hormone (alpha-MSH) by CALLA/endopeptidase 24.11 expressed by human melanoma cells in culture, *Int J Cancer* (1990) **46**:1124–30.
16. Autelitano DJ, Blum M, Lopingco M et al., Corticotropin-releasing factor differentially regulates anterior and intermediate pituitary lobe proopiomelanocortin gene transcription, nuclear precursor

RNA and mature mRNA in vivo, *Neuroendocrinology* (1990) **51**:123–30.

17. Slominski A, Wortsman J, Luger T et al., Corticotropin releasing hormone and proopiomelanocortin involvement in the cutaneous response to stress, *Physiol Rev* (2000) **80**:979–1020.
18. Lu D, Willard D, Patel IR et al., Agouti protein is an antagonist of the melanocyte-stimulating-hormone receptor, *Nature* (1994) **371**:799–802.
19. Cone RD, Lu D, Koppula S et al., The melanocortin receptors: agonists, antagonists, and the hormonal control of pigmentation, *Recent Prog Horm Res* (1996) **51**:287–317.
20. Wintzen M, Gilchrest BA, Proopiomelanocortin, its derived peptides, and the skin, *J Invest Dermatol* (1996) **106**:3–10.
21. Schauer E, Trautinger F, Köck A et al., Proopiomelanocortin derived peptides are synthesized and released by human keratinocytes, *J Clin Invest* (1994) **93**:2258–62.
22. Chakraborty A, Slominski A, Ermak G et al., Ultraviolet B and melanocyte-stimulating hormone (MSH) stimulate mRNA production for alpha MSH receptors and proopiomelanocortin-derived peptides in mouse melanoma cells and transformed keratinocytes, *J Invest Dermatol* (1995) **105**:655–9.
23. Dissanayake NS, Mason RS, Modulation of skin cell functions by transforming growth factor β1 and ACTH after ultraviolet irradiation, *J Endocrinol* (1998) **159**:153–63.
24. Brzoska T, Scholzen T, Becher E et al., Effect of UV light on the production of proopiomelanocortin-derived peptides and melanocortin receptors in the skin. In: Altmeyer P, Hoffmann K, Stücker M, eds, *Skin Cancer and UV-radiation* (Springer-Verlag: Berlin, 1997) 227–37.
25. Fisbeck T, Schiller M, Kalden DH et al., Human skin cells in vitro express the neuroendocrine-specific prohormone convertase 2 cofactor 7B2, *J Invest Dermatol* (1999) **112**:600.
26. Brzoska T, Scholzen T, Becher E et al., UVB irradiation regulates the expression of proopiomelanocortin, prohormone convertase 1 and melanocortin receptor 1 by human keratinocytes, *J Invest Dermatol* (1997) **108**:622.
27. Luger TA, Schwarz T, Kalden DH et al., Role of epidermal cell-derived α-melanocyte stimulating hormone in ultraviolet light mediated local immunosuppression, *Ann N Y Acad Sci* (1999) **885**:209–16.
28. Kalden DH, Brzoska T, Schwarz T et al., UV-induced production of immunosuppressive mediators in human skin: prevention by a broadspectrum sunscreen, *J Invest Dermatol* (1999) **113**:468.
29. Holzmann A, Altmeyer P, Stohr L et al., Modification of αMSH by UVA irradiation of the skin, *Hautarzt* (1983) **34**:294–7.
30. Mugridge KG, Perretti M, Ghiara P et al., Alpha-melanocyte-stimulating hormone reduces interleukin-1 beta effects on rat stomach preparations possibly through interference with a type I receptor, *Eur J Pharmacol* (1991) **197**:151–5.
31. Brzoska T, Kalden DH, Scholzen T et al., Molecular basis of α-MSH/IL-1 antagonism, *Ann N Y Acad Sci* (1999) **885**:230–8.
32. Cannon JG, Tatro JB, Reichlin S et al., Alpha melanocyte stimulating hormone inhibits immunostimulatory and inflammatory actions of interleukin 1, *J Immunol* (1986) **137**:2232–6.
33. Daynes RA, Robertson BA, Cho BH et al., Alpha-melanocyte-stimulating hormone exhibits target cell selectivity in its capacity to affect interleukin 1-inducible responses in vivo and in vitro, *J Immunol* (1987) **139**:103–9.
34. Bhardwaj RS, Becher E, Mahnke K et al., Evidence for the differential expression of the functional alpha melanocyte stimulating hormone receptor MC-1 on human monocytes, *J Immunol* (1997) **158**:3378–84.
35. Star RA, Rajora N, Huang J et al., Evidence of autocrine modulation of macrophage nitric oxide synthase by alpha-MSH, *Proc Natl Acad Sci U S A* (1995) **92**:8016–20.
36. Becher E, Mahnke K, Brzoska T et al., Human peripheral blood-derived dendritic cells express functional melanocortin receptor MC-1R, *Ann N Y Acad Sci* (1999) **885**:188–95.
37. Genedani S, Bernardi M, Baldini MG et al., Influence of CRF and alpha-MSH on the migration of human monocytes in vitro, *Neuropeptides* (1992) **23**:99–102.
38. Rajora N, Ceriani G, Catania A et al., alpha-MSH production, receptors, and influence on neopterin in a human monocyte/macrophage cell line, *J Leukoc Biol* (1996) **59**:248–53.
39. Bhardwaj RS, Schwarz A, Becher E et al., Proopiomelanocortin-derived peptides induce IL-10 production in human monocytes, *J Immunol* (1996) **156**:2517–21.
40. Lipton JM, Catania A, Mechanisms of antiinflammatory action of the neuroimmunomodulator peptide α-MSH, *Ann NY Acad Sci* (1998) **840**:373–80.
41. Huang QH, Hruby VJ, Tatro JB, Systemic alpha-MSH suppresses LPS fever via central melanocortin receptors independently of its sup-

pression of corticosterone and IL-6 release, *Am J Physiol* (1998) **275(2 Pt 2)**:R524–30.
42. Brzoska T, Schwarz A, Moeller M et al., Treatment of murine BMDC with α-MSH results in the generation of T-suppressor cells, *J Invest Dermatol* (2001) **117**.
43. Baeuerle PA, Baltimore D, NF-kappa B: ten years after, *Cell* (1996) **87**:13–20.
44. Manna SK, Aggarwal BB, α-melanocyte-stimulating hormone inhibits the nuclear transcription factor NF-κB activation induced by various inflammatory agents, *J Immunol* (1998) **161**:2873–80.
45. Kalden DH, Scholzen T, Brzoska T et al., Mechanisms of the antiinflammatory effects of α-MSH: Role of transcription factor NF-κB and adhesion molecule expression, *Ann N Y Acad Sci* (1999) **885**:254–61.
46. Grabbe S, Bhardwaj RS, Steinert M et al., Alpha-melanocyte stimulating hormone induces hapten-specific tolerance in mice, *J Immunol* (1996) **156**: 473–8.
47. Taylor AW, Streilein JW, Cousins SW, Alpha-melanocyte-stimulating hormone suppresses antigen-stimulated T cell production of gamma-interferon, *Neuroimmunomodulation* (1994) **1**: 188–94.
48. Luger TA, Schauer E, Trautinger F et al., Production of immunosuppressing melanotropins by keratinocytes, *Ann N Y Acad Sci* (1993) **680**:567–70.
49. Luger TA, Köck A, Schauer E et al., Cytokine neuropeptide interactions in the skin. In: Van Vlothen WA, Lambert WC, eds, *Basic Mechanism of Psysiological and Aberrant Lymphoproliferation in the Skin* (Plenum Press: New York, 1994) 95–102.
50. Catania A, Airaghi L, Garofalo L et al., The neuropeptide alpha-MSH in HIV infection and other disorders in humans, *Ann N Y Acad Sci* (1998) **840**:848–56.
51. Aebischer I, Stämpfli MR, Zürcher A et al., Neuropeptides are potent modulators of human in vitro immunoglobulin E synthesis, *Eur J Immunol* (1994) **24**:1908–13.
52. Grutzkau A, Henz BM, Kirchhof L et al., Alpha-melanocyte stimulating hormone acts as a selective inducer of secretory functions in human mast cells, *Biochem Biophys Res Commun* (2000) **278**: 14–19.
53. Raap U, Brzoska T, Päth G et al., α-Melanocyte stimulating hormone (α-MSH) is a modulator of immune responses in allergen-induced airway inflammation in vivo, *Allergy* (2001) **56**:21.
54. Hartmeyer M, Scholzen T, Becher E et al., Human microvascular endothelial cells (HMEC-1) express the melanocortin receptor type 1 and produce increased levels of IL-8 upon stimulation with αMSH, *J Immunol* (1997) **159**:1930–7.
55. Böhm M, Schulte U, Kalden DH et al., Alpha-melanocyte-stimulating hormone modulates activation of NF-κB and AP-1 and secretion of IL-8 in human dermal fibroblasts, *Ann N Y Acad Sci* (1999) **885**:277–86.
56. Butcher EC, Leukocyte-endothelial cell recognition: three (or more) steps to specificity and diversity, *Cell* (2000) **67**:1033–6.
57. Scholzen T, Hartmeyer M, Fastrich M et al., Ultraviolet light and interleukin-10 modulate expression of cytokines by transformed human dermal microvascular endothelial cells (HMEC-1), *J Invest Dermatol* (1998) **111**:50–6.
58. Swerlick RA, Lawley TJ, Role of microvascular endothelial cells in inflammation, *J Invest Dermatol* (1993) **100**:111S–15S.
59. Sunderkötter C, Kalden DH, Brzoska T et al., α-MSH reduces vasculitis in the local Shwartzman reaction, *Ann N Y Acad Sci* (1999) **885**:414–18.

12

Melanocortin peptides and their control of skin pigmentation

Janis Ancans, Marina Tsatmali, Martin J. Hoogduijn and Anthony J. Thody

Introduction

Skin colour is determined by the relative amounts of eumelanin and phaeomelanin produced by epidermal melanocytes.[1,2] The mechanisms involved in regulating the production of these pigments are not fully understood. Recent interest has focused on the role of the melanocortin signaling system, as it is well recognized that melanocortin peptides, such as α-melanocyte stimulating hormone (α-MSH) and adrenocorticotrophin (ACTH), increase skin darkening in humans.[3,4] It is also clear that these peptides increase melanogenesis and, more specifically, eumelanin production in cultured human melanocytes.[5–8] More recently, it has been suggested that the melanocortin-1 receptor (MC-1R) is a key control point in the regulation of pigmentation phenotype. Thus, there are reports of MC-1R variants in red-haired individuals and persons with poor tanning ability.[9–11] More than 30 allelic variants have now been identified[12,13] and three of these, Arg151Cys, Arg160Trp and Asp294His, were found to be associated with red hair. These three alleles were shown to be loss-of-function mutants,[14,15] and this would explain the lack of responsiveness to α-MSH previously observed in melanocytes from red-haired persons.[16] These mutations have little effect on receptor binding but disrupt receptor coupling to the cAMP pathway. Loss-of-function mutations of pro-opiomelanocortin (POMC), the melanocortin precursor, have also been shown to be associated with red hair and pale skin phenotypes.[17]

As well as being involved in controlling constitutive skin pigmentation, there is evidence that the melanocortin signaling system is important for facultative pigmentation and may mediate the pigmentary effects of UVR. Thus, it has been shown that UVR stimulates the secretion of α-MSH by keratinocytes,[18,19] and the expression of MC-1R on melanoma cells and human melanocytes.[20,21] This may explain why the skin-darkening effects of the melanocortins are especially pronounced in areas of the skin normally exposed to the sun.[3,4,22]

How the melanocortin signaling system functions to regulate skin pigmentation is uncertain, and numerous questions remain. For instance, although the acetylated form of α-MSH is a potent agonist at the human MC-1R (hMC-1R), other POMC cleavage products could serve as naturally occurring ligands at this receptor. It is also possible that the hMC-1R couples to other intracellular signaling pathways as well as the cAMP pathway. Another question concerns the actions of α-MSH and whether these are confined to melanogenesis or can affect other processes associated with the pigmentary response. We should also recognize that skin pigmentation is not regulated solely by the melanocortin signaling system, and consider that several systems are involved acting both independently and through interactions with the melanocortins. We have been addressing these questions during the last few years and, in this article, present some of our recent findings.

The origin of the hMC-1R ligands

The melanocortins are produced from the proteolytic cleavage of the 31–36 kDa POMC. The main site of POMC production is the pituitary, although it is expressed and undergoes cleavage at other sites, including the skin. α-MSH was the first melanocortin to be identified in the skin[23] but other melanocortins, including several ACTH peptides, are present in the skin and at concentrations exceeding those of α-MSH.[24] One of the most abundant of these is ACTH1-17. This peptide not only serves as an intermediate during the cleavage of ACTH to α-MSH[25,26] but, as discussed later, also functions as a potent agonist at the hMC-1R.[27,28]

Keratinocytes are a major source of these peptides, although α-MSH is also abundant in melanocytes.[24] The predominant form of α-MSH in the skin, as in other extrapituitary sites, is desacetyl MSH.[23,24] There are reports that γ-MSH peptides are present in human skin, but whether they are produced there or are of neural origin is unclear.[29] β-lipotrophin has also been found in the skin[30] but there is no evidence to suggest that this is cleaved to β-MSH, as occurs in the pituitary. Local mechanisms are important in skin homeostasis and it is not unreasonable that melanocytes would be regulated by melanocortins that are locally produced. The presence of local control mechanisms may help to explain why there are regional differences in skin pigmentation. The fact that melanocytes produce α-MSH suggests that this peptide may function as an autocrine mediator.

Actions at the MC-1R

Acetylated α-MSH is a potent agonist at the hMC-1R. Desacetyl α-MSH, on the other hand, the most abundant α-MSH in the skin, is a relatively weak agonist.[27] ACTH peptides also bind and activate the hMC-1R. Of these, the full-length ACTH peptide, ACTH1-39, binds with an affinity considerably lower than that of acetylated α-MSH, but ACTH1-17 shows comparable binding to that of acetylated α-MSH and is equipotent with acetylated α-MSH in stimulating cyclic AMP (cAMP) production.[24,27] It has been reported that, unlike the α-MSH peptides, ACTH1-17 also increases the production of inositol trisphosphate (IP3).[27] This suggests that ACTH1-17 causes the MC-1R to couple to both the cAMP and the IP3/DAG pathways. Thus, while α-MSH acts selectively via protein kinase A, ACTH1-17 will, in addition, activate protein kinase C and should stimulate the release of intracellular calcium. We have currently shown that ACTH1-17 increases Ca^{2+} in human melanocytes (Hoogduijn MJ, unpublished work). Since α-MSH had a similar effect, we would postulate that the increases in intracellular Ca^{2+} that occur in response to MC-1R activation are not necessarily mediated via IP3.

Desacetyl α-MSH is a partial agonist at the hMC-1R

As mentioned above, desacetyl α-MSH is a relatively weak agonist at the hMC-1R and a weak activator of cAMP production. However, we have found that desacetyl α-MSH can function as a partial agonist at the hMC-1R and is capable of blocking the stimulatory actions of acetylated α-MSH and ACTH1-17[31] (Tsatmali M, unpublished work). Interestingly, desacetyl α-MSH acts in the same way to inhibit the actions of α-MSH in *Anolis* melanophores.[32] Therefore, while desacetyl α-MSH may be of little importance as a stimulator of melanocyte function, it could have significance by modulating the actions of potent MC-1R agonists, such as acetylated α-MSH and ACTH1-17. The way in which POMC is cleaved and the resulting profile of melanocortin peptides could have an important bearing on melanocyte function.

Antagonists of MC-1R signaling

In many mammals, hair pigmentation is regulated by interactions involving the melanocortins and the product of the *agouti* locus. Evidence suggests that the agouti signal protein (ASP) is produced in the hair papilla and acts to downregulate the functioning of the MC-1R in the murine hair follicular melanocytes.[33] In this way, ASP inhibits the effects of α-MSH on coat pigmentation. It has been also reported that ASP can antagonize the actions of MSH on human melanocytes *in vitro*.[34] However, this mechanism may not have the same importance in the regulation of human epidermal melanocytes as in the murine hair follicle. In the first place, human ASP is not produced locally and, secondly, the human ASP receptor lacks the cytoplasmic domain present in its mouse counterpart.[35] Moreover, there are no indications that human ASP has a pigmentary function *in vivo*. It therefore remains speculative as to whether the

ASP has any relevance in the regulation of the skin pigmentation in humans.

Whether other α-MSH antagonists are present and functional in human skin is not yet clear. One possible candidate is the melanin-concentrating hormone (MCH). This peptide was first identified for its ability to antagonize the effects of α-MSH on the melanophores of teleosts.[36] We have recently shown that MCH and its receptor are expressed in human skin.[37] Sequence analysis of the pro-MCH revealed the full-length transcript as well as a spliced variant lacking exon 2. In the same study, it was shown that human melanocytes expressed the MCH receptor, SLC-1, and, when activated by MCH, it antagonized the pigmentary actions of α-MSH. Our findings suggest that the MCH/SLC-1 signaling system is present in human skin and may function as a negative regulator of pigmentation (Hoogduijn et al, not yet published).

How do the melanocortins act to bring about a pigmentary response?

It is now well accepted that the melanocortins act to stimulate melanogenesis and, more specifically, the synthesis of eumelanin.[38,39] This involves upregulation of tyrosinase enzymatic activity and there is evidence that α-MSH can increase both *de novo* expression of tyrosinase and activity of pre-existing enzyme (see later).[8,40] A successful pigmentary response is, however, not solely dependent upon the production of melanin. Other processes, such as dendrite formation and the transfer of melanin from the melanocyte into the keratinocyte, are also important and are likely to represent additional control points for pigmentation. Whether the melanocortins regulate melanin transfer is unclear. Nevertheless, they are capable of stimulating melanocyte dendricity[7,8,16] and this will ensure contact with neighbouring keratinocytes and permit the transfer of melanin.[41]

cAMP is the key second messenger that mediates the actions of melanocortins on melanocyte dendricity and melanogenesis[8,16] (Fig. 12.1). However, whilst some melanocyte cultures fail to show a melanogenic response to α-MSH, they often respond morphologically, which suggests that melanogenesis and dendricity are controlled independently.[16,42] It is likely that there is divergence in the downstream signaling pathways that control these two processes. In support of this, it has been shown that, while cAMP-induced melanogenesis and dendricity can involve an inhibition of the PI3-kinase/ p70S6-kinase pathway, inhibition of p706S6-kinase induces melanogenesis without affecting melanocyte morphology.[43]

Control of melanogenesis at the melanosomal level

There now seems little doubt that the MC-1R is a control point for pigmentation. However, even if the melanocortin signaling system is functioning, melanogenesis will ultimately depend upon the level of tyrosinase activity. As discussed above, α-MSH stimulates expression of tyrosinase and can also promote increases in tyrosinase activity without affecting enzyme abundance.[44,45] It has been suggested that a pool of inactive tyrosinase exists in melanocytes and that one of the actions of MSH is to increase the activity of this pre-existing pool.[46–49] This post-translational activation of tyrosinase would provide an important control point of action for MSH and represent a regulatory mechanism for melanin synthesis. Whilst the stimulation of tyrosinase expression by MC-1R and cAMP signaling pathway has been characterized,[42] it is unclear as to how MSH brings about an activation of tyrosinase. There have been several suggestions and we have recently considered the possibility that one mechanism could include the regulation of melanosomal pH.

Since the catalytic domains of tyrosinase are located on the inner side of the melanosomal membrane, its activity will be dependent upon the melanosomal environment. There are several reports that melanosomes are acidic organelles and, when mature, can have a pH as low as 4.[52,53] However, tyrosinase is relatively inactive at $pH<5$ and shows optimal activity at neutral pH.[49,54,55] This led us to propose that, although melanosomal pH can be acidic, such conditions do not favour melanogenesis and that this process will be stimulated as melanosomal acidity is reduced.[50,51] In support of this, there is evidence that neutralization of acidic organelle pH, using the weak base ammonium chloride, increases melanogenesis in mouse melanoma cells[48] and melanocytes.[46,56]

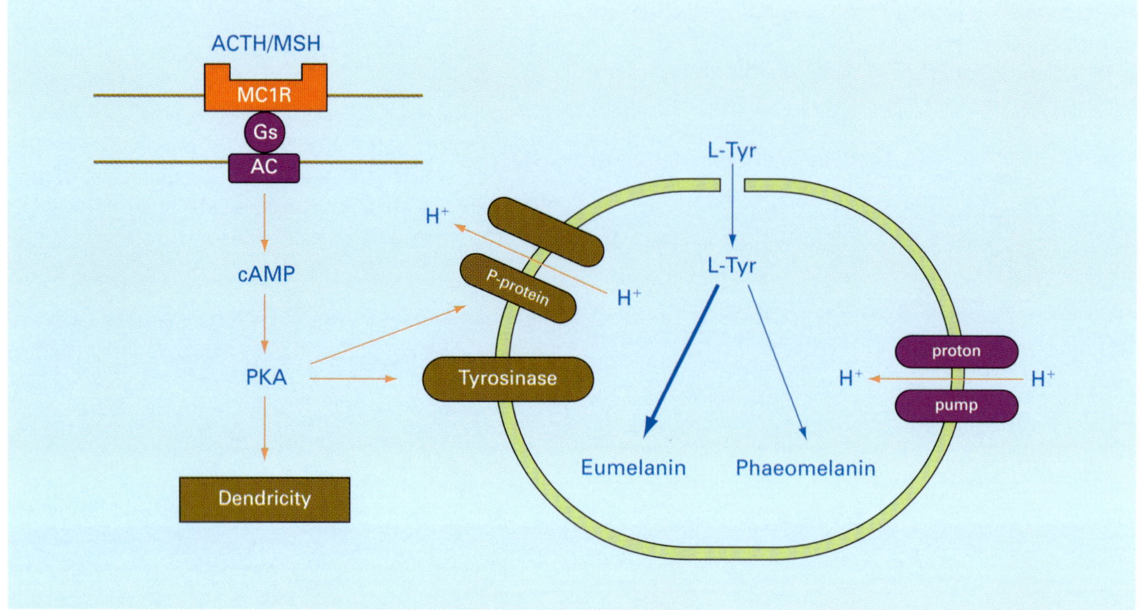

Figure 12.1

The melanocortin signaling system regulates melanocyte dendricity and melanogenesis. Whilst regulation of tyrosinase abundance is an important control point, eumelanin production will depend upon the catalytic activity of tyrosinase. Tyrosinase activity depends upon melanosomal pH which is controlled by the v-type proton pump and P-protein. We propose that the melanocortin signaling system stimulates eumelanogenesis by modulating melanosomal pH through an increase in P-protein expression.

Similar results have been obtained using selective vacuolar type H^+-ATPase inhibitors (bafilomycin A1 and concanamycin A), which were effective in inducing melanogenesis in amelanotic but tyrosinase-positive mouse and human melanoma cells.[51] These effects were not inhibited by cycloheximide and this is consistent with a non-genomic mechanism of activation.

We have recently extended these observations to human melanocytes from different Caucasian skin types.[57] All melanocyte cultures showed rapid (within 24 hours) increases in melanogenesis and melanosomal maturation in response to neutralization of melanosomal pH, suggesting that the low melanosomal pH in Caucasian melanocytes is sub-optimal for tyrosinase activity and, thus, suppresses melanin production.

How melanosomal pH is controlled is not yet clear, but our recent results would implicate the P-locus protein.[57,58] Thus, we have shown that neutralization of acidic organelle pH restores melanogenesis in P-protein-negative mouse and human pigment cells. In the light of our findings, and the fact that the P-locus protein is homologous to the *E.coli* Na^+/H^+ anti-porter, we would propose that the P-protein functions as a channel which acts to reduce the proton concentration inside the melanosome and, in this way, regulates tyrosinase activity. Indeed, it has been shown that transfection of B16 mouse melanoma cells with P-gene cDNA results in increased tyrosinase activity and melanogenesis, but with no corresponding changes in the amounts of tyrosinase, or TRP-1 and TRP-2.[59] The same workers reported that increases in the catalytic activity of tyrosinase in response to α-MSH correlate with P-protein expression in human melanocytes. Furthermore, *in situ* hybridization has revealed that UVR also increases the expression of P-locus in melanocytes in human skin.[60] It has been shown that the presence of P-protein is essential for eumelanin production,[61,62] and this is of interest because, as mentioned above, an increase in eumelanin production is a characteristic of pigmentary response to melanocortin peptides. Finally, it has been reported that skin of the extremities of P-locus-deficient mice was unable to pigment in response to UVR, although melanocyte numbers, proliferation rate and dendricity were the same as in wild-type P-locus-strain skin.[63] There is, therefore, increasing evidence that the P-protein is involved in the regulation of tyrosinase catalytic activity, and we would suggest that the P-locus is a potential target for the melanocortin signaling pathway and UVR (Fig. 12.1).

Conclusions

There seems little doubt that the melanocortin signaling system is of importance for human skin pigmentation. It seems reasonable to suppose that this involves local mechanisms and will depend upon the processing of POMC and the actions of the resulting peptides at the hMC-1R. Several POMC-derived peptides have been shown to function as ligands at the hMC-1R and one of the most potent is ACTH1-17. Interestingly, the most abundant form of α-MSH in the skin, desacetyl α-MSH, functions as a partial agonist at the hMC-1R. The way in which POMC is processed in the skin is, therefore, likely to be of importance in the regulation of this receptor and, hence, pigmentation. At the present time, little is known about the control mechanisms that regulate POMC expression, although there is evidence that UVR is involved and this has led to the view that melanocortins serve as mediators of UV- induced pigmentation. Whether UV affects the processing of POMC and can alter the way in which the melanocortins act at the hMC-1R is unknown. To what extent other locally produced factors affect melanocortin signaling is also unclear. One such peptide, MCH, has been shown to antagonize the pigmentary actions of α-MSH in cultured human melanocytes and it would be of interest to know whether this action has any significance in the skin.

There is increasing evidence to suggest that the pigmentary actions of α-MSH and other melanocortins are not confined to melanogenesis. It is now recognized that these peptides stimulate melanocyte dendricity and, as we have previously proposed, could play a key role in maintaining the integrity of the epidermal-melanin unit. This is obviously essential for the transfer of melanin into the keratinocytes. There is no evidence, at present, that melanocortins can affect melanin transfer but this is a possibility that needs investigation.

During recent years, there has been considerable interest in MC-1R mutations and the presence of loss-of-function alleles underlines the importance of the hMC-1R in the regulation of pigmentation. However, the MC-1R is not the only control point for pigmentation, and MC-1R mutations cannot account for all cases of red hair and poor tanning ability. Whilst a loss of POMC expression will affect pigmentation,[17] other control points downstream of the melanocortin signaling system are likely to be important. For instance, melanosomal pH is a critical factor for melanogenesis and its control could be an inherited feature that is vital for pigmentation. If, as we suspect, melanosomal pH is regulated by the P-locus, then the latter could serve as a rate-limiting gene for melanogenesis that determines the wide range of constitutive skin pigmentation. Furthermore, P-protein expression is upregulated by the UVR and melanocortin signaling system, and this would provide an important control point for facultative pigmentation (Fig. 12.1). It follows that pigmentary responses to the melanocortin peptides could be affected not only by MC-1R mutations, but also by the numerous P-protein alleles that have been reported.[64–67] These two factors could account for the many different levels of tanning ability seen in Caucasian populations.

Acknowledgement

We are pleased to acknowledge the generous support of Stiefel International.

References

1. Thody AJ, Higgins EM, Wakamatsu K et al., Pheomelanin as well as eumelanin is present in human epidermis, *J Invest Dermatol* (1991) **97**:340–4.
2. Smit NP, Kolb RM, Lentjes EG et al., Variations in melanin formation by cultured melanocytes from different skin types, *Arch Dermatol Res* (1998) **290**:342–9.

3. Lerner AB, McGuire JS, Melanocyte-stimulating hormone and adrenocorticotropic hormone. Their relation to pigmentation, *N Engl J Med* (1964) **270**:539–46.
4. Lerner AB, McGuire JS, Effect of alpha and beta-melanocyte stimulating hormone on skin colour of man, *Nature* (1961) **169**:176–9.
5. Hunt G, Kyne S, Ito S et al., Eumelanin and phaeomelanin contents of human epidermis and cultured melanocytes, *Pigment Cell Res* (1995) **8**:202–8.
6. Abdel-Malek Z, Swope VB, Suzuki I et al., Mitogenic and melanogenic stimulation of normal human melanocytes by melanotropic peptides, *Proc Natl Acad Sci U S A* (1995) **92**:1789–93.
7. Hunt G, Todd C, Cresswell JE et al., Alpha-melanocyte stimulating hormone and its analogue Nle4DPhe7 alpha-MSH affect morphology, tyrosinase activity and melanogenesis in cultured human melanocytes, *J Cell Sci* (1994) **107**:205–11.
8. Hunt G, Donatien PD, Lunec J et al., Cultured human melanocytes respond to MSH peptides and ACTH, *Pigment Cell Res* (1994) **7**:217–21.
9. Box NF, Wyeth JR, O'Gorman LE et al., Characterisation of melanocyte stimulating hormone receptor variant alleles in twins with red hair, *Hum Mol Genet* (1997) **6**:1891–7.
10. Koppula SV, Robbins LS, Lu D et al., Identification of common polymorphisms in the coding sequence of the human MSH receptor (MCIR) with possible biological effects, *Hum Mutat* (1997) **9**:30–6.
11. Valverde P, Healy E, Jackson I et al., Variants of the melanocyte-stimulating hormone receptor gene are associated with red hair and fair skin in humans, *Nat Genet* (1995) **11**:328–30.
12. Flanagan N, Healy E, Ray A et al., Pleiotropic effects of the melanocortin 1 receptor (MC1R) gene on human pigmentation, *Hum Mol Genet* (2000) **9**: 2531–7.
13. Rees JL, The melanocortin 1 receptor (MC1R): more than just red hair, *Pigment Cell Res* (2000) **13**:135–40.
14. Frandberg PA, Doufexis M, Kapas S et al., Amino acid residues in third intracellular loop of melanocortin 1 receptor are involved in G-protein coupling, *Biochem Mol Biol Int* (1998) **46**:913–22.
15. Schioth HB, Phillips SR, Rudzish R et al., Loss of function mutations of the human melanocortin 1 receptor are common and are associated with red hair, *Biochem Biophys Res Commun* (1999) **260**: 488–91.
16. Hunt G, Todd C, Thody AJ, Unresponsiveness of human epidermal melanocytes to melanocyte-stimulating hormone and its association with red hair, *Mol Cell Endocrinol* (1996) **116**:131–6.
17. Krude H, Biebermann H, Luck W et al., Severe early-onset obesity, adrenal insufficiency and red hair pigmentation caused by POMC mutations in humans, *Nat Genet* (1998) **19**:155–7.
18. Chakraborty AK, Funasaka Y, Slominski A et al., Production and release of proopiomelanocortin (POMC) derived peptides by human melanocytes and keratinocytes in culture: regulation by ultraviolet B, *Biochim Biophys Acta* (1996) **1313**:130–8.
19. Schauer E, Trautinger F, Kock A et al., Proopiomelanocortin-derived peptides are synthesised and released by human keratinocytes, *J Clin Invest* (1994) **93**:2258–62.
20. Chakraborty AK, Orlow SJ, Bolognia JL et al., Structural/functional relationships between internal and external MSH receptors: modulation of expression in Cloudman melanoma cells by UVB radiation, *J Cell Physiol* (1991) **147**:1–6.
21. Thody AJ, Hunt G, Donatien PD et al., Human melanocytes express functional melanocyte-stimulating hormone receptors, *Ann N Y Acad Sci* (1993) **680**:381–90.
22. Levine N, Sheftel SN, Eytan T et al., Induction of skin tanning by subcutaneous administration of a potent synthetic melanotropin, *JAMA* (1991) **266**:2730–6.
23. Thody AJ, Ridley K, Penny RJ et al., MSH peptides are present in mammalian skin, *Peptides* (1983) **4**:813–16.
24. Wakamatsu K, Graham A, Cook D et al., Characterisation of ACTH peptides in human skin and their activation of the melanocortin-1 receptor, *Pigment Cell Res* (1997) **10**:288–97.
25. Benjannet S, Rondeau N, Paquet L et al., Comparative biosynthesis, covalent post-translational modifications and efficiency of prosegment cleavage of the prohormone convertases PC1 and PC2: glycosylation, sulphation and identification of the intracellular site of prosegment cleavage of PC1 and PC2, *Biochem J* (1993) **294**:735–43.
26. Seidah NG, Day R, Chretien M, The family of pro-hormone and pro-protein convertases, *Biochem Soc Trans* (1993) **21**:685–91.
27. Tsatmali M, Yukitake J, Thody AJ, ACTH1–17 is a more potent agonist at the human MC1 receptor than alpha-MSH, *Cell Mol Biol* (1999) **45**:1029–34.
28. Tsatmali M, Ancans J, Yukitake J et al., Skin POMC peptides: their actions at the human MC-1 receptor and roles in the tanning response, *Pigment Cell Res* (2000) **13** (Suppl 8):125–9.
29. Johansson O, Ljungberg A, Han SW et al., Evidence

for gamma-melanocyte stimulating hormone containing nerves and neutrophilic granulocytes in the human skin by indirect immunofluorescence, *J Invest Dermatol* (1991) **96**:852–6.

30. Wintzen M, Gilchrest BA, Proopiomelanocortin, its derived peptides, and the skin, *J Invest Dermatol* (1996) **106**:3–10.
31. Yukitake J, Tsatmali M, Ancans J et al., Desacetyl α-MSH is a partial agonist at the human MC1-R, *Pigment Cell Res* (1999) **12**:72 (abst).
32. McCormack AM, Carter RJ, Thody AJ et al., Desacetyl MSH and gamma-MSH act as partial agonists to alpha-MSH on the Anolis melanophore, *Peptides* (1982) **3**:13–16.
33. Abdel-Malek Z, Scott M, Furumura M et al., The melanocortin 1 receptor is the principal mediator of the effects of agouti signaling protein on mammalian melanocytes, *J Cell Sci* (2001) **114**:1019–24.
34. Suzuki I, Tada A, Ollmann MM et al., Agouti signalling protein inhibits melanogenesis and the response of human melanocytes to alpha-melanotropin, *J Invest Dermatol* (1997) **108**:838–42.
35. Gunn TM, Miller KA, He L et al., The mouse mahogany locus encodes a transmembrane form of human attractin, *Nature* (1999) **398**:152–6.
36. Baker BI, The role of melanin-concentrating hormone in colour change, *Ann N Y Acad Sci* (1993) **680**:279–89.
37. Hoogduijn MJ, Ancans J, Thody AJ, Mammalian pigment cells express the MCH receptor, *Pigment Cell Res* (2000) **13**:400 (abst).
38. Burchill SA, Thody AJ, Ito S, Melanocyte-stimulating hormone, tyrosinase activity and the regulation of eumelanogenesis and phaeomelanogenesis in the hair follicular melanocytes of the mouse, *J Endocrinol* (1986) **109**:15–21.
39. Hunt G, Kyne S, Wakamatsu K et al., Nle4DPhe7 alpha-melanocyte-stimulating hormone increases the eumelanin:phaeomelanin ratio in cultured human melanocytes, *J Invest Dermatol* (1995) **104**:83–5.
40. Suzuki I, Cone RD, Im S et al., Binding of melanotropic hormones to the melanocortin receptor MC1R on human melanocytes stimulates proliferation and melanogenesis, *Endocrinology* (1996) **137**:1627–33.
41. Thody AJ, alpha-MSH and the regulation of melanocyte function, *Ann N Y Acad Sci* (1999) **885**:217–29.
42. Busca R, Ballotti R, Cyclic AMP a key messenger in the regulation of skin pigmentation, *Pigment Cell Res* (2000) **13**:60–9.
43. Busca R, Bertolotto C, Ortonne JP et al., Inhibition of the phosphatidylinositol 3-kinase/p70(S6)-kinase pathway induces B16 melanoma cell differentiation, *J Biol Chem* (1996) **271**:31824–30.
44. Wong G, Pawelek J, Melanocyte-stimulating hormone promotes activation of pre-existing tyrosinase molecules in Cloudman S91 melanoma cells, *Nature* (1975) **255**:644–6.
45. Jimenez M, Kameyama K, Maloy WL et al., Mammalian tyrosinase: biosynthesis, processing, and modulation by melanocyte-stimulating hormone, *Proc Natl Acad Sci U S A* (1988) **85**:3830–4.
46. Fuller BB, Rungta D, Iozumi K et al., Hormonal regulation of melanogenesis in mouse melanoma and in human melanocytes, *Ann N Y Acad Sci* (1993) **680**:302–19.
47. Iozumi K, Hoganson GE, Pennella R et al., Role of tyrosinase as the determinant of pigmentation in cultured human melanocytes, *J Invest Dermatol* (1993) **100**:806–11.
48. Saeki H, Oikawa A, Stimulation of tyrosinase activity of cultured melanoma cells by lysosomotropic agents, *J Cell Physiol* (1983) **116**:93–7.
49. Saeki H, Oikawa A, Stimulation by ionophores of tyrosinase activity of mouse melanoma cells in culture, *J Invest Dermatol* (1985) **85**:423–5.
50. Ancans J, Tobin DJ, Thody AJ, Melanosomal pH: non-genomic regulatory mechanism of melanogenesis, *Pigment Cell Res* (2000) **13**:400 (abst).
51. Ancans J, Thody AJ, Activation of melanogenesis by vacuolar type H(+)-ATPase inhibitors in amelanotic, tyrosinase positive human and mouse melanoma cells, *FEBS Lett* (2000) **478**:57–60.
52. Bhatnagar V, Anjaiah S, Puri N et al., pH of melanosomes of B 16 murine melanoma is acidic: its physiological importance in the regulation of melanin biosynthesis, *Arch Biochem Biophys* (1993) **307**:183–92.
53. Moellmann GA, Slominski A, Kuklinska E et al., Regulation of melanogenesis in melanocytes, *Pigment Cell Res* (1987) (Suppl 1):79–87.
54. Hearing VJ, Ekel TM, Mammalian tyrosinase. A comparison of tyrosine hydroxylation and melanin formation, *Biochem J* (1976) **157**:549–57.
55. Townsend D, Guillery P, King RA, Optimised assay for mammalian tyrosinase (polyhydroxyl phenyloxidase), *Anal Biochem* (1984) **139**:345–52.
56. Fuller BB, Spaulding DT, Smith DR, Regulation of the catalytic activity of pre-existing tyrosinase in black and Caucasian human melanocyte cell cultures, *Exp Cell Res* (2001) **262**:197–208.
57. Ancans J, Tobin DJ, Hoogduijn MJ et al., Melanosomal pH controls rate of melanogenesis, eumelanin/

phaeomelanin ratio and melanosome maturation rate in melanocytes and melanoma cells, *Exp Cell Res* (2001) **268**:26–35.

58. Ancans J, Hoogduijn MJ, Thody AJ, Melanosomal pH, pink locus protein and their roles in melanogenesis, *J Invest Dermatol* (2001) **117**:158–9.
59. Suzuki I, Yokoyama K, Abdel-Malek ZA et al., P-gene product may play an important role in α-MSH induced pigmentation in human melanocytes, *Pigment Cell Res* (1997) **10**:328 (abst).
60. Suzuki I, Kato T, Motokawa Y et al., Messenger RNA levels of melanogenesis-associated genes *in vivo* and their responses to UV irradiation, *Pigment Cell Res* (2000) **13**:406 (abst).
61. Ito S, Fujita K, Takahashi H et al., Characterisation of melanogenesis in mouse and guinea pig hair by chemical analysis of melanins and of free and bound DOPA and 5-S-cysteinyldopa, *J Invest Dermatol* (1984) **83**:12–14.
62. Rinchik EM, Bultman SJ, Horsthemke B et al., A gene for the mouse pink-eyed dilution locus and for human type II oculocutaneous albinism, *Nature* (1993) **361**:72–6.
63. Quevedo WCJ, Smith JA, Studies on radiation-induced tanning of skin, *Ann N Y Acad Sci* (1963) **100**:364–88.
64. Lee ST, Nicholls RD, Bundey S et al., Mutations of the P gene in oculocutaneous albinism, ocular albinism, and Prader-Willi syndrome plus albinism, *N Engl J Med* (1994) **330**:529–34.
65. Lee ST, Nicholls RD, Schnur RE et al., Diverse mutations of the P gene among African-Americans with type II (tyrosinase-positive) oculocutaneous albinism (OCA2), *Hum Mol Genet* (1994) **3**:2047–51.
66. Lee ST, Nicholls RD, Jong MT et al., Organization and sequence of the human P gene and identification of a new family of transport proteins, *Genomics* (1995) **26**:354–63.
67. King RA, Genetic hypomelanoses: disorders characterised by generalised hypomelanoses. In: Norlund JJ, Boissy RE, Hearing VJ et al., eds, *The Pigmentary System: Physiology and Pathophysiology* (Oxford University Press: New York, 1998) 553–75.

13

The role of *Agouti* and *Mahogany* in the control of melanogenesis

Zalfa Abdel-Malek

Human pigmentation and skin cancer risk

Interest in investigating the regulation of human pigmentation stems primarily from the significance of melanin in protection against the photodamaging effects of solar ultraviolet radiation (UVR).[1,2] The most drastic effects of excessive sun exposure are photoaging and skin cancer.[3] The magnitude of the cutaneous responses to UVR are determined, to a large extent, by constitutive pigmentation.[4] A hallmark of sun exposure is increased skin pigmentation, *i.e.* tanning. Stimulation of melanogenesis is perceived as a response to DNA damage and as a mechanism to protect against subsequent exposure to UVR. In general, there is a direct correlation between constitutive skin pigmentation and the ability to tan.[4] This correlation exists *in situ* as well as *in vitro*.[5,6] Individuals who have lightly-pigmented skin and hair, and blue eyes, have a poor tanning ability, a high sensitivity to UVR-induced DNA damage and increased risk for skin cancer.[3] On the other hand, individuals with dark skin color who tan readily following sun exposure do not have extensive DNA damage in their skin, and, generally, have a low risk for developing skin cancer. *In vitro*, melanocytes cultured from lightly-pigmented skin fail to respond to UVB radiation with a significant increase in melanin content, and form extensive cyclobutane pyrimidine dimers in their DNA.[5] In comparison, melanocytes cultured from dark skin exhibit a marked increase in melanin content and less DNA photoproducts following UVB exposure.

Constitutive pigmentation is a complex genetic trait that is regulated by a large number of genes and many environmental factors. Those genes code for a variety of proteins, including regulatory enzymes for melanin synthesis, melanosome structural proteins, transcription factors, and melanogenic factors and their receptors that affect the rate of eumelanin or pheomelanin synthesis.[7–12] During the past two decades, significant advances have been made to elucidate the genetic and biochemical basis for the differences in constitutive pigmentation among humans. Human melanocytes, similar to other mammalian melanocytes, synthesize eumelanin, the black/brown pigment, and pheomelanin, the red/yellow pigment.[13] Total melanin content and the relative eumelanin-to-pheomelanin contents are important determinants of human skin color. Melanocytes in dark skin synthesize more melanin and have a higher eumelanin-to-pheomelanin ratio than melanocytes in lightly-pigmented skin.[14,15] These differences are detectable *in vitro* and *in situ*. Hence, a direct correlation exists between total melanin content and the ratio of eumelanin to pheomelanin. The activity of tyrosinase, the rate-limiting enzyme in the melanogenic pathway, as well as the protein levels of tyrosinase, tyrosinase-related protein (TRP)-1 and -2, correlate directly with total melanin content of human melanocytes.[16] High levels of tyrosinase, TRP-1, and TRP-2 are associated with stimulation of eumelanin synthesis, while low levels of those enzymes are involved in the synthesis of pheomelanin.[17–21]

Individuals with the pigmentary phenotype characterized by low melanin content and eumelanin-to-pheomelanin ratio represent a population that is at a high risk for skin cancer.[3] In dark skin *in situ*, melanosomes, which are presumably rich in eumelanin, form supranuclear caps in keratinocytes and remain intact throughout the epidermal layers.[22,23] In contrast, in light-colored skin, intact melanosomes, presumably containing mostly pheomelanin, are not visible, even in the suprabasal layer of the epidermis. This allows for more penetration of harmful UV rays through the epidermal layers. These observations suggest differences in the photoprotective capacities of eumelanin and pheomelanin, a notion supported by the findings that purified eumelanin is superior to purified pheomelanin in its photoprotective properties. Eumelanin is more resistant to photodegradation and is more efficient in scavenging reactive oxygen species than pheomelanin.[24] Pheomelanin itself seems to be capable of generating superoxide anions and hydroxyl radicals, thus possibly contributing to oxidative stress in the skin. These differences between eumelanin and pheomelanin have only been demonstrated *in vitro*, and studies comparing the photoprotective effects of those melanins in melanocytes with different eumelanin-to-pheomelanin contents still need to be carried out.

Genetic regulation of pheomelanin and eumelanin synthesis in mouse follicular melanocytes

Regulation of pheomelanin and eumelanin synthesis in human melanocytes is relatively poorly understood. With the cloning of various pigmentary genes, including the human *melanocortin 1 receptor* (*MC1R*) and *Agouti*, it became evident that extensive homology exists between the respective human and mouse genes.[11,25] So far, in the mouse, three principal regulators of eumelanin and pheomelanin synthesis have been identified, *MC1R*, *Agouti*, and *mahogany*. Other genes also affect the production of these melanins in melanocytes. Particularly, the murine *pink-eyed dilution* is important for eumelanin synthesis, since mutations in this gene reduce eumelanin synthesis without affecting the production of pheomelanin.[26] The mouse MC1R, the receptor for α-MSH, is coded for by the *Extension* locus, and its activation results in increased eumelanin synthesis.[27,28] Agouti signaling protein (ASP), the product of the *Agouti* locus, is a soluble factor that functions as the physiological antagonist of MC1R.[29] ASP is temporally expressed in dermal papilla cells during the mid-portion of the hair growth cycle, where it functions as a paracrine regulator of mouse follicular melanocytes and competes with α-MSH for binding to the MC1R. The dorsal–ventral variation in hair coloration occurs due to the complex *Agouti* regulatory regions. Distinct regulatory elements direct the expression of exon 1A of *Agouti* to the ventral region, while regulatory elements specific for the mid-portion of the hair growth cycle control exons 1B and 1C.[29] The *mahogany* gene is the latest pigmentary gene to be cloned and its product (mahogany/attractin) identified.[30,31] It is expressed in many cell types and tissues, including melanocytes and in the hypothalamus.[30] This gene was first described in 1960 as a recessive umbrous gene.[32] Mahogany protein is thought to function as a low-affinity receptor for ASP, concentrating it in the vicinity of the MC1R, thus facilitating its role as a competitive inhibitor of α-MSH binding to the MC1R.[30,31]

In mouse follicular melanocytes, the MC1R plays a central role in regulating eumelanin/pheomelanin synthesis. Genetic and biochemical studies on mouse coat color revealed that activation of the MC1R by its ligand, α-melanocyte stimulating hormone (α-MSH), stimulates the synthesis of eumelanin, and inhibition of MC1R activation by ASP stimulates the synthesis of pheomelanin.[28,33] The coat color of the wild-type agouti mouse is characterized by black hairs with a subapical band that is yellow in color. The black portion of the hair is indicative of eumelanin synthesis in response to α-MSH, while the yellow band represents the abrupt switch from eumelanin to pheomelanin synthesis due to the stringently controlled spacial and temporal expression of *Agouti*.[34] The loss of function mutation in *MC1R*, *recessive yellow* (*e/e*), results in a yellow coat color due to lack of eumelanin synthesis, thus lending evidence for the significance of functional MC1R in regulating this process.[27] Dominant mutations in *Agouti*, such as *lethal yellow* (A^y), result in ectopic expression of ASP that leads to a yellow coat color (due to antagonism of MC1R), obesity (due to antagonism of MC4R in the hypothalamus) and increased longitudinal growth.[35,36] Agouti mice expressing *mg* mutation in the *mahogany* gene have significantly darker central dorsal hairs with reduced yellow bands, gray ventral hairs with no yellow band, and darker ears and tails than wild-type mice.[32] In mice carrying the gain-of-function *Agouti* mutation A^y, mutations in *mahogany* (*mg*, or mg^{3J}) suppressed the pleiotropic effects of ubiquitously-expressed agouti protein, including increased pheomelanin synthesis and obesity.[37] On the other hand, in mice homozygous for *recessive yellow* (*e/e*), the effects of *mg* or mg^{3J} are suppressed, and the mouse is yellow in color. These observations indicate that *mahogany* lies upstream of the *MC1R* and downstream of *Agouti*. In humans and other primates, there is no expression of the agouti phenotype.[38] However, human melanocytes synthesize eumelanin and pheomelanin, and are responsive to both α-MSH and ASP.[13,18,20]

Regulation of eumelanin and pheomelanin synthesis in human epidermal melanocytes

The role of melanocortins and MC1R

In humans, skepticism about the role of α-MSH as a physiological regulator of human pigmentation lasted until the early 1990s.[39] α-Melanocyte stimulating hormone was presumed to function exclusively as an endocrine factor, and the low serum levels of α-MSH in humans minimized its significance for human pigmentation.[40] The cloning of the *MC1R* from human melanocytes and the demonstration that this receptor is functional and that melanocortins are synthesized in the skin ended this long-lasting controversy.[11,41] The MC1R belongs to a family of five distinct G-protein coupled receptors with seven transmembrane domains, each of which is the product of a distinct gene.[11,42–45] These receptors differ in their tissue distribution and in their affinity for the various melanocortins. Activation of these receptors by ligand binding increases cAMP formation and activates the cAMP-dependent signaling pathway.[46–48] The effects of melanocortins are mimicked by agents that elevate intracellular cAMP levels, such as forskolin and cholera toxin, confirming that the cAMP pathway is the main signaling pathway that mediates the effects of melanocortins.[49] As in the mouse, NDP-α-MSH, the potent synthetic analog of α-MSH, stimulates eumelanin synthesis in cultured human melanocytes.[50] Interestingly, the human MC1R has a higher affinity for α-MSH than the mouse MC1R.[51] Additionally, the human MC1R, unlike the mouse counterpart, binds ACTH with a similar affinity as α-MSH, suggesting that, potentially, both hormones are physiologically effective in regulating eumelanin synthesis in human melanocytes.[48]

The significance of the human MC1R in regulating human pigmentation is further supported by the tremendous variation of the gene, and by the association of specific allelic variants with the red-hair and fair-skin phenotype.[52,53] So far, about 30 allelic variants of the *MC1R* have been identified in Northern European and Australian populations. In particular, four allelic variants, Arg142His, Arg151Cys, Arg160Trp, and Asp294His, represent loss of function mutations, while others, such as Val92Met, are polymorphisms that do not cause a significant alteration in receptor function.[54–56] The impact of most of the allelic variants on MC1R function is still unknown. Interestingly, variants of the *MC1R* are not common in African populations, where the wild-type gene is predominantly expressed.[57] This lends further support for the role of this gene in regulating the synthesis of eumelanin in human skin.

Not only normal expression of MC1R, but also availability of melanocortins, are important for determining constitutive human pigmentation and the magnitude of eumelanin synthesis. The melanocortins α-, β-, γ-MSH, and ACTH are all derived from a 31-Kd precursor peptide, proopiomelanocortin (POMC).[58] In humans, the *POMC* gene consists of 7.8 kb and three exons.[59] Almost all the genomic DNA information of POMC is contained within exon 3. Post-translational processing of POMC results in the generation of various bioactive peptides, including melanocortins, β-lipotropic hormone, and β-endorphin. In humans, mutations that disrupt the expression of *POMC* result in red hair, obesity, and adrenal insufficiency.[60] In mice, there are no known mutations in *POMC*. Proopiomelanocortin and its derivatives were generally known to be synthesized by the pituitary gland and to function as endocrine factors. It is now recognized that *POMC* is expressed in many human peripheral tissues, including the skin, gonads, and gastrointestinal tract.[61] In the human epidermis, α-MSH and ACTH are synthesized by melanocytes and keratinocytes and thus can function as autocrine/paracrine regulators of melanocytes.[41,62] It is not yet known whether the processing of POMC and the rate of production of melanocortins is the same or different in different pigmentary phenotypes. Investigating this issue will further clarify the basis for the diversity of human pigmentation.

The role of ASP as MC1R antagonist

In mice, expression of *Agouti* results in the switch to pheomelanin synthesis in follicular melanocytes.[29] The human *Agouti* gene has been cloned and its product, a 132 amino acid peptide, has been purified. The human and mouse ASPs have 80% homology in their amino acid sequences.[63] Like the mouse protein, the human ASP contains all the structural characteristics of a secreted protein, with a hydrophobic signal sequence and lack of transmembrane domains.[34] The mature protein has a highly basic amino terminus, a proline-rich central domain, and a cysteine-rich carboxyl terminus, which is the active site of the protein and is sufficient for its action as an antagonist of MC1R. To determine the function of human ASP, transgenic mice expressing the human *Agouti* gene were generated.[25] The phenotype of these mice mimicked that of mice with mutations that result in overexpression of mouse agouti protein.

The human MC1R is activated by binding of α-MSH or ACTH, and is antagonized by ASP.[20,48] There is compelling evidence for the role of ASP as a competitive inhibitor of α-MSH binding to the MC1R. Expression of functional MC1R is required for the action of ASP on melanocytes.[64] Evidence for this comes from studies showing that mouse melanoma cells that lack the expression of MC1R do not respond to ASP.[65] Recently, we showed that primary mouse melanocyte cultures established from the skins of recessive yellow or sombre mice, with loss of function *MC1R* mutations, cannot respond to ASP.[21] In contrast, melanocyte cultures established from congenic wild-type mouse skins responded to ASP with reduction in tyrosinase, TRP-1 and TRP-2, and complete inhibition of the melanogenic effect of α-MSH. These observations clearly suggest that the MC1R is the principal mediator of the effects of ASP. Furthermore, the function of MC1R as the binding site for α-MSH and ASP makes it a main regulator of eumelanin and pheomelanin synthesis in mammalian melanocytes. The exact role for ASP in regulating human pigmentation is not understood. Cultured human melanocytes respond to ASP with complete abrogation of the melanogenic effect of α-MSH due to displacement of α-MSH from its receptor, and by acting as an inverse agonist.[20] Similar results were obtained in mouse melanocytes.[19,21] Our preliminary studies suggest that ASP increases pheomelanin synthesis in human melanocytes, resulting in a 20–25% increase in the ratio of pheomelanin to eumelanin (Abdel-Malek ZA and Ito S, unpublished results). These results suggest a role for ASP in regulating pheomelanin synthesis in human melanocytes.

Recent studies on the pigmentary effects of α-MSH and ASP on mammalian melanocytes shed new light on the biochemical regulation of eumelanin and pheomelanin synthesis. Treatment of either mouse or human melanocytes with α-MSH significantly increased tyrosinase activity and the protein levels of tyrosinase, TRP-1 and TRP-2.[18,19,21] In contrast, treatment with ASP decreased tyrosinase activity and drastically reduced the protein levels of tyrosinase, TRP-1, and TRP-2.[19,20] Studies on mouse hair follicles demonstrated that high levels of tyrosinase, TRP-1 and TRP-2 are associated with eumelanin synthesis, while very low levels of these enzymes are associated with pheomelanin synthesis.[17] From this, it can be concluded that eumelanin synthesis that is stimulated by α-MSH requires high expression of tyrosinase, TRP-1 and TRP-2, while pheomelanin synthesis in response to ASP proceeds in the presence of very low activities and protein levels of these enzymes.

Possible effects of *mahogany*

Mahogany codes for a 1428 amino acid protein, with a single transmembrane domain.[31] The extracellular domain of mahogany is the orthologue of human attractin that was purified from serum and found to be produced by activated T-cells and to mediate T-lymphocyte and macrophage interaction.[31,66] Attractin causes monocyte spreading and T-cell clustering. At least two mRNA species have been identified in humans, a 4-Kb transcript that codes for a secreted protein, and an 8.5-Kb transcript that codes for a membrane-bound protein.[30,31] Attractin is expressed and highly conserved in many species, such as *Drosophila, C. elegans,* mouse and human.[67] The membrane-type attractin/mahogany protein has a large extracellular component that contains three EGF domains, two laminin-like EGF repeats, a CUB domain, two plexin-like repeats, a c-type lectin and seven consecutive Kelch repeats.[30] The multiple EGF domains are characteristic of membrane proteins that are involved in cell adhesion and receptor–ligand interactions.

Recently, it was reported that the rat zitter (*zi*) mutation, which induces hypomyelination and vacuolization in the central nervous system, resulting in early onset tremors, is an 8-bp deletion at a splice site of *attractin* that markedly reduces the *attractin* mRNA in the brain.[68] Rats with the *zi* mutation have darker coat colors than agouti rats. It was discovered that *mg* mice and *zi* rats have similar neurological abnormalities.[67] The pigmentary and neurological abnormalities of *zi* rats could be complemented by the membrane type, but not the secreted attractin. These observations define a new and critical role for *mahogany/attractin* in myelination of the central nervous system, and suggest that the pleiotropic effects of this gene are mediated by the membrane-type product.

Based on the structure and the pleiotropic effects of mahogany/attractin, several models for its function have been proposed. The most plausible model is that mahogany acts as an 'accessory' receptor that allows for increased accessibility of extracellular factors to their high-affinity receptors. In mouse melanocytes, mahogany seems to act as an MC1R antagonist by serving as a low-affinity receptor for ASP (Fig. 13.1).[30,31] Interestingly, mahogany/attractin is not a low-affinity receptor for the neuropeptide agouti-related protein (AGRP), which is homologous to ASP and acts as the physiologic antagonist of MC4R.[67] It is not known whether mahogany interacts with ASP independently of MC1R or with ASP and MC1R to form a ternary complex.[67] An alternative model for

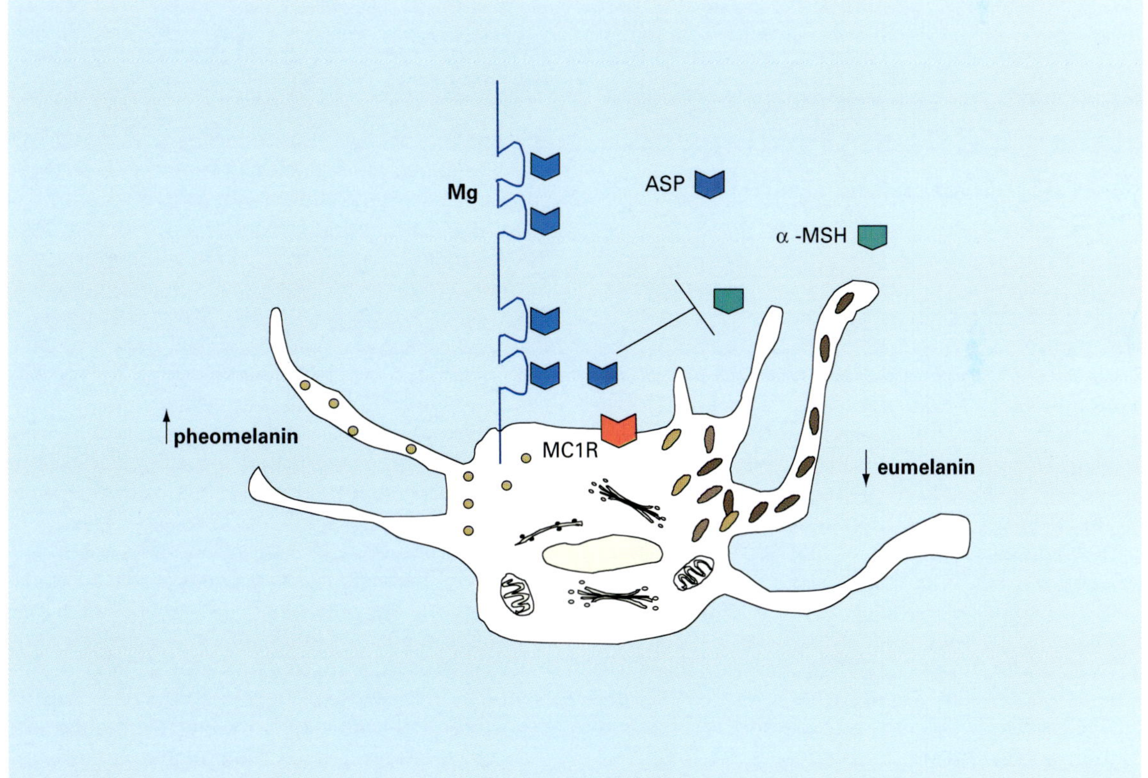

Figure 13.1

Proposed mechanism of action of *mahogany/attractin* in melanocytes. Membrane-type mahogany/attractin is thought to function as a low-affinity accessory receptor for ASP, concentrating it and facilitating its binding to MC1R. This is expected to block α-MSH binding and allow for stimulation of pheomelanin synthesis.

mahogany action is sequestration of melanocortins away from MC1R, or desensitization of the MC1R, for example, by enhancing agonist-induced internalization.[30,31]

The role of *mahogany* in human pigmentation has not yet been investigated. Based on the effect of this gene on mouse coat color, it can be speculated that it serves a similar function in human skin. Assuming that ASP regulates pheomelanin synthesis in human melanocytes, mahogany will be expected to enhance this effect by facilitating the accessibility of ASP to the MC1R. In this regard, mahogany may indirectly inhibit the activation of the MC1R by melanocortins, thus reducing eumelanin synthesis. Since *mahogany* is expressed in human melanocytes, it would be interesting to determine the level of its expression in melanocytes from different pigmentary phenotypes, and correlate that with their relative eumelanin-to-pheomelanin content.

Regulation of expression of the human *MC1R*: Implications on the response of melanocytes to UVR

A model for the regulation of *MC1R* expression by UVR-induced factors is presented in Figure 13.2. The pigmentary effect of UVR is mediated to a large extent by increased synthesis of paracrine/autocrine factors that regulate melanocyte function. Exposure to UVR increases α-MSH and ACTH production by human epidermal cells *in vitro* and *in vivo*.[41,62] Also, UVR increases the synthesis of endothelin-1, which functions as a mitogen and a melanogenic modulator of human melanocytes, by human keratinocytes.[69] The expression of human MC1R is subject to regulation by its ligands and by other epidermal paracrine factors. α-Melanocyte stimulating hormone and ACTH, as well as endothelin-1, upregulate the mRNA levels of *MC1R*, an effect that is expected to increase eumelanin synthesis in response to UVR.[48,70] These factors seem to maintain the expression of the MC1R and sustain the ability of melanocytes to respond to melanocortins following UV exposure.

Activation of the MC1R seems to be critical for the melanogenic response to UVR. This is supported by the observations that loss-of-function mutations in *MC1R* are associated with poor tanning ability.[71] We have reported that stimulation of the cAMP pathway, the principal mediator of the effects of α-MSH, is pivotal for UVB-stimulated melanogenesis in human melanocytes.[72] These results emphasize the central role for MC1R in regulating human pigmentation and in the response of human melanocytes to UVR. So far, the regulation of *Agouti* expression by UVR or UVR-induced factors is not known. Similarly, the effects of UVR on the expression of *mahogany* have not been explored. It is possible that expression of these genes affects the magnitude of the melanogenic response to UVR, and is important in determining the capacity of melanocytes from different skin types to increase eumelanin synthesis following UV irradiation.

Questions still to be answered

The significance of melanocortins and the MC1R in the regulation of human pigmentation is strongly supported by pigmentary alterations that result from loss-of-function mutations in *POMC* and *MC1R*, respectively.[52,53,60] So far, mutations in the human *Agouti* gene have not been identified, and the role of *mahogany* in human pigmentation is totally unknown. Since *POMC*, *Agouti*, and *mahogany* are potentially significant for human pigmentation, it is important to determine their levels of expression in various pigmentary phenotypes. Besides expression of different *MC1R* allelic variants, differences in constitutive pigmentation may be due to different levels of melanocortins or ASP that are synthesized in the skin of different pigmentary phenotypes. Also, differences in the expression of mahogany may affect the extent of its interaction with ASP, and hence the synthesis of pheomelanin and eumelanin in melanocytes. These possibilities need to be explored in order to clarify the role of ASP and mahogany/attractin in human pigmentation, and to gain more insight into the diversity of human pigmentation.

It is known that exposure to UVR stimulates the synthesis of melanocortins and other paracrine/autocrine factors by keratinocytes and melanocytes.[62,69] In turn, melanocortins will

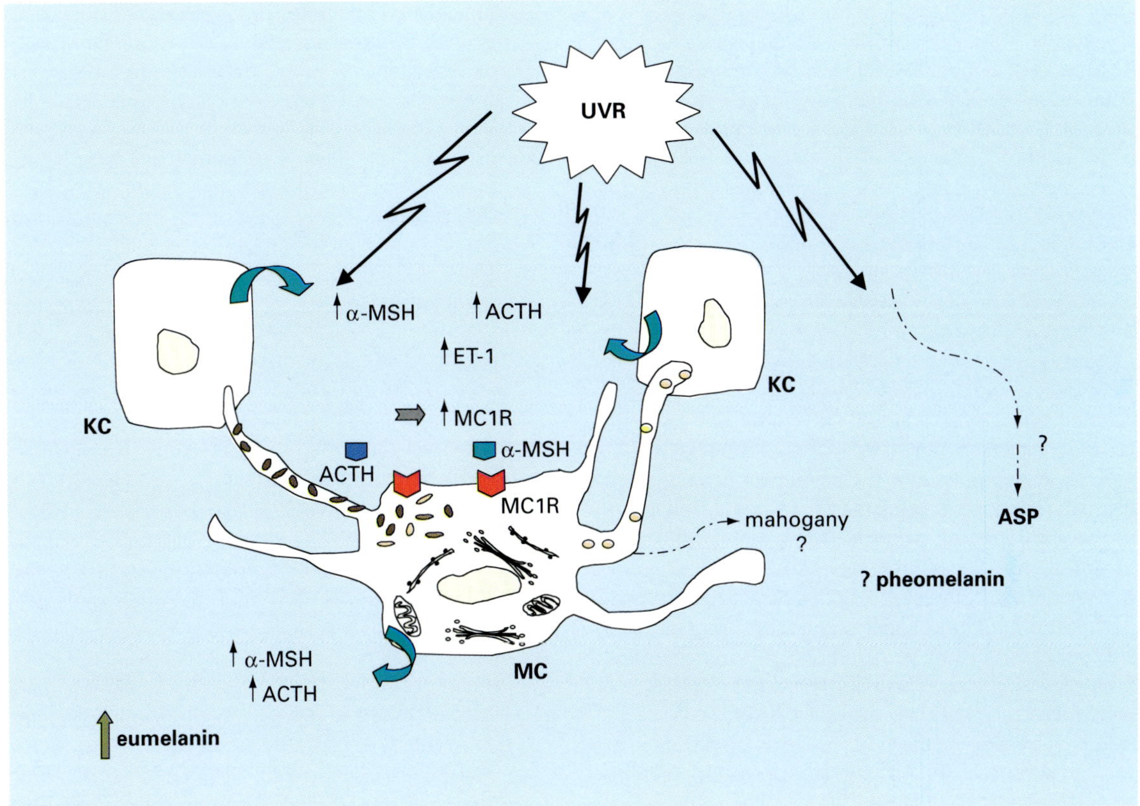

Figure 13.2

Mechanism for regulation of human *MC1R* expression by UVR. Exposure to UVR stimulates the synthesis of α-MSH and ACTH by epidermal melanocytes and keratinocytes, and of endothelin-1 by keratinocytes. Those factors upregulate the expression of *MC1R*, an effect that is expected to maintain the responsiveness of melanocytes to melanocortins and to increase eumelanin synthesis. It is not known whether UVR alters ASP or mahogany levels, leading to changes in pheomelanin synthesis.

upregulate the expression of MC1R on melanocytes and increase the synthesis of eumelanin.[48] This may account for increased eumelanin production following UV exposure. Whether or not the melanogenic response to UVR involves reduction in pheomelanin synthesis is unknown. We speculate that UVR reduces the expression of ASP and/or mahogany/attractin in order to enhance further eumelanin synthesis. Since individuals with different pigmentary phenotypes have different tanning capacities, we expect that, in the presence of functional MC1R, the magnitude of melanocortin production, and of the putative changes in ASP and mahogany/attractin expression, to be more pronounced in dark skin than in lightly-pigmented skin that tans poorly.

Since constitutive pigmentation and the ability to tan in response to sun exposure are regarded as important determinants of an individual's risk for skin cancer, elucidating the regulation of eumelanin and pheomelanin synthesis in human melanocytes is becoming exceedingly important. To achieve this goal, the role of ASP and mahogany/attractin needs to be determined, and the role of melanocortins and MC1R further investigated in human melanocytes. Furthermore, the magnitude of photoprotection afforded by eumelanin versus pheomelanin needs to be delineated.

It has been shown that supranuclear caps that are formed by melanosomes reduce the extent of photoproducts in DNA following UV exposure.[23] Presumably these melanosomes are enriched in eumelanin. Further, melanin is thought to act as an antioxidant, due to its function as a pseudo-superoxide dismutase.[73] A role for α-MSH as an antioxidant has also been proposed.[74] Preliminary results from our laboratory have shown that melanocytes produce substantial numbers of reactive oxygen species in response to irradiation with UVB or UVA. Potentially, oxidative stress may result in mutagenesis and malignant transformation. In comparison to keratinocytes and fibroblasts, melanocytes have lower antioxidant enzyme activities, and thus might be more vulnerable to UV-induced oxidative stress.[75] Comparing the ability of eumelanin versus pheomelanin to scavenge reactive oxygen species might offer an explanation for the differences in skin cancer risk among individuals with different pigmentary phenotypes. We propose that α-MSH and ASP can potentially be used as experimental tools to manipulate the synthesis of eumelanin and pheomelanin, respectively, in human melanocytes, to determine the respective effects of these melanins on the responses of melanocytes to UVR. An ultimate goal is to identify specific genetic and molecular markers that regulate constitutive and facultative human pigmentation, in order to identify precisely the risk of individuals for skin cancer.

Acknowledgements

Supported in part by a grant from the National Institutes for Environmental Health Sciences (R01 ES09110).

Special thanks go to Itaru Suzuki and Sungbin Im, and to collaborators in these studies: Vincent Hearing, Greg Barsh, Lynn Lamoreux and Shosuke Ito.

References

1. Kaidbey KH, Poh Agin P, Sayre RM et al., Photoprotection by melanin—a comparison of black and Caucasian skin, *J Am Acad Dermatol* (1979) **1**:249–60.
2. Pathak MA, Functions of melanin and protection by melanin. In: Zeise L, Chedekel MR, Fitzpatrick TB, eds, *Melanin: Its Role in Human Photoprotection* (Valdenmar Publishing Company: Overland Park, 1995) 125–33.
3. Fitzpatrick TB, Sober AJ, Pearson BJ et al., Cutaneous carcinogenic effects of sunlight in humans. In: Castellani A, ed, *Research in Photobiology* (Plenum Press: New York, 1976): 485–90.
4. Pathak MA, Jimbow K, Fitzpatrick T, Photobiology of pigment cells. In: Seiji M, ed *Phenotypic Expression in Pigment Cells* (University of Tokyo Press: Tokyo, 1980): 655–70.
5. Barker D, Dixon K, Medrano EE et al., Comparison of the responses of human melanocytes with different melanin contents to ultraviolet B irradiation, *Cancer Res* (1995) **55**:4041–6.
6. Bessou-Touya S, Picardo M, Maresca V et al., Chimeric human epidermal reconstructs to study the role of melanocytes and keratinocytes in pigmentation and photoprotection, *J Invest Dermatol* (1998) **111**:1103–8.
7. Kwon BS, Haq AK, Pomerantz SH et al., Isolation and sequence of a cDNA clone for human tyrosinase that maps at the mouse c-albino locus, *Proc Natl Acad Sci U S A* (1987) **84**:7473–7.
8. Yokoyama K, Yasumoto K, Suzuki H et al., Cloning of the human DOPAchrome tautomerase/tyrosinase-related protein 2 gene and identification of two regulatory regions required for its pigment cell-specific expression, *J Biol Chem* (1994) **269**:27080–7.
9. Tachibana M, Perez-Jurado LA, Nakayama A et al., Cloning of *MITF*, the human homolog of the mouse *microphthalmia* gene, and assignment to human chromosome 3, region p14.1–p12.3, *Hum Mol Genet* (1994) **3**:553–7.
10. Brannan CI, Lyman SD, Williams DE et al., *Steel-Dickie* mutation encodes c-kit ligand lacking transmembrane and cytoplasmic domains, *Proc Natl Acad Sci U S A* (1991) **88**:4671–4.
11. Mountjoy KG, Robbins LS, Mortrud MT et al., The cloning of a family of genes that encode the melanocortin receptors, *Science* (1992) **257**:1248–51.
12. Rosemblat S, Durham-Pierre D, Gardner JM et al., Identification of a melanosomal membrane protein encoded by the pink-eyed dilution (type II oculocutaneous albinism) gene, *Proc Natl Acad Sci U S A* (1994) **91**:12071–5.
13. Thody AJ, Higgins EH, Wakamatzu K et al., Pheomelanin as well as eumelanin is present in human epidermis, *J Invest Dermatol* (1991) **97**:340–4.

14. Abdel-Malek ZA, Swope VB, Nordlund JJ et al., Proliferation and propagation of human melanocytes in vitro are affected by donor age and anatomical site, *Pigment Cell Res* (1994); **7**:116–22.
15. Hunt G, Kyne S, Ito S et al., Eumelanin and pheomelanin contents of human epidermis and cultured melanocytes, *Pigment Cell Res* (1995) **8**:202–8.
16. Abdel-Malek Z, Swope V, Collins C et al., Contribution of melanogenic proteins to the heterogeneous pigmentation of human melanocytes, *J Cell Sci* (1993) **106**:1323–31.
17. Kobayashi T, Vieira WD, Potterf B et al., Modulation of melanogenic protein expression during the switch from eu- to pheomelanogenesis, *J Cell Sci* (1995) **108**:2301–9.
18. Abdel-Malek Z, Swope VB, Suzuki I et al., Mitogenic and melanogenic stimulation of normal human melanocytes by melanotropic peptides, *Proc Natl Acad Sci U S A* (1995) **92**:1789–93.
19. Sakai C, Ollmann M, Kobayashi T et al., Modulation of murine melanocyte function *in vitro* by agouti signal protein, *EMBO J* (1997) **16**:3544–52.
20. Suzuki I, Tada A, Ollmann MM et al., Agouti signaling protein inhibits melanogenesis and the response of human melanocytes to α-melanotropin, *J Invest Dermatol* (1997) **108**:838–42.
21. Abdel-Malek ZA, Scott MC, Furumura M et al., The melanocortin 1 receptor is the principal mediator of the effects of agouti signaling protein on mammalian melanocytes, *J Cell Sci* (2001) **114**:1019–24.
22. Pathak MA, Hori Y, Szabó G et al., The photobiology of melanin pigmentation in human skin. In: Kawamura T, Fitzpatrick TB, Seiji M, eds, *Biology of Normal and Abnormal Melanocytes* (University Park Press: Baltimore, 1971) 149–69.
23. Kobayashi N, Nakagawa A, Muramatsu T et al., Supranuclear melanin caps reduce ultraviolet induced DNA photoproducts in human epidermis, *J Invest Dermatol* (1998) **110**:806–10.
24. Menon IA, Persad S, Ranadive NS et al., Photobiological effects of eumelanin and pheomelanin. In: Bagnara JT, Klaus SN, Paul E et al., eds, *Biological, Molecular and Clinical Aspects of Pigmentation* (University of Tokyo Press: Tokyo, 1985) 77–86.
25. Wilson BD, Ollmann MM, Kang L et al., Structure and function of *ASP*, the human homolog of the mouse *agouti* gene, *Hum Mol Genet* (1995) **4**:223–30.
26. Lamoreux ML, Zhou B-K, Rosemblat S et al., The pinkeyed-dilution protein and the eumelanin/pheomelanin switch: In support of a unifying hypothesis, *Pigment Cell Res* (1995) **8**:263–70.
27. Robbins LS, Nadeau JH, Johnson KR et al., Pigmentation phenotypes of variant extension locus alleles result from point mutations that alter MSH receptor function, *Cell* (1993) **72**:827–34.
28. Geschwind II, Huseby RA, Nishioka R, The effect of melanocyte-stimulating hormone on coat color in the mouse, *Rec Prog Hormone Res* (1972) **28**:91–130.
29. Vrieling H, Duhl DMJ, Millar SE et al., Differences in dorsal and ventral pigmentation result from regional expression of the mouse *agouti* gene, *Proc Natl Acad Sci U S A* (1994) **91**:5667–71.
30. Nagle DL, McGrail SH, Vitale J et al., The *mahogany* protein is a receptor involved in suppression of obesity, *Nature* (1999) **398**:148–52.
31. Gunn TM, Miller KA, He L et al., The mouse *mahogany* locus encodes a transmembrane form of human attractin, *Nature* (1999) **398**:152–6.
32. Lane PW, Green MC, Mahogany, a recessive color mutation in linkage group V of the mouse, *J Hered* (1960) **51**:228–30.
33. Tamate HB, Takeuchi T, Action of the *e* locus of mice in the response of phaeomelanic hair follicles to α-melanocyte-stimulating hormone in vitro, *Science* (1984) **224**:1241–2.
34. Miller MW, Duhl DMJ, Vrieling H et al., Cloning of the mouse *agouti* gene predicts a secreted protein ubiquitously expressed in mice carrying the *lethal yellow* mutation, *Genes Dev* (1993) **7**:454–67.
35. Yen TT, Gill AM, Frigeri LG et al., Obesity, diabetes, and neoplasia in yellow A^{vy}/- mice: Ectopic expression of the *agouti* gene, *FASEB J* (1994) **8**:479–88.
36. Fan W, Boston BA, Kesterson RA et al., Role of melanocortinergic neurons in feeding and the *agouti* obesity syndrome, *Nature* (1997) **385**:165–8.
37. Miller KA, Gunn TM, Carrasquillo MM et al., Genetic studies of the mouse mutation *mahogany* and *mahoganoid*, *Genetics* (1997) **146**:1407–15.
38. Searle AG, *Comparative Genetics of Coat Colour in Mammals* (Academic Press: New York, 1968).
39. Halaban R, Tyrrell L, Longley J et al., Pigmentation and proliferation of human melanocytes and the effects of melanocyte-stimulating hormone and ultraviolet B light, *Ann N Y Acad Sci* (1993) **680**:290–301.
40. Eberle AN, Secretion, distribution and inactivation of MSH. In: Eberle AN, ed, *The Melanocortins* (Karger: Basel, 1998) 171–209.
41. Wakamatsu K, Graham A, Cook D et al., Characterization of ACTH peptides in human skin and their activation of the melanocortin-1 receptor, *Pigment Cell Res* (1997); **10**:288–97.

42. Chhajlani V, Muceniece R, Wikberg JES, Molecular cloning of a novel human melanocortin receptor, *Biochem Biophys Res Commun* (1993) **195**: 866–73.
43. Gantz I, Konda Y, Tashiro T et al., Molecular cloning of a novel melanocortin receptor, *J Biol Chem* (1993) **268**:8246–50.
44. Gantz I, Miwa H, Konda Y et al., Molecular cloning, expression, and gene localization of a fourth melanocortin receptor, *J Biol Chem* (1993) **268**:15174–9.
45. Labbé O, Desarnaud F, Eggerickx D et al., Molecular cloning of a mouse melanocortin 5 receptor gene widely expressed in peripheral tissues, *Biochemistry* (1994) **33**:4543–9.
46. Wong G, Pawelek J, Sansone M et al., Response of mouse melanoma cells to melanocyte stimulating hormone, *Nature* (1974) **248**:351–4.
47. Fuller BB, Lunsford JB, Iman DS, Alpha-melanocyte-stimulating hormone regulation of tyrosinase in Cloudman S91 mouse melanoma cell cultures, *J Biol Chem* (1987) **262**:4024–33.
48. Suzuki I, Cone R, Im S et al., Binding capacity and activation of the MC1 receptors by melanotropic hormones correlate directly with their mitogenic and melanogenic effects on human melanocytes, *Endocrinology* (1996) **137**:1627–33.
49. O'Keefe E, Cuatrecasas P, Cholera toxin mimics melanocyte stimulating hormone in inducing differentiation in melanoma cells, *Proc Natl Acad Sci U S A* (1974) **71**:2500–4.
50. Hunt G, Kyne S, Wakamatsu K et al., Nle^4DPhe^7 α-Melanocyte-stimulating hormone increases the eumelanin: Phaeomelanin ratio in cultured human melanocytes, *J Invest Dermatol* (1995) **104**:83–5.
51. Mountjoy KG, The human melanocyte stimulating hormone receptor has evolved to become "super-sensitive" to melanocortin peptides, *Mol Cell Endocrinol* (1994) **102**:R7–R11.
52. Smith R, Healy E, Siddiqui S et al., Melanocortin 1 receptor variants in Irish population, *J Invest Dermatol* (1998) **111**:119–22.
53. Box NF, Wyeth JR, O'Gorman LE et al., Characterization of melanocyte stimulating hormone receptor variant alleles in twins with red hair, *Hum Mol Genet* (1997) **6**:1891–7.
54. Frändberg P-A, Doufexis M, Kapas S et al., Human pigmentation phenotype: A point mutation generates nonfunctional MSH receptor, *Biochem Biophys Res Commun* (1998) **245**:490–2.
55. Schiöth HB, Phillips SR, Rudzish R et al., Loss of function mutations of the human melanocortin 1 receptor are common and are associated with red hair, *Biochem Biophys Res Commun* (1999) **260**:488–91.
56. Koppula SV, Robbins LS, Lu D et al., Identification of common polymorphisms in the coding sequence of the human MSH receptor (MC1R) with possible biological effects, *Hum Mutat* (1997) **9**:30–6.
57. Harding RM, Healy E, Ray AJ et al., Evidence for variable selective pressures at MC1R, *Am J Hum Genet* (2000) **66**:1351–61.
58. Smith AI, Funder JE, Proopiomelanocortin processing in the pituitary, central nervous system and peripheral tissues, *Endocrinol Rev* (1988); **9**:159–79.
59. Takahashi H, Hakamata Y, Watanabe Y et al., Complete nucleotide sequence of the human corticotropin-β-lipotropin precursor gene, *Nucleic Acids Res* (1983) **11**:6847–58.
60. Krude H, Biebermann H, Luck W et al., Severe early-onset obesity, adrenal insufficiency and red hair pigmentation caused by *POMC* mutations in humans, *Nat Genet* (1998) **19**:155–7.
61. DeBold CR, Menefee JK, Nicholson WE et al., Proopiomelanocortin gene is expressed in many normal human tissues and in tumors not associated with ectopic adrenocorticotropin syndrome, *Mol Endocrinol* (1988) **2**:862–70.
62. Chakraborty AK, Funasaka Y, Slominski A et al., Production and release of proopiomelanocortin (POMC) derived peptides by human melanocytes and keratinocytes in culture: regulation by ultraviolet B, *Biochim Biophys Acta* (1996) **1313**:130–8.
63. Kwon HY, Bultman SJ, Löffler C et al., Molecular structure and chromosomal mapping of the human homolog of the agouti gene, *Proc Natl Acad Sci U S A* (1994) **91**:9760–4.
64. Lu D, Willard D, Patel IR et al., Agouti protein is an antagonist of the melanocyte-stimulating-hormone receptor, *Nature* (1994) **371**:799–802.
65. Siegrist W, Willard DH, Wilkison WO et al., Agouti protein inhibits growth of B16 melanoma cells in vitro by acting through melanocortin receptors, *Biochem Biophys Res Commun* (1996) **218**:171–5.
66. Duke-Cohan JS, Gu J, McLaughlin DF et al., Attractin (DPPT-L), a member of the CUB family of cell adhesion and guidance proteins, is secreted by activated human T lymphocytes and modulates immune cell interactions, *Proc Natl Acad Sci U S A* (1998) **95**:11336–41.
67. He L, Gunn TM, Bouley DM et al., A biochemical function for attractin in agouti-induced pigmentation and obesity, *Nat Genet* (2001) **27**:40–7.

68. Kuramoto T, Kitada K, Inui T et al., Attractin/Mahogany/Zitter plays a critical role in myelination of the central nervous system, *Proc Natl Acad Sci U S A* (2001) **98**:559–64.
69. Imokawa G, Yada Y, Miyagishi M, Endothelins secreted from human keratinocytes are intrinsic mitogens for human melanocytes, *J Biol Chem* (1992) **267**:24675–80.
70. Tada A, Suzuki I, Im S et al., Endothelin-1 is a paracrine growth factor that modulates melanogenesis of human melanocytes and participates in their responses to ultraviolet radiation, *Cell Growth Differ* (1998) **9**:575–84.
71. Healy E, Flannagan N, Ray A et al., Melanocortin-1 receptor gene and sun sensitivity in individuals without red hair, *Lancet* (2000) **355**:1072–3.
72. Im S, Moro O, Peng F et al., Activation of the cAMP pathway by α-melanotropin mediates the response of human melanocytes to UVB light, *Cancer Res* (1998) **58**:47–54.
73. Bustamante J, Bredeston L, Malanga G et al., Role of melanin as a scavenger of active oxygen species, *Pigment Cell Res* (1993) **6**:348–53.
74. Haycock JW, Rowe SJ, Cartledge S et al., α-Melanocyte-stimulating hormone reduces impact of proinflammatory cytokine and peroxide-generated oxidative stress on keratinocyte and melanoma cell lines, *J Biol Chem* (2000) **275**:15629–36.
75. Yohn JJ, Norris DA, Yrastorza DG et al., Disparate antioxidant enzyme activities in cultured human cutaneous fibroblasts, keratinocytes, and melanocytes, *J Invest Dermatol* (1991) **97**:405–9.

14

The role of SOX10 in melanocyte development and function

Corine Bertolotto and Robert Ballotti

The embryonic neural crest gives rise to multipotent cells originating in the dorsal part of the neural tube and then differentiating into several lineages, including the peripheral nervous system, glial, bone, cartilage, adrenomedullary cells and melanocytes of the skin, hair and inner ears. The mechanisms governing the development of neural crest-derived melanocytes and how alterations in these pathways lead to hypopigmentation are not fully understood.

Melanoblasts migrate along a dorsolateral pathway before taking up their final positions in the hair follicles and epidermis.[1,2] Subsequently, the melanoblasts differentiate to melanin-producing melanocytes by acquiring a specific enzymatic machinery responsible for pigment production. Three melanocyte-specific enzymes: tyrosinase, tyrosinase-related protein 1 (tyrp1) and Dopa-Chrome tautomerase/tyrosinase-related protein 2 (DCT), are involved in the enzymatic process that converts tyrosine to melanin pigments that are responsible for the skin color.[3–7]

Waardenburg syndrome-associated proteins

Microphthalmia-associated transcription factor (MITF) is a basic helix-loop-helix leucine zipper transcription factor that plays a crucial role in the survival and differentiation of melanocytes. In mice, mutations in *Mitf* gene lead to hypopigmentation due to absence of melanocytes, supporting the involvement of MITF in melanocyte development and survival.[8,9] MITF has also been demonstrated to control pigmentation by up-regulating the expression of tyrosinase, tyrp1 and DCT through the binding and activation of their promoter sequences demonstrating its role in melanocyte differentiation.[10–12] In humans, mutations within the *MITF* gene have been associated with the Waardenburg syndrome type 2a. Waardenburg syndrome, of which four types exist (WS 1–4), is a rare disorder (1 in 40 000 live births) characterized by distinctive facial features, cochlear deafness and pigmentary defects due to the failure of melanoblasts to develop normally.[13–15] The Waardenburg syndrome types 1 and 3 result from mutations in the *PAX3* gene, which encodes a paired domain and homeodomain transcription factor (Tassabehji, 1992 #85; 95 hum mol genet). PAX3 has been shown to bind and transactivate the MITF promoter while PAX3 mutant forms, found in patients with WS fail to do so. These results demonstrate an epistatic relationship between MITF and PAX3 that can explain the pigmentary defects observed in WS 1 and 3.[16,17] Patients with WS 4, also called Waardenburg–Hirschsprung's disease or Shah–Waardenburg syndrome, show, during the neonatal period, an aganglionic megacolon that leads to an intestinal obstruction characteristic of the Hirschsprung's disease.[18] Mutations in three different genes have been identified in WS 4. These genes include the endothelin-B receptor gene, the gene coding for its ligand, the endothelin-3, and the gene encoding the transcription factor *SOX10*.[19–22]

Structure and function of the SOX10 transcription factor

SOX10 is a member of the sex determining factor (SRY)-like, high mobility group (HMG) DNA binding

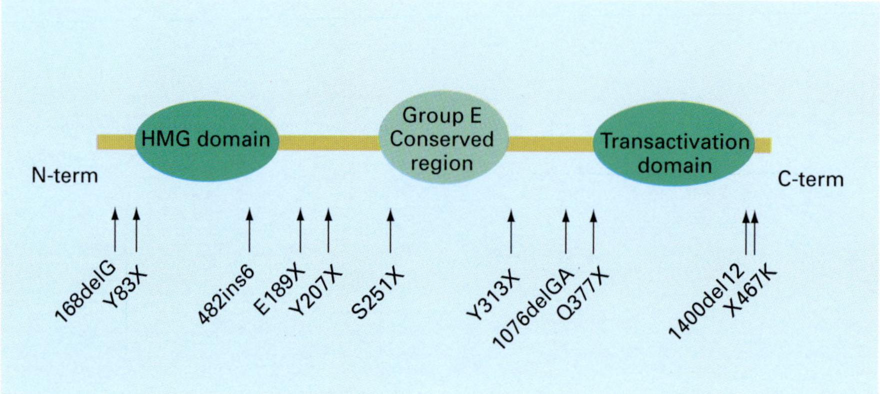

Figure 14.1

Structure of SOX10 and mutations of this gene identified in WS4 patients.

transcription factors that possess a transactivation domain in their C-terminal part (Fig. 14.1).[23] To date, more than 20 members of the SOX10 gene family have been identified in mammals. Their binding to a 7 bp consensus DNA element (AT)(AT)CAA(AT)G as monomers or dimers, induces a strong DNA bend.[24–26] This generates a conformational change of the promoters and their associated proteins therefore constituting an enhanceosome-like structure.[27] SOX proteins play important roles in diverse developmental processes such as sex determination, chondrogenic differentiation, hematopoiesis and melanocyte development.[17,28] In the mouse, the expression of Sox10 is initiated in neural crest cells as they dissociate from the neural tube and is maintained during migration of neural crest cells. Then, Sox10 expression continues in the glial and melanocyte lineages, but is turned off in many other neural crest-derived cells.[29–31] In mice, in the heterozygous state, the spontaneous mutation of *Sox10*, identified as the dominant megacolon mutation (*Sox10^{Dom}*/+), causes intestinal aganglionosis and spotted pigmentation.[32,33] This homozygous mutation of *Sox10* (*Sox10^{Dom}*/*Sox10^{Dom}*) is lethal and the embryos fail to produce melanoblasts. In zebrafish, mutations at the *colourless* locus lead to an extensive loss of pigment cells and cells of the enteric nervous system, as well as large reductions in sensory and sympathic neurones, resembling the WS 4 phenotype.[35,35] Recently, a zebrafish *Sox10* homologue has been mapped to the *colourless* locus. Moreover, mutations in this *Sox10* homologue have been identified in the *colourless* zebrafish and Sox10 expression rescues the wild type zebrafish phenotype.[36] These observations indicate that Sox10 plays a critical role in the early development of the melanocyte lineage in different species.

Involvement of SOX10 in the regulation of MITF

The fact that mutations within the *Mitf*, *Pax3* or *Sox10* genes give similar phenotypes suggest a potential relationship between these transcription factors in melanocyte development. Recently, a genetic interaction between Sox10 and Mitf has been demonstrated *in vivo*. Mice with mutations in either *Sox10* (*Sox10^{Dom}*/+) or *Mitf* (Mitf^{mi}/+) are almost completely pigmented with some hypopigmented ventral spot. On the other hand, double heterozygote mice (*Sox10^{Dom}*/+; Mitf^{mi}/+) show extensive hypopigmentation thereby indicating that both Sox10 and Mitf act synergistically to govern the development of neural crest-derived melanocytes (Fig. 14.2).[17] Furthermore, in homozygous *Sox10* mutant embryos (*Sox10^{Dom}*/*Sox10^{Dom}*) no Mitf-positive cells can be detected.[37] As Mitf expression follows that of Sox10 in melanoblasts migrating along the dorsolateral embryonic pathway, this suggests that Sox10 might be involved in the regulation of Mitf.[8,38] This

$Mitf^{mi}$/+ *$Soc10^{Dom}$/+*

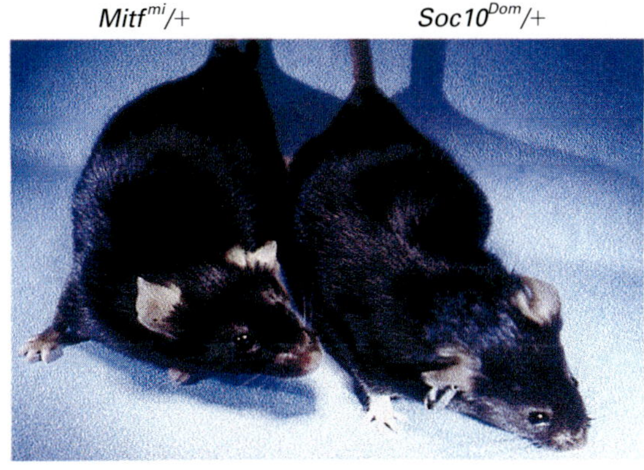

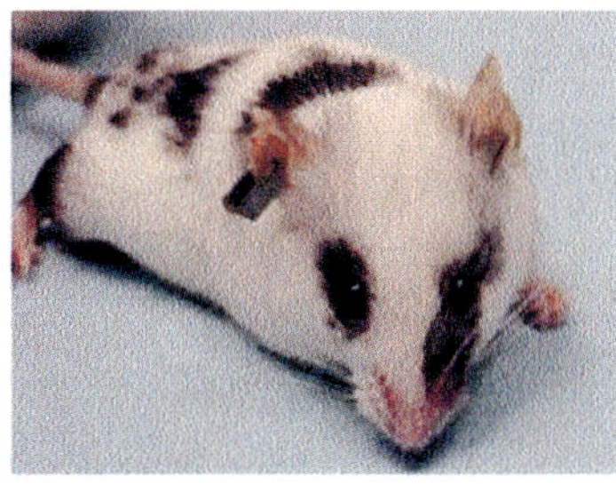

$Mitf^{mi}$/+; $Soc10^{Dom}$/+

Figure 14.2

Synergistic interaction between SOX10 and MITF *in vivo. (from Potterfet al, Hum. Genet. 2000, 107: 1–6)*

hypothesis is supported by the identification of four potential Sox binding sites in the proximal region of the *MITF* promoter.[17,39,40] Analysis of the *MITF* promoter activity in melanoma (B16 and Mel501 cells) or in non-melanocyte (Hela or NIH3T3 cells) cell lines that do not express Sox10, reveals that SOX10 strongly stimulates the transcriptional activity of the *MITF* promoter.[17,39–41] Additionally, a mutation in the HMG domain abolishes the ability of SOX10 to activate the *MITF* promoter indicating that SOX10 DNA binding is required for its activity.[40] SOX4, another member of the SRY-related transcription factors does not affect the *MITF* promoter activity either in B16 or NIH3T3 cells, which suggests a specific role of SOX10 in regulating the *MITF* promoter activity.[40] As mentioned before, PAX3 has been shown to stimulate the activity of the *MITF* promoter.[42] Interestingly, the SOX10 binding sequences are adjacent to the PAX3 site in the *MITF* promoter. Moreover, previous observations have reported that SOX10 can act in partnership with PAX3 in glial cells[43] and in the formation of the enteric nervous system.[44] In agreement with these observations, SOX10 and PAX3, together lead to a better stimulation of the *MITF* promoter activity compared to their respective independent action. Further, a SOX10 mutant, lacking the transactivation domain, fails to stimulate the *MITF* promoter and the synergism with PAX3 is lost. This data show that SOX10 and PAX3 functionally cooperate to fully transactivate the *MITF* promoter.[17,41] It should be mentioned that the concerted action of PAX3 and SOX10 has been observed in non-melanocyte cells such as Hela and NIH3T3 cells. However, other experiments, performed in B16 melanoma cells, indicate that SOX10 and PAX3 do not synergize to up-regulate the *MITF* promoter.[40] This result is consistent with the previous observation that SOX10 and PAX3 do not interact *in vitro* and that mutation of the PAX3 sequence in the *MITF* promoter does not impair the SOX10 responsiveness of the promoter.[39,40] Thus, it remains to clearly establish whether PAX3 and SOX10 synergism is required, *in vivo*, to fully stimulate the *MITF* promoter. Whatever the case, mutants of SOX10 found in WS 4 failed to activate the *MITF* promoter and dramatically reduced the expression of endogenous MITF (Fig. 14.3).[17,39,40] It has been suggested that the developmental defects, observed in WS 4 disease, are caused by a dominant-negative action of the SOX10 mutant protein.[17,21,22,33,39] Interestingly, the expression of DCT, the enzyme involved in melanin synthesis, is dramatically reduced in heterozygous Sox10 mutant mouse, and is completely absent in homozygous animals.[37,45] Further, transient transfection experiments confirm that SOX10 stimulates the activity of the DCT promoter, while a mutant of SOX10, in which the transactivation domain has been deleted, fails to activate the promoter.[45] These results demonstrate that SOX10 may have a direct role in the regulation of melanocyte differentiation by regulating the expression of DCT. However, at least in mice, the

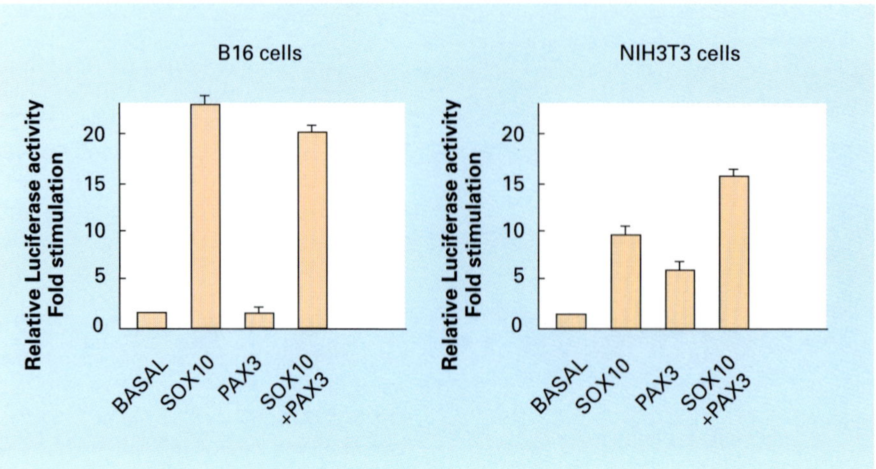

Figure 14.3

Effects of SOX10 and PAX3 on the MITF promoter activity in melanoma cells (B16 mouse melanoma) and in non-melanocyte cell type (NIH3T3 cells). *(from Verastegui et al, J. Biol. Chem. 2000, 275: 30757–30760)*

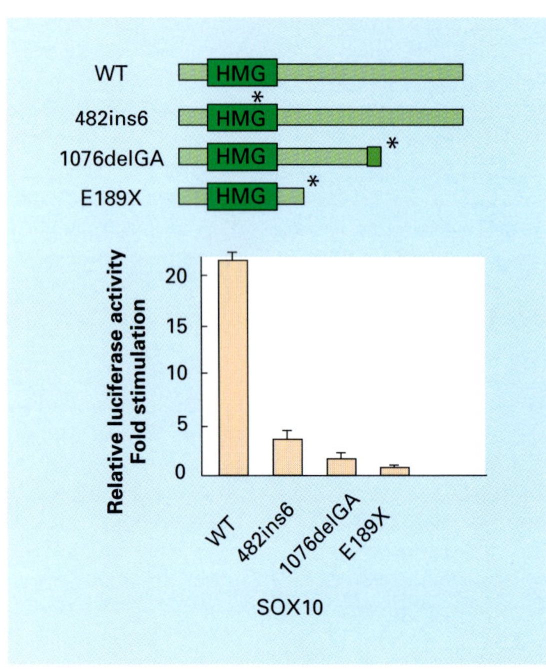

Figure 14.4

Mutations found in WS4 patients (Figure 1) invalidate the transcriptional activity of SOX10. *(from Verastegui et al, J. Biol. Chem. 2000, 275: 30757–30760)*

regulation of DCT by Sox10 is transient and restricted to early phases. Indeed, later stages of melanocyte development show a normal expression of DCT, indicating that Sox10 has a selective spatio-temporal action on DCT expression.[45] Additional studies are now required to determine the mechanisms allowing an expression of DCT during later stages of melanocyte development.

Together, these data provide compelling evidence that one consequence of SOX10 invalidation is to reduce the expression of MITF. Because MITF plays a key role in the melanocyte development and differentiation, these observations give new clues to the auditory-pigmentary symptoms in Waardenburg type 4 syndrome that results from the absence of melanocytes in the affected organs.

References

1. Hall BK, *New York: Springer*, (1999).
2. Le Douarin NM, Kalcheim C, *Cambridge, UK: Cambridge University Press*, (1999)
3. Jackson IJ, *Proc Natl Acad Sci U S A* (1988) **85**:4392–6.
4. Jackson IJ, Chambers DM,, Tsukamoto K et al., *Embo J* (1992) **11**:527–35.

5. Shibahara S, Tomita Y., Sakakura T et al., *Nucleic Acids Res* (1986) **14**:2413–27.
6. Tanaka S, Yamamoto H, Takeuchi S, Takeuchi T, *Development* (1990) **108**:223–7.
7. Tsukamoto K, Jackson IJ, Urabe K et al., *Embo J* (1992) **11**:519–26.
8. Hodgkinson CA, Nakayama A, Li H et al.,*Hum Mol Genet* (1998) **7**:703–8.
9. Steingrimsson E, Moore KJ, Lamoreux ML et al., *Nat Genet* (1994) **8**:256–63.
10. Bertolotto C, Busca R, Abbe P et al., *Mol Cell Biol* (1998) **18**:694–702.
11. Lowings P, Yavuzer U, Goding CR, *Mol Cell Biol* (1992) **12**:3653–62.
12. Yokoyama K, Yasumoto K, Suzuki H, Shibahara S, *J Biol Chem* (1994) **269**:27080–7.
13. Tachibana M, Perez-Jurado LA, Nakayama A et al., *Hum Mol Genet* (1994) **3**:553–7.
14. Tachibana M, *J Investig Dermatol Symp Proc* (1999) **4**:126–9.
15. Tassabehji M, Newton VE, Read AP, *Nature Genet* (1994) **8**:251–5
16. Watanabe A, Takeda K, Ploplis B, Tachibana M, *Nat Genet* (1998) **18**:283–6.
17. Potterf SB, Furumura M, Dunn KJ et al., *Hum Genet* (2000) **107**:1–6.
18. Badner JA, Chakravarti A, *Am J Med Genet* (1990) **35**:100–4.
19. Attie T, Till M, Pelet A et al., *Hum Mol Genet* (1995) **4**:2407–9.
20. Edery P, Attie T, Amiel J et al., *Nat Genet* (1996) **12**:442–4.
21. Kuhlbrodt K, Schmidt C, Sock E et al., *J Biol Chem* (1998) **273**:23033–8.
22. Pingault V, Bondurand N, Kuhlbrodt K et al., *Nat Genet* (1998) **18**:171–3.
23. Pevny LH, Lovell-Badge R, *Curr Opin Genet Dev* (1997) **7**:338–44.
24. Kamachi Y, Cheah KS, Kondoh H, *Mol Cell Biol* (1999) **19**:107–20.
25. McDowall S, Argentaro A, Ranganathan S et al., *J Biol Chem* (1999) **274**:24023–30.
26. Peirano RI, Wegner M, *Nucleic Acids Res* (2000) **28**:3047–55.
27. Prior HM, Walter MA, *Mol Med* (1996) **2**:405–12.
28. Wegner M, *Nucleic Acids Res* (1999) **27**:1409–20.
29. Herbarth B, Pingault V, Bondurand N et al., *Proc Natl Acad Sci U S A* (1998) **95**:5161–5.
30. Kuhlbrodt K, Herbarth B, Sock E et al., *J Neurosci* (1998) **18**:237–50.
31. Pusch C, Hustert E, Pfeifer D et al., *Hum Genet* (1998) **103**:115–23.
32. Southard-Smith EM, Kos L, Pavan WJ, *Nat Genet* (1998) **18**:60–4.
33. Southard-Smith EM, Angrist M, Ellison JS et al., *Genome Res* (1999) **9**:215–25.
34. Kelsh RN, Eisen JS, *Development* (2000) **127**:515–25.
35. Kelsh RN, Schmid B, Eisen JS, *Dev Biol* (2000) **225**:277–93.
36. Dutton KA, Pauliny A, Lopes SS et al., *Development* (2001) **128**:4113–25.
37. Britsch S, Goerich DE, Riethmacher D et al.,*Genes Dev* (2001) **15**:66–78.
38. Nakayama A, Nguyen MT, Chen CC et al., *Mech Dev* (1998) **70**:155–66.
39. Lee M, Goodall J, Verastegui C et al., *J Biol Chem* (2000) **275**:37978–83.
40. Verastegui C, Bille K, Ortonne JP, Ballotti R, *J Biol Chem* (2000) **275**:30757–60.
41. Bondurand N, Pingault V, Goerich DE et al., *Hum Mol Genet* (2000) **9**:1907–17.
42. Watanabe K, Takeda K, Katori Y et al., *Brain Res Mol Brain Res* (2000) **84**:141–5.
43. Kuhlbrodt K, Herbarth B, Sock E et al., *J Biol Chem* (1998) **273**:16050–7.
44. Lang D, Chen F, Milewski R et al., *J Clin Invest* (2000) **106**:963–71.
45. Potterf SB, Mollaaghababa R, Hou L et al., *Dev Biol* (2001) **237**:245–57.

15
Crosstalk between the cAMP and the MAPK pathways in melanocytes

Roser Buscà

Melanocytes and the cAMP regulation of melanogenesis

Melanocytes are specialized epidermal cells, which derive from the neural crest. During embryonic development, non-differentiated melanocytes (melanoblasts) migrate to reach the basal layer of the epidermis, where they differentiate to mature melanocytes possessing the complete machinery to ensure melanin synthesis and distribution within the skin.[1,2] Melanin synthesis takes place within specialized intracellular organelles named melanosomes, which move from the perinuclear region to the dendrite extremities and are then transferred to keratinocytes by a still not well-characterized mechanism. These events, which ensure uniform distribution of melanin pigments in the epidermis, are responsible for skin and hair color in humans and animals. The rate-limiting enzymes controlling melanogenesis are tyrosinase, Tyrp-1 and DCT, which play a regulatory part in a complex enzymatic cascade ending in melanin synthesis.[3–5]

Melanogenesis can be induced by UV light directly acting on melanocytes (see reference 6 for a review). As observed by the group of B. Gilchrest, this involves membrane phospholipids modification leading to phospholipase C, diacylglycerol and PKC signaling (reviewed in references 7 and 8). Roméro-Graillet et al.[9] have shown that nitric oxide (NO) can also be a UV-induced melanocyte factor involved in melanogenesis. DNA damage and DNA repair also seem to play relevant roles in melanocyte UV direct melanogenesis induction.[10] Nevertheless, most of the melanogenic response is a result of paracrine effects of UV-induced keratinocyte-released factors acting on melanocytes. Among keratinocyte-secreted factors which induce melanocyte activation, we find prostaglandins PGE2,[11] the pro-opiomelanocortin peptides, α-MSH and ACTH, which activate the cAMP pathway,[12] endothelin-1,[13,14] and NO, which activates the cGMP pathway.[15] On the other hand, in response to UV, keratinocytes secrete specific factors that inhibit melanogenesis, such as interleukin-1α, TNF-α, interferons and bFGF. The balance between the actions of these multiple keratinocyte factors results in the activation or inhibition of distinct molecular mechanisms, finely regulating melanocyte growth, differentiation and survival, thereby controlling skin pigmentation.

The pro-opiomelanocortin peptide, α-MSH, is a strong melanogenic agent which binds to a particular receptor, MC1R, specifically present at the surface of melanocytes. MC1R is a seven-transmembrane domain receptor, coupled to an αs G-protein that activates adenylyl cyclase and upregulates the cAMP content in melanocytes. Several compelling genetic and epidemiologic data have pointed to the pivotal role of melanocortin peptides and the cAMP upregulation in melanogenesis. For example, skin hyperpigmentation has been reported in patients suffering from Addison's disease[16] or Cushing's syndrome, characterized by an overproduction of ACTH. A case of skin hyperpigmentation due to α-MSH hypersecretion has been reported.[17] Similarly to the observation made in mice, in humans, the pro-opiomelanocortin peptide and receptor system is also involved in control of melanin quality. Indeed, the red hair phenotype, which is due to pheomelanin instead of eumelanin synthesis, is associated with mutations in the MC1R receptor, some of which decrease the affinity of the receptor for its ligand.[18] More recently, mutations in the pro-opiomelanocortin gene, interfering with α-MSH and ACTH synthesis, have been found in patients with severe obesity and red hair pigmentation.[19] Administration of α-MSH analogs to humans induces skin pigmentation in the absence of UV exposure.[20–21] Furthermore, in cultured human melanocytes and in mouse melanoma cells, α-MSH and ACTH upregulate melanogenesis and dendricity.[22] These effects can be mimicked by pharmacological cAMP-elevating agents, such as forskolin (FK), cholera toxin (CT), and isobutylmethylxantine (IBMX).[23–24] These compelling observations clearly corroborate the essential role of the cAMP pathway in the regulation of melanogenesis.

The molecular mechanisms involved in the cAMP regulation of melanogenesis are developed in detail in Chapter 8, and they will not be discussed here. Just in summary, cAMP, by activating the protein kinase A, activates the CREB family of transcription factors. Once activated, CREB factors bind to their CRE consensus sequences found in specific gene promoters. A CRE sequence is found in the promoter of Microphthalmia (MITF), a tissue-specific and melanocyte-expressed transcription factor, which plays a crucial role in melanocyte development and survival,[25] as well as in melanogenesis, as described in Chapter 8. cAMP upregulation clearly increases MITF expression.[26] MITF is a basic helix-loop-helix transcription factor, containing a leucin zipper domain, and it binds to M-box and E-box sequences contained in the promoters of the melanogenic enzymes, tyrosinase, Tyrp-1 and DCT.[27,28] In consequence, when MITF expression is increased by the cAMP pathway, the MITF binding to its target sequences is enhanced, and, therefore, the transcriptional upregulation of these melanogenic genes takes place. Therefore, cAMP highly increases the melanogenic enzyme expression in an MITF-dependent manner and this results in melanin synthesis.

Very interestingly, in the melanocyte cell system, the cAMP second messenger regulates several signaling pathways, such as the PI3K/p70S6K[29] and PI3K/Akt pathways (unpublished results), the pathways commanded by the Rho family of small GTP-binding proteins[24] and the MAP-kinase pathway, on which we will focus in this chapter.

The MAPK pathway

The mitogen-activated protein kinases (MAP-kinases) ERK1 and ERK2 are serine threonin kinases activated upon dual phosphorylation by the MAPK kinase (MAPKK) MEK which, in its turn, is phorphorylated and, therefore, activated by the MAPKKK of the Raf family (reviewed in references 30 and 31). Raf kinases are activated after their interaction with the GTP-bound form of p21 Ras (reviewed in reference 32). Ras is a small, GTP-binding protein which is activated by its specific exchange factors, of which Son of Sevenless (SOS) is the most ubiquitous and widely studied.[33,34] The MAPK pathway links the cell-surface-mediated signals to expression of specific genes. It transmits signaling from tyrosine kinase receptor, some G-protein-coupled receptors, cytokine receptors, and integrins, through the above-described cascade of events. MAP-kinases are able to phosphorylate multiple substrates found in various subcellular localizations: membrane-associated, such as epidermal growth-factor receptor (EGFr),[35] and cytoplasmic, such as c-PLA2,[36] but most of the MAPK subtrates are transcription factors, such as Elk-1/TCF[37–39] or c-myc.[40] MAPK also phosphorylates and activates p90Rsk,[41] which is also involved in the transcriptional regulation of several genes, as well as in protein translation. The nuclear translocation of MAP-kinase is a crucial event for the regulation of its function. MAP-kinases have been shown to be involved in proliferation, differentiation, and survival, depending on the cell type.

Connecting cAMP to MAP-kinases in melanocytes

In melanocytes, as in other cell systems, MAP-kinases ERK1 and ERK2 are activated by multiple stimuli, including growth factors, such as the Steel factor (Sl/mast/stem cell growth factor), nerve growth factor (NGF), epidermal growth factor (EFG), fibroblast growth factor (FGF), TPA which acts through PKC activation, and hormones like endothelin-1. But what makes melanocytes a relevant cell system here is that MAP-kinases are also activated by the cAMP stimulus (α-MSH and pharmacological cAMP-elevating agents) in a cell-specific manner. cAMP activates MAP-kinases in B16 mouse melanoma cells[23] and in normal human melanocytes.[6] To date, cAMP has been reported to activate MAP-kinases in a very limited number of other cell types, including T-cells[42] and PC12 rat phaeochromocytoma.[43,44] By the time a cAMP activation of MAPK in melanocyte cells was first observed, a cAMP-dependent activation of MAPK had only been found in PC12 cells, and the fact that both PC12 cells and melanocytes derive from the neural crest led to the hypothesis of a neuronal-like specificity of this activation. Thus, elucidating the role of MAPK pathway and the cell-specific mechanisms of MAPK activation by cAMP in melanocyte cells became interesting subjects of study.

The role of the MAPK pathway in melanocytes, MAPK and melanogenesis

Initially, the strong melanogenic effects of cAMP, and the finding that cAMP activates the MAPK cascade in melanocytes, suggested that MAPK activation could mediate at least some of the cAMP-induced melanogenesis. Furthermore, cAMP activates the AP-1 transcription factor in mouse melanoma cells, suggesting that AP-1 could also be involved in the cAMP-induced melanogenesis. In contrast to these initial hypotheses, further experiments added important information to these findings. The inhibition of the MAP-kinase pathway in mouse melanoma cells, by using the MEK inhibitor PD98059, resulted in increased tyrosinase activity and expression. Additionally, overexpression of dominant-negative mutants of p21Ras and MEK acting upstream of MAPK, together with a 2.2 Kb fragment of the mouse tyrosinase promoter cloned upstream of the luciferase reporter gene, showed an increase in the tyrosinase promoter activity, thus revealing a melanogenesis induction.[45] Moreover, the overexpression of a constitutive active mutant of p21Ras or MEK inhibited the melanogenic promoter activity, thus indicating a melanogenesis inhibition.[45] Thus, MAPK pathway activation in melanocyte cells inhibits melanogenesis. Taking these findings together, cAMP upregulation plays a dual role in melanogenesis: on the one hand, it activates PKA, thus increasing MITF and melanogenic enzyme expression, and on the other, it activates the MAPK pathway which inhibits melanogenesis. We could speculate that this constitutes a fine retrocontrol process that prevents the overproduction of melanin that is toxic for melanocytes.

Very interesting studies have connected the MAPK pathway and melanocyte behavior. Specific pigmentation anomalies, found in syndromes such as piebaldism and Waardenburg type II, have put much attention on c-Kit and MITF as transducers of melanocyte lineage development and, therefore, melanogenic response. The receptor tyrosine kinase, c-Kit, and its ligand, the Steel factor (Sl, mast/stem cell growth factor), have been found mutated in piebaldism, characterized by patchy depigmentation. MITF has been found mutated in Waardenburg syndrome type II, characterized by marked depigmentation and deafness due to the absence of melanocytes in skin and the inner ear (reviewed in reference 46). In 1998, the group of Dr Fisher reported a biochemical link between c-Kit signaling, the MAPK pathway and melanogenesis. In response to the Sl factor, the activated c-Kit receptor activates the MAPK cascade. Activated MAP-kinase rapidly phosphorylates MITF at its Ser73 and this phosphorylation increases the MITF-dependent transcriptional reporter activity (Fig. 15.1). Nevertheless, this phosphorylation does not significantly alter MITF subcellular localization nor DNA binding or dimerization. The dissection of the molecular events leading to this MAPK-dependent increase in MITF transcriptional activity have revealed that MITF phosphorylation by MAPK at Ser73 enhances the recruitment of p300/CBP (CREB-binding protein),[46] an MITF coactivator that interacts with and modulates the transcriptional activity of the factor.[47]

Later on, Xu et al.[48] added new insights into the understanding of the role of MITF phosphorylation by MAPK. By the two-hybrid system, they demonstrated that MITF interacts with the ubiquitin-conjugating enzyme, hUBC9, and suggested that MITF phosphorylation at Ser73 mediates this interaction. Overexpression of hUBC9 in transfected melanocyte cells promoted proteosome-mediated degradation of phosphorylated MITF that was abolished by mutation of the MAPK phosphorylation site Ser73 to alanine. The conclusion from this work was that phosphorylation of MITF by MAPK promotes ubiquitinilation of the transcription factor on K201 and its subsequent targeting to the proteasome for degradation. This was further complicated when Wu et al.[49] found that Ser409 at the C-terminus of MITF is likely to be a target of p90Rsk, which is an MAPK target.

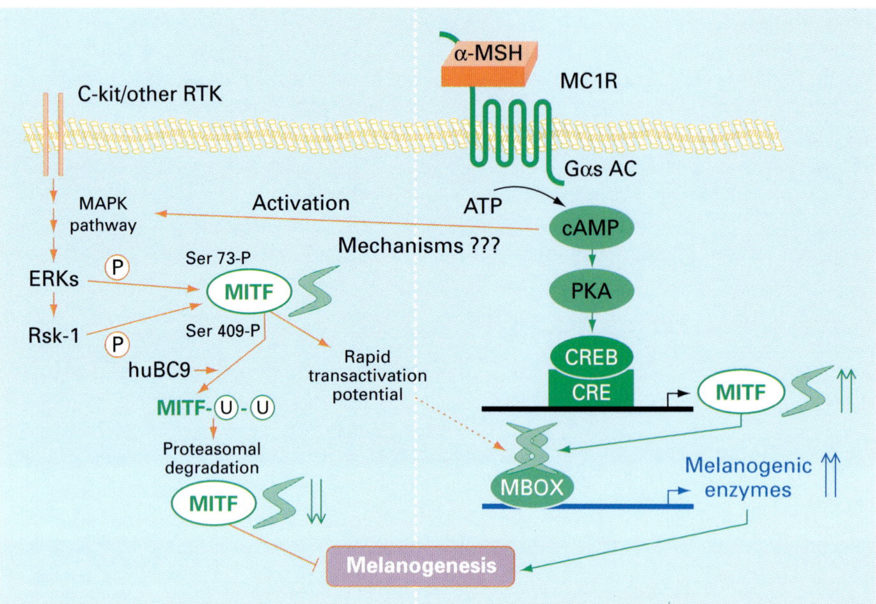

Figure 15.1

Model for the dual role of cAMP in melanogenesis. The MAPK pathway appears to be a very important regulatory point in melanocyte biology as well as in the cAMP-induced melanogenesis. MITF is the central melanogenic point where the cAMP-CREB and cAMP-MAPK-Rsk-1 pathways converge. Multiple signals regulate MITF expression and activity. Rapid expression and activation versus the stability of the transcription factor by these different signals are critical steps for the proper function of MITF, the control of melanocyte development, proliferation, survival and, finally, melanogenesis, which leads to pigmentation. RTK, receptor tyrosine kinase; MC1R, melanocortin 1 receptor; AC, adenylyl cyclase.

These authors report that the stability of MITF is dependent on a dual phosphorylation event: the MAPK phosphorylation of Ser73 on MITF, and the p90Rsk phosphorylation of the transcription factor on Ser409. They show that the stability of MITF is unaffected in the presence of the c-Kit signaling, only when both residues are substitued by an alanine, but the transcription factor loses its transactivation potential. Thus, the signals that produce transcriptional activation and protein degradation of MITF are functionally coupled in melanocytes.

In any case, considering the effects of the MAPK pathway on MITF, we can clearly explain why a melanogenesis inhibition is observed when the MAPK pathway is switched on in a sustained manner. MAPK phosphorylation of MITF on Ser73, even though rapidly increasing the MITF transactivation potential, acts as a relevant degradation signal for the transcription factor. In addition, the Rsk phosphorylation of MITF on Ser409 produces the same effect on MITF stability, all these events resulting in MITF degradation. MITF being degraded and, therefore, reduced in amount, it cannot bind to the regulatory consensus sequences found in the melanogenic enzyme promoters. This results in a reduced melanogenic enzyme transcription and, therefore, decreased melanogenesis (Fig. 15.1).

In summary, the MAPK pathway appears to be a very important regulatory point in melanocyte biology, as well as in cAMP-induced melanogenesis (Fig. 15.1). MITF is, to date, the central melanogenic point where the cAMP-CREB and cAMP-MAPK-Rsk-1 pathways converge. Since MITF plays several roles in 'melanocyte life', it seems obvious to consider that multiple signals must regulate its expression and activity. Rapid expression and activation versus the stability of the transcription factor by these different signals are critical steps for the proper function of MITF, the control of melanocyte development, proliferation, survival and, finally, melanogenesis, which leads to pigmentation.

In view of this critical role of the MAPK pathway in melanocytes and the fact that this pathway is specifically activated by the cAMP signal in these cells, great interest has been focused on the specific mechanisms by which cAMP activates MAPK in melanocyte cells.

Mechanisms of cAMP-dependent activation of MAPK in melanocytes

It is clear that cAMP upregulation, by the physiological stimulus of α-MSH or by pharmacological cAMP-elevating agents, activates the MAP-kinases ERK1 and ERK2 in normal human melanocytes and melanoma cells (Fig. 15.2).[50] This activation seems to be quite cell specific, since it takes place in very few cell types, such as melanocyte cells and PC12 cells, which both possess a neural origin.

In melanocyte cells, cAMP also activates the MAPK-kinase MEK-1 and the MEK-kinase B-Raf that function upstream of ERKs in the classical MAPK pathway. B-Raf is a Raf isoform which is highly expressed in neuronal cells, and such a high expression has also been found in melanocytes (unpublished data). Raf-1, which is the ubiquitously expressed form of MEK-kinase, is not activated by cAMP in melanocyte cells. Raf-1 is rather inhibited by the cAMP signaling in melanocytes and other cell systems. These results strongly suggest that B-Raf mediates the cAMP-dependent activation of MAP-kinases in melanocytes. Studies using dominant-negative mutants of Raf-1 and B-Raf have shown that the cAMP activation of ERKs involves B-Raf, and not Raf-1 activation. Further, Raf-1 cannot transmit the cAMP effects, since the kinase is inhibited by cAMP itself. How B-Raf is activated by cAMP in melanocytes remains to be elucidated. Is there a cell-specific mechanism

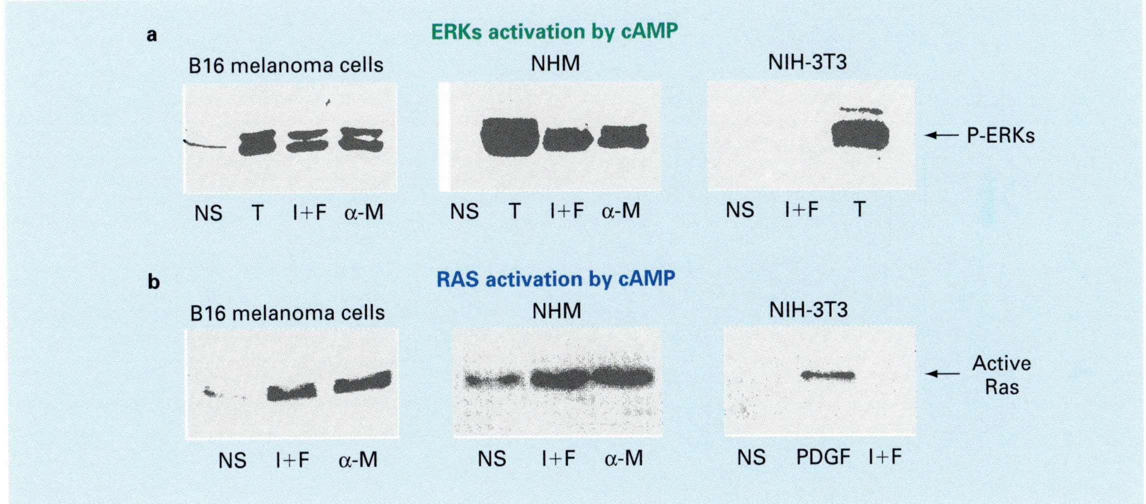

Figure 15.2

(a) cAMP activates ERKs in melanocyte cells. Lysates from non-stimulated cells (NS), cells stimulated for 10 minutes with the cAMP-elevating agents, forskolin plus IBMX (I+F), α-MSH (α-M) or with the protein kinase C activator, TPA (T) were subjected to Western blot analysis with an anti-phospho-ERKs antibody to detect the activated forms of ERKS. (b) cAMP activates Ras in melanocyte cells. B16 cells, normal human melanocytes or NIH-3T3 fibroblasts were treated with IBMX plus forskolin (I+F) or with α-MSH (α-M) for the indicated times. Cells were lysed and subjected to 'pull-down' experiments using a B-Raf RBD GST fusion protein to detect activated Ras. NIH-3T3 fibroblasts were also stimulated for 5 minutes with PDGF as a positive control. Precipitated proteins were subjected to Western blotting using an anti-Ras monoclonal antibody.

leading to this B-Raf activation? In PC12 cells, it has been shown that the small GTP-binding protein, Rap-1, in a PKA-dependent manner, activates B-Raf and ERKs,[51] but in melanocytes this does not seem to be the case, since Rap-1 mutants do not exercise any effect on the activation of ERKs. In melanocytes, cAMP activates Ras and this activation is crucial for downstream ERKs phosphorylation, since a dominant-negative mutant of Ras blocks the cAMP-dependent activation of ERKs in B16 melanoma cells. Moreover, a cAMP activation of Ras had never been found in other cell systems. Very recently, Tsygankova et al.,[52] and Ambrosini et al.,[53] have observed a Ras activation by cAMP in thyroid cells and cortical neurons, respectively. In melanocyte cells, the cAMP activation of Ras is not mediated by the classical Ras exchange factor SOS, and, very interestingly, Ras activation is independent of PKA activation, since neither a specific PKA inhibitor nor the overexpression of the PKA catalytic subunit affects the cAMP regulation of ERKs activity. So far, most of the described effects of cAMP undergo PKA activation; however, cAMP interacts directly with some ion channels[54,55] and PKA has not been clearly implicated in the cAMP regulation of some neural functions.[56–58] The mechanisms of cAMP activation of Ras are still unkown. In 1998, two independent groups cloned several exchange factors for the small GTP-binding protein Rap-1, containing a cAMP-binding sequence and which are directly activated by cAMP.[59,60] Nevertheless, these exchange factors do not function on Ras. Interestingly, in the HUGE (human unidentified gene-encoded) large proteins, a new protein, named KIAA0313, can be found, which possesses a cAMP-binding domain and a nucleotid exchange domain for Ras. The function of this protein has been recently analyzed by two separate groups: De Rooij et al.,[61] who have named the protein PDZ-GEF1, have described an ubiquitous expression of the protein and have found that it acts as a cAMP-regulated exchange factor for Rap-1 and Rap-2; and Pham et al.,[62] who have named the protein CNrasGEF, and report that the factor has a cAMP-dependent nucleotid exchange activity for

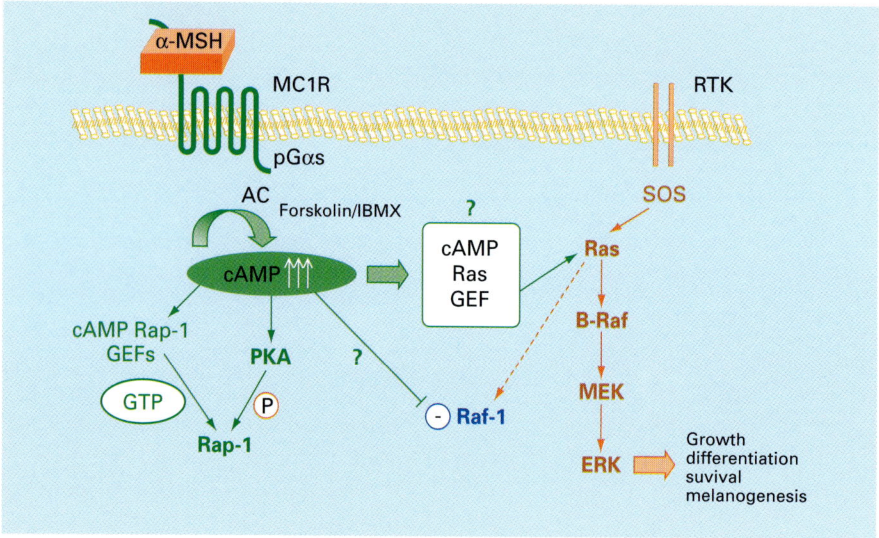

Figure 15.3

Model for the cAMP-dependent activation of the MAP-kinase pathway in melanocyte cells. α-Melanocyte-stimulating hormone (α-MSH) binds the melanocyte receptor (MC1R) and activates adenylyl cyclase (AC), leading to an increase in intracellular cAMP content. cAMP activates Rap-1 through phosphorylation by PKA by a cAMP-dependent Rap-1 GEFs (Epac/cAMP Rap-1 GEFs). In melanocytes, cAMP could also directly activate a still unidentified cell-specific cAMP-dependent Ras GEF ('cAMP Ras GEF') which would activate Ras in response to cAMP. Ras activates Raf-1 and B-Raf, but Raf-1 is inhibited by an unknown mechanism; therefore, activated B-Raf mediates the Ras activation of MEK and ERKs.

Ras. However, KIAA0313 does not act as an exchange factor for Ras in melanocyte cells, and, therefore, cannot be the candidate molecule mediating the cAMP activation of Ras in these cells (unpublished results). According to this, the hypothesis of the existence of a melanocyte-specific exchange factor for Ras directly activated by cAMP is worth considering and analyzing. The melanocyte-specific expression of such an exchange factor would explain the specific Ras, and therefore, MAPK, cascade activation by cAMP in melanocyte cells (Fig. 15.3). The identification of this factor and the study of its regulation would bring a much better understanding of the mechanisms of control of MAPK activation in melanocytes, a signaling pathway which participates in the melanogenic process.

References

1. Fitzpatrick TD, Szabo G, Seiji M et al., *Biology of the Melanin Pigmentary System* (1979) 131–63.
2. Le Douarin N, *The Neural Crest* (Cambridge University Press, 1982).
3. Hearing VJ, Jimenez M, Mammalian tyrosinase—the critical regulatory point in melanocyte pigmentation, *Int J Biochem* (1987) **19:**1141–7.
4. Kobayashi T, Urabe K, Winder A et al., Tyrosinase related protein 1 (TRP1) functions as a DHICA oxidase in melanin biosynthesis, *EMBO J* (1994) **13:** 5818–25.
5. Kameyama K, Takemura T, Hamada Y et al., Pigment production in murine melanoma cells is regulated by tyrosinase, tyrosinase-related protein1 (TRP-1), DOPAchrome tautomerase (TRP2) and a melanogenic inhibitor, *J Invest Dermatol* (1993) **100:**126–31.
6. Buscà R, Ballotti R, Cyclic AMP a key messenger in the regulation of skin pigmentation, *Pigment Cell Res* (2000) **13:**60–9.
7. Gilchrest BA, Park HY, Eller MS et al., Mechanisms of ultraviolet light-induced pigmentation, *Photochem Photobiol* (1996) **93:**1–10.
8. Park HY, Perez JM, Laursen R et al., Protein kinase C-beta activates tyrosinase by phosphorylating serine residues in its cytoplasmic domain, *J Biol Chem* (1999) **274:**16470–8.
9. Roméro-Graillet C, Aberdam E, Biagoli N et al., Ultraviolet B radiation acts through the nitric oxide and cGMP signal transduction pathway to stimulate melanogenesis in human melanocytes, *J Biol Chem* (1996) **271:**28052–6.
10. Eller MS, Maeda T, Magnoni C et al., Enhancement of DNA repair in human skin cells by thymidine dinucleotides: evidence for a p53–mediated mammalian SOS response, *Proc Natl Acad Sci U S A* (1997) **94:**12627–32.
11. Abdel-Malek A, Swope BV, Amornsiripanitch N et al., In vitro modulation of proliferation and melanization of S91 melanoma cells by prostaglandins, *Cancer Res* (1987) **47:**3141–6.
12. Hunt G, Donatien PD, Lunec J et al., Cultured human melanocytes respond to MSH peptides and ACTH, *Pigment Cell Res* (1994) **7:**217–21.
13. Hara M, Yaar M, Gilchrest BA, Endothelin-1 of keratinocyte origin is a mediator of melanocyte dendricity, *J Invest Dermatol* (1995) **105:**744–8.
14. Yohn JJ, Morelli JG, Walchack SJ et al., Cultured human keranocytes synthesize and secreted endothelin-1, *J Invest Dermatol* (1993) **100:**23–6.
15. Roméro-Graillet C, Aberdam E, Clement M et al., Nitric oxide produced by ultraviolet-irradiated keratinocytes stimulates melanogenesis, *J Clin Invest* (1997) **99:**1–8.
16. Lamerson CL, Norlund JJ, Pigmentary changes in Addison's disease with adrenal insufficiency. In: Norlund J J, Boissy R E, Hearing V J et al., eds, *The Pigmentary System: Physiology and Pathophysiology* (Oxford University Press: Oxford, 1998): 875–7.
17. Pears JS, Jung RT, Bartlett W et al., A case of skin hyperpigmentation due to alpha-MSH hypersecretion, *Br J Dermatol* (1992) **126:**286–9.
18. Valverde P, Healy E, Jackson I et al., Variants of the melanocyte-stimulating hormone receptor gene are associated with red hair and fair skin in humans, *Nat Genet* (1995) **11:**328–30.
19. Krude H, Biebermann H, Luck W et al., Severe early-onset obesity, adrenal insufficiency and red hair pigmentation caused by POMC mutations in humans, *Nat Genet* (1998) **19:**155–7.
20. Lerner AB, McGuire JS, Effect of α- and β-melanocyte stimulating hormone on the skin colour of the man, *Nature* (1961) **189:**176–9.
21. Levine N, Sheftel SN, Eytan T et al., Induction of skin tanning by subcutaneous administration of a potent synthetic melanotropin, *JAMA* (1991) **226:**2730–6.
22. Abdel-Malek Z, Swope V, Suzuki I et al., Mitogenic and melanogenic stimulation of normal human melanocytes by melanotropic peptides, *Proc Natl Acad Sci U S A* (1995) **92:**1789–93.
23. Englaro W, Rezzonico R, Durand-Clément M et al., Mitogen-activated protein kinase pathway and AP-1

are activated during cAMP-induced melanogenesis in B-16 melanoma cells, *J Biol Chem* (1995) **270:** 24315–20.

24. Buscà R, Bertolotto C, Abbe P et al., Inhibition of Rho is required for cAMP-induced melanoma cell differentiation, *Mol Biol Cell* (1998) **9**:1367–78.
25. Goding CR, Mitf from neural crest to melanoma: signal transduction and transcription in the melanocyte lineage, *Genes Dev* (2000) **14**:1712–28.
26. Bertolotto C, Abbe P, Hemesath TJ et al., Microphthalmia gene product as a signal transducer in cAMP-induced differentiation of melanocytes, *J Cell Biol* (1998); **142:** 827–35.
27. Bertolotto C, Bille K, Ortonne JP, Ballotti R, Regulation of tyrosinase gene expression by cAMP in B16 melanoma cells involves two CATGTG motifs surrounding the TATA box: implication of the microphthalmia gene product, *J Cell Biol* (1996) **134:**747–55.
28. Bertolotto C, Buscà R, Abbe P et al., Different cis-acting elements are involved in the regulation of TRP1 and TRP2 promoter activities by cyclic AMP: pivotal role of M boxes (GTCATGTGCT) and of microphthalmia, *Mol Cell Biol* (1998b) **18:**694–702.
29. Buscà R, Bertolotto C, Ortonne J-P et al., Inhibition of the phosphatidylinositol 3-kinase/p70^{S6}-kinase pathway induces B16 melanoma cell differentiation, *J Biol Chem* (1996) **271**:31824–30.
30. Robinson MJ, Cobb MH, Mitogen-activated protein kinase pathways, *Curr Opin Cell Biol* (1997) **9**:180–6.
31. Moodie SA, Willumsen BM, Weber MJ et al., Complexes of Ras.GTP with Raf-1 and mitogen-activated protein kinase, *Science* (1993) **260:**1658–61.
32. Morrison DK, Cutler Jr RE, The complexity of Raf-1 regulation, *Curr Opin Cell Biol* (1997) **9**:174–9.
33. Buday L, Downward J, Epidermal growth factor regulates p21ras through the formation of a complex of receptor, Grb2 adapter protein, and Sos nucleotide exchange factor, *Cell* (1993) **73:**611–20.
34. Li N, Batzer A, Daly R et al., Guanine-nucleotide-releasing factor hSos1 binds to Grb2 and links receptor tyrosine kinases to Ras signalling, *Nature* (1993) **363:**85–8.
35. Northwood IC, Gonzalez FA, Wartmann M et al., Isolation and characterization of two growth factor-stimulated protein kinases that phosphorylate the epidermal growth factor receptor at threonine 669, *J Biol Chem* (1991) **266:**15266–76.
36. Lin LL, Wartmann M, Lin AY et al., cPLA2 is phosphorylated and activated by MAP kinase, *Cell* (1993) **72:**269–78.
37. Gille H, Sharrocks AD, Shaw PE, Phosphorylation of transcription factor p62TCF by MAP kinase stimulates ternary complex formation at c-fos promoter, *Nature* (1992) **358:**414–17.
38. Janknecht R, Ernst WH, Pingoud V et al., Activation of ternary complex factor Elk-1 by MAP kinases, *EMBO J* (1993) **12:**5097–104.
39. Marais R, Wynne J, Treisman R, The SRF accessory protein Elk-1 contains a growth factor-regulated transcriptional activation domain, *Cell* (1993) **73:**381–93.
40. Seth A, Gonzalez FA, Gupta S et al., Signal transduction within the nucleus by mitogen-activated protein kinase, *J Biol Chem* (1992) **267:**24796–804.
41. Grove JR, Price DJ, Banerjee P et al., Regulation of an epitope-tagged recombinant Rsk-1 S6 kinase by phorbol ester and erk/MAP kinase, *Biochemistry* (1993) **32:**7727–38.
42. Saxena M, Williams S, Tasken K et al., Crosstalk between cAMP-dependent kinase and MAP kinase through a protein tyrosine phosphatase, *Nat Cell Biol* (1999) **1:**305–11.
43. Frodin M, Peraldi P, Van Obberghen E, Cyclic AMP activates the mitogen-activated protein kinase cascade in PC12 cells, *J Biol Chem* (1994) **269:** 6207–14.
44. Young SW, Dickens M, Tavare JM, Differentiation of PC12 cells in response to a cAMP analogue is accompanied by sustained activation of mitogen-activated protein kinase. Comparison with the effects of insulin, growth factors and phorbol esters, *FEBS Lett* (1994) **338:**212–16.
45. Englaro W, Bertolotto C, Busca R et al., Inhibition of the mitogen-activated protein kinase pathway triggers B16 melanoma cells differentiation, *J Biol Chem* (1998) **273:**1–5.
46. Price ER, Ding HF, Badalian T et al., Lineage-specific signaling in melanocytes. C-kit stimulation recruits p300/CBP to microphthalmia, *J Biol Chem* (1998) **273:**17983–6.
47. Sato S, Roberts K, Gambino G et al., CBP/p300 as a co-factor for the Microphthalmia transcription factor, *Oncogene* (1997) **14:**3083–92.
48. Xu W, Gong L, Haddad MM et al., Regulation of microphthalmia-associated transcription factor MITF protein levels by association with the ubiquitin-conjugating enzyme hUBC9, *Exp Cell Res* (2000) **255:**135–43.
49. Wu M, Hemesath TJ, Takemoto CM et al., c-Kit triggers dual phosphorylations, which couple activation and degradation of the essential melanocyte factor Mi, *Genes Dev* (2000) **14:**301–12.
50. Buscà R, Abbe P, Mantoux F et al., Ras mediates the cAMP-dependent activation of extracellular signal- regulated kinases (ERKs) in melanocytes, *EMBO J* (2000) **19:**2900–10.

51. Vossler MR, Yao H, York RD et al., cAMP activates MAP kinase and Elk-1 through a B-Raf and Rap1-dependent payhway, *Cell* (1997) **89:**73–82.
52. Tsygankova OM, Kupperman E, Wen W et al., Cyclic AMP activates Ras, *Oncogene* (2000) **19:** 3609–15.
53. Ambrosini A, Tininini S, Barassi A et al., cAMP cascade leads to Ras activation in cortical neurons, *Brain Res Mol Brain Res* (2000) **75:**54–60.
54. Zufall F, Leinders-Zufall T, Identification of a long-lasting form of odor adaptation that depends on the carbon monoxide/cGMP second-messenger system, *J Neurosci* (1997) **17:**2703–12.
55. Santoro B, Liu DT, Yao H et al., Identification of a gene encoding a hyperpolarization-activated pacemaker channel of brain, *Cell* (1998) **93:**717–29.
56. Huang NN, Wang DJ, Heller E et al., Homologous desensitization of ATP-stimulated mitogenesis: mechanism involves desensitization of arachidonic acid release and cAMP elevation but not the activation of protein kinase A, *J Cell Physiol* (1995) **165:** 667–75.
57. Liu FC, Takahashi H, McKay RD et al., Dopaminergic regulation of transcription factor expression in organotypic cultures of developing striatum, *J Neurosci* (1995) **15:**2367–84.
58. Brandon EP, Idzerda RL, McKnight GS, PKA isoforms, neural pathways, and behaviour: making the connection, *Curr Opin Neurobiol* (1997) **7:**397–403.
59. De Rooij J, Zwartkruis FJ, Verheijen MH et al., Epac is a Rap1 guanine-nucleotide-exchange factor directly activated by cyclic AMP, *Nature* (1998) **396:**474–7.
60. Kawasaki H, Springett GM, Mochizuki N et al., A family of cAMP-binding proteins that directly activate Rap1, *Science* (1998) **282:**2275–9.
61. De Rooij J, Boenink NM, van Triest M et al., PDZ-GEF1, a guanine nucleotide exchange factor specific for Rap1 and Rap2, *J Biol Chem* (1999) **274:**38125–30.
62. Pham N, Cheglakov I, Koch CA et al., The guanine nucleotide exchange factor CNrasGEF activates ras in response to cAMP and cGMP, *Curr Biol* (2000) **10:**555–8.

16 The involvement of the protein kinase C pathway in melanogenesis

Hee-Young Park and Barbara A. Gilchrest

Introduction

Murine melanoma cells have, for a long time, been used to elucidate cellular and molecular mechanisms involved in pigmentation. In the past two decades, the availability of human melanocyte cultures[1,2] has allowed mechanistic studies of human pigmentation as well. However, dissection of intracellular signaling pathways regulating tyrosinase activity in cultured human primary melanocytes was initially hindered by media supplements required to stimulate or maintain melanocyte growth in the absence of, as yet unidentified, key mitogens.[1,3] The suspected role of agents acting through the cAMP pathway, such as α-melanocyte-stimulating hormone (α-MSH), could not be demonstrated in the presence of cholera toxin or similar additives that maintained high intracellular cAMP levels; and, in particular, the role of protein kinase C (PKC) in the regulation of human melanogenesis was marked by the confounding presence of phorbol esters in most culture media. The known ability of chronic phorbol ester treatment to deplete PKC[4,5] was eventually discovered to severely downregulate tyrosinase activity.[6,7] Maintaining human melanocytes in the absence of phorbol esters has been critical in elucidating the role of the PKC signal transduction pathway in regulating pigmentation. The general biochemical properties of PKC and phorbol esters, as well as the specific role of PKC in melanogenesis, are reviewed below.

Biochemical properties of PKC

PKC is a serine/threonine kinase involved in diverse biological functions, including growth, transformation and differentiation.[8,9] It is a monomer, consisting of regulatory and catalytic domains.[8] PKC resides in an inactive form in the cytoplasm and is translocated to the membrane part of the cells when activated by diacylglycerol (DAG).[8] Extensive studies have revealed that PKC is a family of proteins with at least 12 isoforms (Table 16.1).[10,11] The PKC isoforms are categorized into three groups: classical (c), novel (n), and atypical (a). All isoforms share identical catalytic subunits, but the regulatory subunits vary among the isoforms in their dependency on Ca^{++} and phospholipids for activation.[11] The classical PKC isoforms require phospholipids and Ca^{++} for activation, whereas novel PKC isoforms are activated by phospholipids only, and do not require Ca^{++}.[11] The atypical isoforms can be activated independently of Ca^{++} and phospholipids.[11]

The mechanisms by which PKC transmits signals are diverse. PKC can phosphorylate its cytoplasmic or membrane-associated substrates, such as epidermal growth factor receptors,[12,13] or regulate gene expression through modulating the interaction between the 12-*O*-tetradecanoylphorbol-13-acetate (TPA) response element (TRE), TGAGTCA, and its transcription factors.[14,15] One of the major transcription factors known to interact with TRE is AP-1, a heterodimer of c-fos/c-jun.[15] It is not well established whether these transcription factors are directly phosphorylated by PKC *in vivo*, although the reported nuclear translocation of PKC[16] suggests that this may occur in some cases.

There is differential expression of PKC isoforms among tissues, and it has been speculated that each isoform of PKC has a unique biological function.[17] The mechanisms by which each PKC isoform exerts its unique biological function have not been well elucidated. Subcellular localization

Table 16.1 Protein kinase C isoforms

	Activation requirements	*Isoform*	*Distribution*
Conventional	Ca^{++} and phospholipids	α	Widespread,[17] melanocytic cells[19–21]
		βI/βII	Widespread,[17] melanocytic cells[19–21]
		γ	Brain[17]
Novel	Phospholipids only	δ	Widespread,[17] melanocytic cells[19–21]
		ε	Brain,[17] hematopoietic tissue,[61,62] melanocytic cells[17,18]
		η	Heart,[63] skin,[64] lung[63]
		θ	Hematopoietic tissue,[65] skeletal muscle,[65] brain,[17]
		μ	Lung,[65] epithelial cells[66]
Atypical	Neither Ca^{++} nor phospholipids	ζ	Widespread,[17] melanocytic cells[19–21]
		ι/λ	Ovary,[9] testis[9]

within specific compartments of cells has been implicated in determining the physiological function of each PKC isoform. cAMP has been shown to translocate PKC to the nucleus,[18] and association of PKC with the Golgi membrane has been observed,[17] although, to date, few isoform-specific functions have been identified. Cultured human melanocytes expressed at least α, β, δ, ε, and ζ isoforms of PKC,[19,20] as do murine S91 Cloudman melanoma cells.[21] Specifically, the β isoform of PKC has been demonstrated to be involved in melanogenesis,[22] as described below, in physical association with melanosomes. Interestingly, in skin and skin-derived cultured cells, PKC-β expression can be detected only in melanocytes (Park and Gilchrest, unpublished observations). Oka and colleagues have suggested that activation of ζ isoforms of PKC are involved in the growth regulation of normal human melanocytes,[23] whereas Brooks et al.[24] have suggested that depletion of α, δ, and ε isoforms of PKC play a role in growth of Mel-ab murine melanocytic cells.

Compartmentalization of PKC isoforms with a specific organelle has been shown to be mediated, in part, by receptors for activated-C kinase (RACK1).[25,26] Cloning of the intracellular receptor for PKC revealed that it has homology to the β subunit of G-protein.[27] To date, at least two types are identified and characterized: RACK-I and COP-I.[26] It appears that RACK-I has the highest affinity for PKC-β[26,28] and COP-I has the highest affinity for PKC-ε.[29] A specific anchoring site on PKC-β for RACK has been identified using the inhibitor dequalinium (DECA),[30] which binds to the C2 region of PKC-β and prevents it from interacting with RACK-I.[30]

Phorbol esters

Phorbol esters are naturally-occurring tumor promoters. TPA is a product of the medicinal plant *Croton tiglium*.[31] TPA binds to PKC reversibly and competes for the same binding site on PKC as DAG,[32] thus substituting for DAG in activating PKC.[33,34] DAG is very short lived and metabolized within minutes,[35,36] but phorbol esters are long lived in the cell and continuously activate PKC by translocating the enzyme from the cytosol to the membrane fraction of the cell. The continuous activation of PKC by chronic exposure to TPA was shown to downregulate or, more correctly, deplete PKC.[4,5] Therefore, TPA displays a biphasic effect in all cell types: it acutely activates PKC, usually within minutes to hours,[6,7,37,38] and subsequently downregulates or depletes PKC, usually after hours to days.[6,7,37,38]

The initially-reported culture conditions for growth of normal human melanocytes relied on phorbol ester as a key agent.[1] Addition of pituitary extract[2] or basic fibroblast growth factor,[39] the major melanocyte mitogen in this extract, to culture medium removes the requirement for phorbol ester,[40] but many laboratories have since, nevertheless, routinely used TPA to grow human melanocytes. Under these conditions, the physiologic role of the PKC pathway cannot be appreciated.

Role of PKC in pigmentation

A role for PKC in the differentiation or proliferation of melanocytic cells has been suggested by many studies, and the differentiation state is generally conceded to influence melanogenesis, the major differentiated function of melanocytes. In normal human melanocytes, the active ξ isoform of PKC was suggested to be important for growth, because the incorporation of ^{3}H-tymidine correlated specifically with the level of active PKC-ξ.[23] In mouse melanocytic Mel-ab cells, the TPA-induced proliferation of Mel-ab cells was shown to be due to the depletion of PKC-α, -δ, and -ε isoforms.[24,41] Retinoic-acid-induced differentiation of mouse melanoma cells was shown to rely on PKC-α.[42]

In the past decade, a critical role of PKC in pigmentation has become clear. It was first observed that addition of DAG, the endogenous activator of PKC, to cultured human melanocytes in the absence of TPA caused a rapid 3–4 increase in total melanin content,[43] and this increase was blocked by a PKC inhibitor.[43] Moreover, topical application of active DAG species to guinea pig skin increased melanogenesis, while a DAG species not capable of activating PKC failed to do so.[44] In cultured human melanocytes, total PKC activity was found to correlate with total melanin content in melanocytes cultured from several donors of different complexion, and the activity of tyrosinase paralleled the activity of PKC.[7] Primary human melanocytes grown in the absence of TPA and then stimulated with TPA show an initial modest increase in melanin content, followed by a progressive decrease, over 24–48 hours, in melanin content to very low levels. Melanin is regenerated after chronic TPA exposure within 2 weeks when TPA is removed (Fig. 16.1), suggesting that presence of active PKC is critical for optimal

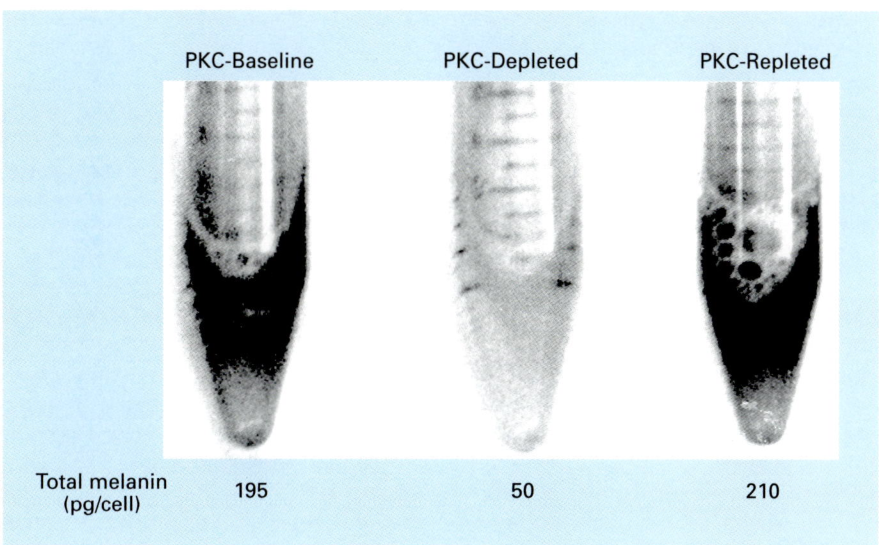

Figure 16.1

The TPA effect on total melanin level is profound but completely reversible in cultured human melanocytes. Paired cultures of primary human melanocytes were treated with DMSO (vehicle) alone or 10^{-7} M TPA for 2 weeks, a time sufficient for PKC depletion.[7] Equal numbers of cells were pelleted from vehicle-treated (PKC-Baseline) and TPA-treated (PKC-Depleted) cultures and the total melanin level was determined in each plate as previously described.[43] TPA was then removed from one of the plates treated with TPA, and cells were allowed to grow for an additional 2 weeks to regenerate PKC and the total melanin level was then determined (PKC-Repleted).

melanogenesis. In human melanocytes, cholera-gen fails to induce pigmentation in the presence of TPA, while removal of TPA allows a significant increase in total melanin.[45]

PKC also plays a critical role in melanogenesis in murine melanoma cells, in that depletion of PKC inhibits α-MSH-induced pigmentation.[6] Similarly, treatment of B16 mouse melanoma cells with TPA for 48 hours, sufficient for PKC depletion to occur,[38] inhibits forskolin-induced increases in melanogenesis.[46]

Specific role of PKC-β in melanogenesis

Elucidation of the specific role of PKC-β in melanogenesis resulted from experiments using human melanocytes and melanoma cells. Immunoblots of human melanocyte proteins revealed that the level of PKC-β, but not the comparably expressed PKC-α, correlated with the total pigment content.[7] An amelanotic subclone (NP-MM4) of a pigmented human melanoma cell line (P-MM4) was found to lack the expression of PKC-β, while the parental line expressed PKC-β. Both lines contained equal and abundant tyrosinase protein.[7] Transfection of PKC-β cDNA into NP-MM4 cells activated tyrosinase,[7] suggesting that PKC-β is required to activate tyrosinase.

Because, by definition, kinases act by phosphorylating substrate proteins, to explore the mechanism by which PKC-β activates tyrosinase, *in vivo* phosphorylation experiments were performed. Intact melanocytes were preincubated with ^{32}P-ortho-phosphate, followed by activation of PKC by phorbol ester treatment and subsequent immunoprecipitation of tyrosinase.[47] There was incorporation of ^{32}P-ortho-phosphate into tyrosinase in cells in which PKC was activated but no incorporation of radioactive phosphate in untreated control cells,[47] establishing that tyrosinase is a phosphoprotein and, potentially, a PKC substrate. Tyrosinase was similarly phosphorylated in NP-MM4 cells transfected with PKC-β, whereas tyrosinase remained unphosphorylated in non-transfected and amelanotic NP-MM4 cells.[47] Moreover, PKC-β was shown to be associated with the melanosomes,[47] and melanosomes were subsequently shown to have membrane-associated RACK-I,[48] the receptor for the activated PKC-β.[26,28]

To determine whether PKC-β directly phosphorylates tyrosinase, an *in vitro* assay was employed. When purified melanosomes were incubated with purified and activated PKC-β, there was a marked increase in tyrosinase activity, whereas incubation with inactive PKC-β caused no change in activity.[49] Moreover, addition of phosphatase prevented PKC-β-induced activation of tyrosinase.[49] The deduced amino acid sequences of human tyrosinase reveal that the cytoplasmic domain of tyrosinase contains no threonine, but two serine residues at amino acid positions of 505 and 509,[50] candidate sites for phosphorylation by this serine/threonine kinase. In purified melanosomes, removal of the cytoplasmic domain completely abolishes phosphorylation of tyrosinase by PKC-β,[47] suggesting that only the cytoplasmic domain of tyrosinase is phosphorylated by PKC-β. Subsequent two-dimensional gel-electrophoresis analysis of peptide fragments generated from the cytoplasmic domain of tyrosinase demonstrated that both serines, at amino acid positions 505 and 509, are phosphorylated by PKC-β.[47]

The critical role of the cytoplasmic domain in determining the activity of tyrosinase implied by the above experiments is further supported by mutations identified in patients with oculocutaneous albinism. Although this disease is most commonly attributable to deletions or amino acid substitutions that disturb the catalytic function of tyrosinase residing in the intramelanosomal portion of the protein,[51] mutations leading to premature termination of tyrosinase with deletion of the 20–22 terminal amino acids from the cytoplasmic domain, including the serines at 505 and 509, also abolish all tyrosinase activity,[51] despite the fact that the inner and membrane domains are intact.

PKC-β appears to be equally important in regulating murine pigmentation. Experiments using the S91 murine melanoma line, known to spontaneously lose its ability to make melanin during serial passage,[21] revealed that the expression of PKC-β is lost in parallel to loss in melanogenic activity, while the expression of tyrosinase and PKC-δ remains unchanged.[21] PKC was also shown to be required in α-MSH-induced pigmentation in murine melanoma cells, in that depletion of PKC completely blocked α-MSH-induced pigmentation.[6] Indeed, the α-MSH-induced increases in tyrosinase mRNA, protein and activity were all blocked either by depletion of PKC or by PKC inhibitors.[6]

Interestingly, α-MSH treatment of melanoma cells increases the level of PKC-β, but not of PKC-α.[6]

It is unlikely that the PKC- and cAMP-dependent pathways in pigmentation act independently of each other, in that blocking either pathway blocks pigmentation.[6,52] Rather, it is likely that the two pathways cross-talk, as shown for other cell functions in other cell types.[53–55] One possibility is that the cAMP-dependent pathway regulates the expression of PKC-β, as suggested by induction of PKC-β by α-MSH.[6] To address whether there is a role for PKC-β in cAMP-induced pigmentation, human melanocyte culture conditions were modified to remove agents that elevate cAMP. Subsequent treatment with isobutyl methyl xanthine caused an increase in tyrosinase activity and tyrosinase protein,[56] as expected. However, the IBMX-induced increase in tyrosinase activity occurred days after the IBMX-induced increase in tyrosinase protein,[56] and closely correlated with the IBMX-induced increase in the PKC-β level. Furthermore, the IBMX-induced increase in tyrosinase activity was inhibited by a selective PKC inhibitor.[56] These data suggest that the cAMP pathway may influence the protein level of PKC-β and, hence, the phosphorylation (activation) of tyrosinase.

Role of PKC in UV-induced pigmentation

Ultraviolet (UV) light, a major physiological inducer of pigmentation,[57] is shown to affect the PKC-dependent pathway. In cultured human epithelioid P3 cells, natural solar radiation (5 minutes of midday exposure in mid-July, latitude 42°N) induced total PKC mRNA twofold within 1–2 hours.[58] UVA irradiation (320–400) of mouse fibroblasts activates PKC within 1–3 hours.[59] Activation of PKC by UV irradiation is also implied by the finding that UV

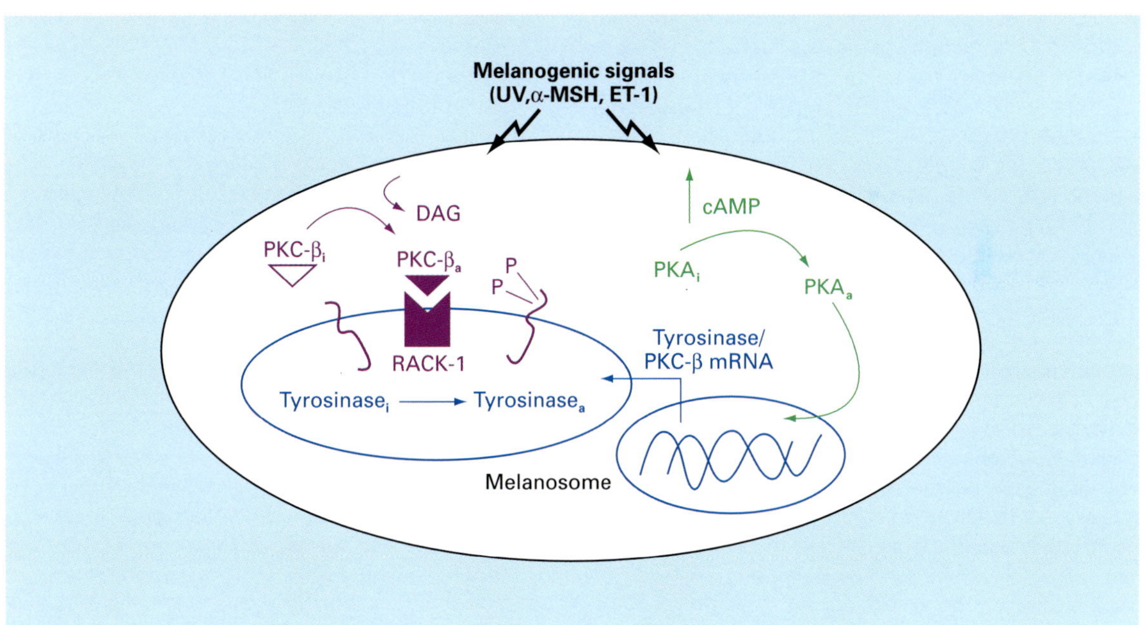

Figure 16.2

Diagram of PKC-β pathways regulating melanogenesis. Extracellular signals release DAG from the plasma membrane to activate otherwise inactive PKC-β_i. Active PKC-β (PKC-β_a) then moves to the melanosomal membrane, is anchored by RACK-1, and phosphorylates tyrosinase, leading to its activation. Extracellular signals may also increase cAMP levels. The cAMP/cAMP-dependent protein kinase (PKA) pathway then, presumably, alters the transcription rate of key genes, including tyrosinase and PKC-β, with an eventual increase in tyrosinase protein activity.

irradiation increases the intracellular level of DAG in keratinocytes.[60] UV was shown to induce enthothelin-1 (ET-1) production by keratinocytes and ET-1 was shown to act, in part through the PKC pathway, in mediating UV-induced melanogenesis.[61] Effects of UV on PKC activity in human melanocytes are less well studied, but DAG was shown to augment UV-induced melanogenesis in human melanocytes.[62] UV also elevated the expression of PKC-β in cultured human melanocytes within 1 hour after irradiation.[49] Thus, UV may enhance pigmentation in part through affecting both the level and the activity of PKC-β.

Summary

The role of PKC, particularly the β isoform, is now well documented in human and murine melanogenesis. In response to stimuli, such as UV irradiation or receptor-ligand binding, DAG is released and activates PKC-β (Fig. 16.2). Active PKC-β then activates tyrosinase by phosphorylating two serine residues on the cytoplasmic domain of this transmembrane, melanosomal protein, increasing melanogenesis. Specificity for the β isoform appears to be conferred by the presence, on the melanosome's cytoplasmic surface, of RACK-1, a PKC-anchoring protein with selective affinity for PKC-β. In addition, cross-talk between the PKC and cAMP pathways may further amplify other melanogenic signals at the level of gene transcription. Loss of PKC-β-mediated phosphorylation of tyrosinase by PKC depletion or inhibition, or by loss of the phosphorylation sites on tyrosinase, as in some patients with oculocutaneous albinisms, completely blocks melanogenesis. Identification of PKC-β as a critical regulator of melanogenesis provides a novel target for pharmacologic manipulation of skin and hair color.

References

1. Eisinger M, Marko O, Selective proliferation of normal human melanocytes in vitro in the presence of phorbol ester and cholera toxin, *Proc Natl Acad Sci U S A* (1982) **79**:2018–22.
2. Gilchrest BA, Vrabel MA, Flynn E et al., Selective cultivation of human melanocytes from newborn and adult epidermis, *J Invest Dermatol* (1984) **83**:370–6.
3. Yaar M, Gilchrest BA, Human melanocyte growth and differentiation: a decade of new data, *J Invest Dermatol* (1991) **97**:611–17.
4. Grove DS, Mastro A, Prevention of the TPA-mediated down-regulation of protein kinase C, *Biochem Biophys Res Commun* (1988) **151**:94–9.
5. Ballester R, Rosen O, Fate of immunoprecipitable protein kinase C in GH_3 cells treated with phorbol 12-myristate 13-acetate, *J Biol Chem* (1985) **260**:15194–9.
6. Park HY, Russakovsky V, Ao Y et al., α-melanocyte stimulating hormone-induced pigmentation is blocked by depletion of protein kinase C, *Exp Cell Res* (1996) **227**:70–9.
7. Park HY, Russakovsky V, Ohno S et al., The beta isoform of protein kinase C stimulates human melanogenesis by activating tyrosinase in pigment cells, *J Biol Chem* (1993) **268**:11742–9.
8. Nishizuka Y, Turnover of inositol phospholipids and signal transduction, *Science* (1984) **225**:1365–70.
9. Nishizuka Y, Intracellular signaling by hydrolysis of phospholipids and activation of protein kinase C, *Science* (1992) **258**:607–14.
10. Liscovitch M, Cantley LC, Lipid second messengers, *Cell* (1994) **77**:329–34.
11. Dekker LV, Parker PJ, *Protein Kinase C—A Question of Specificity* (Elsevier Science Ltd: 1994) 94.
12. Cochet C, Gill GN, Meisenhelder J et al., C-kinase phosphorylates the epidermal growth factor receptor and reduces its epidermal growth factor-stimulated tyrosine protein kinase activity, *J Biol Chem* (1984) **259**:2553–8.
13. Hunter T, Ling N, Cooper JA, Protein kinase C phosphorylation of the EGF receptor at a threonine residue close to the cytoplasmic face of the plasma membrane, *Nature* (1994) **311**:480–3.
14. Fisch TM, Prywes R, Roeder RG, c-fos sequences necessary for basal expression and induction by epidermal growth factor, 12-O-tetradecanol phorbol-13-acetate, and the calcium ionophore, *Mol Cell Biol* (1987) **7**:34900–5000.
15. Curran T, Franza Jr BR, Fos and jun: the AP-1 connection, *Cell* (1988) **55**:395–7.
16. Buchner K, Protein kinase C in the transduction of signals toward and within the cell nucleus, *Eur J Biochem* (1995) **228**:211–21.
17. Nishizuka Y, The molecular heterogeneity of protein kinase C and its implications for cellular regulation, *Nature* (1988) **334**:661–5.
18. Cambier JC, Newell MK, Justement LB et al., Ia bind-

ing ligands and cAMP stimulate nuclear translocation of PKC in B lymphocytes, *Nature* (1987) **327**:629–32.

19. Park HY, Rubeiz N, Fernandez E et al., Expression of protein kinase C isoforms in cultured human melanocytes, *J Invest Dermatol* (1994) **102**:440.
20. Yamanishi DT, Graham M, Buckmeier JA et al., The differential expression of protein kinase C genes in normal human neonatal melanocytes and metastatic melanomas, *Carcinogenesis* (1991) **12**:105–9.
21. Park HY, Gilchrest BA, Reduction of melanogenic activity and responsiveness to α-melanocyte stimulating hormone during serial passage of melanoma cells, *J Cut Med Surg* (1996) **1**:4–9.
22. Park HY, Perez JM, Laursen R et al., Protein kinase C-β activates tyrosinase by phosphorylating serine residues in its cytoplasmic domain, *J Biol Chem* (1999) **274**:16470–8.
23. Oka M, Ogita K, Ando H et al., Differential down-regulation of protein kinase C subspecies in normal human melanocytes: possible involvement of the ζ subspecies in growth regulation, *J Invest Dermatol* (1995) **105**:567–71.
24. Brooks G, Goss MW, East JE et al., Growth of melanocytic cells is associated with down-regulation of protein kinase C α, δ, and ε, *J Biol Chem* (1993) **268**:23868–75.
25. Csukai M, Mochley-Rosen D, Pharmacologic modulation of protein kinase C isozymes: the role of RACKs and subcellular localisation, *Pharmacol Res* (1999) **39**:253–9.
26. Mochley-Rosen D, Localization of protein kinases by anchoring proteins: a theme in signal transduction, *Science* (1995) **268**:247–51.
27. Ron D, Chen CH, Caldwell J et al., Cloning of an intracellular receptor for protein kinase C: a homolog of the β subunit of G proteins, *Proc Natl Acad Sci U S A* (1994) **91**:839–43.
28. Ron D, Jiang Z, Yao L et al., Coordinated movement of RACK1 with activated βIIPKC, *J Biol Chem* (1999) **274**,38:27039–46.
29. Csuka M, Chen CH, De Matteis M et al., The coatomer protein β′-COP, a selective binding protein (RACK) for protein kinase Cε, *J Biol Chem* (1997) **272**:29200–6.
30. Rotenberg SA, Sun XG, Photoinduced inactivation of protein kinase C by Dequalinium identifies the RACK-1-binding domain as a recognition site, *J Biol Chem* (1998) **273:**2390–5.
31. Rouhi AM, Crystal structure sheds light on binding of tumor promoters to key enzyme, *C&EN* (1995) **October 23**:21–5.
32. Sharkey NA, Leach KL, Blumberg PM, Competetive inhibition by diaclyglycerol of specific phorbol ester binding, *Proc Natl Acad Sci USA* (1984) **81**:607–10.
33. Castagna M, Takai Y, Kaibuchi K et al., Direct activation of calcium-activated, phospholipid-dependent protein kinase by tumor-promoting phorbol esters, *J Biol Chem* (1982) **257**:7847–51.
34. Ashendel CL, The phorbol ester receptor: A phospholipid-regulated protein kinase, *Biochim Biophys Acta* (1985) **822:**219–42.
35. Bishop WR, Bell RM, Attenuation of sn-1, 2-diacylglycerol second messengers. Metabolism of exogenous diacylglycerols by human platelets, *J Biol Chem* (1986) **261**:12513–19.
36. Florin-Christensen J et al., Metabolic fate of plasma membrane diacylglycerols in NIH 3T3 fibroblasts, *J Biol Chem* (1992) **267**:14783–9.
37. Park HY, Campisit J, Posttranslational control of cyclic AMP-dependent protein kinase by phorbol ester in normal but not in chemically transformed 3T3 cells, *Cancer Res* (1990) **50**:7145–52.
38. Ludwig KW, Niles RM, Suppression of cyclic-AMP dependent protein kinase activity in murine melanoma cells by 12-*O*-tetradecanoyl-phorbol-13-acetate, *Biochemistry* (1980) **95**:269–303.
39. Halaban R, Ghosh S, Baird A, bFGF is the putative natural growth factor for human melanocytes, *In Vitro Cell Dev Biol* (1987) **23**:47–52.
40. Gilchrest BA, Friedmann PS, A culture system for the study of human melanocyte physiology. In: Jimbow K, ed, *Structure and Function of Melanin* (Sapporo: Japan, 1987) 4.
41. Brooks G, Wilson RE, Dooley TP et al., Protein kinase C down-regulation, and not transient activation, correlates with melanocyte growth, *Cancer Res* (1991) **51**:3281–8.
42. Gruber JR, Ohno S, Niles RM, Increased expression of protein kinase C_α plays a key role in retinoic acid-induced melanoma differentiation, *J Biol Chem* **267**:13356–60.
43. Gordon PR, Gilchrest BA, Human melanogenesis is stimulated by diacylglycerol, *J Invest Dermatol* (1989) **93**:700–2.
44. Allan AE, Archambault M, Messana E et al., Topically applied diacylglycerols increase pigmentation in guinea pig skin, *J Invest Dermatol* (1995) **105**: 687–92.
45. Medrano EE, Yang F, Boissy R et al., Terminal differentiation and senescence in the human melanocyte: Repression of tyrosinase-phosphorylation of the extracellular signal-regulated kinase 2 selectively defines the two pheontypes, *Mol Biol Cell* (1994) **5**:497–509.

46. Bertolotto C, Bille K, Ortonne JP et al., In B16 melanoma cells, the inhibition of melanogenesis by TPA results from PKC activation and diminution of microphthalmis binding to the M-box of the tyrosinase promoter, *Oncogene* (1998) **16**:1665–70.
47. Park HY, Perez JM, Laursen R et al., Protein kinase C-β activates tyrosinase by phosphorylating serine residues in its cytoplasmic domain, *J Biol Chem* (1999) **274**:16470–8.
48. Park HY, Hu HW, Young D et al., PKC-β is associated with its receptor RACK-1 at the melanosomal surface in human melanocytes, *J Invest Dermatol* (2000) **114**:787.
49. Park HY, Gilchrest BA, Signaling pathways mediating melanogenesis, *Cell Mol Biol* (1999) **45**:919–30.
50. Shibahara S, Tomita Y, Tagami H et al., Molecular basis for the heterogeneity of human tyrosinase, *Tohoku J Exp Med* (1988) **156**:403–14.
51. King RA, Townsend D, Oetting WS, Inherited hypopigmented disorders. In: Levine N, ed, *Pigmentation and Pigmentary Disorders* (CRC Press: Boca Raton, FL, 1993) 297–336.
52. Ao Y, Park HY, Olaizola-Horn S et al., Activation of cAMP-dependent protein kinase is required for a-melanocyte stimulating hormone-induced pigmentation, *Exp Cell Res* (1998) **244**:117–24.
53. Yoshimasa T, Sibley DR, Bouvier M et al., Cross-talk between cellular signaling pathways suggested by phorbol-ester-induced adenylate cyclase phosphorylation, *Nature* (1987) **327**:67–70.
54. Shirakawa F, Mizel SB, In vitro activation and nuclear translocation of NF-κB catalyzed by cyclic AMP-dependent protein kinase and protein kinase C, *Mol Cell Biol* (1989) **9**:2424–30.
55. Vaello M-L, Ruiz-Gomez A, Lerma J et al., Modulation of inhibitory glycine receptors by phosphorylation by protein kinase C and cAMP-dependent protein kinase, *J Biol Chem* (1994) **269**:2002–8.
56. Park HY, Murphy MM, Gilchrest BA, Increasing PKC-β is the rate limiting step in cAMP-induced human melanogenesis, *J Invest Dermatol* (1999) **112**:540.
57. Gilchrest BA, Park HY, Eller MS et al., The photobiology of the tanning response. In: Nordlund JJ, Boissy RE, Hearing VJ et al., eds, *The Pigmentary System: Physiology and Pathophysiology* (Oxford University Press: New York, 1998) 359–73.
58. Peak JG, Woloschak GE, Peak MJ, Enhanced expression of protein kinase C gene caused by solar radiation, *Photochem Photobiol* (1991) **53**:395–7.
59. Matsui MS, DeLeo VA, Induction of protein kinase C activity by ultraviolet radiation, *Carcinogenesis* (1990) **11**:229–34.
60. Punnonen K, Yuspa SH, Ultraviolet light irradiation increases cellular diacylglycerol and induces translocation of diacylglycerol kinase in murine keratinocytes, *J Invest Dermatol* (1992) **99**:221–6.
61. Imokawa G, Yada Y, Miyagushi M, Endothelins secreted from human keratinocytes are intrinsic mitogens for human melanocytes, *J Biol Chem* (1992) **267**:24675–80.
62. Friedmann PS, Wren FE, Matthews JNS, Ultraviolet stimulated melanogenesis by human melanocytes is augmented by di-acyl glycerol but not TPA, *J Cell Physiol* (1990) **142**:334–41.
63. Li Y, Davis KL, Sytkowski AJ, Protein kinase C-ε is necessary for erythropoietin's up-regulation of c-myc and for factor-dependent DNA synthesis, *J Biol Chem* (1996) **271**:27025–30.
64. Moriya S, Kazlauskas A, Akimoto K et al., Platelet-derived growth factor activates protein kinase C-ε through redundant and independent signaling pathways involving phospholipase C-γ or phosphatidylinositol 3-kinase, *Proc Natl Acad Sci U S A* (1996) **93**:151–5.
65. Osada S, Hashimoto Y, Nomura S et al., Predominant expression of nPKC eta, a $CA^{(++)}$ independent isoform of protein kinase C in epithelial tissues, in association with epithelial differentiation, *Cell Growth Differ* (1993) **4**:167–75.
66. Murakami A, Chida K, Suzuki Y et al., Absence of down-regulation and translocation of the η isoform of protein kinase C in normal human melanocytes, *J Invest Dermatol* (1996) **106**:790–4.
67. Smith BL, Krushelnycky BW, Mochly-Rosen et al., The HIV Nef protein associates with protein kinase C theta, *J Biol Chem* (1996) **271**:16753–7.
68. Monick M, Staber J, Thomas K et al., Respiratory syncytial virus infection results in activation of multiple protein kinase C isoforms leading to activation of mitogen-activated protein kinase, *J Immunol* (2001) **166**:2681–7.

Section V

MELANOSOME BIOGENESIS AND TRANSPORT

17 The biology and disorders of melanosome biogenesis: The Hermansky–Pudlak and Chediak–Higashi syndromes

Richard A. Spritz

Introduction

Over the past three decades, a group of intriguing genetic diseases has been defined, in which diverse, yet characteristic, clinical features are associated with defects in the biogenesis of multiple cellular organelles—melanosomes, lysosomes, and cytoplasmic granular elements. These disorders include the various forms of Hermansky–Pudlak syndrome (HPS; 203300), the Chediak–Higashi syndrome (CHS; MIM #214500), as well as the Griscelli syndrome (MIM #214450), all of which are characterized clinically by hypopigmentation or albinism (the result of defects of melanosomes), platelet dysfunction (the result of defects of platelet granules), in some cases immune deficiencies (the result of defects of lysosomes and cytoplasmic granules), as well as other manifestations of uncertain pathogenesis.[1–6] A similar series of 'multi-organellar' disorders has been characterized in the mouse, involving at least 18 different genetic loci, in which hypopigmentation and other phenotypic manifestations are likewise associated with defects of melanosomes, lysosomes, and platelet granules.[7,8] Many of the genes associated with these human and mouse disorders have recently been identified and found to encode components of cellular systems that direct the sorting of organelle-specific proteins to their cytoplasmic destinations, whereas others encode entirely novel proteins whose functions are not yet known but which are, presumably, similarly involved in organellar protein trafficking or organellar transport (Table 17.1).

Comparison of these human and murine genes, and searches for mutations in both human patients and in the mutant mice, have made it clear that there is close correspondence between the human and mouse multi-organellar disorders (Table 17.1). Indeed, the story of these disorders provides one of the best illustrations of how cross-species genotype–phenotype comparisons between human and mouse can alternately leapfrog each field ahead, over the back of the other, providing a much richer and deeper understanding than would have resulted from the study of either species alone. Indeed, the number of multi-organellar defects known in the mouse is much larger than in the human, and it is evident that the three original eponymic human disorders mentioned above will be considerably subdivided as patients with atypical phenotypes are found to have mutations in different genes first identified in these mutant mice. This has already occurred in Hermansky–Pudlak syndrome, and will certainly continue as additional patients are better characterized clinically and subjected to detailed molecular study.

Trafficking of organelle-specific proteins to melanosomes, lysosomes, and cytoplasmic granules

The molecular and biochemical mechanisms by which newly synthesized organelle-specific proteins are sorted into specific cytoplasmic

Table 17.1 Human and mouse genes with melanosome/lysosome/platelet granule multi-organellar phenotypes.

Human	*Mouse*	*Function*
Unknown	Buff (*bf*)	Unknown
Chediak–Higashi syndrome (*CHS1*)	Beige (*bg*)	Unknown; 429 kDa cytoplasmic protein
Unknown	Cappuccino (*cno*)	Unknown
Hermansky–Pudlak syndrome 3 (*HPS3*)	Cocoa (*coa*)	Unknown; novel cytoplasmic protein
Griscelli syndrome (*MYO5A*)	Dilute (*d*)	Organellar motor
Hermansky–Pudlak syndrome 1 (*HPS1*)	Pale-ear (*ep*)	Unknown; 79 kDa cytoplasmic protein
Unknown	Gunmetal (*gm*)	Rab geranylgeranyl transferase α subunit
Hermansky–Pudlak syndrome 4 (*HPS4*)	Light-ear (*le*)	Unknown; novel cytoplasmic protein
Unknown	Mocha (*mh*)	AP-3 δ subunit
Unknown	Muted (*mu*)	Unknown; novel protein
Unknown	Pallid (*pa*)	Syntaxin-13 interacting protein; vesicle docking
Hermansky–Pudlak syndrome 2 (*AP3B1*)	Pearl (*pe*)	AP-3 β3A subunit
Unknown	Reduced pigmentation (*rp*)	Unknown
Unknown	Ruby eye (*ru*)	Unknown
Unknown	Ruby eye-2 (*ru2*)	Unknown
Unknown	Sandy (*sdy*)	Unknown
Unknown	Sepia (*sea*)	Unknown
Unknown	Subtle gray (*sut*)	Unknown

compartments are not yet known in detail, and our knowledge of melanosome biogenesis remains rudimentary. As shown in Figure 17.1, in general, proteins destined for ultimate delivery to specific cytoplasmic organelles are synthesized in the endoplasmic reticulum, and enter the secretory pathway through the Golgi apparatus. In the *trans*-Golgi network, these organelle-specific proteins are then packaged into transport vesicles for eventual transport to endosomes, some via intermediate endosomal compartments and others, perhaps, directly. Formation of one class of transport vesicles is mediated by cytosolic 'adaptor protein complexes', which concentrate proteins that are to be sorted to organelles into clathrin-coated vesicles recognizing tyrosine- and dileucine-based sorting signals contained in these proteins. The coated vesicles then transport organelle-specific proteins to late endosomes, and, eventually, to nascent organelles.[9–14] Other pre-organellar transport systems may involve non-coated vesicles, and might transport proteins to organellar precursors directly, rather than via endosomal intermediates. Alternative pathways of protein transport from the *trans*-Golgi network to organelles via the plasma membrane and late endosomes also exist.

The adaptor protein complex that appears to be most important in trafficking proteins to melanosomes, lysosomes, and platelet granules, is AP-3, a heterotrimeric protein complex consisting of δ (160 kDa), β3A (120 kDa), μ3 (47 kDa), and σ3 (22 kDa) subunits and perhaps alternative proteins in some cases.[15–17] As will be discussed below, several of the multi-organellar disorders of humans and of mouse have been found to result from defects in the AP-3-mediated pathway. Others of the multi-organellar disorders involve proteins whose functions do not appear to be directly related to the AP-3-mediated pathway, and likely involve different pathways of multi-organellar protein trafficking.

Multi-organellar disorders of pigmentation

Hermansky–Pudlak syndrome 1 (HPS1; MIM 203300)

Hermansky–Pudlak syndrome (HPS) is a group of rare autosomal recessive genetic disorders characterized by oculocutaneous albinism, bleeding tendency, and a poorly defined ceroid-lipofuscin lysosomal storage disease.[2,4,18–24] Life-threatening manifestations typically develop during adulthood, including progressive pulmonary fibrosis,[19–21] granulomatous colitis,[19,20,22] and, occasionally, cardiomyopathy and renal failure.[19,20] Unlike in CHS and Griscelli syndrome, discussed below, there is no immune deficit in HPS.[23] At present, there is no

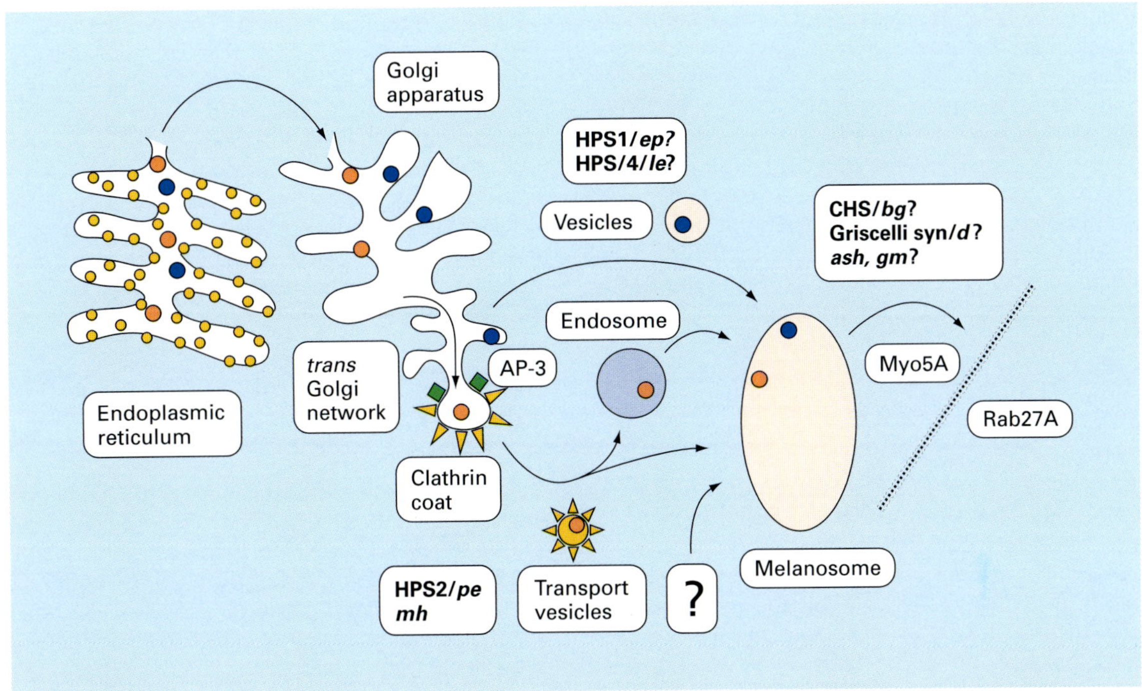

Figure 17.1

Pathways of melanosome biogenesis and protein trafficking. Newly synthesized 'cargo' proteins are translated in the endoplasmic reticulum and transported to the *cis*-Golgi and, subsequently, to the *trans*-Golgi network. In the AP-3 pathway, cargo proteins are then packaged into clathrin-coated vesicles, in a process that involves the AP-3 adaptor protein complex, and are then trafficked to organelles and cytoplasmic granules, either via an endosomal intermediate or directly. In the HPS-related pathway, cargo proteins are packaged into non-coated vesicles and trafficked to organelles and granules, again, either directly or via an endosomal intermediate.

specific or effective treatment for HPS, and average survival is only 30–50 years, death usually resulting from restrictive lung disease (68%), hemorrhage (17%), or colitis (15%).[19,20]

Hypopigmentation in HPS is associated with quantitatively reduced and qualitatively abnormal melanosomes in skin melanocytes, with resultant defective pigment biosynthesis.[24–26] Bleeding in HPS varies in severity, but is usually clinically mild, and results from almost total absence of (or empty) platelet-dense (δ) granules, and consequent 'storage pool deficiency' and defective platelet aggregation.[20,27–30] Lysosomal storage in HPS is less well characterized, principally involving accumulation of ceroid-lipofuscin-like material in the lysosomes of reticuloendothelial cells, bone marrow, lung macrophages, and many other cell types,[18–20,31–33] suggesting possible lysosomal dysfunction. Nevertheless, patients with HPS exhibit none of the progressive neurologic, hepatic, or skeletal manifestations of the classical neuronal ceroid-lipofuscinosis.

HPS is rare in most populations, but it is the most common genetic disorder in Puerto Rico, where it occurs with an estimated incidence of 1:1800,[19,20] and in an isolated village in the Swiss Alps.[24,25,30] The *HPS1* gene is located in chromosome segment 10q23,[34,35] and consists of 55 exons[36] encoding a ubiquitously expressed, 700 amino acid, 79.3 kDa polypeptide that is not related to any other known proteins and that contains no motifs that might provide clues to its function.[37] The HPS protein has been highly conserved during mammalian evolution, with 81% amino acid sequence identity among the human,[37] mouse,[38,39] and rat[40] HPS polypeptides. The HPS protein is a non-glycosylated, non-membrane protein that is a component of two distinct high-molecular-weight complexes. In non-melanotic cells, the HPS protein is contained in a ~200 kDa cytosolic complex, whereas in melanotic cells, about half of the HPS protein is contained in a >500 kDa complex that is associated with organellar membranes. The HPS protein appears to be located in small, non-coated vesicles and tubulovesicular structures in the peri-Golgi region, and with early-stage melanosomes, suggesting that the HPS complex is involved in trafficking proteins to early melanosomes.[41,42] Nevertheless, cells from patients with HPS show no evident abnormalities in the expression or distribution of the AP-3 adaptor protein complex.[41]

A number of pathologic mutations of the *HPS1* gene have now been identified (Fig. 17.2),[37,43–45] the most clinically important of which is a frameshift resulting from a 16-base duplication that is found in virtually all Puerto Rican patients with HPS.[37] Thus far, all but one of the HPS mutations that have been identified have been protein-nulls, and no missense mutant alleles have been found at all. This suggests that amino acid substitution or other mild mutations of the *HPS1* gene might result in a phenotype that is not readily recognized on clinical grounds. Indeed, about half of non-Puerto Rican HPS patients lack identifiable mutations in the *HPS1* gene,[43] and it is apparent that at least some cases of HPS must result from mutations of genes other than *HPS1*.[43]

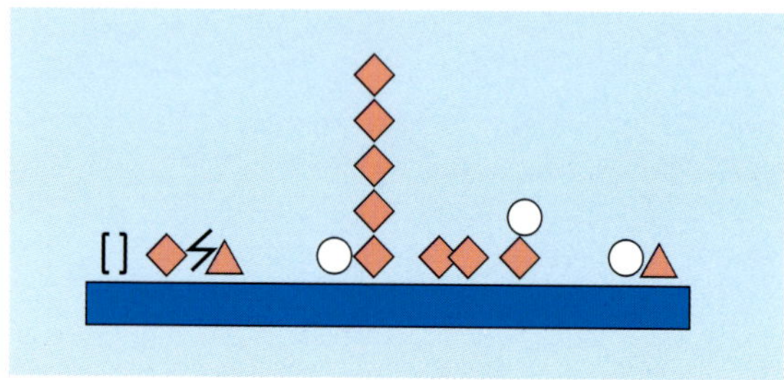

Figure 17.2

Mutations of the *HPS1* gene. Blue box denotes coding region. Red diamonds represent frameshifts; triangles, nonsense mutations; zigzag, a splice junction mutation; brackets, a single-codon deletion. Open circles denote non-pathological amino acid substitutions. Multiple diamonds at one site indicate a hot spot for recurrent, independent frameshift mutations.[43]

Finally, mutation analysis showed that the murine *Hps* gene is defective in pale-ear (*ep*) mutant mice[38,39] (Table 17.1), which exhibit mild hypopigmentation associated with structural abnormalities of melanosomes, platelet storage pool deficiency associated with absent dense granules, abnormal lysosomal function, and reduced NK cell function.[46,47] In this last respect, in particular, mouse pale-ear (*ep*) is more similar to human Chediak–Higashi syndrome than it is to human HPS *per se*.

Hermansky–Pudlak syndrome 2 (HPS2; MIM 603401)

Analyses of non-Puerto-Rican patients with HPS showed that only about half have identifiable mutations in the *HPS1* gene, and, in at least some cases, mutations in the 10q23 *HPS1* locus could be excluded on genetic grounds, indicating the existence of locus heterogeneity for HPS.[43,46] Because of the likely involvement of the HPS1 polypeptide in organellar protein trafficking, by screening HPS patients lacking identifiable *HPS1* gene mutations for defective expression of the AP-3 protein trafficking adaptor complex, Dell'Angelica et al.[49] identified compoundly heterozygous pathologic mutations in the gene encoding the β3A subunit of AP-3 (*AP3B1*) in two brothers with a variant HPS phenotype that included hip dysplasia, recurrent upper respiratory infections, and neutropenia.[50] Although the specific clinical features of these patients were not quite the same as those of classical HPS, this finding would seem to warrant subdividing Hermansky–Pudlak syndrome into at least two entities: HPS1, the disorder prevalent in Puerto Rico, and HPS2, the disorder in these two brothers and perhaps other patients. It appears that mutations in the *AP3B1* gene account for only a very small fraction of those patients with HPS who lack mutations in the *HPS1* gene, and it thus seems likely that additional HPS genes remain to be identified.

Interestingly, *pearl* (*pe*) mutant mice also have defects of the *Ap3b1* gene encoding the AP-3 β3A subunit,[51] resulting in melanomal abnormalities and hypopigmentation, abnormal secretion of lysosomal enzymes, and storage pool deficiency of platelets in *pe*/*pe* homozygous mice. Pearl is thus the murine homologue of human HPS2. Similarly, the mouse *mocha* (*mh*) gene, which also is associated with a multi-organellar hypopigmentation phenotype, results from mutations in the gene encoding the AP-3 δ subunit (*Ap3d1*), although no human HPS patients have yet been found to have mutations in the *AP3D1* gene. The human HPS2 and the mouse pearl and mocha defects involve a relatively early step in organelle-specific protein sorting (Fig. 17.3), and it seems likely that the *HPS1* gene product may likewise involve in an early step in organellar protein trafficking, although its specific role has yet to be determined.

Chediak–Higashi syndrome (CHS; MIM 214500)

CHS is an autosomal-recessive disorder in which moderate hypopigmentation to oculocutaneous albinism is accompanied by bleeding tendency, severe cellular immunologic deficiency with neutropenia and frequent bacterial infections, and slowly progressive neurologic dysfunction.[1–5,52–58] About 85–90% of patients with CHS eventually develop a so-called 'accelerated' lymphoproliferative phase, characterized by generalized lymphohistiocytic infiltrates, fever, jaundice, hepatosplenomegaly, lymphadenopathy, pancytopenia, and bleeding. There is no specific treatment for CHS. Management of the accelerated phase is quite difficult, and chemotherapy provides only transient benefit, most patients ultimately requiring bone marrow transplantation.[59] Of the patients who do not develop an accelerated phase, most have relatively few significant infections, although some may develop progressive neurological manifestations, including seizures, progressive intellectual decline, and progressive peripheral neuropathy, with tremor, muscle weakness, clumsiness, and wide-based gait.[60,61]

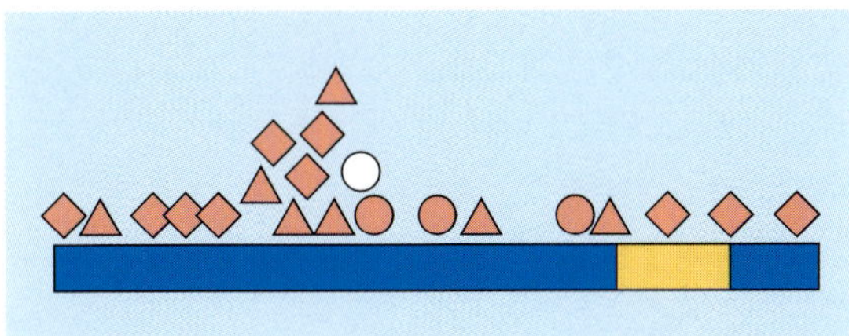

Figure 17.3

Mutations of the *CHS1* gene. Blue box denotes coding region; BEACH domain is indicated by yellow. Diamonds represent frameshifts; triangles, nonsense mutations; filled circle, missense substitution; open circle, a non-pathological amino acid substitution.

The ultrastructural hallmark of CHS is the occurrence of giant granular inclusion bodies, giant lysosomes, and giant melanosomes. Giant inclusions are seen in virtually all granulated cells, and histochemical and electron micrographic studies indicate that these inclusions are derived from lysosomes, secretory granules, and melanosomes, many of which have undergone promiscuous fusion, apparently accounting for defective function.[62–69]

The principal immunologic defects of CHS are neutropenia and lack of natural killer (NK) cytotoxicity activity, resulting in recurrent pyogenic infections.[70–72] NK cell number and target binding are normal, but effector function is defective,[73] perhaps due to the inability of CHS T-cells to secrete cytolytic proteins stored in their giant granules, defective granular secretion resulting from abnormal vesicular membrane fusion.[74] Bleeding tendency in CHS, manifesting principally by bruisability, is associated with prolonged bleeding time and reduced platelet aggregation, due to storage pool deficiency[75,76] and a greatly reduced number of platelet-dense (δ) granules.[77–80]

Disorders similar to human CHS occur in many mammalian species,[81–88] most importantly the beige (*bg*) mouse (Table 17.1).[89,90] Beige-mutant mice exhibit hypopigmentation of the coat and eye, bacterial infections due to greatly reduced NK function,[91] platelet storage pool deficiency,[92] and giant melanosomes and lysosomes.[91,93] The mouse *bg* gene was identified by positional cloning.[94–96] The human *CHS1* gene is located in chromosome segment 1q42–q43,[97,98] in a region of conserved synteny with the region of mouse chromosome 13 that contains the *bg* locus. Analysis of the human homologue of the mouse *bg* gene led to identification of pathologic gene mutations in patients with CHS (Fig. 17.3).[94,99–103] The *CHS1* gene product is a 3801 amino acid, 429 kDa polypeptide of unknown function.[99] The CHS1 protein does not contain extensive regions of homology or polypeptide functional motifs that provide clear clues to its possible function, although the so-called BEACH (*Be*ige *A*nd *Ch*ediak–Higashi) domain, first identified in the CHS1 protein,[99] has subsequently been found in a number of novel proteins of unknown functions. The CHS1 protein is cytoplasmic in location,[104] and seems likely to be involved in either fusion or reversal of fusion of biomembranes, perhaps in one of the later steps of organellogenesis (Fig. 17.1).

Analysis of the *CHS1* gene in patients with the various clinical forms of CHS has shown a straightforward genotype–phenotype correlation. Most patients with severe, childhood CHS are homozygous for null mutant alleles of the *CHS1* gene.[94,99–103] However, the situation is quite different for patients with milder forms of CHS. Patients with 'adult' CHS, who show no evidence of accelerated phase, are usually homozygous for missense mutant alleles that result in nonconservative amino acid substitutions.[102] Furthermore, very rare patients with an intermediate, 'adolescent' form of CHS, with occasional severe infections but, again, no accelerated phase, are compound heterozygotes, each with one null mutant allele and one missense mutant allele.[103] Unfortunately, the very large size and great genomic complexity of the *CHS1* gene makes clinical mutation analysis of patients with CHS quite problematic. Furthermore, it has been possible to identify any mutations of the *CHS1* gene at all in only about half of patients with CHS. Among those patients in whom mutations have not been found, genetic analysis has excluded the *CHS1* gene in several, indicating the likely existence of additional genes that result in CHS-like mutant phenotypes in humans.[103] 'Pseudo-Chediak–Higashi anomaly' in patients with acute leukemia has been associated with a translocation, t(15;17),[105] and, thus, it may be that a gene for a novel form of CHS is located on either chromosome 15 or 17.

Perspectives for the future

In recent years, there has been extraordinary progress in understanding the molecular nosology of HPS and CHS, correlating these and similar human disorders with the homologous disorders of mouse, as well as other species, and defining the underlying genetic pathology. Likewise, there has been great progress towards understanding the cell biology of the corresponding proteins and their roles in organellogenesis, including assembly and maturation of melanocytes. It seems likely that this progress will continue and even accelerate, and that HPS, and perhaps also CHS, will continue to undergo subdivision as additional genes are characterized in patients with variant forms of these disorders. Much of this work can be applied to increasingly accurate diagnosis of these disorders. However, there has been, essentially no progress in translating any of these discoveries into improved treatment for patients. This seems especially unfortunate, as, in CHS, and particularly in HPS, medically serious or life-threatening complications are not usually present at birth. In the case of CHS, the immunologic defect can be cured by bone marrow transplantation, and it is possible that gene or pharmacological therapy could achieve a similar outcome. In HPS, most patients do not die from their pulmonary disease until the third or fourth decade of life; hence, there is considerable time during which the underlying disease process might be treated and the fatal outcome prevented. Clearly, improved treatment or prevention of the life-threatening complications of these disorders may well depend on better understanding of the underlying pathogenic processes, and that may, in turn, require better understanding of the normal functions that are defective in these patients. Regardless, it will be of very great importance to eventually focus considerable effort on using this scientific knowledge to benefit patients, and to solve the human problems associated with these terrible diseases.

Acknowledgements

Supported, in part, by NIH R01 AR39892.

References

1. Spritz RA, Genetic defects in Chediak–Higashi syndrome and the beige mouse, *J Clin Immunol* (1998) **18**:97–105.
2. Spritz RA, Molecular genetics of the Hermansky–Pudlak and Chediak–Higashi syndromes, *Platelets* (1998) **9**:21–9.
3. Spritz RA, Multi-organellar disorders of pigmentation: intracellular traffic jams in mammals, flies, and yeast, *TIG* (1999) **15**:337–40.

4. Spritz RA, Multi-organellar disorders of pigmentation: tied up in traffic, *Clin Genet* (1999) **5**:309–17.
5. Spritz RA, Chediak–Higashi syndrome, In: Ochs HD, Smith CIE, Puck JM, eds, *Primary Immunodeficiency Diseases, a Molecular and Genetic Approach*, (Oxford University Press: New York, 1999) 389–96.
6. Spritz RA, Hermansky-Pudlak syndrome and pale ear: melanosome-making for the millennium, *Pigment Cell Res* (2000) **13**:15–20.
7. Bennett D, Genetics, development, and malignancy of melanocytes, *Int Rev Cytol* (1993) **146**:191–260.
8. Swank RT, Novak EK, McGarry MP et al., Mouse models of Hermansky–Pudlak syndrome: a review, *Pigment Cell Res* (1998) **11**:60–80.
9. Mellman I, Endocytosis and molecular sorting, *Annu Rev Cell Dev Biol* (1996) **12**:575–625.
10. Schmid SL, Clathrin-coated vesicle formation and protein sorting: an integrated process, *Annu Rev Biochem* (1997) **66**:511–48.
11. Traub LM, Kornfeld S, The *trans*-Golgi network: a late secretory sorting station, *Curr Opin Cell Biol* (1997) **9**:527–33.
12. Kirchhausen T, Bonifacino JS, Riezman H, Linking cargo to vesicle formation: receptor tail interactions with coat proteins, *Curr Opin Cell Biol* (1997) **9**: 488–95.
13. Robinson MS, Coats and vesicle budding, *Trends Cell Biol* (1997) **7**:99–102.
14. Le Borgne R, Hoflack B, Mechanisms of protein sorting and coat assembly: insights from the clathrin-coated vesicle pathway, *Curr Opin Cell Biol* (1998) **10**:499–503.
15. Dell' Angelica EC, Ohno H, Ooi CE et al., AP-3: an adaptor-like protein complex with ubiquitous expression, *EMBO J* (1997) **16**: 917–28.
16. Simpson F, Peden AA, Christopoulou L et al., Characterization of the adaptor-related protein complex, AP-3, *J Cell Biol* (1997) **137**:835–45.
17. LeBorgne R, Alconada A, Bauer U et al., The mammalian AP-3 adaptor-like complex mediates the intracellular transport of lysosomal membrane glycoproteins, *J Biol Chem* (1998) **273**:29451–61.
18. Hermansky F, Pudlak P, Albinism associated with hemorrhagic diathesis and unusual pigmented reticular cells in the bone marrow, *Blood* (1959) **14**: 162–9.
19. Witkop CJ, Almadovar C, Pineiro B et al., Hermansky–Pudlak syndrome (HPS). An epidemiologic study, *Ophth Paediatr Genet* (1990) **11**: 245–50.
20. Witkop CJ, Babcock MN, Rao GHR et al., Albinism and Hermansky—Pudlak syndrome in Puerto Rico, *Bol Assoc Med P Rico* (1990) **82**:333–9.
21. Garay SM, Gardella JE, Fazzini EP et al., Hermansky–Pudlak syndrome. Pulmonary manifestations of a ceroid storage disorder, *Am J Med* (1979) **6**:737–47.
22. Schinella RA, Greco MA, Cobert BL et al., Hermansky–Pudlak syndrome with granulomatous colitis, *Ann Intern Med* (1980) **92**:20–3.
23. Shanahan F, Randolph L, King R et al., Hermansky–Pudlak syndrome: an immunologic assessment of 15 cases, *Am J Med* (1988) **85**:823–8.
24. Frenk E, Lattion F, The melanin pigmentary disorder in a family with Hermansky–Pudlak syndrome, *J Invest Dermatol* (1982) **78**:141–3.
25. Lattion F, Schneider P, Da Prada M et al., Syndrome d'Hermansky–Pudlak dans un village valaisan, *Helv Paediatr Acta* (1983) **38**:495–512.
26. Boissy RE, Zhao Y, Gahl WA, Altered protein localization in melanocytes from Hermansky–Pudlak syndrome: support for the role of the HPS gene product in intracellular trafficking, *Lab Invest* (1998) **87**:1037–48.
27. White JG, Edson JR, Desnick SJ et al., Studies of platelets in a variant of the Hermansky–Pudlak syndrome, *Am J Pathol* (1971) **63**:319–32.
28. Hardisty RM, Mills CB, Ketsa-Ard K, The platelet defect associated with albinism, *Br J Haematol* (1972) **23**:679–92.
29. Holmsen H, Weiss HJ, Secretable storage pool in platelets. *Blood* (1972) **39**:197–209.
30. Schallreuter KU, Frenk E, Wolfe LS et al., Hermansky–Pudlak syndrome in a Swiss population, *Dermatology* (1993) **187**:248–56.
31. White JG, Witkop CJ, Gerritson SM, The Hermansky–Pudlak syndrome: ultrastructure of bone marrow macrophages, *Am J Pathol* (1973) **70**:329–44.
32. Schinella RA, Greco MA, Garay SM et al., Hermansky–Pudlak syndrome: a clinicopathologic study, *Hum Pathol* (1985) **16**:366–76.
33. Harmon KR, Witkop CJ, White JG et al., Pathogenesis of pulmonary fibrosis: Platelet derived growth factor precedes structural alterations in the Hermansky–Pudlak syndrome, *J Lab Clin Med* (1994) **123**:617–27.
34. Fukai K, Oh J, Frenk E et al., Linkage disequilibrium mapping of the gene for Hermansky–Pudlak syndrome to chromosome 10q23.1–q23.3, *Hum Mol Genet* (1995) **4**:1665–9.
35. Wildenberg SC, Oetting WS, Almodóvar C et al., A

gene causing Hermansky–Pudlak syndrome in a Puerto Rican population maps to chromosome 10q2, *Am J Hum Genet* (1995) **57**:755–65.

36. Bailin T, Oh J, Feng GH et al., Organization and nucleotide sequence of the human Hermansky–Pudlak syndrome (*HPS*) gene, *J Invest Dermatol* (1997) **108**:923–7.
37. Oh J, Bailin T, Fukai K et al., Positional cloning of a gene for Hermansky–Pudlak syndrome, a disorder of cytoplasmic organelles, *Nat Genet* (1996) **14**: 300–6.
38. Feng GH, Bailin T, Oh J et al., Mouse *pale ear* (*ep*) is homologous to human Hermansky–Pudlak syndrome and contains a rare 'AT-AC' intron, *Hum Mol Genet* (1997) 6:793–7.
39. Gardner JM, Wildenberg SC, Keiper NM et al., The mouse pale ear (*ep*) mutation is the homologue of human Hermansky–Pudlak syndrome (HPS), *Proc Natl Acad Sci U S A* (1997) **94**:9238–43.
40. Oh J, LeCras TD, Spritz RA, Characterization and evolutionary comparison of rat *Hps* cDNA and exclusion of red-eyed dilution (*r*) locus, *Mammalian Genome* (2002) **12**: in press.
41. Oh J, Liu Z-X, Feng GH et al., The Hermansky–Pudlak syndrome (HPS) protein is part of a high molecular weight complex involved in biogenesis of early melanosomes, *Hum Mol Genet* (2000) **9**:375–85.
42. Dell'Angelica EC, Aguilar RC, Wolins N et al., Molecular characterization of the protein encoded by the Hermansky–Pudlak syndrome type 1 gene, *J Biol Chem* (2000) **275**:1300–6.
43. Oh J, Ho L, Ala-Mello S et al., Mutation analysis of patients with Hermansky–Pudlak syndrome: A frameshift hot spot in the *HPS* gene and apparent locus heterogeneity, *Am J Hum Genet* (1998) **62**: 593–8.
44. Shotelersuk V, Hazelwood S, Larson D et al., Three new mutations in a gene causing Hermansky–Pudlak syndrome: clinical correlations, *Mol Genet Metab* (1998) **64**:99–107.
45. Spritz RA, Oh J, *HPS* gene mutations in Hermansky–Pudlak syndrome, *Am J Hum Genet* (1999) **64**:658–9.
46. Hazelwood S, Shotelersuk V, Wildenberg SC et al., Evidence for locus heterogeneity in Puerto Ricans with Hermansky–Pudlak syndrome, *Am J Hum Genet* (1997) **61**:1088–94.
47. Silvers WK, *The Coat Colors of Mice* (Springer-Verlag: New York, 1979).
48. Lyon MF, Searle AG, *Genetic Variants and Strains of the Laboratory Mouse*, 2nd edn (Oxford University Press: New York, 1989).
49. Dell' Angelica ED, Shotelersuk V, Aguilar RC et al., Altered trafficking of lysosomal proteins in Hermansky–Pudlak syndrome due to mutations in the β3A subunit of the AP-3 adaptor, *Mol Cell* (1999) **3**:1–20.
50. Shotelersuk V, Dell' Angelica EC, Hartnell L et al., A new variant of Hermansky–Pudlak syndrome due to mutations in a gene responsible for vesicle formation, *Am J Med* (2000) **108**:423–7.
51. Feng L, Seymour AB, Jiang S et al., The β3A subunit gene (*Ap3b1*) of the AP-3 adaptor complex is altered in the mouse hypopigmentation mutant pearl, a model for Hermansky–Pudlak syndrome and night blindness, *Hum Mol Genet* (1999) **8**:323–30.
52. Beguez-Cesar AB, Neutropenia cronica maligna familiar con granulaciones atipicas de los leucocitos, *Bol Soc Cubana Pediatr* (1943) **15**:900–22.
53. Steinbrinck W, Uber eine neue Granulationsanomalie der Leukocyten, *Dtsch Arch Klin Med* (1948) **193**:577–81.
54. Chediak M, Nouvelle anomalie leukocytaire de caractere constitutionnel et familiel, *Rev Hematol* (1952) **7**:362–7.
55. Higashi O, Congenital gigantism of peroxidase granules, *Tohoku J Exp Med* (1954) **59**:315–32.
56. Sato A, Chediak and Higashi's disease: probably identity of 'a new leukocytal anomaly' (Chediak) and 'congenital gigantism of peroxidase granules' (Higashi), *Tohoku J Exp Med* (1955) **61**:201–10.
57. Donohue WL, Bain HW, Chediak–Higashi syndrome: a lethal familial disease with anomalous inclusions in the leukocytes and constitutional stigmata: report of a case with necropsy, *Pediatrics* (1957) **20**:416–30.
58. Blume RS, Wolff SM, The Chediak–Higashi syndrome: studies in four patients and a review of the literature, *Medicine* (1972) **51**:247–80.
59. Bejajoui M, Veber F, Girault D et al., Phase acceleree de la maladie de Chediak–Higashi, *Arch Fr Pediatr* (1989) **46**:733–6.
60. Misra VP, King RHM, Harding AE et al., Peripheral neuropathy in the Chediak–Higashi syndrome, *Acta Neuropathol* (1991) **81**:354–8.
61. Uyama E, Hirano T, Ito K et al., Adult Chediak–Higashi syndrome presenting as parkinsonism and dementia, *Acta Neurol Scand* (1994) **89**:175–83.
62. White JG, The Chediak–Higashi syndrome: a possible lysosomal disease, *Blood* (1966) **28**:143–56.
63. Windhorst DB, Zelickson AS, Good RA, Chediak–Higashi syndrome: hereditary gigantism of cytoplasmic organelles, *Science* (1966) **151**:81–3.
64. Lockman LA, Kennedy WR, White JG, The Chediak–

Higashi syndrome: electrophysiological and electron microscopic observations on the peripheral neuropathy, *J Pediatr* (1967) **70**:942–51.

65. Jones KL, Stewart RM, Fowler M et al., Chediak–Higashi lymphoblastoid cell lines: granule characteristics and expression of lysosome-associated membrane proteins, *Clin Immunol Immunopathol* (1992) **65**:219–26.
66. Burkhardt JK, Wiebel FA, Hester S et al., The giant organelles in *beige* and Chediak–Higashi fibroblasts are derived from late endosomes and mature lysosomes, *J Exp Med* (1993) **178**:1845–56.
67. Windhorst DB, Zelickson AS, Good RA, A human pigmentary dilution based on a heritable subcellular structural defect—the Chediak–Higashi syndrome, *J Invest Dermatol* (1968) **50**:9–18.
68. Zelickson AS, Windhorst DB, White JG et al., The Chediak–Higashi syndrome: formation of giant melanosomes and the basis of hypopigmentation, *J Invest Dermatol* (1967) **49**:575–81.
69. Bedoya V, Pigmentary changes in Chediak–Higashi syndrome, *Br J Dermatol* (1971) **85**:336–47.
70. Haliotis T, Roder J, Klein M et al., Chediak–Higashi gene in humans. I. Impairment of natural-killer function, *J Exp Med* (1980) **151**:1039–48.
71. Klein M, Roder J, Haliotis T et al., Chediak–Higashi gene in humans. II. The selectivity of the defect in natural-killer and antibody-dependent cell-mediated cytotoxicity function, *J Exp Med* (1980) **151**: 1049–58.
72. Roder JC, Haliotis T, Klein M et al., A new immunodeficiency disorder in humans involving NK cells, *Nature* (1980) **284**:553–5.
73. Katz P, Zaytoun AM, Fauci AS, Deficiency of active natural killer cells in the Chediak–Higashi syndrome: Localization of the defect using a single cell cytotoxicity assay, *J Clin Invest* (1982) **69**:1231–8.
74. Baetz K, Isaaz S, Griffiths GM, Loss of cytotoxic T lymphocyte function in Chediak–Higashi syndrome arises from a secretory defect that prevents lytic granule exocytosis, *J Immunol* (1995) **154**: 6122–31.
75. Buchanan GR, Handin RI, Platelet function in the Chediak–Higashi syndrome, *Blood* (1976) **47**:941–8.
76. Boxer GJ, Holmsen H, Robkin L et al., Abnormal platelet function in Chediak–Higashi syndrome, *Br J Haematol* (1977) **35**:521–33.
77. Apitz-Castro R, Cruz MR, Ledezma E et al., The storage pool deficiency in platelets from humans with the Chediak–Higashi syndrome: study of six patients, *Br J Haematol* (1985) **59**:471–83.
78. Costa JL, Fauci AS, Wolff SM, A platelet abnormality in the Chediak–Higashi syndrome of man, *Blood* (1976) **48**:517–20.
79. Parmley RT, Poon MC, Crist WM et al., Giant platelet granules in a child with the Chediak–Higashi syndrome, *Am J Hematol* (1979) **6**:651–60.
80. Rendu F, Breton-Gorius J, Lebret M et al., Evidence that abnormal platelet functions in human Chediak–Higashi syndrome are the result of a lack of dense bodies, *Am J Pathol* (1983) **111**:307–14.
81. Leader RW, Padgett GA, Gorham JR, Studies of abnormal leukocyte bodies in the mink, *Blood* (1963) **22**:477–84.
82. Padgett GA, Leader RW, Gorham JR et al., The familial occurrence of Chediak–Higashi syndrome in mink and cattle, *Genetics* (1964) **49**:505–12.
83. Taylor RF, Farrell RK, Light and electron microscopy of peripheral blood neutrophils in a killer whale affected with Chediak–Higashi syndrome, *Fed Proc* (1973) **32**:822a.
84. Kramer JW, Davis WC, Prieur DJ, The Chediak–Higashi syndrome of cats, *Lab Invest* (1977) **36**: 554–62.
85. Nes N, Lium B, Braend M et al., A Chediak–Higashi-like syndrome in Arctic blue foxes, *Finsk Veterinaertidsskrift* (1983) **89**:313.
86. Nes N, Llium B, Sjaastad O et al., Norsk perlerevmutant med Chediak–Higashi-liknende syndrom, *Norsk Pelsdyrblad* (1985) **59**:325–8.
87. Nishimura M, Inoue M, Nakano T et al., Beige rat: a new animal model of Chediak–Higashi syndrome, *Blood* (1989) **74**:270–3.
88. Ozaki K, Maeda H, Nishikawa T et al., Chediak–Higashi syndrome in rats: light and electron microscopical characterization of abnormal granules in beige rats, *J Comp Pathol* (1994) **110**:369–79.
89. Lutzner MA, Lowrie CT, Jordan HW, Giant granules in leukocytes of the beige mouse, *J Hered* (1966) **58**:299–300.
90. Windhorst DB, Padgett B, The Chediak–Higashi syndrome and the homologous trait in animals, *J Invest Dermatol* (1973) **60**:529–37.
91. Roder JC, The beige mutation in the mouse. I. A stem cell predetermined impairment in natural killer cell function, *J Immunol* (1979) **123**:2168–73.
92. Novak EK, Hui S-W, Swank RT, Platelet storage pool deficiency in mouse pigment mutations associated with several distinct genetic loci, *Blood* (1984) **63**: 536–44.
93. Oliver C, Essner E, Distribution of anomalous lysosomes in the beige mouse: a homologue of

the Chediak–Higashi syndrome, *J Histochem Cytochem* (1973) **21**:218–28.

94. Barbosa MDFS, Nguyen QA, Tchernev VT et al., Identification of the homologous beige and Chediak–Higashi syndrome genes, *Nature* (1996) **382**:262–5.
95. Perou CM, Justice MJ, Pryor RJ et al., Complementation of the beige mutation in cultured cells by episomally replicating murine yeast artificial chromosomes, *Proc Natl Acad Sci U S A* (1996) **93**: 5905–9.
96. Perou CM, Moore KJ, Nagle DL et al., Identification of the murine beige gene by YAC complementation and positional cloning, *Nat Genet* (1996) **13**:303–7.
97. Barrat FJ, Auloge L, Pastural E et al., Genetic and physical mapping of the Chediak–Higashi syndrome on chromosome 1q42–q43, *Am J Hum Genet* (1996) **59**:625–33.
98. Fukai K, Oh J, Karim MA et al., Homozygosity mapping of the gene for Chediak–Higashi syndrome to chromosome 1q42–q44 in a segment of conserved synteny that includes the mouse beige locus (*bg*), *Am J Hum Genet* (1996) **59**:620–4.
99. Nagle DL, Karim MA, Woolf EA et al., Identification and mutation analysis of the complete gene for Chediak–Higashi syndrome, *Nat Genet* (1996) **14**: 307–11.
100. Barbosa MDFS, Barrat FJ, Tchenev VT et al., Identification of mutations in two major mRNA isoforms of the Chediak–Higashi syndrome gene in human and mouse, *Hum Mol Genet* (1997) **6**: 1091–8.
101. Karim MA, Nagle DL, Kandil HH et al., Mutations in the Chediak–Higashi syndrome gene (*CHS1*) indicate requirement for the complete 3801 amino acid CHS protein, *Hum Mol Genet* (1997) **6**:1087–9.
102. Certain S, Barrat F, Pastural E et al., Protein truncation test of LYST reveals heterogeneous mutations in patients with Chediak–Higashi syndrome, *Blood* (2000) **85**:979–83.
103. Karim MA, Suzuki K, Fukai K et al., Apparent genotype–phenotype correlation in childhood, adolescent, and adult Chediak–Higashi syndrome, *Am J Med Genet* (2002) **108**:16–22.
104. Perou CM, Leslie JD, Green W et al., The Beige/ Chediak–Higashi syndrome gene encodes a widely expressed cytosolic protein, *J Biol Chem* (1997) **272**:29790–4.
105. Symes PH, Williams ME, Flessa HC et al., Acute promyelocytic leukemia with the pseudo-Chediak–Higashi anomaly and molecular determination of t(15;17) chromosomal translocation, *Histopathology* (1993) **99**:622–7.

18

A genetic approach to the study of vesicle transport in the mouse

Lydia E. Matesic, Neal G. Copeland and Nancy A. Jenkins

Introduction

Although all visible mammalian pigment is contained within the keratinocytes of the hair and skin to protect the organism from the harmful effects of ultraviolet radiation, it is synthesized within melanocytes inside specialized Golgi-derived organelles, termed melanosomes. Melanocytes are found in the basal layer of the epidermis at the base of the hair shaft and contact surrounding keratinocytes via copious and lengthy dendritic processes, which can be up to 100 μm long.[1] Since new melanosomes form near the center of melanocytes, they have to be transported over a considerable distance to the distal tips of the dendrites, where they are transferred to keratinocytes. The long-range transport of melanosomes from the cell body to the ends of the dendrites is bidirectional and microtubule-dependent.[2] Melanosomes are then concentrated in the periphery by way of a short-range, actin-based transport system that captures the melanosomes for efficient transfer to the keratinocytes.[2]

The identification of the proteins that function in this pathway is facilitated by the availability of a powerful genetic model system for studying vesicle transport in mammals: namely, mutations which affect melanosome transport in the mouse. To date, more than 50 loci that affect coat pigmentation have been identified in the mouse.[3] Three of these, *d*, *ash*, and *ln*, have been grouped together because they are phenotypically indistinguishable (Fig. 18.1). Specifically, all three mutants have normal melanosome synthesis but pigment granule transport is impaired.[4] Mice that are homozygous for any of these recessive mutations display abnormal perinuclear clumping of melanosomes in the melanocyte, resulting in the uneven release of pigment into the hair bulb and a lightened coat color (Fig. 18.2).

Genetic evidence suggests that the proteins encoded by these three genes function in the same or in overlapping pathways. In addition to the fact that these non-allelic mutants have identical phenotypes, we have observed that any double or triple combination of these mutants on a non-*agouti* background have the same appearance (NGC and NAJ, unpublished observations). Further, all three mutations are suppressed by the cell-autonomous, semidominant *dilute suppressor*, *dsu*.[5–7] The recent description of the genes mutated in *d*, *ash*, and *ln* mice has shed some light on the complicated process of melanosome transport and suggests that these proteins may be acting in concert as part of a transport complex.

Identification of the proteins encoded by *dilute, ashen,* and *leaden*

Dilute encodes unconventional myosin VA (*MyoVa*)

Mice homozygous for null mutations at *dilute* have a lightened coat color and die from a neurological defect characterized by ataxia and opisthotonus (arching of the head and neck) 2–3 weeks after birth. Several years ago, mutations in the heavy chain of the unconventional myosin *MyoVa* were shown to cause the vesicle transport defects observed in *dilute* mice.[8] Like all members of this family, MyoVa has a globular head domain that contains the ATP- and actin-binding sites, a 'neck'

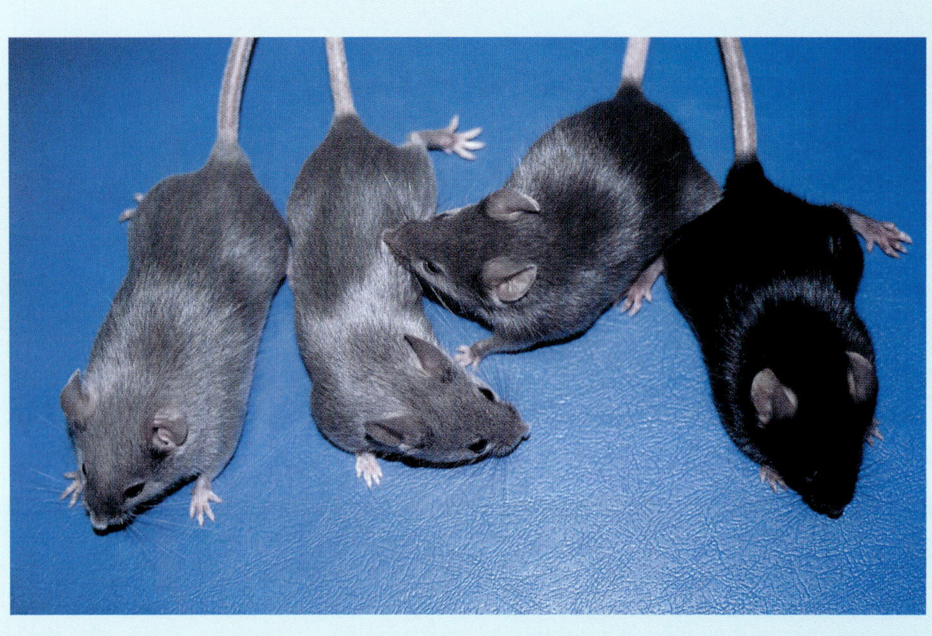

Figure 18.1

Coat-color phenotyes of *dilute*, *ashen*, and *leaden* mice. Pictured from left to right are: *a/a*, *ash/ash*; *a/a*, *ln/ln*; *a/a*, d^n/d^v; and *a/a* (wild type *non-agouti*) mice. All three mutants have nearly identical degrees of coat-color lightening due to impaired melanosome transport.

(the site of calmodulin or light-chain binding), and a tail domain, which is thought to be the cargo-binding region of the protein. Two molecules of MyoVa dimerize to create a plus-end directed motor that moves processively in large steps that approximate the 36 nm pseudorepeat of the actin filament.[9] Thus, in the absence of MyoVa, actin-based transport is impaired, affecting both pigmentation and neurological development.

Normally, MyoVa colocalizes with end-stage melanosomes.[10–12] In melanocytes obtained from homozygous *dilute* animals where there is no MyoVa, pigment synthesis is normal, and long-range, microtubule-dependent movement of melanosomes along the length of the dendrites is unaffected.[2] However, the melanosomes fail to be captured in the actin-rich periphery of the melanocyte, and, instead, become concentrated in the cell center, which is highly enriched in microtubules.[13] This capture model is supported by the observation that a *dilute*-like phenotype can be created in wild-type cells by expressing only the cargo-binding MyoVa tail domain, which causes melanosomes to redistribute to the cell center.[2] Similarly, the neurological defects of *dilute* mice appear to result from failings in the actin-based transport of smooth endoplasmic reticulum (SER). In both the *dilute* mouse and the *dilute* rat, SER is missing from the dendritic spines of cerebellar Purkinje cells, but is present in the dendritic shaft.[14,15] This observation is consistent with the hypothesis that long-range transport from the cell body to the dendritic shaft of neurons is microtubule-dependent, while the short-range transport into the dendritic spines is actin-based.

A human disease corollary of this vesicle transport defect has been identified. Mutations in *MYOVA* have been shown to result in Griscelli syndrome, a rare autosomal disorder characterized by pigment dilution, neurological defects, variable

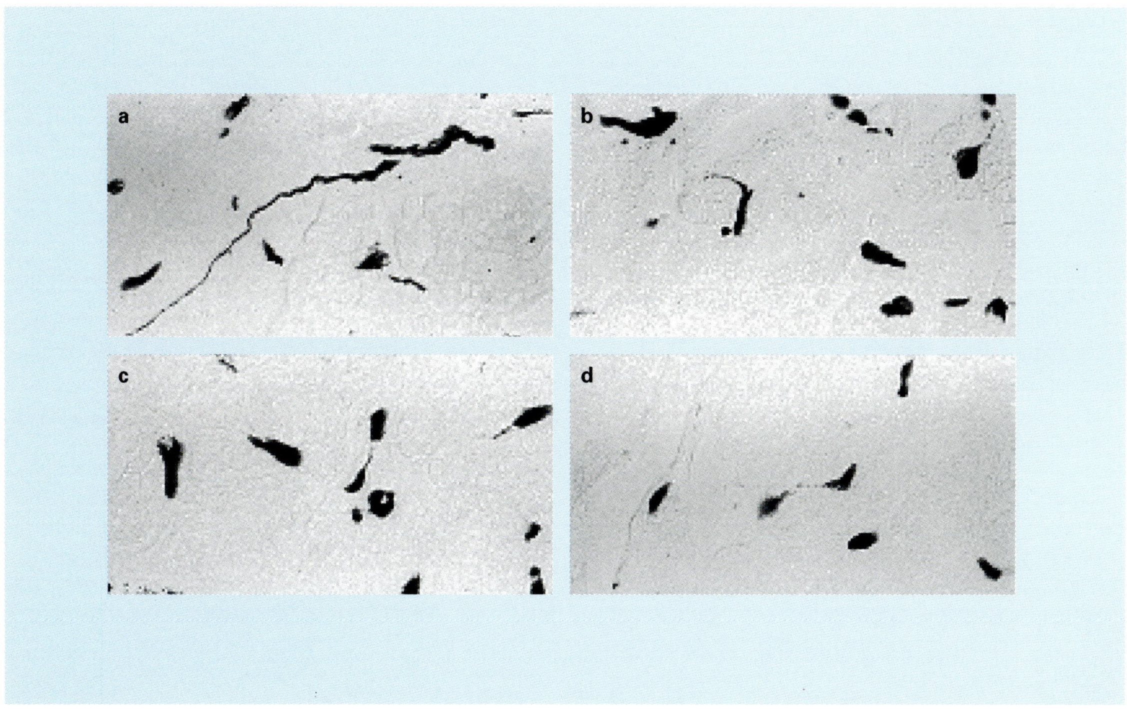

Figure 18.2

Melanocyte phenotypes of *dilute*, *ashen*, and *leaden* mice. Sections of unstained Harderian glands from 10 to 12 days old: (a) *a/a*; (b) *a/a*, d^v/d^v; (c) *a/a*, *ash/ash*; and (d) *a/a*; *ln/ln* mice are shown. All three mutants (b–d) show abnormal perinuclear clumping of melanosomes (black), whereas the normal distribution in the *non-agouti*-derived tissue (a) highlights the long spindle appearance of the melanocyte dendrites, demonstrating peripheral transport and capture of melanosomes.

cellular immunodeficiency, and acute phases of uncontrolled lymphocyte and macrophage activation.[16,17] The pigmentary dilution observed in Griscelli syndrome is characterized by diffuse skin pigmentation, silvery hair (often described as premature graying), large clumps of pigment in the hair shafts, and an abnormal accumulation of melanosomes in melanocytes. This is, of course, reminiscent of the coat-color dilution seen in *dilute* mice, making this mutant an important model for the study of Griscelli syndrome.

Additional insight into important functional domains of MyoVa was gained through a detailed genotype/phenotype analysis of 17 viable, hypomorphic *dilute* alleles, which varied in their effects on coat color and on the nervous system, from mild coat-color lightening to dramatic coat-color dilution associated with some degree of neurological impairment.[2,18,19] There were no identified MyoVa mutations which affected only the nervous system, suggesting that the process of pigmentation is more sensitive to MyoVa levels than is the nervous system (or that there is functional redundancy in the nervous system). Most of these mutations turned out to be missense mutations (seven mapping to the head domain and five mapping to the tail region). For these, the severity of the phenotype correlated with the severity of the mutation (*i.e.* the type of amino acid substitution). However, there were two informative tail-region mutations that represented tissue-specific splicing mutants that lacked one of the exon F-containing MyoVa isoforms, which is normally found in spleen and skin (*i.e.* melanocytes) but not in brain.[20] Phenotypically, the animals with these mutations displayed lightened coat color with no neurological impairments. This suggests that exon F may encode a melanocyte-specific cargo motif.

Identification of MyoVa binding partners has elucidated other possible components of the transport machinery. Yeast two-hybrid studies have demonstrated that the tail domain of MyoVa can interact with the tail region of ubiquitous kinesin heavy chain (Kif5b), a microtubule-based transport motor.[21] These data suggest that these motor molecules act as a complex to coordinate the long-range transport of melanosomes along microtubules (Kif5b-dependent movement) and short-range transport along actin filaments (MyoVa-dependent movement).

MyoVa has also been shown to bind BERP, a novel RING finger protein, in rat brain.[22] BERP contains numerous protein–protein interaction domains that make it a potential adaptor protein for mediating MyoVa cargo transport. These include an N-terminal RING finger (which in many cases acts as an E3 ubiquitin ligase,[23] although this function has not yet been ascribed to BERP), a zinc-binding domain (B-box), a leucine coiled-coil region, and a C-terminal β-propeller through which it binds MyoVa. Interestingly, BERP has also been shown to bind α-actinin-4.[24] Alpha actinin-4 is an actin-binding protein that has been implicated in cell motility and carcinogenesis.[25] While the function of BERP in MyoVa-mediated transport remains to be determined, expression of a dominant-interfering BERP mutant in rat PC12 cells has been shown to prevent neurite outgrowth and to inhibit PC12 cell spreading in response to nerve growth factor.[22] MyoVa also appears to play a role in neurite extension and growth-cone development;[26] thus, it is tempting to speculate that the effects of dominant-interfering mutants of BERP result from its interaction with MyoVa.

Ashen encodes *Rab27a*

Mice homozygous for the *ashen* mutation have a lightened coat color, defects in the formation of platelet-dense granules, and faulty secretion of granules from cytotoxic T-lymphocytes.[22–29] All of these phenotypes are symptomatic of defective vesicle trafficking and, more specifically, of improper sorting of melanosomal and lysosomal proteins. It has recently been recognized that melanosomes and lysosomes share many stages of biogenesis, from entry into the endoplasmic reticulum through sorting at the trans-Golgi network.[30] In this scenario, platelet-dense granules and granules from cytotoxic T-lymphocytes can be viewed as 'specialized secretory lysosomes', which fail to properly form and are, thus, functionally compromised. Mutations in *Rab27a* are responsible for vesicle transport defects observed in *ashen* mice.[27] Rab GTPases are members of the largest branch of the p21 Ras superfamily. All members of this family are known to be geranylgeranylated at their C-terminus, directing their insertion into the cytoplasmic face of the plasma membrane, of organelles, or of vesicles.[31] Each Rab protein identified to date has a specific subcellular localization, which is thought to be crucial to proper vesicular transport and organelle dynamics in eukaryotic cells.[32]

Like MyoVa, Rab27a localizes to end-stage melanosomes in wild-type cells.[33,34] Melanocytes obtained from homozygous *ashen* mice show normal dendrite morphology and normal melanosome biogenesis, rapid bidirectional, microtubule-dependent melanosome movements along the length of the dendrites, and an abnormal accumulation of end-stage melanosomes perinuclearly.[33] This phenotype is consistent with the hypothesis that *ashen* melanocytes, like *dilute* melanocytes, are defective in peripheral melanosome capture and short-range transport. There are experimental observations that support this hypothesis. Introduction of wild-type *Rab27a* cDNA into *ashen* melanocytes restores the peripheral distribution of melanosomes in a microtubule-dependent manner.[33] Conversely, the introduction of a dominant-interfering *Rab27a* cDNA into wild-type melanocytes causes the redistribution of melanosomes to the perinuclear region of the cell.[33,34]

Ashen mice are proving to be valuable models for diseases that affect vesicle transport in humans. Mutations in *RAB27A* were associated with a subset of Griscelli syndrome patients.[17] Specifically, those Griscelli patients that displayed hemophagocytic symptoms (*i.e.* variable cellular immunodeficiency and acute phases of uncontrolled lymphocyte and macrophage activation) had mutations in *RAB27A*, while those patients without this aspect of the disease (but, in one case, with neurological impairment instead) had mutations in *MYOVA*. This is consistent with the phenotypes of the *dilute* and *ashen* mice. While some *dilute* mutants show neurological dysfunction, *ashen* mice do not. However, *ashen* mice do show defects in the formation of platelet-dense granules and faulty secretion of granules from cytotoxic T-lymphocytes, which could be viewed as the equivalent of the hemophagocytic syndrome seen in Griscelli patients with *RAB27A* mutations.

The *ashen* mouse has also provided valuable insight into another vesicle transport disease, Hermansky–Pudlak syndrome (HPS). HPS is an autosomal-recessive disorder, characterized by pigment dilution, decreased visual acuity, a bleeding diathesis, and lysosomal accumulation of ceroid lipofuscin, thought to be caused by improper vesicular trafficking of melansomes and lysosomes.[35] As Rab proteins are recognized as playing an important role in vesicle transport, RAB27A levels are likely affected in HPS. In fact, in a murine model of HPS, *gunmetal*, there is a decrease of Rab27A in platelets as well as decreases in other Rabs in selected tissues.[36] This decrease in Rab levels is caused indirectly by a mutation in the Rab geranylgeranyl transferase alpha subunit that normally acts to prenylate the Rabs. In *gunmetal* mice, Rabs are hypoprenylated and, thus, do not function properly.

Leaden encodes *Melanophilin* (*Mlph*)

The only phenotype associated with *ln/ln* mice to date is a lightened coat color due to abnormal melanosome distribution and consequent inefficient transfer to keratinocytes. As with the two other mutations previously discussed, melanocytes from *leaden* animals show a perinuclear accumulation of melansomes, suggesting that these cells lack the appropriate peripheral capture and short-range transport machinery.[37] Very recently, mutations in *Mlph* were recognized to be responsible for this phenotype.[38] *Mlph* is a previously undescribed member of the Rab effector family. All constituents of this family share a Rab effector domain at the N-terminus of the protein that is approximately 200 amino acids in length. This motif contains two Zn^{2+}-binding $CX_2CX_{13,14}CX_2C$ regions and a short aromatic amino-acid-rich region that is thought to be critical for binding of specific GTP-saturated Rab partners.

Two alleles of *leaden* were analyzed. One (ln^{l1RK3}) was a large deletion on mouse chromosome 1,[39] which removed all the *Mlph* coding sequence.[38] The other allele studied was the original mutation that spontaneously arose in 1933 in the C57BR inbred strain.[40] This allele showed no appreciable difference in transcript size or level of expression.[38] Careful inspection revealed a C-to-T transition that alters splicing of the *Mlph* mRNA, creating an in-frame 21-bp deletion that removes seven acidic amino acids from the Rab effector domain. Since this mutation is a functional null, if stable protein were produced from this message, it likely does not bind to its Rab partner (which is likely to be Rab27a in melanocytes). Precedent for this assertion comes from mutational analysis of Rim, a Rab3A/Rab3C effector molecule associated with neurotransmitter vesicle release.[41] This study determined that one of the critical Rim/Rab3A-binding determinants was a cluster of six acidic amino acid residues in the N-terminal Rab effector domain. This corresponds exactly to the seven amino acids deleted in the *ln* mutant.[38]

Fitting the pieces together: How MyoVa, Rab27a, and Mlph may interact to form a melanosome transport complex

Various studies have shown that Rab27a colocalizes with MyoVa on end-stage melanosomes derived from wild-type cells.[33,34,42] These two proteins can also be co-immunoprecipitated from wild-type melanosome extracts, suggesting a direct or indirect interaction of these two proteins.[34] Further insight into how Rab27a and MyoVa may interact was gleaned by examining the localization of Rab27a in *dilute* melanocytes, as well as the localization of MyoVa in *ashen* melanocytes. Those data showed that, in *dilute* melanocytes, Rab27a could be found on end-stage melanosomes; however, in *ashen* melanocytes, MyoVa does not colocalize with melanosomes, but is, instead, found in the microtubule-organizing center,[33] implying that Rab27a is, or is part of, the melanosome receptor that recruits MyoVa onto melanosomes.

Since antibodies to Mlph have not yet been developed, the precise role of Mlph in melanosome transport is not known at this time. However, hypotheses can be made based on the well-characterized interactions of the Rab effector Rabphilin-3A and its Rab-binding partner, Rab3A. The crystal structure of Rab3a complexed with the effector domain (*i.e.* the N-terminus) of Rabphilin-3A has been determined.[43] Rabphilin-3A contacts Rab3A in two distinct areas. The first interface involves the Rab3A switch I and switch II regions, which are sensitive to the nucleotide-binding state of Rab3A. The second contact point consists of a deep pocket in Rab3A that interacts with a SGAWFF structural motif of Rabphilin-3A. The last three amino acids of this motif are aromatic amino acids that adopt a perpendicular edge-to-plane configuration, which is particularly important for this interaction. Although the parts of the Rabphilin-3A protein that contact switch regions I and II are not particularly well conserved in Mlph, the SGAWFF motif is conserved.[38] Mlph encodes the related SLEWYY motif with the last three residues being aromatic amino acids. The divergence in the first contact region likely reflects the fact that Mlph binds a different Rab, the most likely candidate of which is Rab27a, which is encoded by *ashen*.[27] This leads to the testable hypothesis that Mlph binds to Rab27a via its N-terminus.

As it appears that Rab27a recruits MyoVa to the melanosome, the question of how Mlph fits into this complex arises. There are two possibilities. First, Mlph could localize to the melanosome and, through its interaction with Rab27a, recruit its GTP-bound form to the membrane, which, in turn, or in combination with Mlph, serves as a receptor for MyoVa. Alternatively, upon geranylgeranylation, Rab27a could insert into the melanosome membrane and could then recruit Mlph and MyoVa to the melanosome. The best way to distinguish between these two possibilities is to examine Rab27a localization in *leaden* melanocytes and to look at Mlph localization in *ashen* melanocytes. Such experiments are likely underway. However, there are predictions that can be made at this time, based on the phenotype of Rab3A knockout mice. Homozygous knockout animals display 70% reduction in the protein levels of Rabphilin-3A (although the mRNA level is unchanged), as well as retention of undegraded Rabphilin-3A in the cell body of the neurons (*i.e.* mislocalization of Rabphilin-3A),[44] while homozygous Rabphilin-3A knockout mice show neither mislocalization of Rab3A nor decreases in Rab3A protein levels.[45] Taken together, these observations suggest that Rab3 recruits Rabphilin-3A to the synaptic vesicle. Thus, the hypothesis would be that Rab27a recruits Mlph to the melanosome. These speculations are summarized in the model depicted in Figure 18.3. It will be interesting to see how *dsu* fits into this model after the affected gene is cloned, since *dsu* has been shown to suppress the *dilute* coat-color phenotype to nearly wild type, while it only partially suppresses the coat-color phenotypes of *ashen* and *leaden*.[7]

Conclusions

Mouse genetics has identified three mutants defective in pigment granule transport that have also proven to be valuable model systems for the study of human disease. The identification and biological characterization of those proteins affected by the *dilute*, *ashen*, and *leaden* mutations have provided a scaffold for the intellectual dissection of the transport machinery. Using these proteins as springboards, yeast two-hybrid screens, ENU mutagenesis surveys, and suppressor/enhancer screens can be conducted to search for additional proteins that may function in this pathway. As other key players are identified, we can begin the process of determining how these proteins coordinate the complex, yet crucial, process of melanosome transport. It will also be interesting to see what other roles this transport complex might be playing in the cell. Very recently, this complex has been implicated in contributing to the regulation of apoptosis in response to the loss of cell attachment and of integrin signaling.[46] Certainly, as other components of the transport machinery are identified, the role of this complex in many aspects of cellular homeostasis will be more fully appreciated.

Acknowledgements

We thank Deborah A. Swing for excellent assistance with mouse work. This research was funded by the National Cancer Institute, Department of Health and Human Services.

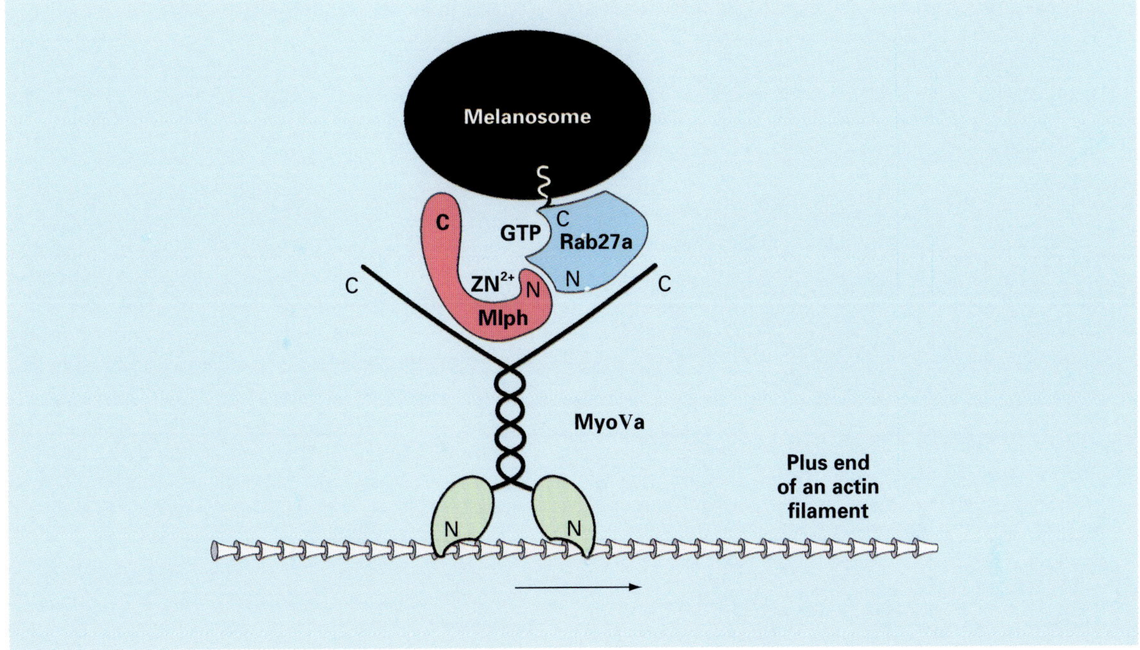

Figure 18.3

Model of melanosome transport machinery. Peripheral capture and transport of melanosomes is likely mediated by a complex theoretically composed of Rab27a, Mlph, and MyoVa. Here, we depict the presumed insertion of the prenyl group of Rab27a into the melanosome membrane. Through its N-terminus, Mlph may bind Rab27a. This unit could then serve as a receptor for MyoVa, the actin-based transport motor.

References

1. Wu X, Hammer JA III, Making sense of melanosome dynamics in mouse melanocytes, *Pigment Cell Res* (2000) **13**:241–7.
2. Wu X, Bowers B, Rao K et al., Visualization of melanosome dynamics within wild-type and dilute melanocytes suggest a paradigm for myosin V function in vivo, *J Cell Biol* (1998) **143**:1899–918.
3. Jackson IJ, Mouse coat colour mutations: a molecular genetic resource which spans the centuries, *Bioessays* (1991) **13**:439–46.
4. Silvers WK, *The Coat Colors of Mice* (Springer: New York, 1979).
5. Sweet HO, Dilute suppressor, a new suppressor gene in the house mouse, *J Hered* (1983) **74**:305–6.
6. Moore KJ, Seperack PK, Strobel MC et al., Dilute suppressor dsu acts semidominantly to suppress the coat color phenotype of a deletion mutation, d^{l20J}, of the murine dilute locus, *Proc Natl Acad Sci U S A* (1988) **85**:8131–5.
7. Moore KJ, Swing DA, Rinchik EM et al., The murine dilute suppressor gene dsu suppresses the coat-color phenotype of three pigment mutations that alter melanocyte morphology, d, ash and ln, *Genetics* (1988) **119**:933–41.
8. Mercer JA, Seperack PK, Strobel MC et al., Novel myosin heavy chain encode by murine dilute coat colour locus, *Nature* (1991) **349**:709–13.
9. Mehta AD, Rock RS, Rief M et al., Myosin-V is a processive actin-based motor, *Nature* (1999) **400**: 590–3.
10. Wu X, Bowers B, Wei Q et al., Myosin V associates with melanosomes in mouse melanocytes: evidence that myosin V is an organelle motor, *J Cell Sci* (1997) **110**:847–59.
11. Nascimento AA, Amaral RG, Bizario JC et al., Subcellular localization of myosin-V in the B16 melanoma cells, a wild-type cell line for the dilute gene, *Mol Biol Cell* (1997) **8**:1971–88.
12. Lambert J, Onderwater J, Vander Haeghen Y et al., Myosin V colocalizes with melanosomes and

subcortical actin bundles not associated with stress fibers in human epidermal melanocytes, *J Invest Dermatol* (1998) **111**:835–40.
13. Wu X, Kocher B, Wei Q et al., Myosin Va associates with microtubule-rich domains in both interphase and dividing cells, *Cell Motil Cytoskeleton* (1998) **40**: 286–303.
14. Dekker-Ohno K, Hayasaka S, Takagishi Y et al., Endoplasmic reticulum is missing in dendritic spines of Purkinje cells of the ataxic mutant rat, *Brain Res* (1996) **714**:226–30.
15. Takagishi Y, Oda S, Hayasaka S et al., The dilute-lethal (dl) gene attacks a Ca^{2+} store in the dendritic spine of Purkinje cells in mice, *Neurosci Lett* (1996) **215**:169–72.
16. Pastural E, Barrat FJ, Dufourcq-Lagelouse R et al., Griscelli disease maps to chromosome 15q21 and is associated with mutations in the myosin-Va gene, *Nat Genet* (1997) **16**:289–92.
17. Pastural E, Ersoy F, Yalman N et al., Two genes are responsible for Griscelli syndrom at the same 15q21 locus, *Genomics* (2000) **63**:299–306.
18. Huang JD, Mermall V, Strobel MC et al., Molecular genetic dissection of mouse unconventional myosin-VA: tail region mutations, *Genetics* (1998) **148**:1963–72.
19. Huang JD, Cope MJ, Mermall V et al., Molecular genetic dissection of mouse unconventional myosin-VA: head region mutations, *Genetics* (1998) **148**:1951–61.
20. Seperack PK, Mercer JA, Strobel MC et al., Retroviral sequences located within an intron of the dilute gene alter dilute expression in a tissue-specific manner, *EMBO J* (1995) **14**:2326–32.
21. Huang JD, Brady ST, Richards BW et al., Direct interaction of microtubule- and actin-based transport motors, *Nature* (1999) **397**:267–70.
22. El-Husseini AE, Vincent SR, Cloning and characterization of a novel RING finger protein that interacts with class V myosins, *J Biol Chem* (1999) **274**: 19771–7.
23. Freemont PS, RING for destruction? *Curr Biol* (2000) **10**:R84–7.
24. El-Husseini AE, Kwasnicka D, Yamada T et al., BERP, a novel ring finger protein, binds to alpha-actinin-4, *Biochem Biophys Res Commun* (2000) **267**:906–11.
25. Honda K, Yamada T, Endo R et al., Actinin-4, a novel actin-bundling protein associated with cell motility and cancer invasion, *J Cell Biol* (1998) **140**:1383–93.
26. Wang FS, Wolenski JS, Cheney RE et al., Function of myosin-V in filopodial extension of neuronal growth cones, *Science* (1996) **273**:660–3.
27. Wilson SM, Yip R, Swing DA et al., A mutation in Rab27a causes the vesicle transport defects observed in ashen mice, *Proc Natl Acad Sci U S A* (2000) **97**:7933–8.
28. Stinchcombe JC, Barral DC, Mules EH et al., Rab27a is required for regulated secretion in cytotoxic T lymphocytes, *J Cell Biol* (2001) **152**:825–34.
29. Haddad EK, Wu X, Hammer JA III et al., Defective granule exocytosis in Rab27a-deficient lymphocytes from ashen mice, *J Cell Biol* (2001) **152**:835–42.
30. Setaluri V, Sorting and targeting of melanosomal membrane proteins: signals, pathways, and mechanisms, *Pigment Cell Res* (2000) **13**:128–34.
31. Farnsworth CC, Seabra MC, Ericsson LH et al., Rab geranylgeranyl transferase catalyzes the geranylgeranylation of adjacent cysteines in the small GTPases Rab1A, Rab3A, and Rab5A, *Proc Natl Acad Sci U S A* (1994) **91**:11963–7.
32. Novick P, Zerial M, The diversity of Rab proteins in vesicle transport, *Curr Opin Cell Biol* (1997) **9**: 496–504.
33. Wu X, Rao K, Bowers MB et al., Rab27a enables myosin Va-dependent melanosome capture by recruiting the myosin to the organelle, *J Cell Sci* (2001) **114**:1091–100.
34. Hume AN, Collinson LM, Rapak A et al., Rab27a regulates the peripheral distribution of melanosomes in melanocytes, *J Cell Biol* (2001) **152**:795–808.
35. Shotelersuk V, Gahl WA, Hermansky–Pudlak syndrome: models for intracellular vesicle formation, *Mol Genet Metab* (1998) **65**:85–96.
36. Detter JC, Zhang Q, Mules EH et al., Rab geranylgeranyl transferase alpha mutation in the gunmetal mouse reduces Rab prenylation and platelet synthesis, *Proc Natl Acad Sci U S A* (2000) **97**:4144–9.
37. Provance DW Jr, Wei M, Ipe V et al., Cultured melanocytes from dilute mutant mice exhibit dendritic morphology and altered melanosome distribution, *Proc Natl Acad Sci U S A* (1996) **93**: 14554–8.
38. Matesic LE, Yip R, Reuss AE et al., Mutations in Mlph, encoding a member of the Rab effector family, cause the melanosome transport defects observed in leaden mice, *Proc Natl Acad Sci U S A* (2001) **98**:10238–43.
39. Roderick TH, Using inversions to detect and study recessive lethals and detrimentals in mice. In: de Serres FJ, Sheridan W, eds, *Utilization of Mammalian Specific Locus Studies in Hazard Evaluation and Estimation of Genetic Risk* (Plenum Press: New York, 1983) 135–67.

40. Murray JM, 'Leaden', a recent color mutation in the house mouse, *Am Nat* (1933) **67**:278–83.
41. Wang X, Hu B, Zimmermann B et al., Rim1 and Rabphilin-3 bind Rab3-GTP by composite determinants partially related through N-terminal alpha-helix motifs, *J Biol Chem* (2001) **276**:32480–8.
42. Bahadoran P, Aberdam E, Mantoux F et al., Rab27a: A key to melanosome transport in human melanocytes, *J Cell Biol* (2001) **152**:843–50.
43. Ostermeier C, Brunger AT, Structural basis of Rab effector specificity: crystal structure of the small G protein Rab3A complexed with the effector domain of rabphilin-3A, *Cell* (1999) **96**:363–74.
44. Li C, Takei K, Geppert M et al., Synaptic targeting of rabphilin-3A, a synaptic vesicle Ca2+/phospholipid-binding protein, depends on rab3A/3C, *Neuron* (1994) **13**:885–98.
45. Schluter OM, Schnell E, Verhage M et al., Rabphilin knock-out mice reveal that rabphilin is not required for rab3 function in regulating neurotransmitter release, *J Neurosci* (1999) **19**:5834–46.
46. Puthalakath H, Villunger A, O'Reilly LA et al., Bmf: a proapoptotic BH3-only protein regulated by interaction with the myosin V actin motor complex, activated by anoikis, *Science* (2001) **293**:1829–32.

19

Rab27a and melanosome transport in human melanocytes

Philippe Bahadoran and Robert Ballotti

Introduction

Normal human pigmentation, providing effective protection against UV light, depends on the uniform distribution of melanosomes in the epidermis. Melanocytes reside in the basal layer of the epidermis and possess long dendritic processes that allow intra- and intercellular transport of melanin-containing melanosomes from the cell body, the site of synthesis, to surrounding keratinocytes. Transfer to and retention of melanosomes at dendrite tips of melanocytes represent the intracellular steps of this complex transport process.

Progress regarding melanosome transport in human melanocytes has benefited from the study of Griscelli syndrome (GS), a genetic hypomelanose with abnormal melanosome distribution. GS is a rare, autosomal-recessive, inherited disease characterized by mild hypopigmentation, manifesting mostly as silvery hair, deficient lymphocyte-mediated cytotoxicity resulting principally in haemophagocytic syndrome, and variable neurological defects. Light microscopy examination of skin sections of GS patients shows the coexistence of heavily-pigmented melanocytes and non-pigmented keratinocytes. Electron microscopy shows that these melanocytes are stuffed with pigmented melanosomes, while adjacent keratinocytes are nearly devoid of these organelles.[1] These microscopic observations have lead to the hypothesis of defective transport of melanosomes in GS. On the other hand, four genetic loci are known in mouse that lighten coat color and disturb melanosome distribution: *dilute, ashen, leaden* and *dilute suppressor, dsu* (see Chapter 18). GS was mapped to 15q21 in a region encompassing the gene of *myosin Va* (*MYOVA*), and *MYOVA* mutations were identified in two GS patients,[2,3] pointing to *MYOVA* as the first gene in GS. In mouse, it had been shown previously that the *dilute* coat color is caused by mutations of *MYOVA*.[4] Following these genetic studies, cell biology studies in human[5] and murine melanocytes[6–8] have confirmed that *myosin Va* is necessary for distal melanosome distribution in melanocytes. In addition, elegant time-lapse videomicroscopy experiments indicate that mammalian melanosomes undergo long-range bidirectional microtubule-based transport, and are retained in peripheral dendrites by interaction with the actin cytoskeleton via *myosin Va*.[9]

Implication of Rab27a in melanosome transport

However, in many patients with GS, despite the mapping of the suspected gene in the 15q21 region, no mutations were found in MYOVA,[3] suggesting the possibility of a second gene in the same region. Interestingly, the human *Rab27a* gene (*RAB27A*) had just been mapped in this 15q21 region,[10] which, knowing the implication of RabGTPases in vesicular trafficking, made *Rab27a* a likely candidate for GS. Indeed, it was demonstrated shortly after, that *RAB27A* is mutated in 16 patients with GS.[11] In mouse, it was shown simultaneously that the *ashen* coat-color dilution is caused by a mutation in *RAB27A*.[12] We studied the melanocytes of a GS patient with a nonsense mutation in *RAB27A* (Fig. 19.1).[11] Immunofluorescence and Western blot analysis indicated that GS melanocytes did not express *Rab27a* (Fig. 19.2). Microscopic examination of cultured GS melanocytes showed normal melanosome

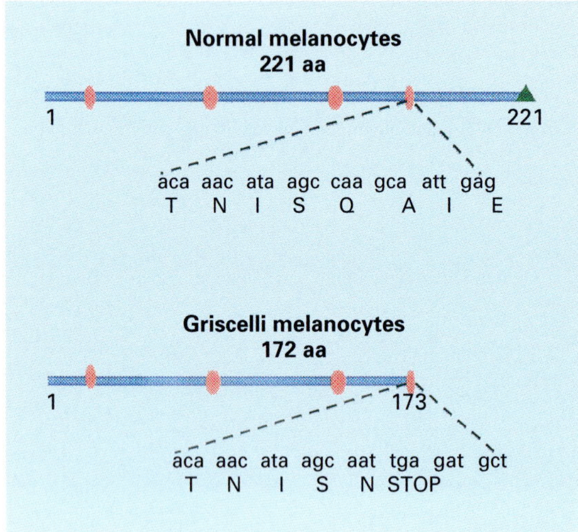

Figure 19.1

RAB27A mutation in a patient with Griscelli syndrome. Rab27a cDNA sequence analysis in normal melanocytes (top) and Griscelli melanocytes (bottom), showing a deletion of five nucleotides in the terminal exon, leading to a premature termination codon in 173, implying that 49 COOH-terminal amino acids are deleted at the protein level.

biogenesis and dendritic morphology, but abnormal melanosome distribution. More precisely, GS melanocytes showed dramatically increased melanosome numbers in the cell centre, contrasting with an extreme scarcity of melanosomes in dendrites, mostly evident at dendrite tips where these organelles should normally accumulate (Fig. 19.3). In addition, the wild-type version of *Rab27a* rescued normal accumulation of melanosomes in GS melanocytes dendrites (Fig. 19.4). These results establish the key role of *Rab27a* in melanosome transport in human melanocytes.[13] In mouse, aberrant melanosome localization and subsequent correction by *Rab27a* expression have been reported in *ashen* melanocytes.[14] Conversely, overexpression of a dominant-negative Rab27a mutant alters melanosome distribution in melan-a melanocytes,[14,15] as well as in B16 melanoma cells (Bahadoran et al., unpublished work).

In addition to pointing to the role of *Rab27a* in melanosome transport, the aforementioned data have yielded interesting genotype/phenotype correlations in human disease. In mouse, it was clear from the beginning that *MYOVA* and *RAB27A* mutations result in two different phenotypes, the *dilute* and *ashen* mouse, respectively, with closely-related pigmentary changes, but neurological impairment only in *dilute* mouse, and defective lymphocyte cytotoxicity only in *ashen* mouse.[16,17] In humans, patients with either *MYOVA* or *RAB27A* mutations have been classified under the term of GS, a disease comprising hypopigmentation, immune deficiency, and neurological symptoms. However, retrospective analysis of patient cases in the light of molecular data showed that mutations of *MYOVA* result in GS with hypopigmentation and severe primary neurological symptoms. This subset of patients probably corresponds to the otherwise-called neuroectodermal melanolysosomal disease or Elejalde syndrome.[18,19] On the other hand, mutations in *RAB27A* account for GS with hypopigmentation and haemophagocytic syndrome (Table 19.1).[11] The frequent occurence of secondary, neurological manifestations caused by haemophagocytic syndrome in the latter subset of patients was probably the confusing factor.[20]

The role of Rab27a in melanosome transport

Having established the crucial role of Rab27a in melanosome transport, studies have aimed to determine the precise role of this Rab in this process. Rab proteins form the largest branch of

Table 19.1 Genotype/phenotype correlation in Griscelli syndrome.

	Griscelli syndrome cutaneous and immunological	**Griscelli syndrome cutaneous and neurological (Elejalde syndrome)**
Albinism with impaired melanosome transport	+	+
Neurological disease (primary)	–	+++
Immunodeficiency	+++	–
Murine model	Ashen	Dilute
Gene	Rab27a	Myosin Va

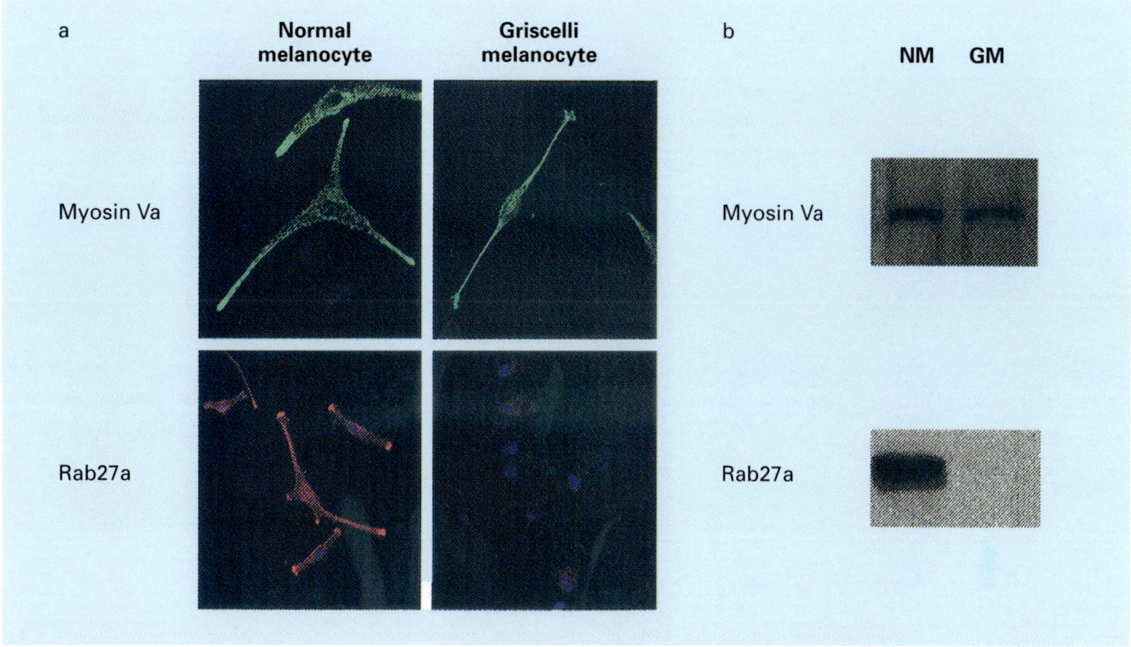

Figure 19.2

Absence of Rab27a expression in Griscelli melanocytes. (a) Immunofluorescence labelling of myosin Va (top) and Rab27a (bottom) in normal (left) and Griscelli (right) melanocytes. (b) Western blot analysis of myosin Va (top) and Rab27a (bottom) in normal (left) and Griscelli (right) melanocytes.

the Ras superfamily of GTPases. Rab proteins are GTPases that control intracellular vesicular transport. Many Rabs have a characteristic subcellular localization and are proposed to regulate specific steps in intracellular vesicle trafficking. The best characterized function of Rabs is to promote targeting, docking and fusion of vesicles with their appropriate acceptor membranes, but recently, several studies have addressed the possibility that Rab proteins may also mediate interactions between intracellular vesicles and cytoskeletal elements, especially molecular motors.[21] In line with these studies, the following results bring compelling evidence to support the idea that Rab27a may interact between melanosomes and myosin Va in melanocytes.

In normal human melanocytes, we have found, by confocal microscopy (Fig. 19.5) and immunoelectron microscopy that Rab27a and melanosomes have the same localization.[13] Furthermore, by immuno-isolation of melanosomes in B16 melanoma cells, we have detected the presence of Rab27a at the surface of these organelles (Bahadoran et al., unpublished work). Similar results have been reported in murine melan-a cells.[14,15] These data indicate that Rab27a interacts with melanosomes.

In normal human melanocytes, we have found that Rab27a and myosin Va exhibit similar patterns of distribution along melanosomes.[13] Moreover, in murine B16 melanoma cells, a GFP-tagged myosin Va tail-domain fusion protein coprecipitates endogenous Rab27a, while a GFP-tagged Rab27a fusion protein coprecipitates endogenous myosin Va (Fig. 19.6) (Bahadoran et al., unpublished work). The colocalization of Rab27a and myosin Va on melanosomes,[14,15] and the coprecipitation of Rab27a and myosin Va,[15] has also been shown in murine melan-a melanocytes. In accordance with the fact that lack of either myosin Va or Rab27a results in a similar misdsitribution of melanosomes, these data suggest that Rab27a and myosin Va interact at the surface of melanosomes.

Previous work has shown that endogenous myosin Va,[5–7] as well as a GFP-tagged myosin

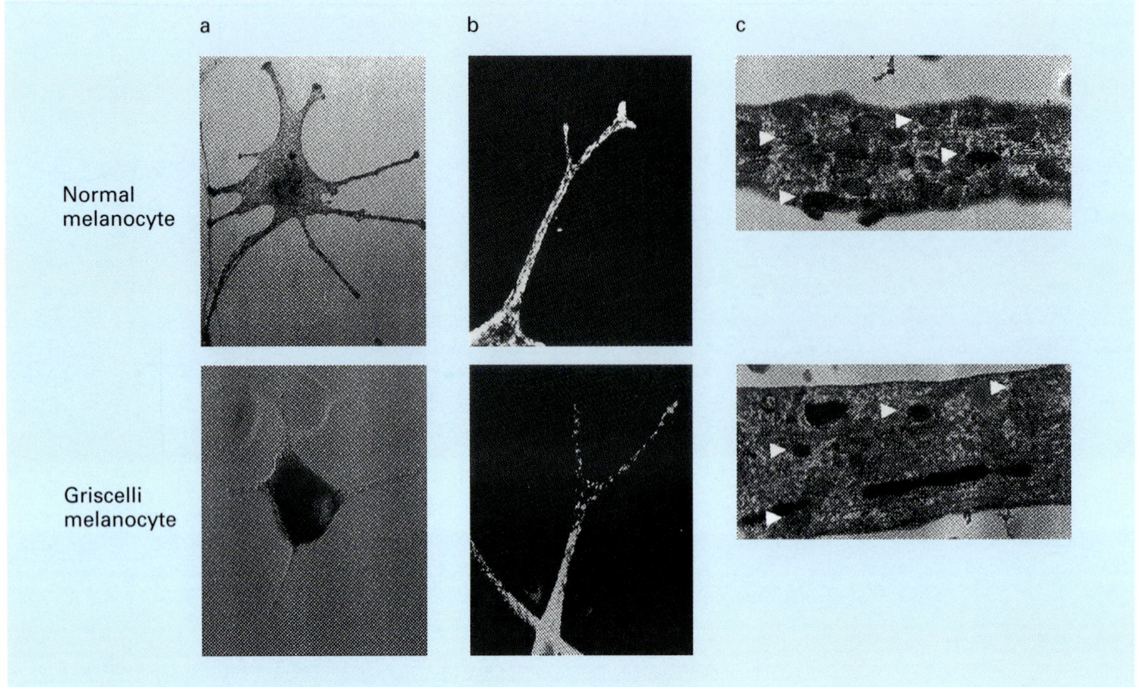

Figure 19.3

Abnormal melanosome distribution in Griscelli syndrome melanocytes. (a) Phase contrast microscopy. (b) Confocal immunofluorescence microscopy after melanosome labelling. (c) Electron microscopy of a dendritic extension of normal (top) and Griscelli (bottom) melanocytes.

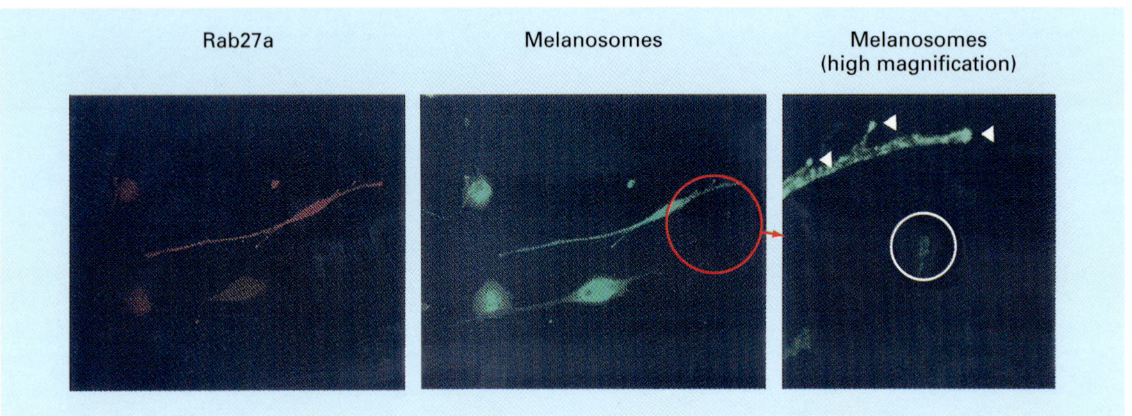

Figure 19.4

Re-expression of Rab27a restores melanosome transport to dendrite tips in Griscelli syndrome melanocytes. Immunofluorescence labelling of GS melanocytes transfected with the normal Rab27a cDNA. The cells were labelled for Rab27a (red) and for melanosomes (green). High magnification clearly shows the accumulation of melanosomes at dendrite tips of a transfected (white arrowhead) but not of an untransfected (white circle) cell.

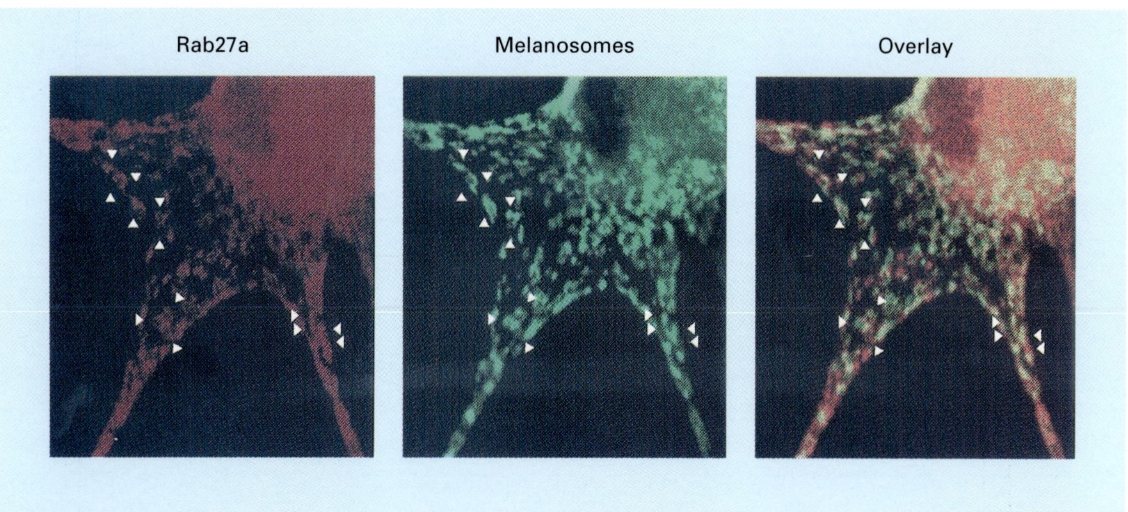

Figure 19.5

Colocalization of Rab27a with melanosomes in normal human melanocytes. Confocal immunofluorescence microscopy of normal human melanocytes labelled for Rab27a (red), melanosomes (green), and image overlay (arrowheads point out to yellow spots representing the colocalization of Rab27a and melanosomes).

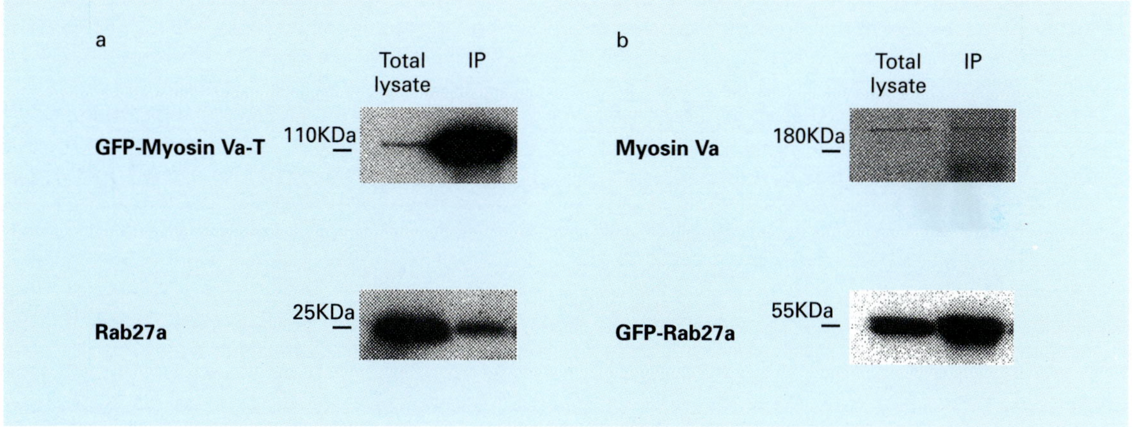

Figure 19.6

Coprecipitation of Rab27a and myosin VA in B16 cells. (a) Coprecipitation of endogenous Rab27a by GFP-tagged myosin Va tail-domain fusion protein. (b) Coprecipitation of endogenous myosin Va by GFP-tagged Rab27a fusion protein.

Va tail-domain fusion protein colocalize with melanosomes in wild-type melanocytes. However, in GS melanocytes that do not express Rab27a, endogenous myosin Va does not seem to colocalize with melanosomes (Bahadoran et al., unpublished work). Similarly, in *ashen* melanocytes that are devoid of Rab27a, endogenous mysoin Va, as well as the aforementioned myosin Va fusion protein, do not seem to colocalize with melanosomes.[14,15] These data are consistent with the idea that Rab27a is required for the association of myosin Va with melanosomes.

Future issues

An important issue will be to determine whether Rab27a is, or is a part of, the melanosome receptor that recruits myosin Va on melanosomes. In the former case, this would mean that there is a direct interaction of Rab27a with myosin Va, an unprecedented situation for a Rab protein. Alternatively, Rab27a could recruit on melanosomes its effector molecules, including the ligand for myosin Va. With this in mind, it is important to point out the most recent identification of *leaden* as being a rabphilin-like member of the Rab effector family.[22] Finally, the identification of the gene encoding *dsu* will probably be the next major step in understanding melanosome transport.

References

1. Griscelli C, Durandy A, Guy-Grand D et al., A syndrome associating partial albinism and immunodeficiency, *Am J Med* (1978) **65**:691–702.
2. Pastural E, Barrat FJ, Dufourcq-Lagelouse R et al., Griscelli disease maps to chromosome 15q21 and is associated with mutations in the myosin-Va gene, *Nat Genet* (1997) **16**:289–92.
3. Pastural E, Ersoy F, Yalman N et al., Two genes are responsible for Griscelli syndrome at the same 15q21 locus, *Genomics* (2000) **63**:299–306.
4. Mercer J, Seperack P, Strobel M et al., Novel myosin heavy chain encoded by murine dilute coat colour locus, *Nature* (1991) **349**:709–13.
5. Lambert J, Onderwater J, Van der Haeghen Y et al., Myosin V colocalizes with melanosomes and subcortical actin bundles not associated with stress fibers in human epidermal melanocytes, *J Invest Dermatol* (1998) **111**:835–40.
6. Wu X, Bowers B, Wei Q et al., Myosin V associates with melanosomes in mouse melanocytes: evidence that myosin V is an organelle motor, *J Cell Sci* (1997) **110**:847–59.
7. Nascimento A, Amaral R, Bizario J et al., Subcellular localization of myosin-V in the B16 melanoma cells, a wild-type cell line for the dilute gene, *Mol Biol Cell* (1997) **8**:1971–88.
8. Provance D, Wei M, Ipe V et al., Cultured melanocytes from dilute mutant mice exhibit dendritic morphology and altered melanosome distribution, *Proc Natl Acad Sci U S A* (1996) **93**: 14554–8.
9. Wu X, Bowers B, Rao K et al., Visualization of melanosome dynamics within wild-type and dilute melanocytes suggests a paradigm for myosin V function in vivo, *J Cell Biol* (1998) **143**:1899–918.
10. Tolmachova T, Ramalho J, Anant J et al., Cloning, mapping and characterization of the human RAB27A gene, *Gene* (1999) **239**:109–16.
11. Menasché G, Pastural E, Feldmann J et al., Mutations in RAB27A cause Griscelli syndrome associated with hemophagocytic syndrome, *Nat Genet.* (2000) **25**:173–6.
12. Wilson S, Yip, Swing D et al., A mutation in *Rab27a* causes the vesicle transport observed in *ashen* mice. *PNAS* (2000) **97**:7933–8.
13. Bahadoran P, Aberdam E, Mantoux F et al., Rab27a: a key to melanosome transport in human melanocytes, *J Cell Biol* (2001) **152**:843–9.
14. Wu X, Rao K, Bowers B et al., Rab27a enables myosin Va-dependant melanosome capture by recruiting the myosin to the organelle, *J Cell Sci* (2001) **114**; 1091–100.
15. Hume A, Collinson L, Rapak A et al., Rab27a regulates the peripheral distribution of melanosomes in melanocytes, *J Cell Biol* (2001) **152**:795–808.
16. Stinchcombe J, Barral D, Mules E et al., Rab27a is required for regulated secretion in cytotoxic T-lymphocytes, *J Cell Biol* (2001) **152**:825–33.
17. Haddad E, Xufeng W, Hammer J et al., Defective granule exocytosis in Rab27a-deficient lymphocytes from ashen mice, *J Cell Biol* (2001) **152**;835–41.
18. Elejalde R, Holguin J, Valencia A et al., Mutations affecting pigmentation in man: neuroectodermal melanolysosomal disease, *Am J Med Genet* (1979) **3**:65–80.
19. Duran-McKinster C, Rodriguez-Jurado R, Ridaura C et al., Elejalde syndrome—A melanolysosomal neurocutaneous syndrome, *Arch Dermatol* (1999) **135**:182–6.
20. Klein C, Philippe N, Le Deist F et al., Partial albinism with immunodeficiency (Griscelli syndrome), *J Pediatr* (1994) **125**:886–95.
21. Segev N, Ypt and Rab GTPases: insight into functions through novel interactions, *J Cell Sci* (2001) **13**:500–11.
22. Matesic LE, Yip R, Reuss EA, Mutations in Mlph, encoding a member of the Rab effector family, cause the melanosome transport defects observed in ashen mice, *PNAS* (2002) in press.

20

The protease-activated receptor-2 regulates pigmentation *via* melanosome phagocytosis

Miri Seiberg and Stanley S. Shapiro

The epidermal-melanin unit, a functional unit that produces and distributes melanin, is composed of one melanocyte and approximately 36 neighboring keratinocytes, working in synchrony. Melanin is synthesized in the melanocyte's melanosomes, and is later translocated from the melanocyte's dendrites into the keratinocytes. The molecular and cellular mechanisms involved in melanosome transfer and the keratinocyte–melanocyte interactions required for this process are not yet completely understood. Recently, we showed that keratinocyte phagocytosis is involved in melanosome transfer. The protease-activated receptor-2 (PAR-2), expressed on keratinocytes but not on melanocytes, was found to affect keratinocyte phagocytosis, control melanosome transfer and, therefore, exert a regulatory role in skin pigmentation. Modulation of PAR-2 activity can enhance or decrease pigmentation both *in vitro* and *in vivo*, but only when keratinocyte–melanocyte contact is established, suggesting a novel mechanism for the regulation of skin pigmentation. Moreover, inhibition of PAR-2 activation results in the prevention of UVB-induced pigmentation, suggesting the involvement of PAR-2 in the mediation of the UV response.

Melanosome transfer

The process of melanogenesis is well documented and the regulation of pigment production by melanocytes is heavily investigated.[1] However, the subsequent transfer of melanosomes into keratinocytes is not well characterized. Pigment-loaded melanosomes move from their site of origin towards the melanocyte dendrite tips, using microtubule-based and actin-based motor proteins,[2–3] and are then translocated into the recipient keratinocytes. Early light and electron microscopy studies documented the membrane layering and organization during melanosome transfer. These studies suggest melanosome transfer mechanisms, such as the release of melanosomes into intercellular spaces followed by endocytosis, direct inoculation ('injection'), keratinocyte–melanocyte membrane fusion and phagocytosis[3–4] (reviewed). Melanosome phagocytosis was first suggested following electron microscopy studies of human hair follicles,[5] and was further supported by time-lapse photography studies of cultured keratinocytes and melanocytes[2] (reviewed). Using three-dimensional keratinocyte–melanocyte cultures, Herlyn and Shih[6] suggested that pigment donation occurs through the uptake of dendrite fragments and phagocytosis of individual melanosomes, theorizing that keratinocyte-produced factors regulate this process.[7]

Phagocytosis

Phagocytosis is the cellular process of internalization of particulate material, of at least 0.5–1 μm in diameter. Phagocytosis is receptor mediated, and receptor activation results in local reorganization of the actin cytoskeleton.[8] The Fcγ receptors, the complement receptor 3, and the fibronectin receptor are known mediators of cellular phagocytosis (reviewed).[8–9] These receptors activate tyrosine and serine/threonine kinases, mobilize Ca^{++} from intracellular storage to the cytoplasm, and activate aracidonate metabolism (reviewed).[10] Phagocytosis is normally associated with 'professional' phagocytes, such as macrophages, neutrophils and monocytes, functioning to eliminate infectious agents, apoptotic cells and cellular debris (reviewed).[11] However, epidermal keratinocytes were shown to have phagocytic capabilities, as they could ingest latex beads in experimental systems.[12] The mechanism and regulation of keratinocyte phagocytosis and its role in epidermal homeostasis are not yet completely understood.

PAR-2

The PAR-2[13] is a seven-transmembrane G-protein-coupled receptor, that is related to, but distinct from, the thrombin receptors (TRs, also named PAR-1, PAR-3 and PAR-4).[14–16] Serine protease cleavage at the extracellular domain of protease-activated receptors results in the exposure of new N-termini, which then act as tethered ligands. Both TRs and PAR-2 could be activated by trypsin, but only TRs are activated by thrombin[13,17] and only PAR-2 is activated by mast cell tryptase.[18] The protease-activated receptors could also be activated without receptor cleavage, using synthetic peptides that correspond to their new N-termini. SLIGRL and SLIGKV, the mouse and human PAR-2-activating peptides, are specific for PAR-2 activation and are equipotent in the specific activation of the human PAR-2 receptor.[19–20] Since the activated receptors are physically coupled to their tethered ligand agonists, efficient mechanisms for signal termination were developed, including cleavage of the tethered ligand, receptor phosphorylation and uncoupling from G-proteins, and endocytosis and degradation of the activated receptors (reviewed).[10,21] PARs are expressed in multiple cells and tissues, and are involved in growth and development, mitogenesis, inflammatory response regulation, malignant transformation, vascular tonus and blood pressure regulation. PAR-1 and PAR-2 are expressed in keratinocytes[22–23] and a role for PAR-2 activation in the inhibition of keratinocyte growth and differentiation has been suggested.[24] Activation of PARs results in Ca^{++} mobilization and IP_3 hydrolysis.[21]

Why look at PAR-2 in pigmentation?

The importance of the balance between serine proteases and their inhibitors in skin homeostasis is documented in our earlier studies. Processes such as epidermal differentiation, hair growth and epidermal-utriculi differentiation were found to be regulated, in part, by serine proteases and their inhibitors.[22,25,26] These studies suggest the involvement of a protease-mediated signal transduction mechanism in the regulation and maintenance of skin homeostasis. Therefore, we looked at potential interactions between G-protein-coupled signaling pathways and serine proteases in skin. Data presented here suggest that the serine-protease-activated receptor, PAR-2, regulates pigmentation by affecting keratinocyte phagocytosis.[27–30] PAR-2 activation increases the ability of keratinocytes to ingest melanosomes, resulting in skin darkening, and inhibition of PAR-2 activation by serine protease inhibitors reduces pigment transfer and leads to depigmentation. Moreover, the inhibition of PAR-2 activation prevents UVB-induced pigmentation and reduces tanning.

PAR-2 modulation affects pigmentation *in vitro*

Multilayered epidermal equivalents containing melanocytes respond to UVB irradiation by darkening, as shown by F&M stained sections and computerized image analysis (Fig. 20.1a). Treatement with trypsin, a serine protease known to activate all PARs, induced pigmentation to a similar level as UVB, while thrombin, a known activator of PAR-1, -3 and -4, but not of PAR-2, failed to induce pigment production in this system (Fig. 20.1a). Trypsin inhibitors (*e.g.* soybean trypsin inhibitor, STI) reduced pigmentation, while thrombin-specific inhibitors (*e.g.* hirudin) had no effect on pigment production, suggesting the involvement of PAR-2 in the process. Of the specific

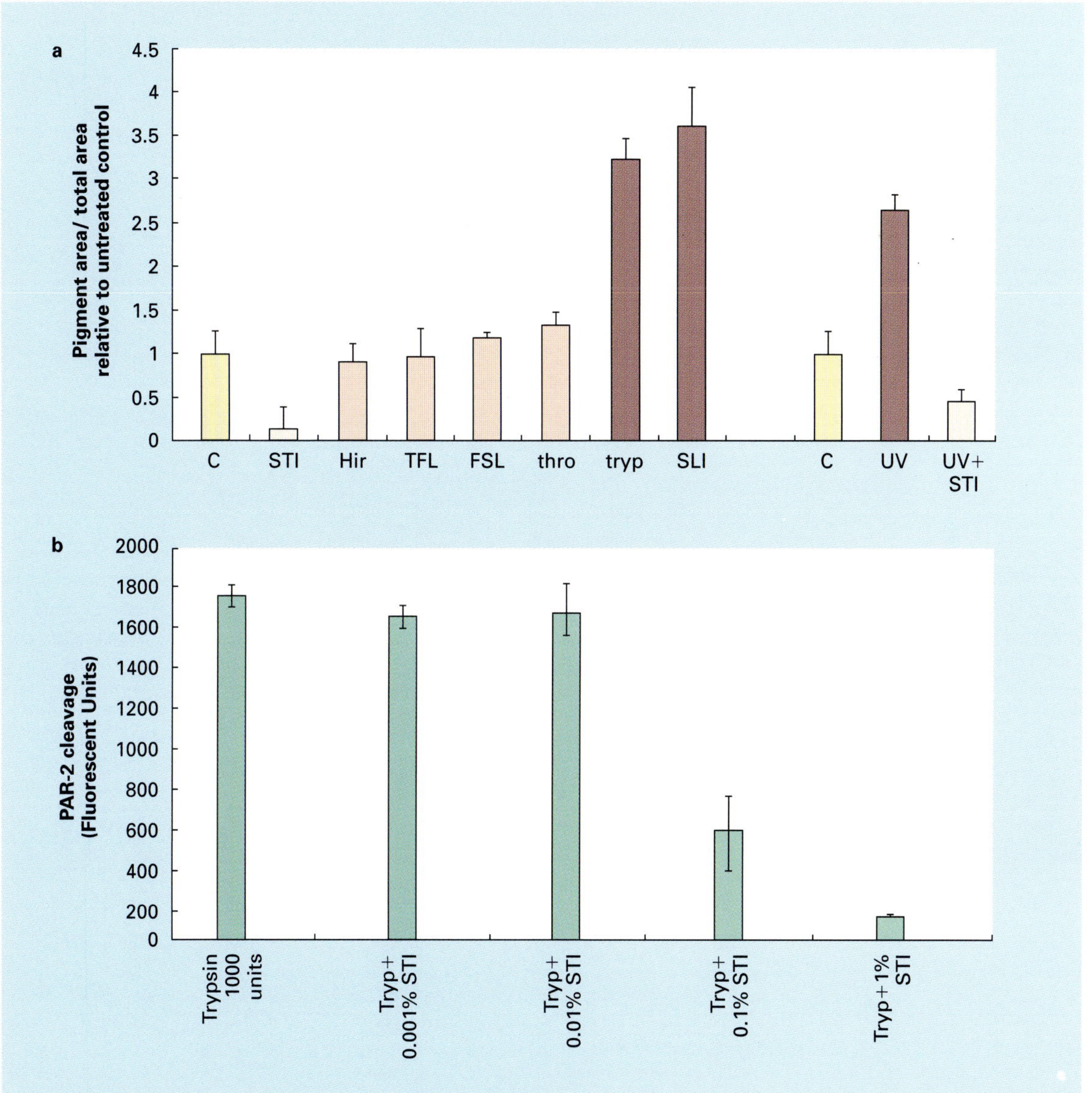

Figure 20.1

PAR-2 modulation affects pigmentation. (a) Epidermal equivalents containing melanocytes were treated daily, for 3 days with test compounds, followed by F&M staining of histological sections. Melanin area relative to total section area was determined using image analysis of F&M-stained sections, and values were normalized to untreated controls. STI is soybean trypsin inhibitor. Hir is hirudin, a specific inhibitor of thrombin. TFL is TFLLRNPNDK, the PAR-1 peptide agonist, which activates PAR-1 only. FSL is FSLLRN, an inactive control peptide. Thro is thrombin, a serine protease that activates PAR-1, -3 and -4. Tryp is trypsin, a serine protease that activates PAR-1–4. SLI is SLIGRL, the PAR-2 peptide agonist which activates PAR-2 only. UVB irradiation (0.11 J/cm^2) was performed on day 1 only. (b) STI inhibits PAR-2 activation. A synthetic peptide, comprising the cleavage site of the human PAR-2, SKGRSLIGK,[31] was labeled with the fluorophore pair Edans/Dabsyl, and was used as a substrate for PAR-2 serine protease activators. The cleavage of this peptide by trypsin (shown as fluorescence units) is inhibited by STI in a dose-responsive manner.

activating peptides for the different PARs, only the PAR-2-activating peptides, SLIGRL and SLIGKV, induced pigmentation. The PAR-1-, -3- and -4-activating peptides, as well as control, scrambled peptides, did not affect pigment production (Fig. 20.1a). This result provided the first evidence that activation of PAR-2 leads to increased pigmentation, while inhibition of PAR-2 activation could result in depigmentation.[27] Treatment with trypsin inhibitors following one exposure to UVB irradiation (100 mJ/cm^2), resulted in a complete inhibition of the UVB-induced pigmentation (Fig. 20.1), suggesting that UVB-induced pigmentation may be, in part, mediated by PAR-2 activation.[27]

STI inhibits PAR-2 activation

To further verify that STI specifically affects the PAR-2 pathway, by inhibiting PAR-2 activation, an enzyme inhibition study was performed. A synthetic fluorescent peptide comprising the cleavage site of the human PAR-2, SKGRSLIGK,[31] was used as a substrate for trypsin, producing dose-dependent increase in fluorescence upon cleavage. Trypsin-induced PAR-2 peptide cleavage was inhibited in the presence of STI in a dose-dependent manner (Fig. 20.1), demonstrating that STI could specifically inhibit PAR-2 activation.[30]

Keratinocyte–melanocyte contact is required for PAR-2-mediated pigmentary effects

Melanocyte-only cultures did not respond to PAR-2 modulation with pigmentary changes. Moreover, cultured monolayer melanocytes grown together with, but not in contact with, epidermal equivalents (containing no melanocytes) were also unaffected by PAR-2 modulation.[27] In contrast, three-dimensional and two-dimensional keratinocyte–melanocyte co-cultures treated with the PAR-2-activating peptide, SLIGRL, or with STI showed an increase or decrease in pigment deposition, respectively (Fig. 20.2). These results suggest that keratinocyte–melanocyte cell contact is required for PAR-2-mediated pigmentary effects.[27] Keratinocytes have previously been shown to express both PAR-1 and PAR-2.[22,23] Our finding that PAR-2 is expressed in keratinocytes, but not in melanocytes,[27] could explain the requirement for keratinocytes for the PAR-2 pigmentary effect.

PAR-2 modulation affects melanosome uptake by keratinocytes

Based on the required keratinocyte–melanocyte contact, we tested the hypothesis that PAR-2 activation affects melanin or melanosome uptake by keratinocytes.[27–28] As shown in Figure 20.3, keratinocytes incubated with isolated melanosomes increased melanosome ingesting following PAR-2 activation. Inhibition of PAR-2 activation by STI resulted in the opposite effect. These results suggest that activation of PAR-2 may increase melanosome ingestion by epidermal keratinocytes, thus increasing the overall pigmentation of the epidermis.[28]

PAR-2 modulates pigmentation *in vivo*

To examine whether modulation of pigmentation by SLIGRL and STI could be reproduced *in vivo*, we used pigmented Yucatan swine and human skins transplanted onto SCID mice. STI treatment of dark-skinned Yucatan swine for 8 weeks induced a dose-dependent visible skin lightening (Fig. 20.4a), which was confirmed histologically (Fig. 20.4b,c). Image analysis of F&M-stained sections, used to quantify the STI effect, showed a statistically significant effect ($p<0.001$, for 0.1 and 1% STI, *t*-test). Treatment of light-skinned Yucatan swine with PAR-2-activating peptides led to increased pigment deposition and enhanced formation of keratinocyte caps (Fig. 20.4d,e). Human Caucasian skin, transplanted onto SCID mice, showed a slight, but visible, increase in pigmentation following SLIGRL treatment, relative to a vehicle-treated transplant from the same donor. An increase in pigment deposition was documented histologically (Fig. 20.5c,d).

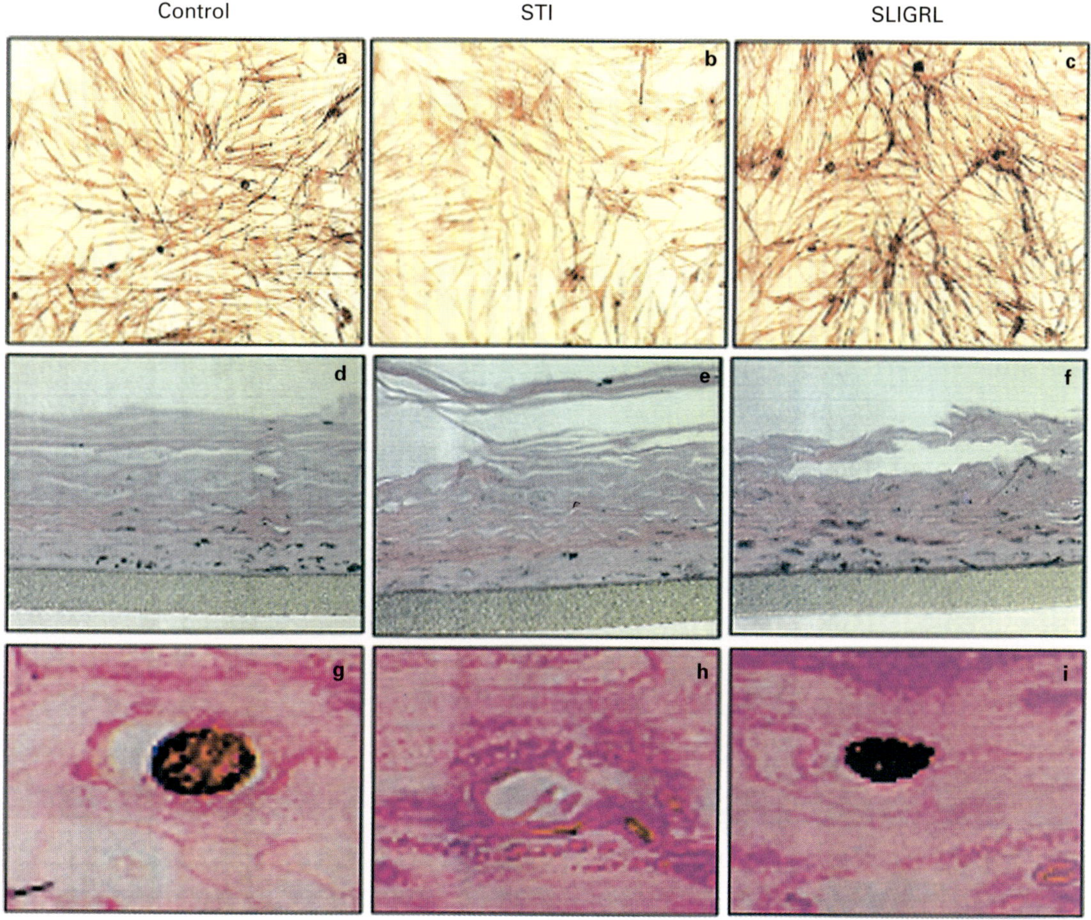

Figure 20.2

PAR-2 modulation affects pigmentation *in vitro*. Keratinocyte–melanocyte monolayer co-cultures and epidermal equivalents containing melanocytes were treated with SLIGRL (10 μM) or with STI (0.01%) for 3 days. On the fourth day, co-cultures were DOPA stained, and histological sections of equivalents were F&M stained. Images shown are of co-cultures (a–c), equivalent sections (d–f) and individual melanocytes within the equivalents (g–i). Untreated controls are a, d, g. STI treatments are b, e, h. SLIGRL treatments are c, f, i.

A hyper pigmented human skin transplanted on SCID mice and treated with STI showed reduced pigment deposition (about 50%), as confirmed histologically (Fig. 20.5a,b). No other changes were observed in the SLIGRL- or STI-treated sites (human or swine), skin architecture was intact and no inflammatory infiltrate was detected histologically. These data suggest that SLIGRL and STI can modulate pigmentation *in vivo*.[27,28,30] The PAR-2-mediated pigmentary effects were reversible.[28] For example, upon termination of STI treatment, darkening of the STI-depigmented skin was visible by the fourth week. Histological analysis revealed a gradual increase in pigment production and distribution, even before the visual observation of re-pigmentation. A 3-week treatment of human mottled skin pigmentation with STI-containing soy extract led to significant skin lightening, indicating that the inhibition of PAR-2 may be a novel way to approach certain pigmentary disorders of the skin.[32]

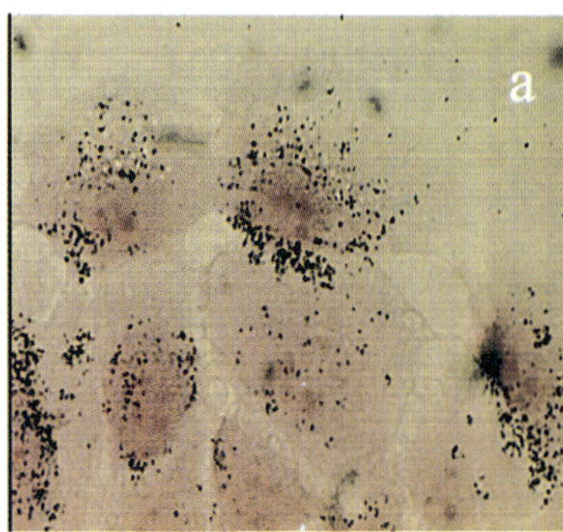

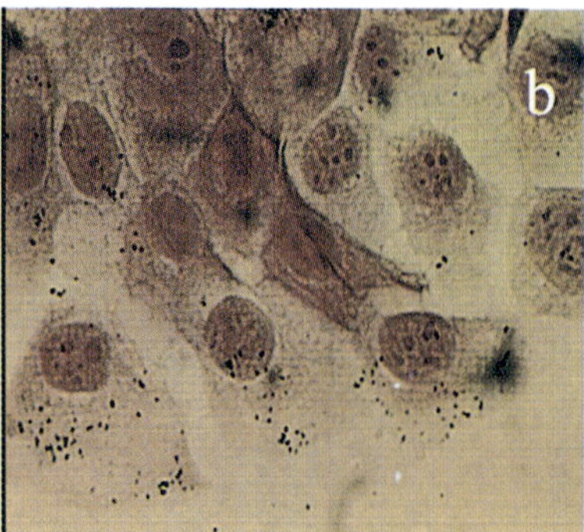

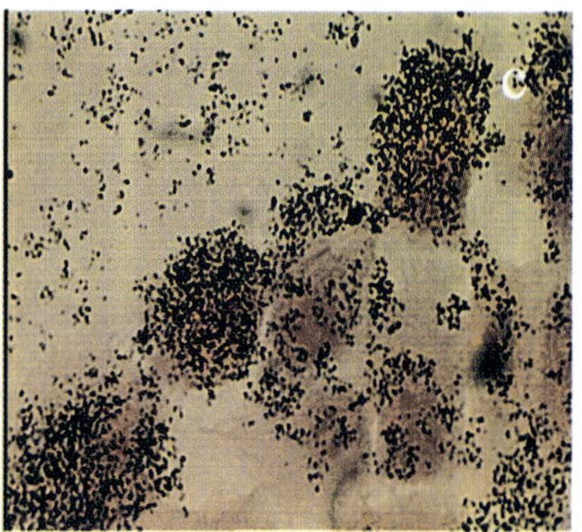

Figure 20.3

PAR-2 affects melanosome ingestion. HaCaT keratinocytes were treated with PBS (a), STI (0.01% (b) or SLIGRL (5 μM (c) for 48 hours and then incubated with isolated melanosomes for 2 hours, followed by an extensive wash and F&M staining. STI inhibits (b) and PAR-2 activation enhances (c) melanosome ingestion by keratinocytes.

Melanosome distribution and dynamics

Epidermal equivalents treated with trypsin inhibitors contained an increased number of melanosomes, which were less mature relative to untreated controls.[28] Higher numbers of dendrites containing mature melanosomes were identified within treated keratinocytes, relative to untreated controls, suggesting abnormal melanosome formation and slow or impaired melanosome transfer into the treated keratinocytes. Yucatan swine skins treated with trypsin inhibitors contained smaller (30–40%) and fewer pigmented melanosomes within their keratinocytes, relative to untreated controls, and the distribution of melanosomes within the treated skin was abnormal. Melanosomes were detected mainly at the epidermal–dermal border, compared to a more random distribution within the untreated sites.[28]

PAR-2 activation increases keratinocyte phagocytosis

Since PAR-2 affects melanosome ingestion and distribution, the possible effect of PAR-2 modulation on keratinocyte phagocytosis was examined.[29] Treated keratinocytes were incubated with fluorescent-labeled *E. coli* K-12 bioparticles, and intracellular fluorescence was measured after trypan-blue quenching of non-internalized fluorescence. As shown in Figure 20.6a,b, PAR-2 activation by SLIGRL or SLIGKV induced a dose-dependent, statistically significant increase in phagocytosis, while their scrambled peptide analogs produced no effect. STI reduced keratinocyte phagocytosis (Fig. 20.6c), but thrombin, PAR-1-activating peptides and scrambled control peptides had minimal or no effect.[29]

Treated keratinocytes were also incubated with fluorescent-labeled microspheres (1 μm diameter). Following incubation, microspheres were ingested by the keratinocytes, and were arranged in a cap-like structure in the perinuclear region, similar to melanin localization in epidermal keratinocytes.[29] STI decreased (Fig. 20.6b) and SLIGRL increased (Fig. 20.6c) microsphere ingestion by the keratinocytes, while the control peptides had no effect. Similar results were obtained using professional phagocytic cells, such as macrophages, and non-phagocytic cells, such as fibroblasts.[29] These data suggest a novel role for PAR-2 in mediating phagocytosis. It is interesting to note that both PAR-2 and the known phagocytic receptors affect intracellular Ca^{++} mobilization.[10,21]

PAR-2 activation induces cytoskeletal reorganization

Phagocytosis is cytoskeleton mediated.[8–11] Therefore, we tested keratinocytes for microsphere

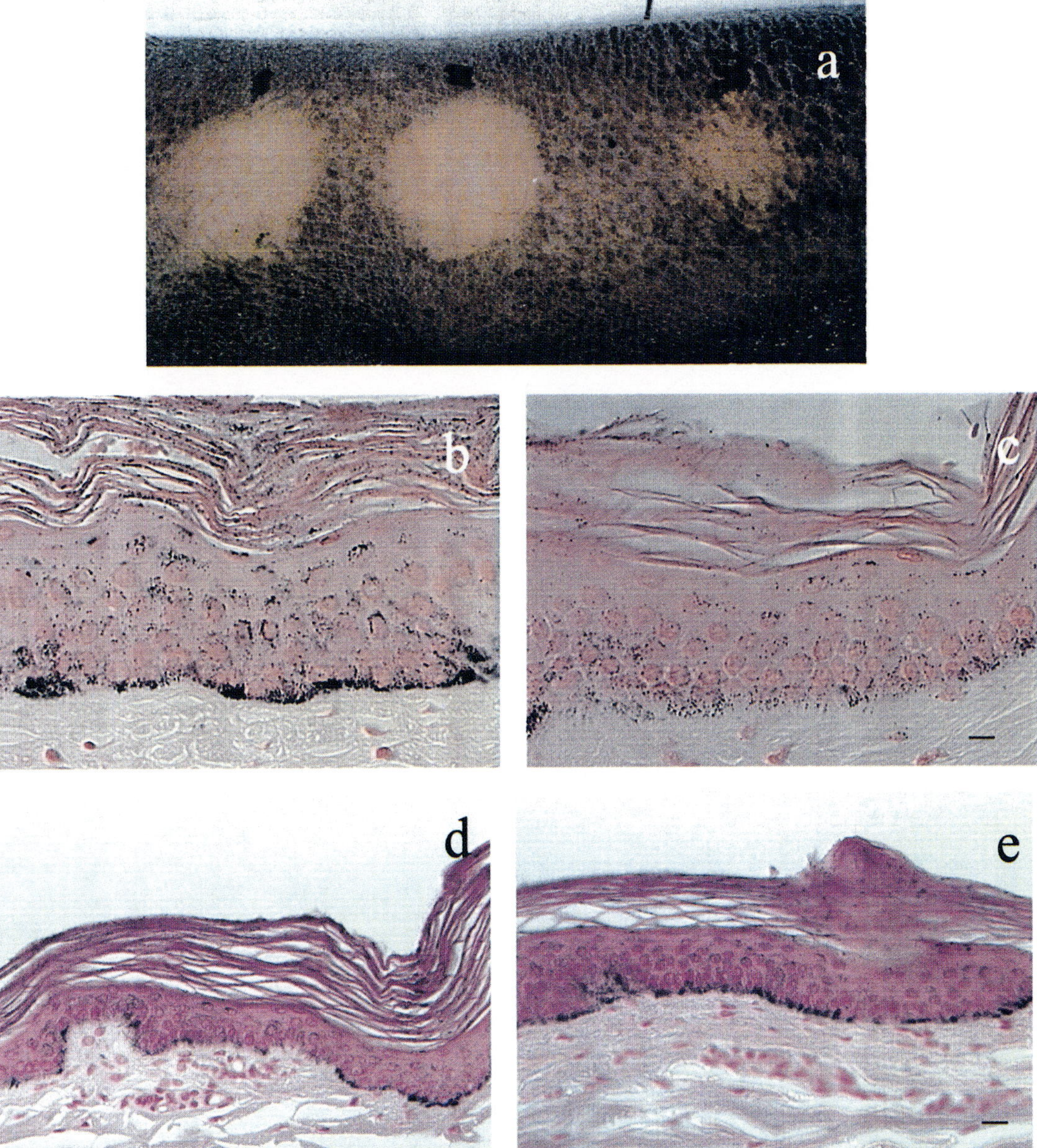

Figure 20.4

PAR-2 modulation affects pigmentation *in vivo*. Yucatan swine treated with STI (1, 0.1, 0.01%, left to right) for 8 weeks showed dose-dependent depigmentation (a). Histological sections stained with F&M (untreated (b), 0.1% STI (c)) demonstrate reduced pigment deposition following STI treatment. Bar = 4 μm. F&M stained sections of Yucatan swine treated with SLIGRL (250 μM) show increased pigment deposition and cap formation (e) relative to control (d). Bar = 8 μm.

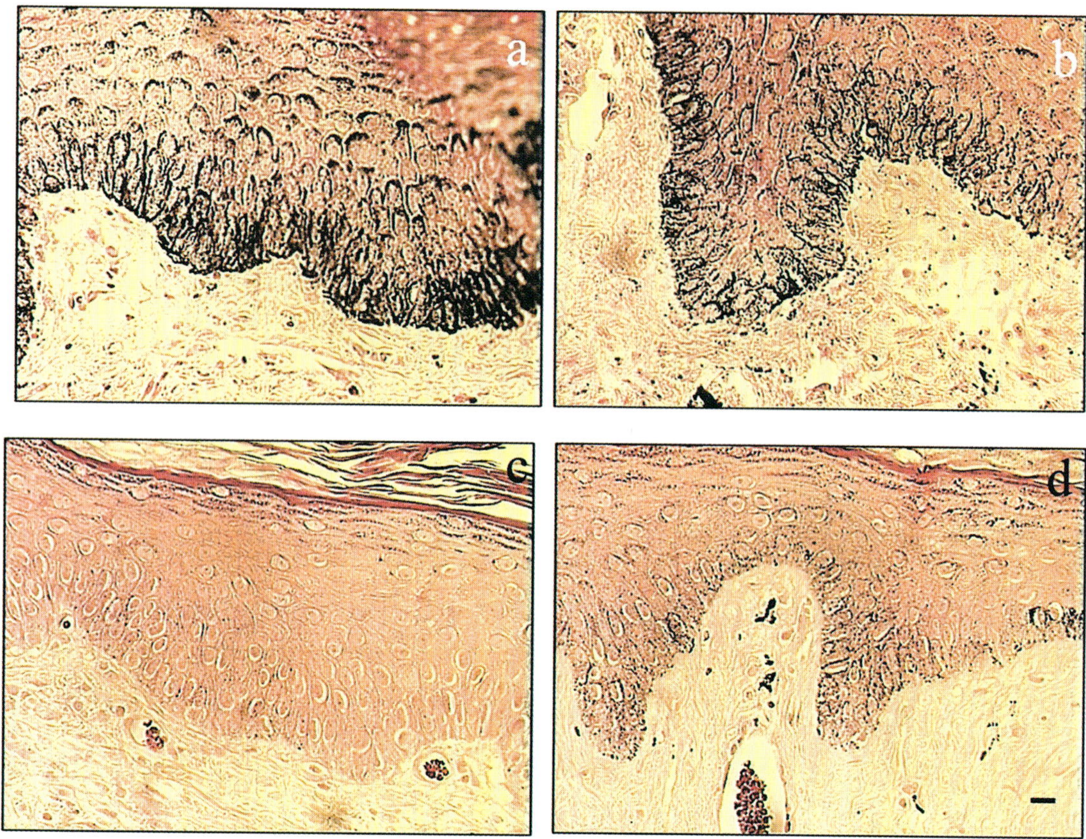

Figure 20.5

PAR-2 modulation affects human skin pigmentation. Heavily pigmented (a, b) and lightly pigmented (c, d) human skins were grafted on SCID mice and were treated with vehicle (a, c), STI (0.1%, (b)) or SLIGRL (50 μM, (d)) for 8 or 9 weeks. F&M-stained histological sections demonstrated reduced pigment deposition following STI treatment. Increased pigment deposition and enhanced cap formation were demonstrated following SLIGRL treatment. Bar = 10 μm.

ingestion in the presence of cytoskeleton-destructive agents. Cytochalasin B and colchicine distrupted PAR-2-mediated keratinocyte phagocytosis,[29] suggesting that active engagement of the cytoskeleton is required for PAR-2-mediated events. Following SLIGRL treatment, F-actin staining showed increased actin polymerization at the core region proximal to the plasma membrane (Fig. 20.8c), as compared to untreated cells (Fig. 20.8a). On the contrary, STI reduced actin polymerization at the plasma membrane (Fig. 20.8b). Similar effects on actin polymerization were documented at the time that microsphere ingestion was affected (Fig. 20.8d–f). Cytoskeletal protein levels were not affected by PAR-2 activation,[29] suggesting that PAR-2-induced keratinocyte phagocytosis is mediated by active cytoskeleton rearrangement.

PAR-2 modulation induces morphological changes of the keratinocyte cell surface

Since PAR-2 modulation affects keratinocyte cytoskeleton reorganization, SLIGRL- and STI-treated keratinocytes were examined by electron

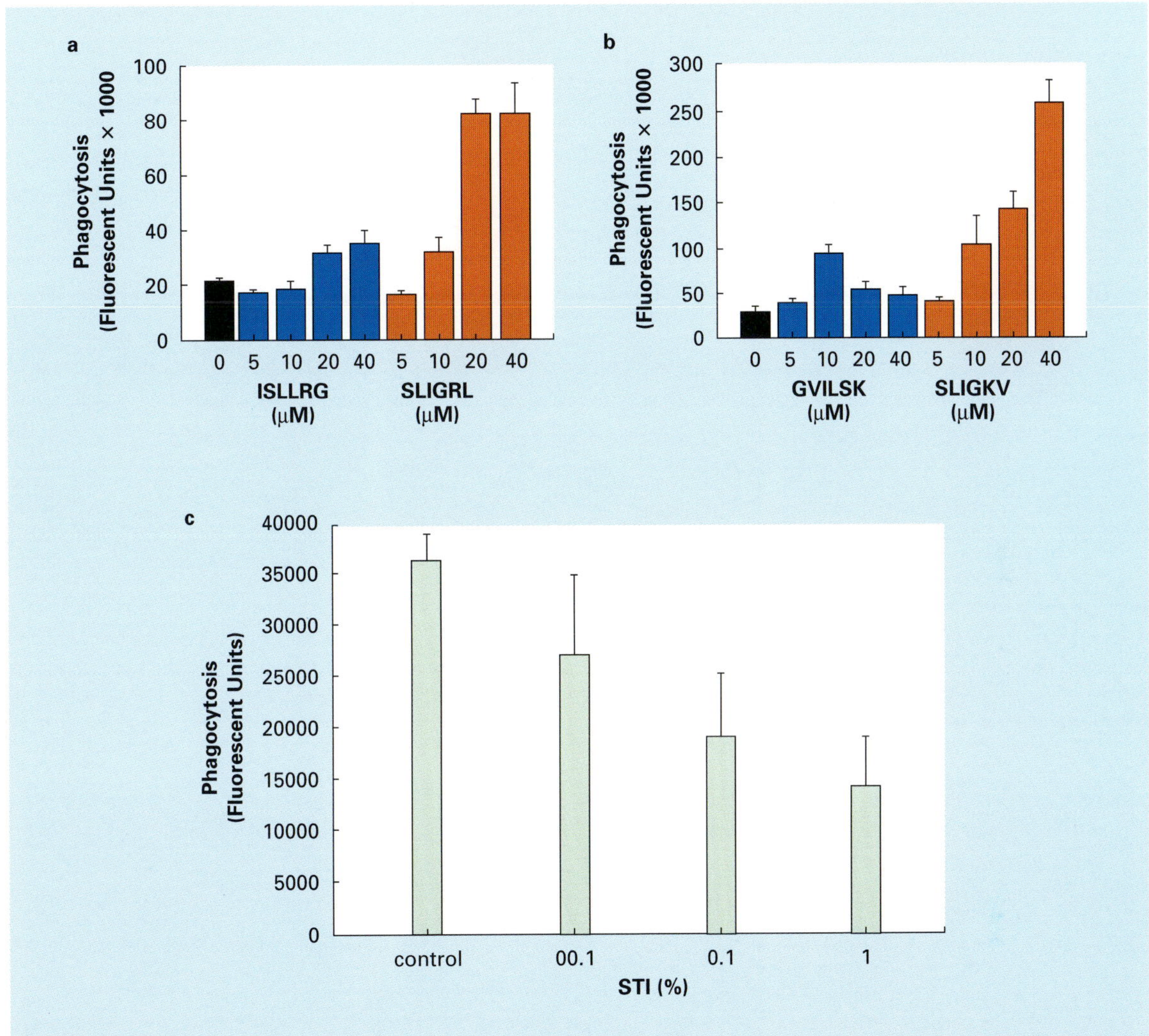

Figure 20.6

PAR-2 modulation affects keratinocyte phagocytosis. HaCaT keratinocytes were treated with the mouse (SLIGRL, (a)) and human (SLIGKV, (b)) PAR-2-activating peptides, their scrambled control peptides (a,b) and STI (c) for 48 hours, followed by a 4-hour incubation with fluorescein-labeled *E. coli* K-12 bioparticles. Fluorescence of ingested particles was measured after trypan-blue quenching of extracellular fluorescence. The PAR-2-activating peptides, but not the control peptides, enhanced HaCaT phagocytosis in a dose-responsive manner, while STI reduced the basal keratinocyte phagocytosis.

microscopy to identify possible PAR-2-affected cell surface morphological changes. SLIGRL-treated keratinocytes (Fig. 20.9c) were found to have increased number, longer and thinner cell projections (podia), while the STI-treated cells (Fig. 20.9b) showed reduced number and shorter length podia, relative to untreated control (Fig. 20.9a). In culture, keratinocyte–keratinocyte contact via these podia was markedly affected by modulation of PAR-2 activity.[29] These suggest that PAR-2 affects cell surface changes that might play an active role in keratinocyte phagocytosis.

PAR-2 activation increases serine protease secretion

Phagocytosis of peripheral blood cells is associated with protease secretion and activation.[33–34] Since PAR-2 was demonstrated to be a phagocytic receptor, we tested the possible release of protease activity following PAR-2 activation in keratinocyte. SLIGRL treatment was found to increase the secretion of serine protease activity into the keratinocytes-conditioned media,[29] with no negative effect on viability. This PAR-2-induced release of serine proteases could provide a positive feedback mechanism for PAR-2 activation.

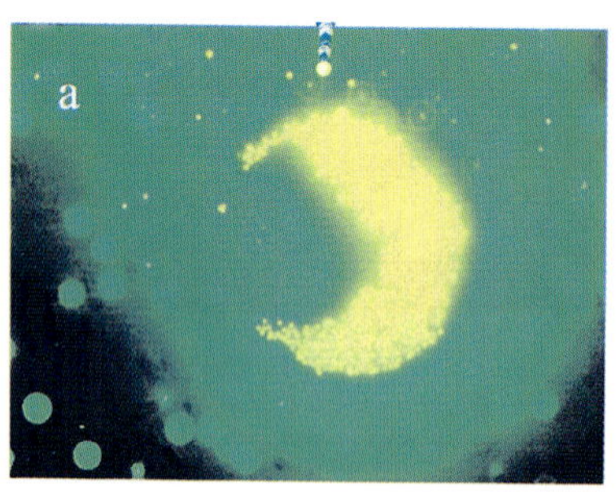

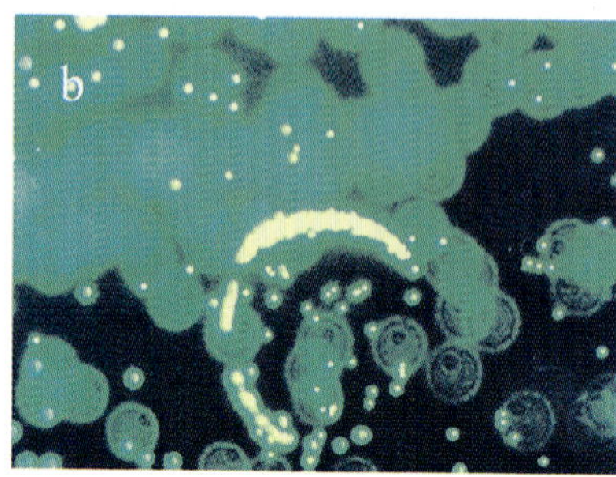

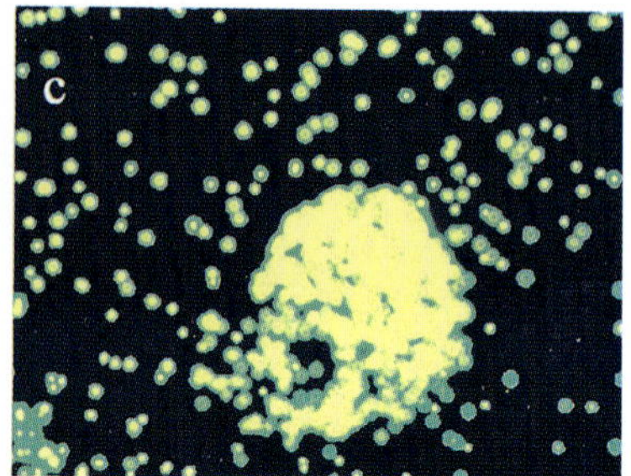

Figure 20.7

PAR-2 modulation affects keratinocyte microsphere ingestion. HaCaT keratinocytes were treated with STI (b) or SLIGRL (c) for 48 hours, followed by incubation with fluorescent-labeled microspheres. (a) is untreated control. PAR-2 activation enhanced, and STI reduced, the ingestion of microspheres.

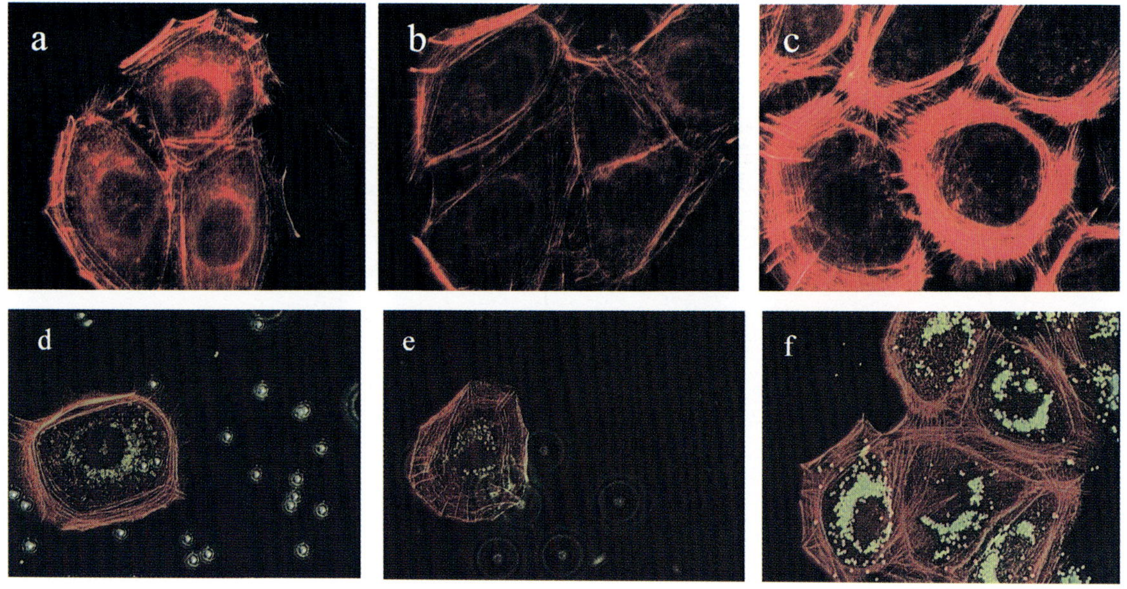

Figure 20.8

PAR-2 modulation affects cytoskeleton reorganization. F-actin (red) staining of control (a, d), STI-treated (b, e) and SLIGRL-treated cells (c, f), in the presence (d–f) or absence (a–c) of fluorescent microspheres (green), shows that enhanced actin polymerization correlates with increased microsphere ingestion.

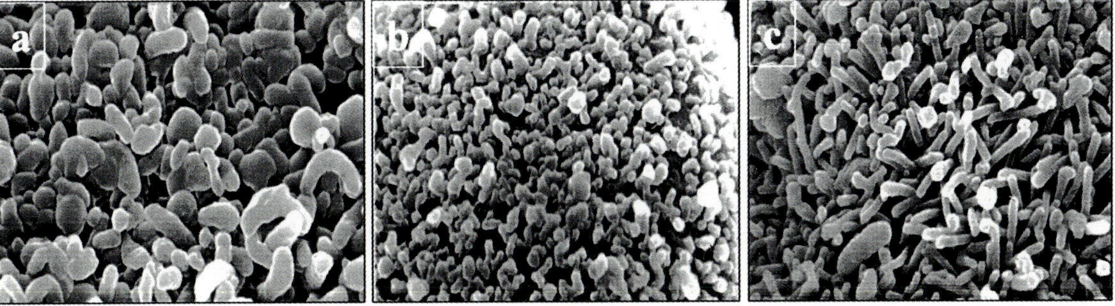

Figure 20.9

PAR-2 activation alters keratinocyte surface morphology. Keratinocytes were treated with STI (b) or SLIGRL (c) for 48 hours, and processed for electron microscopy using standard techniques. SEM analysis shows an increase in cell podia number and a decrease in podia diameter following PAR-2 activation (c). STI treatment results in shorter and altered podia shape (b) relative to untreated control (a). Bar = 0.8125 μm.

UVB irradiation induces PAR-2 activation

The proposed mechanisms for immediate pigment darkening (IPD) include the immediate mobilization of already synthesized melanin, and increased melanosome transfer to keratinocytes.[35] Since the inhibition of PAR-2 activation prevents UVB-induced pigmentation *in vitro*,[27] the possibility that PAR-2 is involved in UV-mediated melanosome ingestion, contributing to IPD, was examined. HaCaT keratinocytes treated with increasing doses of UVB irradiation were found to secrete protease activity. This protease activity was able to cleave a peptide comprising the PAR-2 cleavage site in a dose-dependent manner. Time–response studies demonstrate that this UVB-induced PAR-2 cleaving activity is first increased within the cells and later secreted into the media (Fig. 20.10a). The UVB-induced PAR-2 cleaving activity could be inhibited *in vivo*, using STI-containing compositions,[30] resulting in the prevention of UVB-induced tanning. Yucatan swine treated with UVB, 1 MED, three times during one week, produce visible tanning. Daily treatments with STI prevented this tanning (Fig. 20.10d), while vehicle treatment had no effect on the UVB-increased pigmentation (Fig. 20.10c, compare to untreated control in Fig. 20.10b). Recently, Glynis Scott and colleagues have demonstrated that PAR-2 is upregulated in human skin following UV irradiation.[36] PAR-2 distribution within the epidermis was shown to be UV- and skin-type-dependent, as demonstrated up to 96 hours post UV treatment. Further characterization of the roll of PAR-2 in UV-mediated tanning is ongoing.[36]

Conclusions and future perspectives

Melanin synthesis within the melanosomes and melanosome distribution within the epidermis determine skin pigmentation. The distribution of melanin within the epidermal-melanin unit is regulated, in part, by the keratinocyte receptor, PAR-2. PAR-2 affects melanosome ingestion, and modulation of PAR-2 activation affects melanosome transfer, contributing to the regulation of skin pigmentation. PAR-2 activation induces keratinocyte phagocytosis, affecting cell podia morphology and cytoskeleton reorganization.

In vivo, PAR-2 activation results in increased melanin deposition and enhanced keratinocyte cap formation. Inhibition of PAR-2 activation *in vivo* results in aberrant melanosome processing, abnormal melanosome dynamics and atypical melanosome distribution, resulting in depigmentation. STI-containing soy extracts significantly reduce human skin pigmentation, and may present a novel approach for treatment of certain pigmentary disorders. Inhibition of PAR-2 activation prevents UVB-induced pigmentation *in vitro* and in

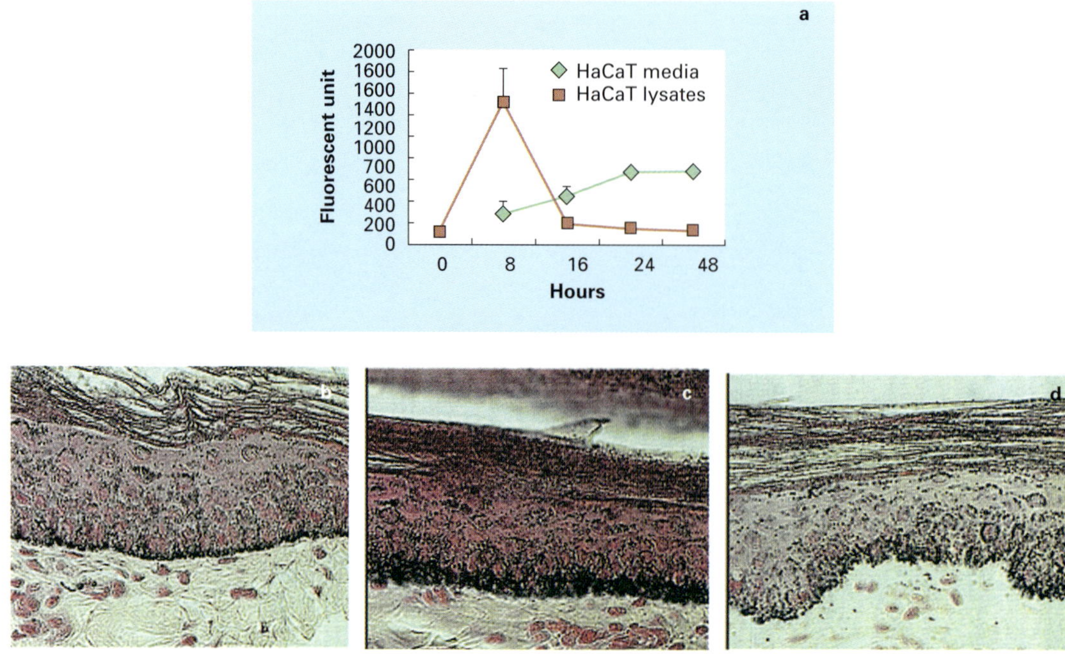

Figure 20.10

PAR-2 is involved in UVB-mediated pigmentation. (a) HaCaT keratinocytes increased their PAR-2-cleaving activity, in cell lysates and conditioned media, at different time points following UVB irradiation. (b–d) STI prevents UVB-induced tanning. F&M-stained sections of UVB and vehicle-treated Yucatan swine skin (c) show increased pigment deposition and cap formation relative to untreated control (b). UVB treatment followed by daily STI treatment (d) prevented the UVB-induced tanning.

swine. Studies are in progress to better understand the role of PAR-2 in UV-mediated skin darkening. The possible involvement of PAR-2 in human skin-type responsiveness remains to be elucidated.

Over the past few years, significant advance has been made towards the understanding of melanosome transfer. Further studies should aim for a comprehensive understanding of the PAR-2 induced events leading to keratinocyte phagocytosis. The regulation of PAR-2 expression and signaling in keratinocytes, the natural activators of PAR-2 in skin and their regulation, and PAR-2 signal termination, all remain to be elucidated. Future studies of the mechanism of melanosome transfer are likely to focus on the identification of key molecules involved in the dendrite–keratinocyte interaction, the 'glue' molecules that enable keratinocyte phagocytosis, and their regulation.

Acknowledgement

We thank our many team members and colleagues who have collaborated with us throughout these studies.

References

1. Levine N, ed, *Pigmentation and Pigmentary Disorders* (CRC Press: Boca Raton, FL, 1993).
2. Lambert J, Vancoillie G, Naeyaert JM et al., Molecular motors and their role in pigmentation, *Cell Mol Biol (Noisy-le-grand)* (1999) **Nov; 45(7):**905–18.
3. Nordlund JJ, Boissy RE, Hearing VJ et al., *The Pigmentary System: Physiology and Pathophysiology* (Oxford University Press: Oxford, 1998).
4. Yamamoto O, Bhawan J, Three modes of

melanosome transfers in Caucasian facial skin: Hypothesis based on an ultrastructural study, *Pigment Cell Res* (1994) **7**:158–69.

5. Birbeck MSC, Mercer EH, Barnicot NA, The structure and formation of pigment granules in human hair, *Exp Cell Res* (1956) **10**:505–14.
6. Herlyn M, Shih IM, Interactions of melanocytes and melanoma cells with the microenvironment, *Pigment Cell Res* (1994) **7**:81–8.
7. Valyi-Nagy IT, Murphy GF, Mancianti ML et al., Phenotypes and interactions of human melanocytes and keratinocytes in an epidermal reconstruction model, *Lab Invest* (1990) **62**:314–24.
8. Kwiatkowski K, Sobota A, Signaling pathways in phagocytosis, *BioEssays* (1999) **21**:422–31.
9. Allen LA, Aderem A, Mechanisms in phagocytosis, *Curr Opin Immunol* (1996) **8**:36–40.
10. Dery O, Bunnett NW, Proteinase-activated receptors: A growing family of heptahelical receptors for thrombin, trypsin and tryptase, *Biochem Soc Trans* (1999) **27**:246–54.
11. Brown EJ, Phagocytosis, *BioEssays* (1995) **17**: 109–17.
12. Wolff K, Konrad K, Phagocytosis of latex beads by epidermal keratinocytes *in vivo*, *J Ultrastruc Res* (1972) **39**:262–80.
13. Nystedt S, Emilsson K, Wahlestedt C et al., Molecular cloning of a proteinase activated receptor, *Proc Natl Acad Sci U S A* (1994) **91**:9208–12.
14. Vu TK, Hung DT, Wheaton VI et al., Molecular cloning of a functional thrombin receptor reveals a novel proteolytic mechanism of receptor activation, *Cell* (1991) **64**:1057–68.
15. Ishihara H, Connolly AJ, Zeng D et al., Protease-activated receptor 3 is a second thrombin receptor in humans, *Nature* (1997) **386**:502–6.
16. Xu WF, Andersen H, Whitmore TE et al., Cloning and characterization of human protease-activated receptor-4, *Proc Natl Acad Sci U S A* (1998) **95**: 6642–6.
17. Nystedt S, Emilsson K, Larsson AK et al., Molecular cloning and functional expression of the gene encoding the human proteinase-activated receptor 2, *Eur J Biochem* (1995a) **232**:84–9.
18. Molino M, Baranthan ES, Numerof F et al., Interactions of mast cell tryptase with thrombin receptors and PAR-2, *J Biol Chem* (1997) **272**:4043–9.
19. Nystedt S, Larsson AK, Aberg H et al., The mouse proteinase-activated receptor-2 cDNA and gene. Molecular cloning and functional expression, *J Biol Chem* (1995b) **270**:5950–5.
20. Bohm SK, Kong W, Bromme D et al., Molecular cloning, expression and potential functions of the human proteinase-activated receptor-2, *Biochem J* (1996) **314**:1009–16.
21. Dery O, Corvera CU, Steinhoff M et al., Proteinase-activated receptors: Novel mechanisms of signaling by serine proteases, *Am J Physiol* (1998) **247**: C1429–52.
22. Marthinuss J, Andrade-Gordon P, Seiberg M, A secreted serine protease can induce apoptosis in Pam12 keratinocytes, *Cell Growth Differ* (1995) **6**:807–16.
23. Santulli RJ, Derian CK, Darrow AL et al., Evidence for the presence of a protease-activated receptor distinct from the thrombin receptor in human keratinocytes, *Proc Natl Acad Sci U S A* (1995) **92**:9151–5.
24. Derian CK, Eckardt AJ, Andrade-Gordon P, Differential regulation of human keratinocyte growth and differentiation by a novel family of protease-activated receptors, *Cell Growth Differ* (1997) **8**:743–9.
25. Seiberg M, Wisniewski S, Cauwenbergh G et al., Trypsin-induced follicular papilla apoptosis results in delayed hair growth and pigmentation, *Dev Dyn* (1997a) **208**:553–64.
26. Seiberg M, Siock P, Wisniewski S et al., The effects of trypsin on apoptosis, utriculi size, and skin elasticity in the Rhino mouse, *J Invest Dermatol* (1997b) **109**:370–6.
27. Seiberg M, Paine C, Sharlow E et al., The protease-activated receptor-2 regulates pigmentation via keratinocyte–melanocyte interactions, *Exp Cell Res* (2000) **254**:25–32.
28. Seiberg M, Paine C, Sharlow et al., Inhibition of melanosome transfer results in skin lightening, *J Invest Dermatol* (2000) **115**:162–7.
29. Sharlow E, Paine C, Eisinger M et al., The protease-activated receptor-2 upregulates keratinocyte phagocytosis, *J Cell Sci* (2000) **113(pt 17)**:3093–101.
30. Paine C, Sharlow E, Liebel F et al., An alternative approach to depigmentation by Soybean extracts via inhibition of the PAR-2 pathway, *J Invest Dermatol*, **116(4)**:587–95.
31. Lourbakos A, Chinni C, Thompson P et al., Cleavage and activation of proteinase-activated receptor-2 on human neutrophils by gingipain-R from Porphyromonas gingivalis, *FEBS Lett* (1998) **435**:45–8.
32. Hermanns JF, Petit L, Martalo O et al., Unraveling the patterns of subclinical pheomelanin-enriched facial hyperpigmentation: effect of depigmenting agents, *Dermatology* (2000) **201**:118–22.
33. Ohlsson K, Lider C, Lundberg E et al., Release of

cytokines and proteases from human peripheral blood mononuclear and polymorphonuclear cells following phagocytosis and LPS and stimulation, *Scand J Clin Lab Invest* (1996) **56:**461–70.

34. Smith ME, van der Maesen K, Somera FP, Macrophage and microglial responses to cytokines in vitro: Phagocytic activity, proteolytic enzyme release, and free radical production, *J Neurosci Res* (1998) **54:**68–78.
35. Honigsmann H, Schuler G, Aberer W et al., Immediate pigment darkening phenomenon. A reevaluation of its mechanisms, *J Invest Dermatol* (1986) **87:**5, 648–52.
36. Scott G, Deng AC, Rodriguez-Burford C et al., Protease-activated receptor-2 (PAR-2), a receptor involved in melanosome transfer, is upregulated in human skin by UV irradiation, *J Invest Dermatol* (2002) **117**:1412–20.

Section VI

APOPTOSIS AND DNA DAMAGE AND REPAIR IN MELANOGENESIS

21 The characteristics of ultraviolet-induced mutations involved in skin carcinogenesis

Giuseppina Giglia-Mari and Alain Sarasin

Introduction

Among all human tumours, skin cancers represent the most frequent human malignancies. Basal cell carcinomas, squamous cell carcinomas (non-melanoma skin cancers) and melanomas mainly represent them. Skin cancers are the ultimate response to repeated sun exposure, especially in light-skinned individuals, and their frequencies have increased constantly over the last couple of decades.[1] Non-melanoma skin cancers are relatively frequent but are easily cured; in contrast, melanomas are very aggressive tumours that metastasize very quickly.

Skin cancers are due to a complex sequence of random events caused and promoted by UV radiation (UVB and UVA and, perhaps, visible light and infrared). The UVB radiation mainly produces DNA lesions between adjacent pyrimidines (TT; CT, TC; CC). Two types of lesions are essentially produced: the cyclobutane pyrimidine dimers (CPDs) and the (6–4) photoproducts (6–4PP).[2] These lesions are normally repaired by the nucleotide excision repair system (NER), which detects the lesions, excises a fragment of DNA of about 30 nucleotides around the lesion, and resynthesizes the lacking DNA fragment in an error-free manner, using the undamaged opposite strand as a template.[3] These UV-induced DNA lesions are very mutagenic in the absence of repair, and they are also at the origin of a temporary UV-induced stress response, such as p53 stabilization or RNA synthesis inhibition.

Even if other factors, such as immunological responses, genetic predisposition, skin phototypes, viruses, etc., are to be taken into account for the development of skin cancer, we will only focus on the mechanisms that lead to mutations, the nature of these mutations and their consequences on skin carcinogenesis. The general dogma in carcinogenesis is the hypothesis of clonal expansion of damaged cells due to activation or inhibition of crucial genes implicated in the control of the cell cycle, maintenance of genetic integrity, proliferation and differentiation. Unrepaired lesions may give rise to mutations, after one or two rounds of replication, in tumour suppressor genes (such as the *p53* gene) or in proto-oncogenes (such as the *ras* family genes) and, therefore, can lead to carcinogenesis.[4]

It appears clear that DNA repair systems play a crucial role in maintaining the genetic integrity against genotoxic attacks and in protecting us from massive tumoral development. This major role is demonstrated by the high incidence of skin cancers in NER-deficient syndromes, such as Xeroderma pigmentosum (XP). In this syndrome, numerous unrepaired UV-lesions will lead to mutations on crucial genes and will start a cellular process of immortalization followed by cell transformation. Ultraviolet light leaves a molecular signature on these genes in all skin cancers (melanomas and non-melanoma skin cancers) in the form of specific mutations, which can help us to understand the pathological history of the tumours.

Skin cancers

Skin cancers are mainly represented by two classes of malignancies: melanomas deriving from melanocytes, and non-melanoma skin cancers (NMSCs) deriving from basal or suprabasal keratinocytes. The role of UV irradiation in skin carcinogenesis has been clearly demonstrated by the fact that skin cancers (essentially NMSCs) are mainly located on sun-exposed parts of the body, are more frequent on light-skinned individuals and increase with low-latitude exposures. Mutations found in the *p53* gene are mainly C to T transitions, located on dipyrimidine sites considered as the UV molecular signature. The XP patients, who are deficient in the pathway of UV-lesions repair, develop, very early in their life, several skin cancers on exposed parts of their bodies.[5]

Malignant melanomas

Malignant melanomas (MMs) represent only 3–5% of total skin cancers, however, they are very aggressive and produce metastasis very rapidly. The role of UV irradiation in the induction of MMs is not very clear. They are not always located on sun-exposed parts of the body, and there is no substantial increase in the number of MMs in individuals who are more sun exposed, except for the elderly.[6] They are often associated with a loss of function of the INK4a locus,[7] and less frequently with a *p53* mutation (10%).[8] However, XP patients develop MMs that are mainly located on sun-exposed parts of the body, which are not as aggressive as the non-XP MMs and show a very high frequency of *p53* mutations (60%); all of these mutations are typically UV induced.[9]

Basal cell carcinomas

Basal cell carcinomas (BCCs) are the most common malignancies in humans, but very rarely lead to metastasis (1 in 10,000). This tumour appears mainly on exposed parts of the body of light-skinned individuals.[10] An inherited disease, Gorlin syndrome, is characterized by a predisposition to developing BCCs. The gene that causes this syndrome is the PTCH tumour suppressor gene.[11,12] In BCCs from XP and non-XP patients, PTCHs and p53 are found to be mutated frequently, and the mutations are clearly UV induced.[13]

Squamous cell carcinomas

Squamous cell carcinomas (SCCs) are not as frequent as BCCs in DNA-proficient individuals, but they eventually metastasize. SCCs are mainly located on chronically sun-exposed parts of the body, and often on pre-existing clinical lesions, such as scars. The pre-malignant lesion is the actinic keratosis (AK); 1 AK in 1000 evolutes towards an SCC, the others may regress spontaneously if there is no more exposure to sun.[14] There is no clearly identified genetically transmitted disease that predisposes to SCCs, apart from the XP syndrome. p53 mutations are found frequently in SCCs and also in AK, indicating that they can be one of the first events in the genesis of SCCs. These mutations are also C to T transitions located on dipyrimidine sites.[15]

XP skin cancers

The most striking difference between NMSCs from XP and non-XP patients is their number and the age of appearance. While non-XP NMSCs appear when the patients are usually older than 50–60 years, XP NMSCs appear very early in life (about 3–5 years old), and with very high frequency, corresponding roughly to a 4000-fold increase compared to the normal population.[5] Usually, these malignancies are less aggressive than the ones found in non-XP patients, at least for melanomas.[16] At the molecular level, another striking difference is the kind of mutation found on different key genes, such as the *p53* gene, the *PTCH* gene or the *INK4a* locus.[17] For both XP and non-XP skin cancers, mutations are located on dipyrimidine sequences, but for non-XP they are mainly C to T transitions, while for XP tumours they are essentially CC to TT tandem mutations. Similarly, the distribution of these mutations on the *p53* gene is not identical for the two types of patients, for still unclear reasons.

NER

The repair system is the way in which the cell deals with injuries on DNA that come from the environment. UV-induced DNA lesions and other bulky lesions are repaired by the most flexible of all the repair systems: the nucleotide excision repair (NER) system. The NER in eukaryotes involves 20–30 proteins. It repairs the damaged strand of

DNA in a cut-and-paste manner, that consists mainly of five steps: recognition of the lesion; opening of the DNA helix; demarcation of the lesion; dual incision of the damaged DNA strand; error-free resynthesis of the gap left by the dual incision and ligation of the newly synthesized DNA strand.[18] A schematic model for NER is shown in Figure 21.1.

Recognition step

Two subpathways of repair have been demonstrated: the rapid transcription coupled repair (TCR) and the slower global genome repair (GGR). TCR repairs a subset of lesions, including UV lesions, on the transcribed strand of active genes, while GGR repairs those lesions on the rest of the genome.[19,20] Mainly, the mechanism of these two pathways is the same, with the exception of the recognition step. In TCR, the signal for the recognition of the lesion is ensured by the blockage of the RNA pol II at the level of the damage.[21] In GGR, the protein XPC, complexed with the homologous protein of Rad 23 in humans (HHR23B), recognizes the distortion of the DNA helix caused by a bulky lesion, and triggers the signal for the rest of the repair machinery on the damaged DNA.[22] Recently, it has been shown that the XPC protein easily recognizes 6–4PP but hardly CPDs, which are less distorting lesions.[23] To be able to recognize CPD, the XPC protein would need the help of another protein, such as the XPE-DDB, or a local opening of the helix (2–4 bases) in the region of the lesion.[24]

Opening of the helix

The presence of the XPC protein on the lesion or the blockage of the RNA pol II are both signals for

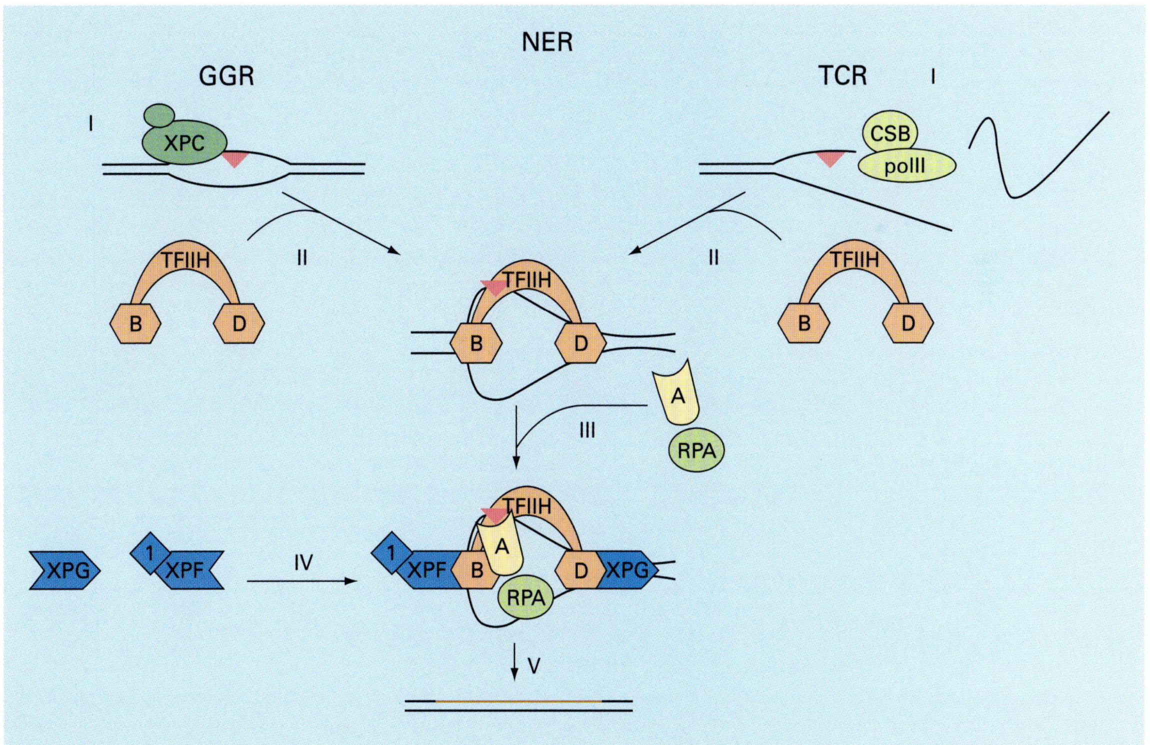

Figure 21.1

Schematic model of the nucleotide excision repair (NER) mechanism. GGR: Global genome repair. TCR: Transcription coupled repair. See text for more details.

the arrival of the multicomplex TFIIH. The helicases XPB and XPD, which are part of the transcription factor TFIIH, open the double strand of DNA around the lesion.[25]

Demarcation of the lesion

The proteins XPA and RPA (replication protein A) may organize the repair machinery around the lesion. XPA is a protein known to bind damaged DNA, and to physically interact with the TFIIH complex and the complex ERCC1–XPF.[26–28] RPA also helps the local unwinding of the DNA with its high affinity to single-strand DNA.[29]

Dual incision

Once the damaged strand has been detected and separated from the undamaged one, an oligonucleotide of 24–32 bases is excised by the concerted activities of two endonucleases: XPG cuts at the 3′ of the lesion[30] and the complex ERCC1–XPF cuts at the 5′.[31] The TFIIH complex could be involved in the positioning of XPG, RPA and PCNA (proliferating cell nuclear antigen), and could be responsible for the polarity of this cut.[32]

Gap filling

Finally, the gap left by the excision of the damaged fragment is filled in by DNA synthesis. Pol δ and/or pol ε, together with RPA, PCNA, RF-C (replication factor C), resynthesise the novel strand[33] and the reaction is completed by the ligation of the newly synthesized strand by the DNA ligase I.[34]

CC to TT tandem mutations

Analysis of mutations found on genes such as *p53*, *PTCH*, *ras* and *INK4* demonstrated that UV lesions cause mainly C to T transitions (always located on dipyrimidine sequences) in non-XP skin cancer and CC to TT tandem mutations in XP skin cancers.[17] CC to TT tandem mutations are absolutely specific to UV irradiation. About 70% of all the mutations found in XP skin cancers are CC to TT tandem mutations, independent of tumoral type.[35] CC to TT mutations seem to be characteristic of XP patients, because only 7% of all mutations found in non-XP skin cancers are CC to TT tandem mutations. This difference is not due to a selective advantage of the mutated proteins bearing the CC to TT tandem mutation versus C to T transition, because, in most cases, the two mutations cause strictly the same amino acid change in p53, hence producing the same mutant p53 protein. Moreover, for both XP and non-XP skin cancers, CC to TT tandem mutations are found more frequently on CpG sequences, known to be methylated at the level of the cytosines at least in the *p53* gene.[36] On the contrary, C to T transitions are more frequently found on non-methylated cytosines. This high frequency of CC to TT tandem mutations in NER-deficient cells and the role of the methylation in the origin of these mutations still remain obscure. We propose a model to try to explain the origin of CC to TT tandem mutations, which is depicted in Figure 21.2.

The UV lesion on the CC*pG site (the C* indicates the 5me-cytosine) could be submitted to a spontaneous or UV-induced desamination of the cytosines, the first one to desaminate would be the 3′ one, because of a high molecular instability of methylated cytosines. The longer the lesion stays in the cell before replication and without being repaired, the more the 5′ cytosine is likely to also be desaminated. Desamination of a 5meC will give rise to a thymine (T), while desamination of a C will lead to a uracile (U). If replication occurs before repair, the DNA polymerase will put an adenine opposite a T or a U, and this will be the cause of the mutations. In a NER-deficient cell, UV lesions stay longer on the DNA, hence, the chance for a second desamination is higher than in a NER-proficient cell. According to this reasoning, it is likely that more CC to TT tandem mutations will be found in UV-damaged cells that in XP skin.

Conclusions

The rare DNA-repair-deficient human syndromes represent very interesting models to understand cancer development in humans, and have led to the discovery and isolation of more than 20 genes and proteins involved in the process of DNA repair. This has permitted the development of the knock-out transgenic mouse, representing a good model

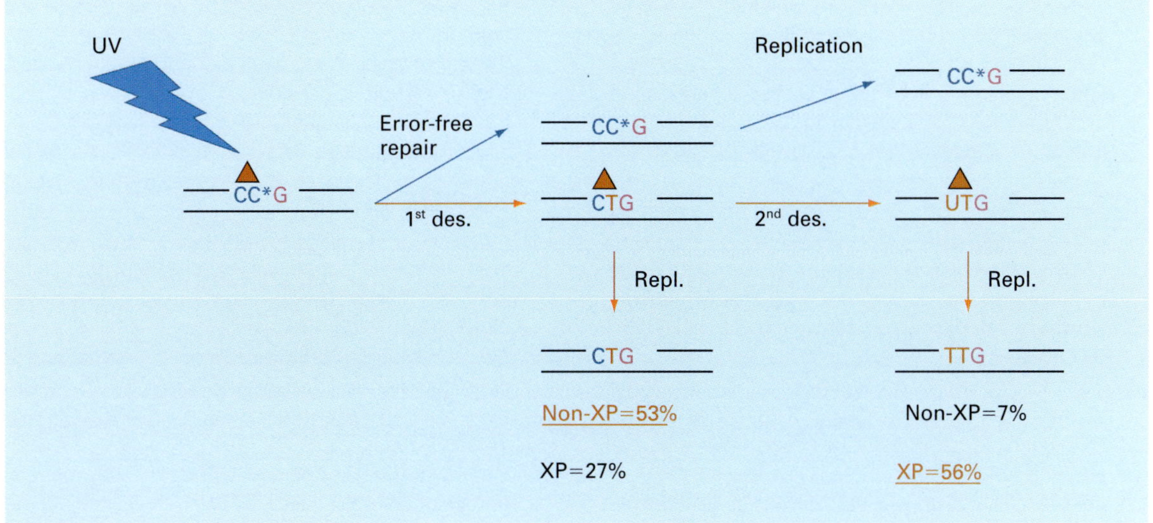

Figure 21.2

Model proposed to explain the origin of the CC to TT tandem mutations. C* indicates 5me-cytosine. The numbers correspond to the percentage of C to T or CC to TT mutations in XP and non-XP skin cancers, all types of cancers included. des.: Desamination. Repl.: Replication.

for human diseases, thus allowing experiments which would be impossible to perform on human patients, for obvious ethical reasons.

The vast majority of the human population has, fortunately, normal or subnormal DNA-repair efficacy that protects them from skin cancers for at least 50–60 years. However, some individuals develop multiple skin cancers and/or cancers at early ages, as compared to the general population. If one excludes all possible sources of variations (skin phototype, UV exposure, lifestyle, virus infections, working conditions), it is plausible that small variations in the efficiency of UV-induced DNA lesion repair could be partially associated with early or late onset of skin cancers. Several reports are trying to correlate kinds of repair markers, tumour incidence and/or age of appearance.[37]

Among the 20 genes and proteins implicated in the NER pathway, the XPD gene, coding for a DNA helicase involved in both DNA repair and initiation of transcription, has been studied in terms of correlation between some single nucleotide polymorphisms and the frequency of skin tumours, including melanomas.[38] Up until now, results of these studies have not been fully convincing because of the limitation of the small number of individuals involved. However, the knowledge of all single nucleotide polymorphisms for all genes involved directly or indirectly in the regulation of genetic stability and fidelity should allow a better way to analyse these relationships and, eventually, detect the individuals at risk.

References

1. Black HS, deGruijl FR, Forbes PD et al., Photocarcinogenesis: an overview, *J Photochem Photobiol B* (1997) **40**:29–47.
2. Mullenders LH, Hazekamp-van Dokkum AM, Kalle WH et al., UV-induced photolesions, their repair and mutations, *Mutat Res* (1993) **299**:271–6.
3. Balajee AS, Bohr VA, Genomic heterogeneity of nucleotide excision repair, *Gene* (2000) **250**:15–30.
4. Dumaz N, Stary A, Soussi T et al., Can we predict solar ultraviolet radiation as the causal event in human tumours by analysing the mutation spectra of the p53 gene?, *Mutat Res* (1994) **307**:375–86.
5. Kraemer KH, Lee MM, Scotto J, Xeroderma pigmentosum. Cutaneous, ocular, and neurologic abnormalities in 830 published cases, *Arch Dermatol* (1987) **123**:241–50.
6. Rivers JK, Melanoma, *Lancet* (1996) **347**:803–6.

7. Hussussian CJ, Struewing JP, Goldstein AM et al., Germline p16 mutations in familial melanoma, *Nat Genet* (1994) **8**:15–21.
8. Papp T, Jafari M, Schiffmann D, Lack of p53 mutations and loss of heterozygosity in non-cultured human melanocytic lesions, *J Cancer Res Clin Oncol* (1996) **122**:541–8.
9. Spatz A, Giglia-Mari G, Benhamou S et al., Association between DNA-repair deficiency and high level of p53 mutations in melanoma of Xeroderma pigmentosum patients, *Cancer Res* (2001) **61**:2480–6.
10. Goldberg LH, Basal cell carcinoma, *Lancet* (1996) **347**:663–7.
11. Hahn H, Wicking C, Zaphiropoulous PG et al., Mutations of the human homolog of Drosophila patched in the nevoid basal cell carcinoma syndrome, *Cell* (1996) **85**:841–51.
12. Johnson RL, Rothman AL, Xie J et al., Human homolog of patched, a candidate gene for the basal cell nevus syndrome, *Science* (1996) **272**:1668–71.
13. Bodak N, Queille S, Avril MF et al., High levels of patched gene mutations in basal-cell carcinomas from patients with xeroderma pigmentosum, *Proc Natl Acad Sci U S A* (1999) **96**:5117–22.
14. Marks R, Squamous cell carcinoma, *Lancet* (1996) **347**:735–8.
15. Ziegler A, Jonason AS, Leffell DJ et al., Sunburn and p53 in the onset of skin cancer, *Nature* (1994) **372**:773–6.
16. Kraemer KH, Lee MM, Andrews AD et al., The role of sunlight and DNA repair in melanoma and non-melanoma skin cancer. The xeroderma pigmentosum paradigm, *Arch Dermatol* (1994) **130**:1018–21.
17. Soufir N, Daya-Grosjean L, de La Salmoniere P et al., Association between INK4a-ARF and p53 mutations in skin carcinomas of Xeroderma pigmentosum patients, *J Natl Cancer Inst* (2000) **92**:1841–7.
18. de Boer J, Hoeijmakers JH, Nucleotide excision repair and human syndromes, *Carcinogenesis* (2000) **21**:453–60.
19. Bohr VA, Smith CA, Okumoto DS et al., DNA repair in an active gene: removal of pyrimidine dimers from the DHFR gene of CHO cells is much more efficient than in the genome overall, *Cell* (1985) **40**:359–69.
20. Mellon I, Spivak G, Hanawalt PC, Selective removal of transcription-blocking DNA damage from the transcribed strand of the mammalian DHFR gene, *Cell* (1987) **51**:241–9.
21. Mu D, Sancar A, Model for XPC-independent transcription-coupled repair of pyrimidine dimers in humans, *J Biol Chem* (1997) **272**:7570–3.
22. Sugasawa K, Ng JM, Masutani C et al., Xeroderma pigmentosum group C protein complex is the initiator of global genome nucleotide excision repair, *Mol Cell* (1998) **2**:223–32.
23. Kasumoto R, Masutani C, Sugasawa K et al., Diversity of the damage recognition step in the global genomic nucleotide excision repair in vitro, *Mutat Res* (2001), **485**:219–27.
24. Sugasawa K, Okamoto T, Shimizu Y et al., A multistep damage recognition mechanism for global genomic nucleotide excision repair, *Genes Dev* (2001) **15**:507–21.
25. Evans E, Moggs JG, Hwang JR et al., Mechanism of open complex and dual incision formation by human nucleotide excision repair factors, *EMBO J* (1997) **16**:6559–73.
26. Park CH, Mu D, Reardon JT et al., The general transcription-repair factor TFIIH is recruited to the excision repair complex by the XPA protein independent of the TFIIE transcription factor, *J Biol Chem* (1995) **270**:4896–902.
27. Park CH, Sancar A, Formation of a ternary complex by human XPA, ERCC1, and ERCC4(XPF) excision repair proteins, *Proc Natl Acad Sci U S A* (1994) **91**:5017–21.
28. Li L, Elledge SJ, Peterson CA et al., Specific association between the human DNA repair proteins XPA and ERCC1, *Proc Natl Acad Sci U S A* (1994) **91**:5012–16.
29. de Laat WL, Appeldoorn E, Sugasawa K et al., DNA-binding polarity of human replication protein A positions nucleases in nucleotide excision repair, *Genes Dev* (1998) **12**:2598–609.
30. O'Donovan A, Davies AA, Moggs JG et al., XPG endonuclease makes the 3′ incision in human DNA nucleotide excision repair, *Nature* (1994) **371**:432–5.
31. Sijbers AM, de Laat WL, Ariza RR et al., Xeroderma pigmentosum group F caused by a defect in a structure- specific DNA repair endonuclease, *Cell* (1996) **86**:811–22.
32. Iyer N, Reagan MS, Wu KJ et al., Interactions involving the human RNA polymerase II transcription/nucleotide excision repair complex TFIIH, the nucleotide excision repair protein XPG, and Cockayne syndrome group B (CSB) protein, *Biochemistry* (1996) **35**:2157–67.
33. Shivji MK, Podust VN, Hubscher U et al., Nucleotide excision repair DNA synthesis by DNA polymerase epsilon in the presence of PCNA, RFC, and RPA, *Biochemistry* (1995) **34**:5011–17.
34. Barnes DE, Tomkinson AE, Lehmann AR et al., Mutations in the DNA ligase I gene of an individ-

ual with immunodeficiencies and cellular hypersensitivity to DNA-damaging agents, *Cell* (1992) **69**: 495–503.
35. Giglia G, Dumaz N, Drougard C et al., p53 mutations in skin and internal tumors of xeroderma pigmentosum patients belonging to the complementation group C, *Cancer Res* (1998) **58**:4402–9.
36. Tornaletti S, Pfeifer GP, Complete and tissue-independent methylation of CpG sites in the p53 gene: implications for mutations in human cancers, *Oncogene* (1995) **10**:1493–9.
37. Benhamou S, Sarasin A, Variability in nucleotide excision repair and cancer risk: a review, *Mutat Res* (2000) **462**:149–58.
38. Tomescu D, Kavanagh G, Ha T et al., Nucleotide excision repair gene XPD polymorphisms and genetic predisposition to melanoma, *Carcinogenesis* (2001) **22**:403–8.

22

The role of DNA damage and telomeres in melanogenesis

Mark S. Eller, Ina M. Hadshiew and Barbara A. Gilchrest

Perhaps the best known and most widely recognized inducer of melanogenesis (tanning) in human skin is solar UV irradiation. Although the regulation of melanogenesis is complex and incompletely understood, several lines of evidence suggest that UV-induced DNA photodamage and/or a repair intermediate is at least one of the initial signals that stimulates melanogenesis in response to UV irradiation.[1] First, the action spectrum for the tanning response in human skin is the same as that for the induction of the major DNA photoproducts.[2,3] Second, enhancing DNA repair by treatment of UV-irradiated melanocytic cells with the prokaryotic DNA repair enzyme T4 endonuclease V approximately doubles the melanin content of these cells as compared with irradiated cells treated with either heat-inactivated enzyme or diluent alone.[4] In addition, treatment of unirradiated S91 cells with DNA-damaging agents, such as methyl methanesulfonate and the restriction endonuclease PvuII also increases their melanin content.[5]

We and others have also shown that treatment of normal human skin cells, human and murine melanoma cells or intact rodent skin with specific small DNA fragments, particularly thymidine dinucleotide, pTT* and, more recently, other larger oligonucleotides (such as a 9mer, pGAGTATGAG), leads to the induction of DNA damage responses, including increased melanogenesis (Fig. 22.1),[5–8] cell growth arrest,[7–9] enhanced DNA repair capacity,[9,10] and transient immunosuppression.[11] These responses are accomplished, at least in part, through induction of p53 and p53-regulated genes, such as p21.[9,10] The increase in pigmentation in S91 cells is preceded by an increase in the level of tyrosinase mRNA and protein, the rate-limiting enzyme in melanin biosynthesis.[5,6] Furthermore, treatment of these cells with pTT, as well as with DNA-damaging radiomimetic drugs or restriction enzymes, enhances the binding of α-MSH, a peptide hormone known to induce tyrosinase expression and pigmentation, to the surface of these cells, as does UV irradiation.[5,12–15,33] More recently, using melanoma cells permanently transfected with a dominant-negative mutant form of p53, we have shown that tyrosinase mRNA is induced by p53 activation in response to UV irradiation or treatment with the oligonucleotides.[16,17]

The melanogenic activity of these oligonucleotides generally increases with an increase in their molecular size, although sequence also has a major influence on this activity (Fig. 22.2). For example, the dinucleotide pTT induces a sevenfold increase in melanin content in S91 cells,[5,6] whereas the dinucleotide pdApdA is inactive;[6] and the 5-nucleotide sequence pGTATG is a more potent stimulator than pTT, whereas pCATAC (a truncated form of the 9mer described above), an oligonucleotide of identical size, is completely inactive.[7] In addition, the largest oligonucleotide tested to date, a 20mer, fails to stimulate pigmentation above control, diluent-treated cells (Fig. 22.3).[7]

A phosphate on the 5′ end of the oligonucleotide is also necessary for their melanogenic activity (Fig. 22.3), and it is critical for these oligonucleotides to be internalized by the cells, as demonstrated by confocal microscopy analysis using fluorescently labeled oligonucleotides (Fig. 22.4).[7] Similarly, confocal analysis suggested that the more active oligonucleotides accumulate preferentially in the cell nucleus, compared to the less active pTT (Fig. 22.4). These data strongly imply

* Previously designated pTpT; in the designation used here, 'p' refers to a 5′ phosphate group; all other bases are joined by phosdiester linkages.

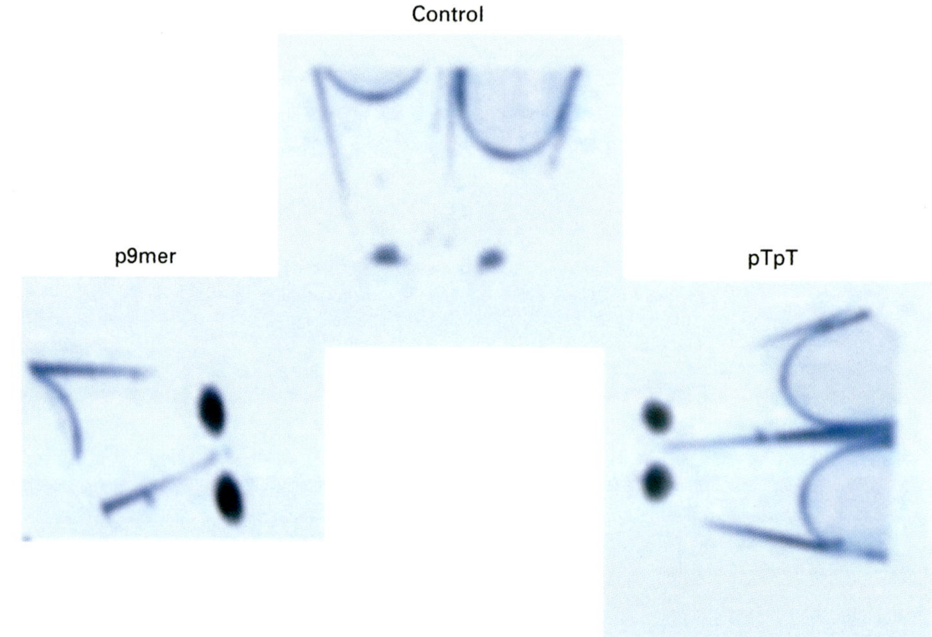

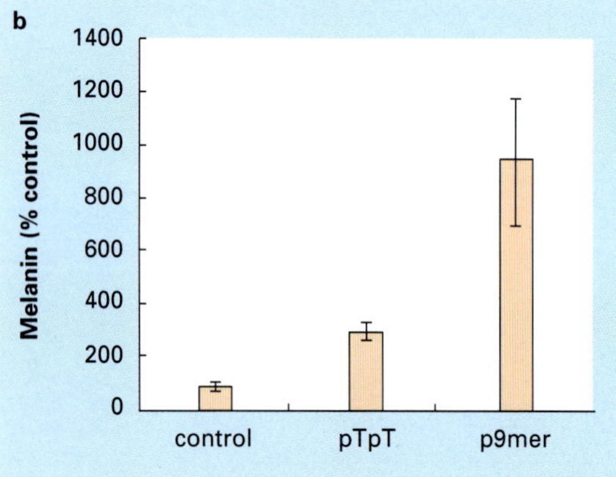

Figure 22.1

Multiple oligonucleotides induce melanogenesis. Duplicate cultures of S91 cells were treated with 100 μM oligonucleotide or diluent as a control. (a) Cell pellets of an equal number of cells from duplicate cultures of one representative experiment. (b) Melanin content (OD 495 nm) graphed as percentage of diluent-treated controls (mean ± SD) for three independent experiments (from Hadshiew et al., reference 7).

that these oligonucleotides act intracellularly, most likely in the cell nucleus.

The observation that these oligonucleotides stimulate multiple responses also stimulated by DNA damage suggested that they are detected within the cell as damaged DNA or as some consequence of this damage and, in this way, trigger these responses.[1] Recent findings linking the disruption of telomeres with DNA damage-like responses have provided evidence for a more detailed and provocative hypothesis.[18]

Most mammalian cells, including melanocytes, have a tightly regulated program of replicative senescence, suggested to be a fundamental defense against cancer.[19] Cell senescence is controlled, in large part, by the length of telomeres, tandem repeats of the DNA sequence TTAGGG, several thousand base pairs long.[20] In germ-line cells and most cancer cells, immortality is associated with maintenance of telomere length by the reverse transcriptase subunit of the enzyme telomerase, TERT, that adds repeats of TTAGGG

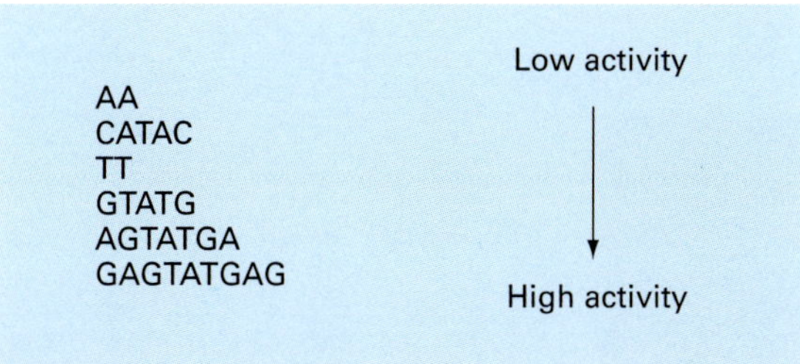

Figure 22.2

Melanogenic activity of oligonucleotides depends on size and sequence. Multiple oligonucleotides are arranged in order of their melanogenic activity. Generally, the activity increases with molecular size, but sequence also has a major influence.

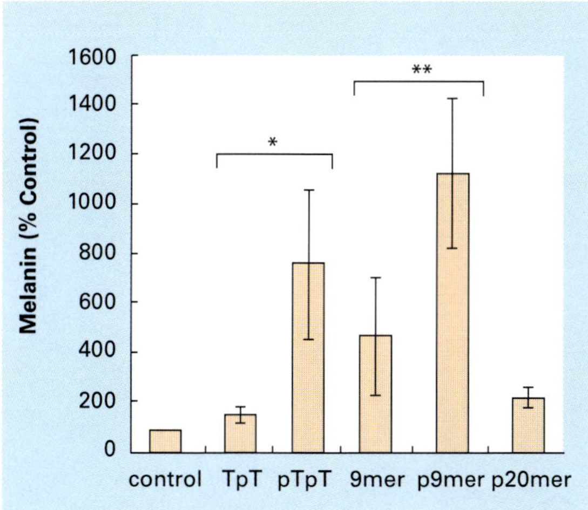

Figure 22.3

Melanogenic activity of the oligonucleotides is greatly enhanced by a 5′ phosphate and depends on base sequence. pTpT and the p9mer were constructed with and without the 5′ phosphate and were added to triplicate S91 cell cultures at a concentration of 100 μM. In addition, a p20mer was also tested at 100 μM. The values were calculated as percentage of diluent-treated control. The graphed values represent three independent experiments. $^{*}p<0.004$, $^{**}p<0.03$, two-tailed Student's *t* test (from Hadshiew et al., reference 7).

residues to the 3′ ends of chromosomes.[22,23] TERT is generally not expressed in normal somatic cells,[20] so telomeres become shorter with each round of DNA replication and, when critically shortened, trigger either replicative senescence or massive genomic instability and, eventually, cell death.[24] Although the molecular mechanisms that mediate these responses are not fully understood, evidence strongly suggests that p53 and the p53-regulated cyclin-dependent kinase inhibitor, p21, are major mediators of the induction of cellular senescence.[25–27] In this respect, the cellular responses to telomere shortening are similar to those induced by a variety of DNA-damaging agents, such as UV irradiation.[28]

The 3′ end of each telomere consists of a . . . TTAGGG . . . single-stranded overhang that has been proposed to stabilize a loop structure at the chromosome ends by base-parting within the telomere double helix (Fig. 22.5).[29] In addition, mammalian telomeres are associated with two proteins, telomere repeat factors 1 and 2 (TRF1 and -2), which regulate telomere length and integrity, respectively.[30] Disruption of the telomere–TRF structure by expression of a dominant-negative mutant version of TRF2 results in the exposure and degradation of the 3′ telomere overhang, as well as the induction of p53 and p53-dependent apoptosis in certain cell types (Fig. 22.6).[31] Recently, Blackburn[32] proposed that telomere function is governed not simply by length, but also by an equilibrium between a 'capped', or silent, state and an 'uncapped' state that triggers cell cycle arrest and other DNA damage responses. The exact molecular nature of these two states and how they initiate DNA damage responses have not been described.

Inspection of the base sequence of the active, melanogenic oligonucleotides reveals that these DNAs show a substantial homology to the telomere 3′ overhang repeat sequence, TTAGGG (Fig. 22.7), ranging from having one-third to two-thirds identity. Furthermore, oligonucleotide sequences that did not induce the DNA damage responses, such as pAA and pCATAC, are not represented in this telomere sequence.

In melanocytes, a differentiated phenotype is characterized by increased melanogenesis, increased expression of the micropthalmia transcription factor, and a cell cycle arrest resulting from decreased activity of the cyclin-dependent kinases which mediate progression through the cell cycle.[33] These characteristics can be induced not only by telomere shortening,[20] but also by oxidative[34] and genotoxic stress,[28] certain oncogenic stimuli,[35,36] and exposure to high levels of cyclic AMP.[33]

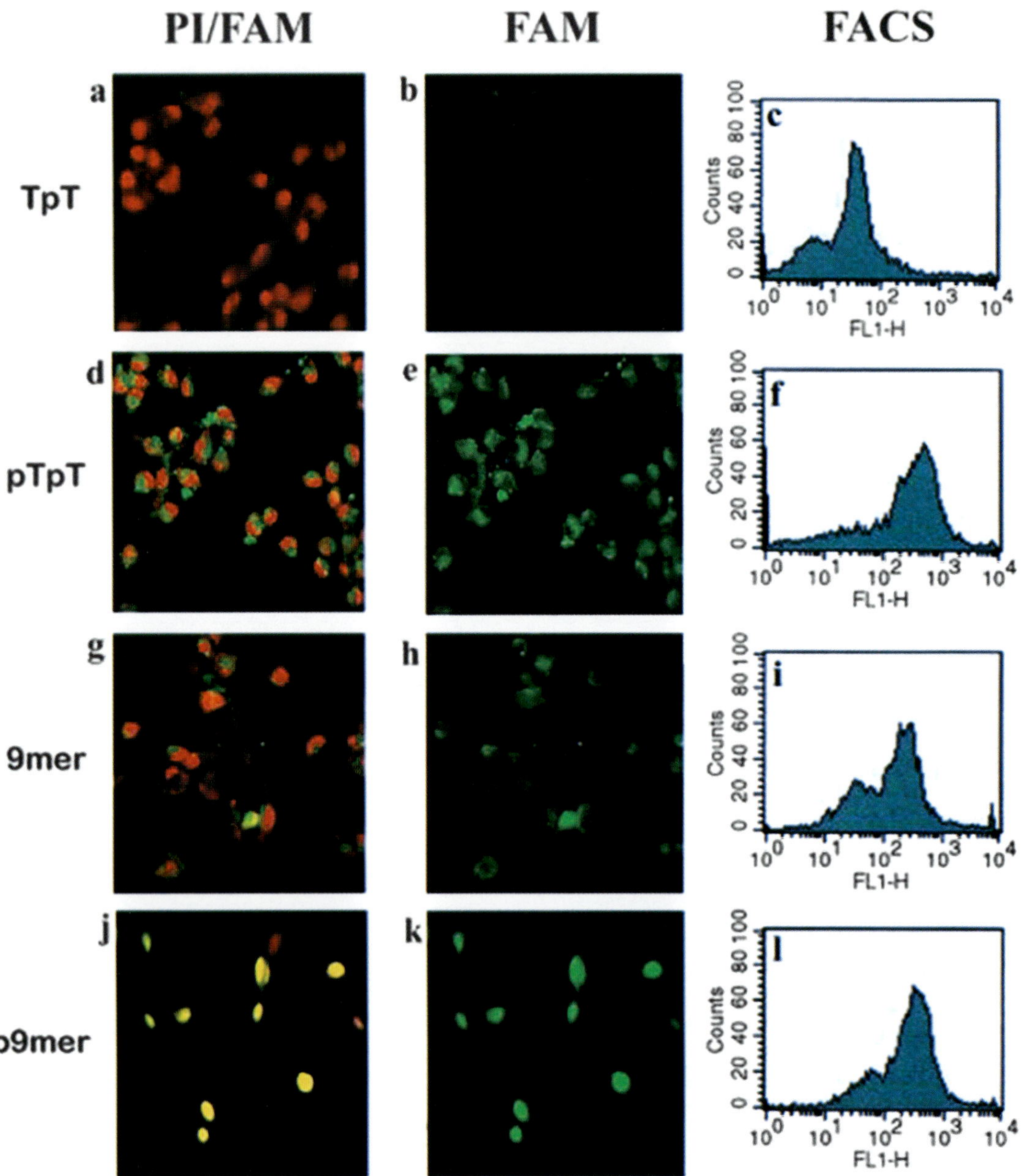

Figure 22.4

Confocal microscopy and fluorescent-activated cell sorter (FACS) analysis demonstrates FAM-labeled oligonucleotides accumulate intracellularly. Cultures of S91 cells were treated with FAM-labeled oligonucleotides for 4 hours and then processed for confocal microscopy or FACS analysis. Images a, d, g and j show both propidium iodide (red) and FAM-oligonucleotide (green) fluorescence. Co-localization of the two fluorescent molecules produces a yellow color. Images b, e, h and k show only the green FAM fluorescence. FACS analysis of FAM-labeled oligonucleotide-treated cells is presented in c, f, i and l (from Hadshiew et al., reference 7).

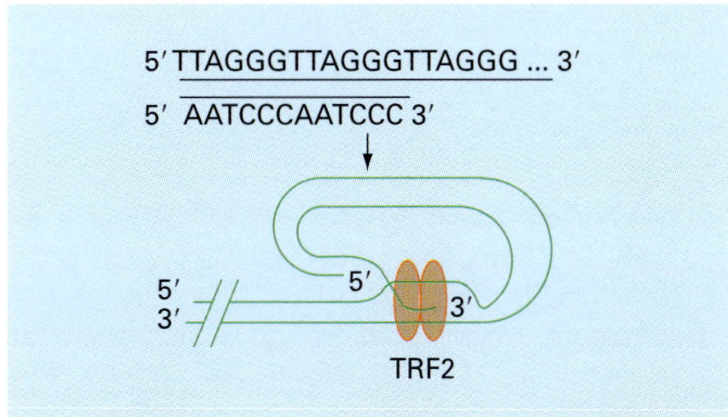

Figure 22.5

Telomeres cap ends of eukaryotic chromosomes. Telomeres, repeats of TTAGGG, contain a single-stranded 3′ overhang sequence that likely facilitates the formation of a loop structure. This structure is further stabilized by telomere repeat factor (TRF) proteins, particularly TRF2.

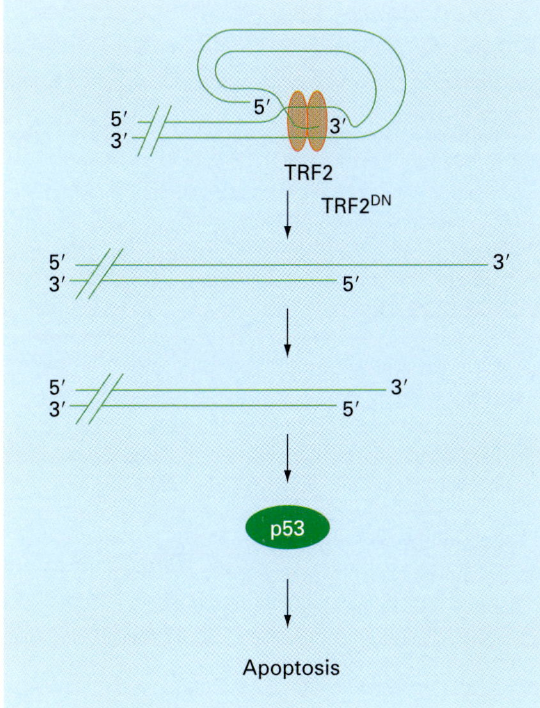

Figure 22.6

Telomere disruption leads to p53-induction of apoptosis. Disruption of the telomere loop structure by expression of a dominant-negative mutant form of TRF2 leads to the exposure of the 3′ overhang and induction of p53 and p53-dependent apoptosis in certain cell types.[31]

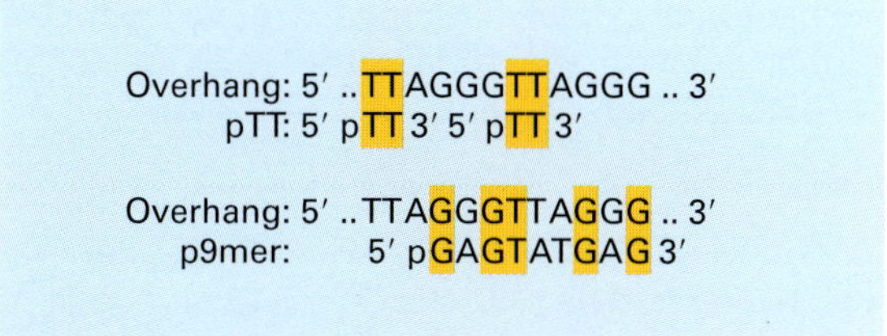

Figure 22.7

Melanogenic oligonucleotides and telomere 3′ overhang show sequence homology. PTT and the 9mer oligonucleotide, both active stimulators of melanogenesis, are compared to the telomere 3′ overhang.

Because critical telomere shortening during aging,[37] experimental telomere disruption,[31] and treatment with these DNA oligonucleotides[9,10] all lead to p53 induction, DNA damage responses and differentiation, and because all the active but none of the inactive oligonucleotides studied[6,7,11] have partial sequence homology to the telomere overhang, we hypothesize that exposure of single-stranded telomeric DNA is a primary physiologic signal that leads to p53 induction and subsequent DNA damage responses, such as cell senescence, apoptosis or melanogenesis, depending on the cell type and signal intensity. Furthermore, we speculate that the DNA oligonucleotides mimic the exposed telomeric DNA in the cell nucleus and, thus, trigger the same responses in the absence of DNA damage or telomere disruption.

Together, these data suggest a model whereby exposure of the single-stranded 3′ telomeric DNA is a critical signal for the induction of DNA damage responses such as cell cycle arrest/replicative senescence, a more differentiated phenotype (such as enhanced melanogenesis) or apoptosis, depending on cell type and/or signal intensity. Exposure of this DNA could occur during normal DNA replication or from destabilization of the telomere loop structure due to critical telomere shortening or from DNA damage, such as thymine dimers formed as a result of UV irradiation. In this respect, telomeres in mammalian cells may not only serve as a measure of replicative age but also of genotoxic stress, and may contribute to the generation of DNA damage responses. Additional experiments, using inhibitors of these telomere responses, will further define their role in constitutive as well as UV-induced pigmentation.

References

1. Gilchrest BA, Eller MS, DNA photodamage stimulates melanogenesis and other photoprotective responses, *J Invest Dermatol Symp Proc* (1999) **4**:35–40.
2. Parrish JA, Jaenicke KF, Anderson RR, Erythema and melanogenesis action spectra of normal human skin, *Photochem Photobiol* (1982) **36**:187–91.
3. Freeman SE, Hacham H, Gange RW et al., Wavelength dependence of pyrimidine dimer formation in DNA of human skin irradiated in situ with ultraviolet light, *Proc Natl Acad Sci U S A* (1989) **86**:5605–9.
4. Gilchrest BA, Zhai S, Eller MS et al., Treatment of human melanocytes and S91 melanoma cells with the DNA repair enzyme T4 endonuclease V enhances melanogenesis after ultraviolet irradiation, *J Invest Dermatol* (1993); **101**:666–72.
5. Eller MS, Ostrom K, Gilchrest BA, DNA damage enhances melanogenesis, *Proc Natl Acad Sci U S A* (1996) **93**:1087–92.
6. Eller MS, Yaar M, Gilchrest BA, DNA damage and melanogenesis, *Nature* (1994) **372**:413–14.
7. Hadshiew IM, Eller MS, Gasparro FP et al., Stimulation of melanogenesis by DNA oligonucleotides: effect of size, sequence and 5′ phosphorylation, *J Dermatol Sci* (2001) **25**:127–38.
8. Pedeux R, Al-Irani N, Mateau C et al., Thymidine dinucleotides induce S phase cell cycle arrest in addition to increased melanogenesis in human melanocytes, *J Invest Dermatol* (1998) **111**: 472–7.
9. Eller MS, Maeda T, Magnoni C et al., Enhancement of DNA repair in human skin cells by thymidine dinucleotides: Evidence for a p53-mediated mammalian SOS response, *Proc Natl Acad Sci U S A* (1997) **94**:12627–32.
10. Maeda T, Eller MS, Hedayati M et al., Enhanced repair of benzo(a)pyrene-induced DNA damage in human cells treated with thymidine dinucleotides, *Mutat Res* (1999) **433**:137–45.
11. Cruz PD Jr, Leverkus M, Dougherty I et al., Thymidine dinucleotides inhibit contact hypersensitivity and activate the gene for tumor necrosis factor α, *J Invest Dermatol* (2000) **114**:253–8.
12. Hadley ME, Levine N, eds *Pigmentation and Pigmentary Disorders* (CRC: Boca Raton, FL, 1993) 95–114.
13. Fuller BB, Lunsford JB, Iman DS et al., Alpha-melanocyte-stimulating hormone regulation of tyrosinase in Cloudman S-91 mouse melanoma cell cultures, *J Biol Chem* (1987) **262**:4024–33.
14. Donatien PD, Hunt G, Pieron C, The expression of functional MSH receptors on cultured human melanocytes, *Arch Dermatol Res* (1992) **284**: 424–6.
15. Bolognia J, Murray M, Pawelek J, UVB-induced melanogenesis may be mediated through the MSH-receptor system, *J Invest Dermatol* (1989) **92**:651–6.
16. Khlgatian M, Asawanonda P, Eller MS et al., Tyrosinase expression is regulated by p53, *J Invest Dermatol* (1999) **112**:548.
17. Khlgatian MK, Hadshiew IM, Asawanonda P et al., Tyrosianse gene expression is regulated by p53, *J Invest Dermatol* (in press).
18. Eller MS, Hadshiew IM, Puri N et al., The single-stranded telomeric DNA induces DNA damage responses, *J Invest Dermatol* (2000) **114**:756.
19. Campisi J, Replicative senescence: an old lives tale?, *Cell* (1996) **84**:497–500.
20. Greider CW, Telomere length regulation, *Annu Rev Biochem* (1996) **65**:337–65.
21. Feng J, Funk WD, Wang SS et al., The RNA component of human telomerase, *Science* (1995) **269**:1236–41.
22. Harrington L, McPhail T, Mar V et al., A mammalian telomerase-associated protein, *Science* (1997) **275**:973–7.
23. Nakamura TM, Morin GB, Chapman KB et al., Telomerase catalytic subunit homologs from fission yeast and human, *Science* (1997) **277**:955–7.
24. de Lange T, Telomeres and senescence: ending the debate, *Science* (1998) **279**:334–5.
25. Dimri GP, Itahana K, Acosta M et al., Regulation of a senescence checkpoint response by the E2F1 transcription factor and p14ARF tumor suppressor, *Mol Cell Biol* (2000) **20**:273–85.
26. Atadja P, Wong H, Garkavtsev I, Increased activity of p53 in senescing fibroblasts, *Proc Natl Acad Sci U S A* (1995) **92**:8348–52.
27. Campisi J, Dimri GP, Hara E, Control of replicative senescence. In: Schneider E, Rowe J, eds, *Handbook of the Biology of Aging*, 4th edn (Academic Press: New York, NY, 1996) 121–49.
28. DiLeonardo A, Linke SP, Clarkin K et al., DNA damage triggers a prolonged p53-dependent GI

arrest and long-term induction of Cip1 in normal human fibroblasts, *Genes Dev* (1994) **8**:2540–51.

29. Griffith JD, Comeau L, Rosenfeld S et al., Mammalian telomeres end in a large duplex loop, *Cell* (1999) **97**:503–14.
30. van Steensel B, Smogorewska A, de Lange T, TRF2 protects telomeres from end-to-end fusions, *Cell* (1998) **92**:401–13.
31. Karlseder J, Broccoli D, Dai Y et al., p53- and ATM-dependent apoptosis induced by telomeres lacking TRF2, *Science* (1999) **283**:1321–5.
32. Blackburn E, Telomere states and cell fates, *Nature* (2000) **408**:53–6.
33. Haddad MM, Xu W, Schwahn DJ et al., Activation of a cAMP pathway and induction of melanogenesis correlate with association of p16(INK4) and p27(KIP1) to CDKs, loss of E2F-binding activity, and premature senescence of human melanocytes, *Exp Cell Res* (1999) **253**:561–72.
34. Chen QM, Bartholomew JC, Campisi J et al., Molecular analysis of H2O2-induced senescent-like growth arrest in normal human fibroblasts: p53 and Rb control G1 arrest but not cell replication, *Biochem J* (1998) **332**:43–50.
35. Serrano M, Lin AW, McCurrach ME et al., Oncogenic ras provokes premature cell senescence associated with accumulation of p53 and p16INK4a, *Cell* (1997) **88**:593–602.
36. Zhu J,Woods D, McMahon M et al., Senescence of human fibroblasts induced by oncogenic Raf, *Genes Dev* (1998) **12**:2997–3007.
37. Stein GH, Drullinger LF, Soulard A et al., Differential roles for cyclin-dependent kinase inhibitors p21 and p16 in the mechanisms of senescence and differentiation in human fibroblasts, *Mol Cell Biol* (1999) **19**:2109–17.
38. Dimri GP, Lee X, Basile G et al., A biomarker that identifies senescent human cells in culture and in aging skin in vivo, *Proc Natl Acad Sci U S A* (1995) **92**:9363–7.

23

The genotoxicity of simulated solar UV and UVA on normal human Caucasian melanocytes

Laurent Marrot, Jean-Roch Meunier, Jean-Philippe Belaidi, Philippe Perez and Catherine Agapakis-Causse

Introduction

In order to get a better understanding of the molecular events involved in damaging nuclear DNA of normal human melanocytes exposed to solar UV (290–400 nm) or the whole UVA (320–400 nm), we have used single-cell gel electrophoresis. This test, also named comet assay, is a simple and visual technique for measuring DNA breakage in individual cells.[1] It has been extensively used for the analysis of the genotoxic effects of UV components of the solar spectrum.[2–5] The aim of this study is to investigate the role of intracellular melanin and melanin-related molecules in the induction of DNA photo-oxidative damage. In parallel, cellular proliferation, stimulation of melanogenesis and the status of p53 protein are evaluated as endpoints of cellular response to photoxocity. On the other hand, considering the melanocyte as a very particular target for sunlight, we use this approach to demonstrate that broad-spectrum sunscreens with a high and stable effectiveness in filtering out UVA wavelengths are required to ensure good photoprotection of the skin. Finally, using the same approach to study the impact of the phototoxic drug lomefloxacin,[6,7] we have shown that human melanocytes in culture were particularly sensitive to chemically-induced photogenotoxicity. Thus, pigmentation could constitute an interesting endpoint for safety assessment of compounds likely to undergo sunlight exposure.

Materials and methods

Chemicals: Phosphate-buffered saline (PBS) was from Gibco-BRL. Lomefloxacin was from Sigma. Media for human cells were from Clonetics Inc. Agarose for the comet assay was the low-melting Incert Agarose from FMC. Excell gels SDS from Pharmacia were used for SDS PAGE. Nitrocellulose membranes (Hybond-Cplus, Amersham) were used for protein transfer. Other chemicals were from Sigma. Both sunscreens A and B were prepared and characterized in the laboratories of L'OREAL Applied Research (Centre Zviak, Clichy, France).

Cells and culturing conditions: Cells were normal human melanocytes from neonates (Clonetics Inc.). We used two Caucasian strains with different melanin contents: NHEM 560 (average melanin content in picograms: 20 pg/cell) and NHEM 4528 (average melanin content: 30 pg/cell). Cells were cultured as described by Im et al. (Fig. 23.1).[8]

Light source and spectral measurements: The light source was a solar simulator from ORIEL, equipped with a 1000 W xenon short arc lamp. When solar UV (UVB + UVA) was studied, a WG 320/1.5 mm filter was used. A WG 335/3 mm filter was used for UVA. In both cases, a dichroic mirror removed infrared and the main part of visible light. The beam size was 152 x 152 mm. The nature and fluence of UV reaching the samples were analyzed with spectroradiometer Instaspec III (ORIEL). Figure 23.2 shows the spectral power distribution of solar UV or UVA used in the experiments. Integration of the area under the spectrum gave the following results: with the WG 320 filter,

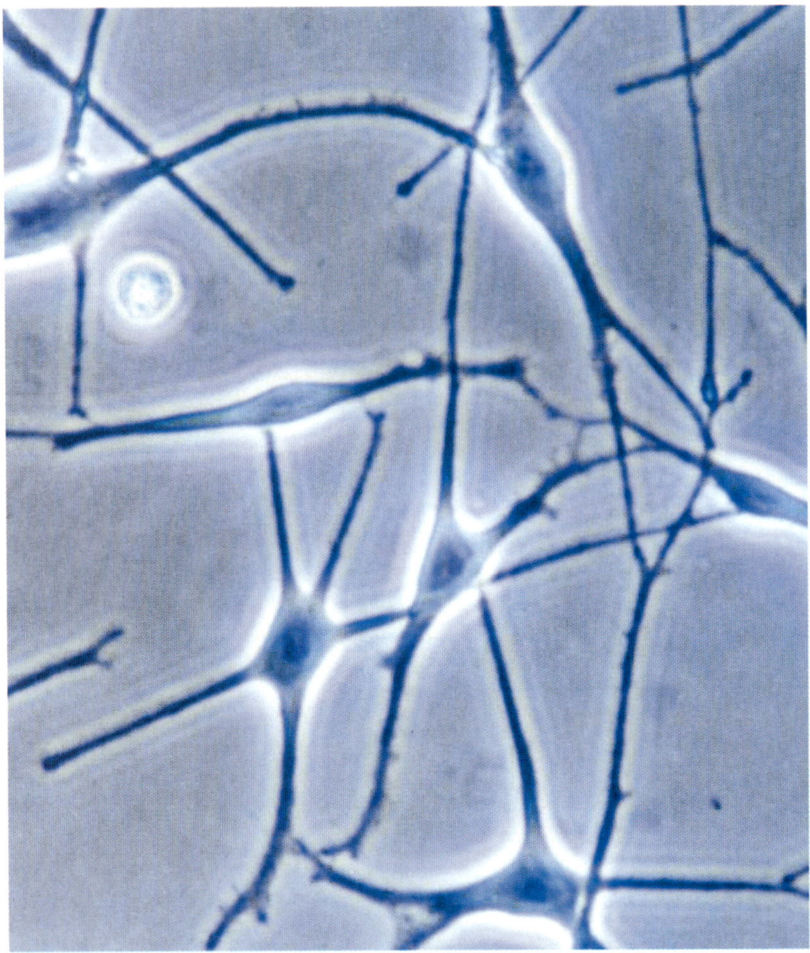

Figure 23.1

Morphological aspect of cultured normal human melanocytes used in the experiments (magnification: x200).

the average irradiance was 10 W/m^2 for UBV (290–320 nm), 20 W/m^2 for UVA2 (320–340 nm) and 72 W/m^2 for UVA1 (340–400 nm). With the WG 335 filter, the average irradiance was 9 W/m^2 for UVA2 and 68.5 W/m^2 for UVAL.

Irradiation procedure: When the comet assay was performed immediately after exposure, melanocytes were first embedded in an agarose–PBS microgel and irradiated in cold PBS (4°C). For photogenotoxicity assessment, lomefloxacin was added to the PBS, incubated for 30 minutes in the dark, and then present during UVA exposure. When exposure was followed by post-treatment incubation in growth medium, cells were incubated in their initial medium after irradiation in cold PBS in 60 mm culture dishes. Sunscreens were spread on a quartz slide with a 20 mm edge (designed for us by HELLMA). In these conditions, the applied amount was around 2 mg/cm^2. The slides were placed over the cells during exposure when photoprotection was assessed (see Figure 23.3).

Comet assay: The comet assay was performed as described by Alapetite et al.[3] Immedately after irradiation, the 0.5% agarose slide, with melanocytes embedded, was placed into the lysis buffer (NaCl 2.5 M; EDTA 100 mM; Triton X100 1%; Tris 10 mM, pH 10) for 75 minutes at 4°C and

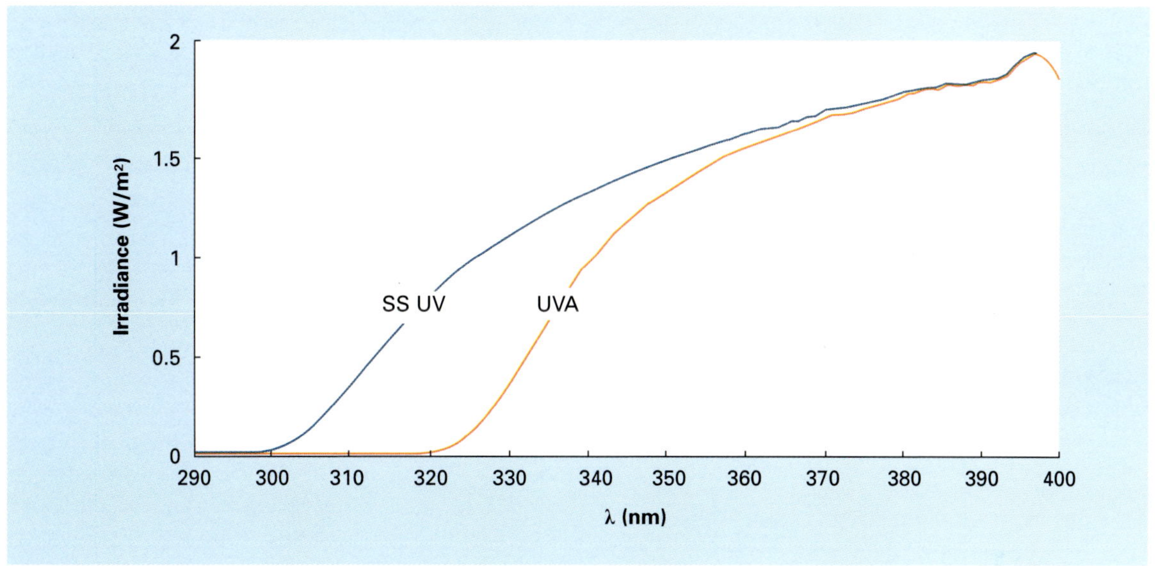

Figure 23.2

Spectral power distribution of solar (SS) UV or UVA from the solar simulator used in the experiments.

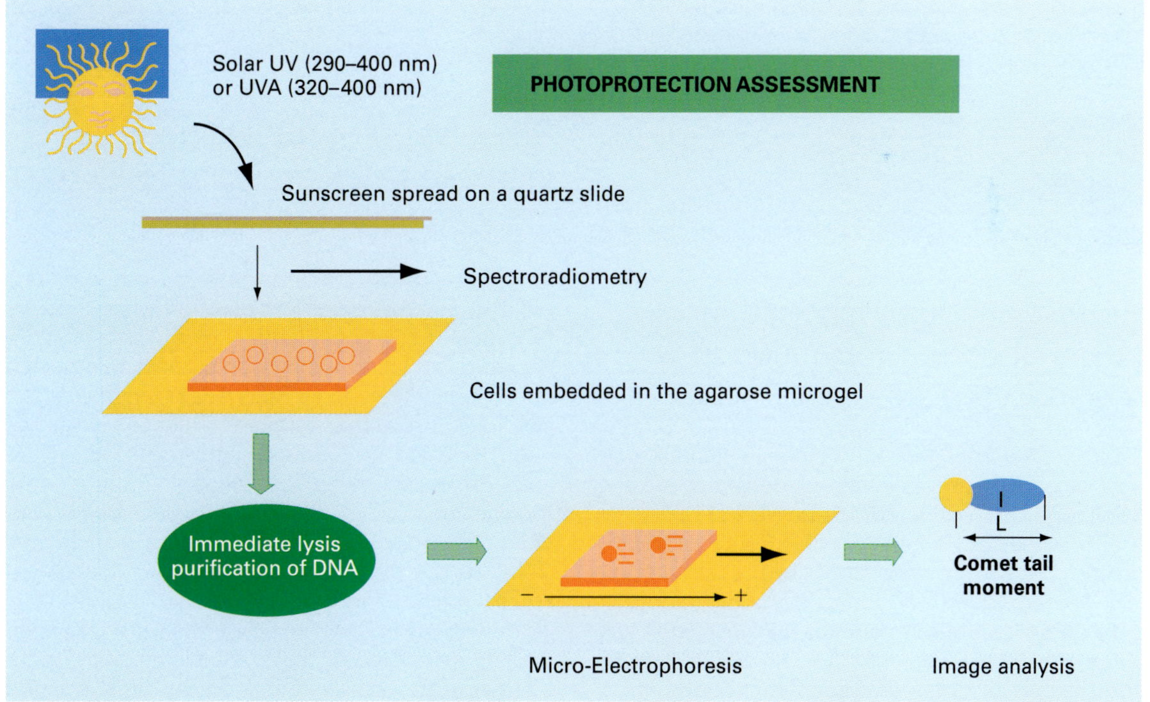

Figure 23.3

Experimental set-up for photoprotection assessment.

then washed and equilibrated in the alkaline buffer (NaOH 0.3 M; EDTA 1 mM) for 20 minutes at room temperature. Alkaline gel electrophoresis was performed for 20 minutes at 25 volts and 300 mA in the same buffer, in the presence of 1% dimethyl sulfoxide. After neutralization in Tris buffer (pH 8), DNA was stained with ethidium bromide (2 mg/ml) and the comets were examined and photographed in a fluorescent microscope. For each experiment, 50 comets were assessed by the measurement of their tail moments, using software image analysis (Comet 3.1, Kinetic Imaging).

Preparation of nuclear extracts and Western blot analysis of p53 protein: Twenty-four hours post-exposure, melanocytes were harvested and proteins of the nucleus were extracted according to Lin and Benchimol.[9]

Melanin content: Experiments were performed with pigment cells in their third to seventh passage. Melanin was solubilized in 0.2 M NaOH and measured spectrophotometrically at an absorbance of 475 nm against a standard curve of known concentrations of synthetic melanin (Sigma).

Tyrosinase activity: Dopa-oxidase activity of tyrosinase was assayed spectrophotometrically by following oxidation of L-dopa to dopachrome at 475 nm. The absorbance values were compared with a standard curve obtained with mushroom tyrosinase (Sigma).

Results

Heterogeneous response in terms of comet formation in melanocytes exposed to UVA

Figure 23.4 shows that the comets obtained with normal human melanocytes immediately after a 30-minute UVA exposure can be very different in shape within the same sample. Some of them, pointed out by arrows in the figure resemble typical comets, generally described for apoptotic cells: DNA is almost totally located in a large tail and the nucleus is restricted to a small fluorescent spot. If one assumes that apoptosis needs more than 30 minutes to develop, this result suggests that some melanocytes within the same population are particularly susceptible to DNA breakage when exposed to UVA.

Modulation of UVA-induced DNA breakage by endogenous melanin

In order to investigate the effects of endogenous melanin and/or its precursors on the response to UVA radiation, we have compared the induction of DNA breaks obtained after a 30-minute UVA exposure in two cell types: normal human fibroblasts, and slightly pigmented normal human melanocytes (strain NHEM 560, with an average melanin content of 20 pg/cell). Figure 23.5 shows the distribution of comet tail moments and confirms the presence of a certain heterogeneity of comet intensities in UVA-exposed melanocytes. Furthermore, there is a clear difference between melanocytes and fibroblasts. In non-pigmented cells, comets are induced by UVA as previously reported,[3] but they appear more homogeneous and significantly less intense. This result is in agreement with the hypothesis that the endogenous pigment in melanocytes can lead to DNA photosensitization.

Stimulation of melanogenesis increases susceptibility to UVA-induced DNA breakage

In order to confirm the role of endogenous melanin (and/or melanin-related molecules) in the breakage of DNA observed when melanocytes are exposed to UVA, experiments were performed after stimulation of melanogenesis in the strain NHEM 560. For this purpose, tyrosine, which has been reported to modulate tyrosinase activity of cultured melanocytes,[10] is added in the culture medium up to 1 mM. In our experimental conditions, the average melanin content increases from 20 to 35 pg/cell after 5 days incubation with tyrosine. Figure 23.6 shows that, after a 15-minute exposure to UVA, comets obtained with tyrosine-treated cells are significantly more intense than comets obtained in the untreated ones.

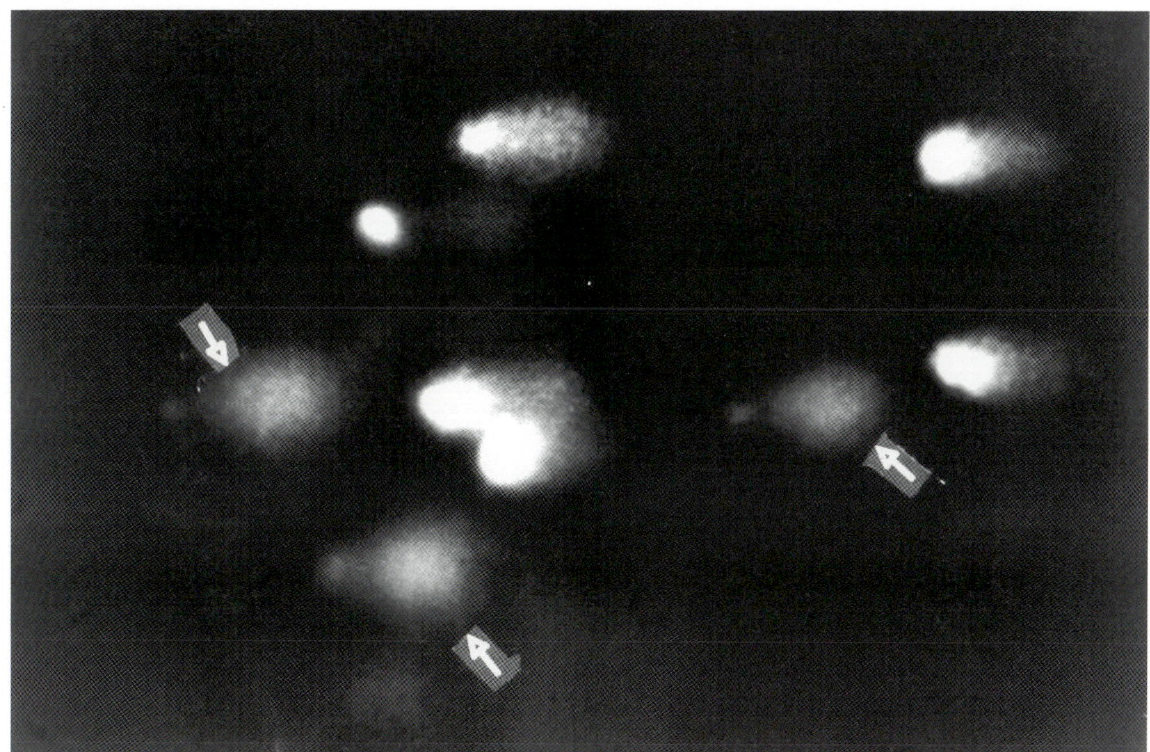

Figure 23.4

Photomicrograph of different DNA migration patterns within the same sample of human melanocytes exposed to UVA for 30 minutes (140 kJ/m^2). Arrows point out 'apoptotic-like' comets showing high cleavage of DNA.

Biological consequences of UVA-induced DNA damage on cultured melanocytes

In order to evaluate the biological impact of UVA when DNA breakage is induced, we also studied the following three complementary endpoints:

- Effect on cellular proliferation as assessed by viable cells number 5 days after exposure.
- Stimulation of melanogenesis as evaluated by tyrosinase activity 5 days after exposure.
- p53 status by measuring p53 protein stabilization and accumulation 24 hours after exposure.

Simulated solar UV that contains UVB was used as a positive control. Figure 23.7 shows that while, as expected, exposure to the whole UV spectrum (290–400 nm) reduces cell proliferation (as assessed by viable cells counts) and triggers tyrosinase activation (assessed by dopa-oxidase activity), the effects observed for UVA alone are less striking than those obtained for solar UV, even if the UVA dose applied is effective in comet induction. Different results are observed with regard to p53 status. As expected, solar UV exposure is followed by the accumulation of this protein 24 hours post-exposure, which is in agreement with previously published results, in particular with those obtained in melanocytes exposed to

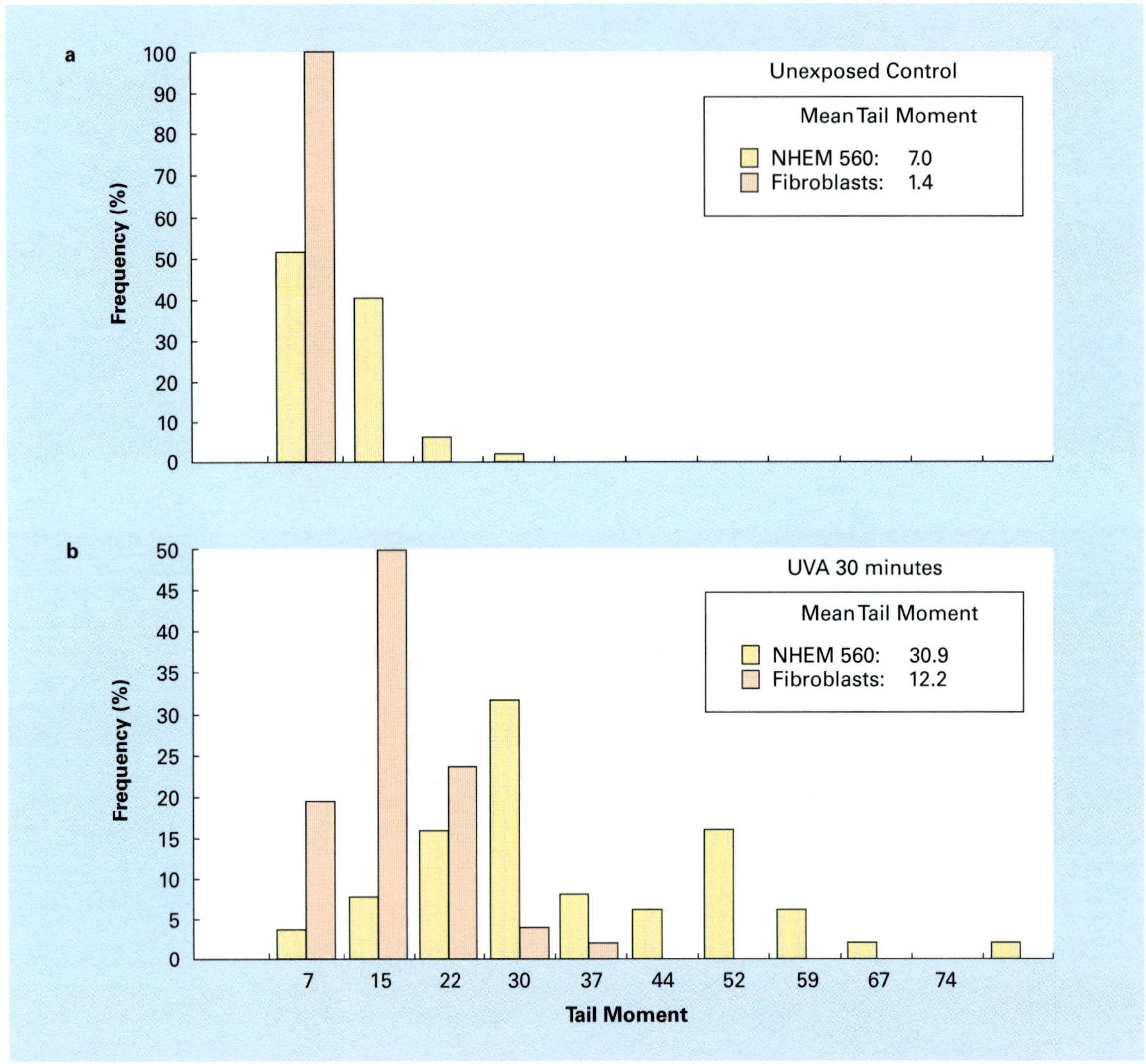

Figure 23.5

Distribution of tail moments of comets from fibroblasts or melanocytes NHEM 560 unexposed (a) or exposed for 30 minutes (140 kJ/m²) to UVA (b) and immediately lysed after exposure.

UVB.[11] Seemingly, with UVA only, longer exposure times and, thus, higher doses, are necessary for triggering p53 stabilization in melanocytes. However, Figure 23.6 shows that UVA response can also be significant, suggesting that the UVA-induced lesions could have reached a critical level in DNA.

Broad-spectrum photoprotection is required for preventing DNA photodamage in melanocytes

Two sunscreens with comparable sun protection factors (SPF) values (approximately 7.5) are compared on their ability to protect melanocytes from UVA-induced DNA breakage in the comet

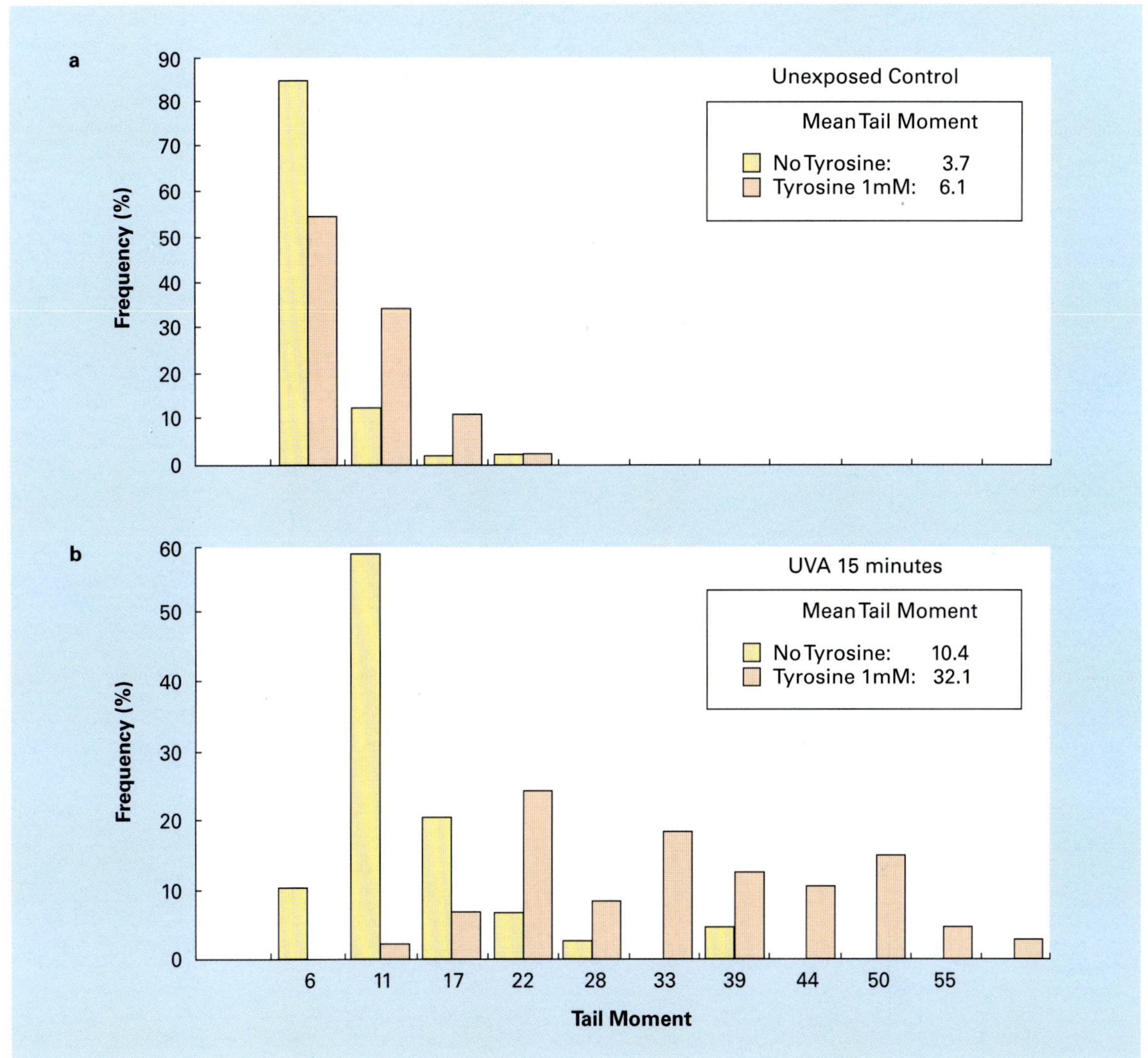

Figure 23.6

Distribution of tail moments of comets obtained with melanocytes NHEM 560 treated or not with tyrosine 1 mM (incubation 5 days) and unexposed (a) or exposed for 15 minutes (70 kJ/m^2) to UVA (b) and immediately lysed after exposure.

assay. The first one (product A) absorbs mostly the UVB part of the solar UV spectrum, while the second one (product B) absorbs broadly from 290 to 380 nm (see Fig. 23.8 for respective absorption characteristics).

In order to compare the photoprotective effects of both products, a 20-mm layer of each sunscreen is spread onto a quartz slide. Solar UV (290–400 nm) is used as incident light; the UV spectra transmitted by each sunscreen is analyzed by spectroradiometry. Figure 23.7 shows that, under our experimental conditions, product A fails to absorb a fraction of UVA, while almost all UV light is effectively absorbed by product B. Melanocytes from strain NHEM 4528, which are more pigmented and, thus, more susceptible to DNA breakage by

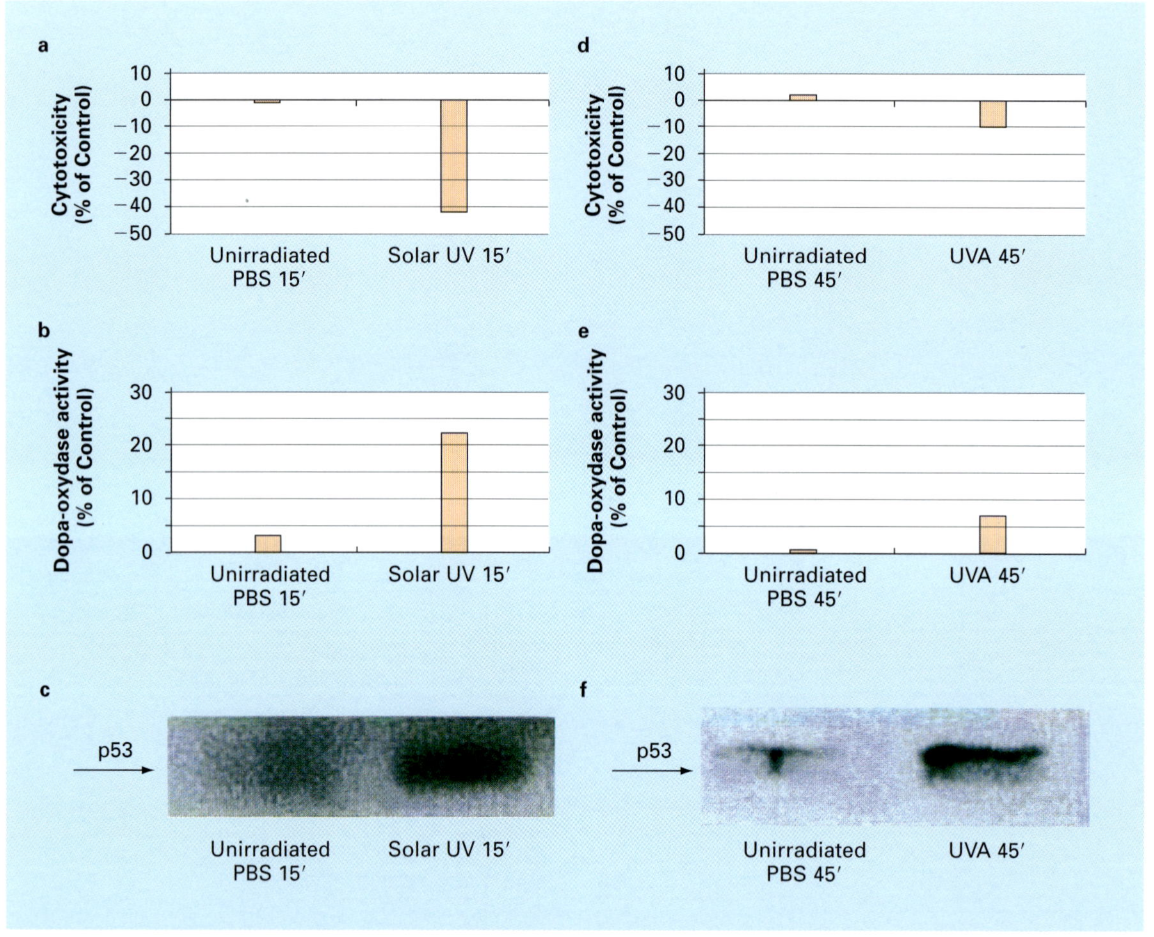

Figure 23.7

Comparison of cellular proliferation, tyrosinase (dopa-oxidase) activity and p53 accumulation in melanocytes exposed for 15 minutes to solar UV (UVB, 9 kJ/m^2 + UVA 83 kJ/m^2) or 45 minutes to UVA alone (210 kJ/m^2). Controls are sham-irradiated samples. (a–c) Solar UV 15 minutes; (d–f) UVA 45 minutes.

UVA, are used here in order to increase the sensitivity of the assay. Cells are embedded in an agarose slide, exposed to solar UV for 45 minutes under a quartz slide, covered or not by one of the sunscreens, and the comet assay is performed immediately after exposure. Figure 23.9 shows that both sunscreens significantly reduce the extent of comet formation. However, a difference can be observed between product A and product B. Product A does not totally abrogate the induction of DNA breaks and, in this case, the mean tail moment remains higher than that of unirradiated control or of the sample protected by product B.

Induction of pigmentation as a consequence of phototoxocity insult

Melanogenesis is considered as a defense mechanism against photo-oxidative stress, and some studies have suggested that DNA damage could trigger pigmentation.[12] Melanin synthesis is under the control of tyrosinase, an enzyme which catalyses the two first steps of this process: tyrosine hydroxylation and oxidation of the resulting dopa.[13] Tyrosinase activity (evaluated here by dopa-oxidase activity)

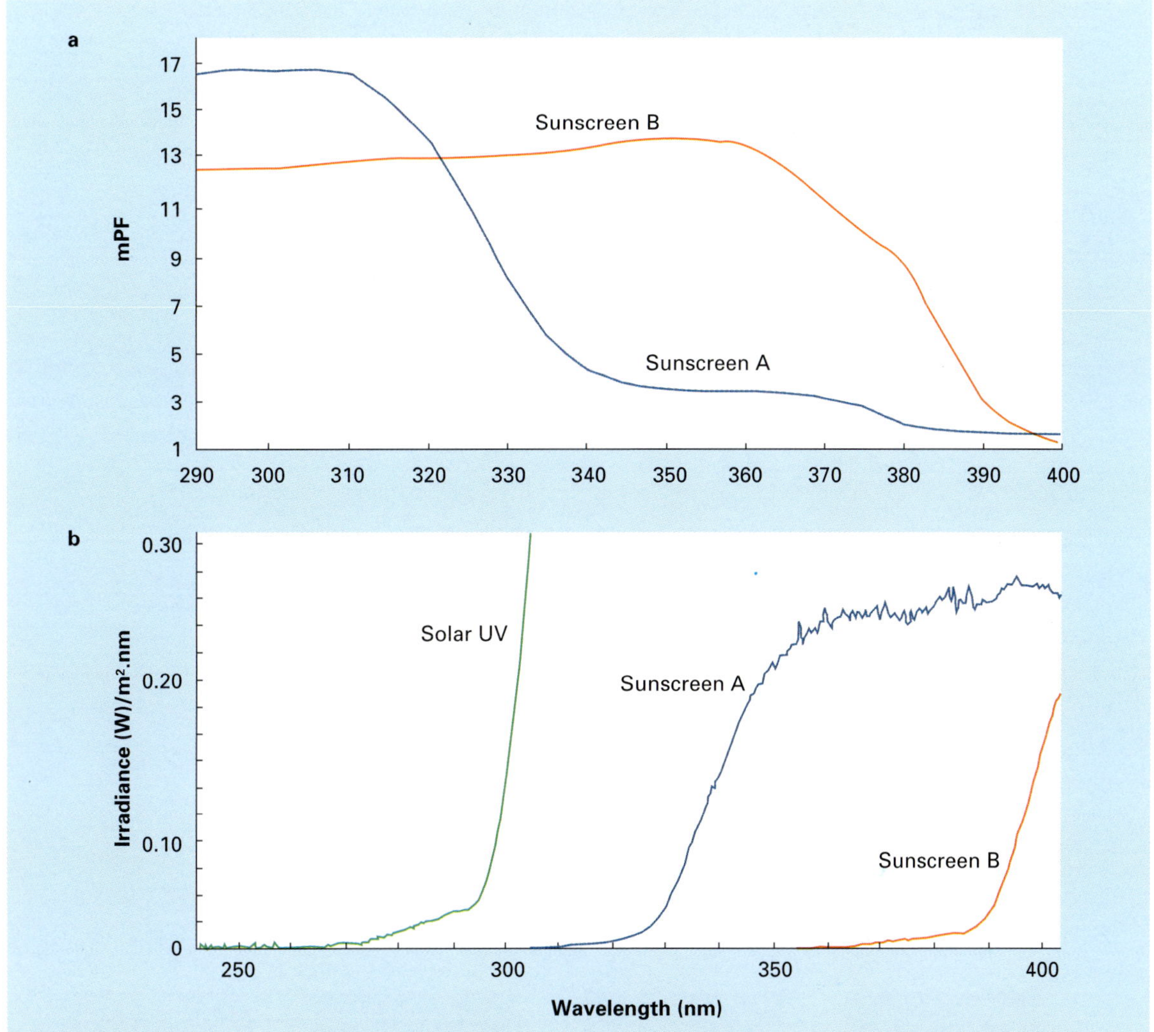

Figure 23.8

(a) Monochromatic protection factor (mPF) of sunscreens A and B. Sun protection factors are 7.5 and 7.4 for products A and B, respectively (data from L'OREAL Applied Research and Development Laboratories). (b) Spectral power distribution of the fraction of solar UV transmitted by a 20-mm thick layer of sunscreens A or B used in the experiments analyzed by spectroradiometry.

can be modulated by post-translational modifications of the enzyme in response to various stresses. Moreover, transcriptional activation of this enzyme was recently reported to be under the control of p53.[14] Tyrosinase status is, thus, an interesting endpoint in order to characterize the impact of a phototoxic molecule through one of its metabolic consequences.

Figure 23.10 shows that lomefloxacin, in contact with melanocytes, could enhace the DNA breakage due to UVA in a concentration-dependant manner.

Figure 23.11 shows that 5 days after treatments by lomefloxacin (5 and 10 mM) and UVA, when no significant cytotoxic effect could be detected (as shown by the MTT test, performed 24 hours

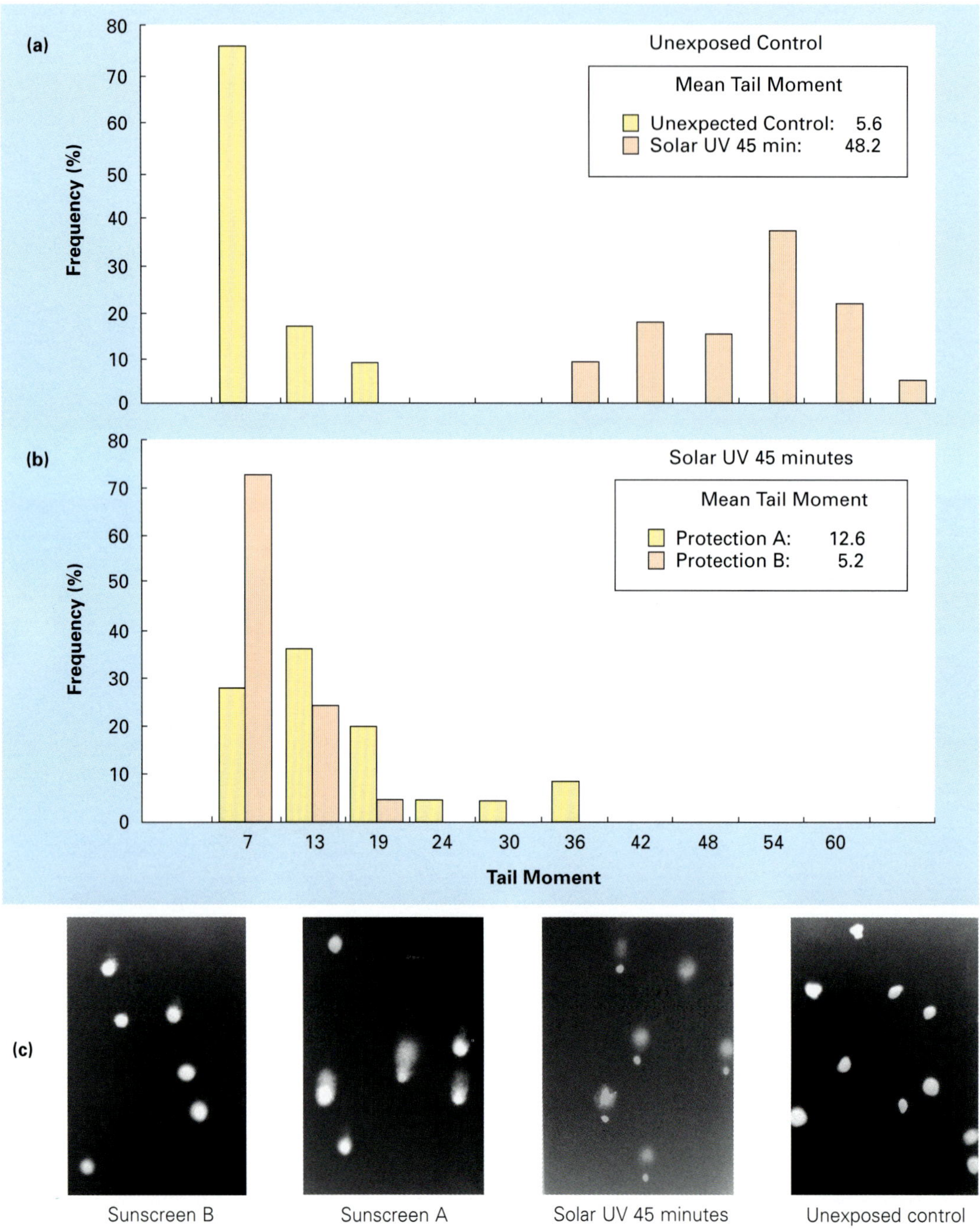

Figure 23.9

Comparison of photoprotection provided by sunscreens A and B using the comet assay applied to melanocytes. Distribution of tail moments of comets from melanocytes NHEM 4528 for unexposed cells or cells exposed for 45 minutes to solar UV (UVB, 27 kJ/m^2 + UVA, 249 kJ/m^2) without protection (a), and for cells exposed for 45 minutes to solar UV protected by a 20-mm thick layer of sunscreen A or B (b). Aspects of the comets without or with protection by sunscreens (c).

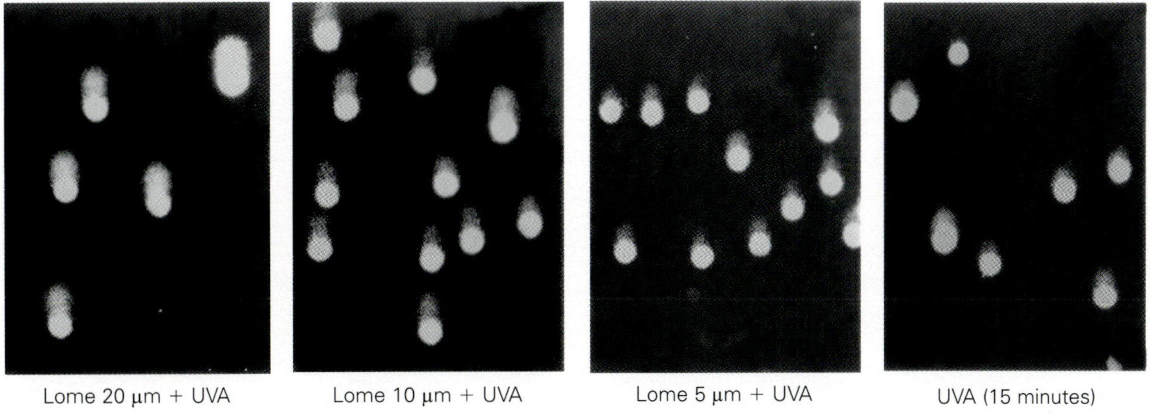

Figure 23.10

Aspects of the comets obtained after treatment of Caucasian melanocytes by lomefloxacin and exposure to UVA (15 minutes).

post-treatment), a dose-dependent stimulation of dopa-oxidase activity of tyrosinase was observed. At the same time, a decrease of melanocyte proliferation rate was also noticed. This result was consistent with the induction of a peculiar defense mechanism of the skin against phototoxicity. At this step, it was, however, difficult to know whether this response was either due to membrane damage or to DNA lesions (or both).

Discussion

Pigmentation is generally considered as a photoprotective process, either for the whole skin or at the level of individual keratinocytes in which melanin is transferred. However, Noz et al.[15] have proposed a role for endogenous melanin in the induction of UVB-induced photodamage in human melanocytes, as detected by the comet assay. Recently, Wenczl et al.[16] have shown that endogenous melanin can induce breaks in the DNA of pigment cells when exposed to UVA, and that stimulation of pigmentation enhances this photosensitization process. Our results confirm that melanocytes must be regarded as a very particular target cell for sunlight and, more specifically, for UVA. Indeed, the pool of reactive intermediates involved in melanogenesis could behave as an endogeneous photosensitizer and generate an oxidative stress when irradiated. Moreover, in the case of Caucasian human melanocytes, the photoinstability of pheomelanin must also be considered as a source of free radicals.[17]

One might also wonder about the biological consequences of UVA-induced DNA strand breaks. In our experiments, at doses where comets are relatively intense, neither cytotoxicity nor melanogenesis stimulation have been detected. However, accumulation of p53 protein is observed, but for a higher dose than when the whole solar UV spectrum is used. This result could suggest that UVA impact is perceived as not negligible by the melanocyte in terms of intracellular signaling, and this response is in agreement with the contribution of UVA to genotoxicity of sunlight. It is also noteworthy that the doses delivered here are relatively low, if one considers the total amount of UVA received by human beings in one day, especially in summer, during extensive sunbathing.

Our results also show that hazard increases when pigmentation is starting, suggesting that skin undergoing tanning could be more exposed to photogenotoxic stress. This raises the question of photoprotection. Sunscreens are generally evaluated by their ability to prevent sunburn and, as a consequence, the SPF is essentially related to UVB effects on the skin. What would be the best protection against solar UVA is often not clearly defined. The experiments reported here, using two sunscreens with comparable SPF but differ-

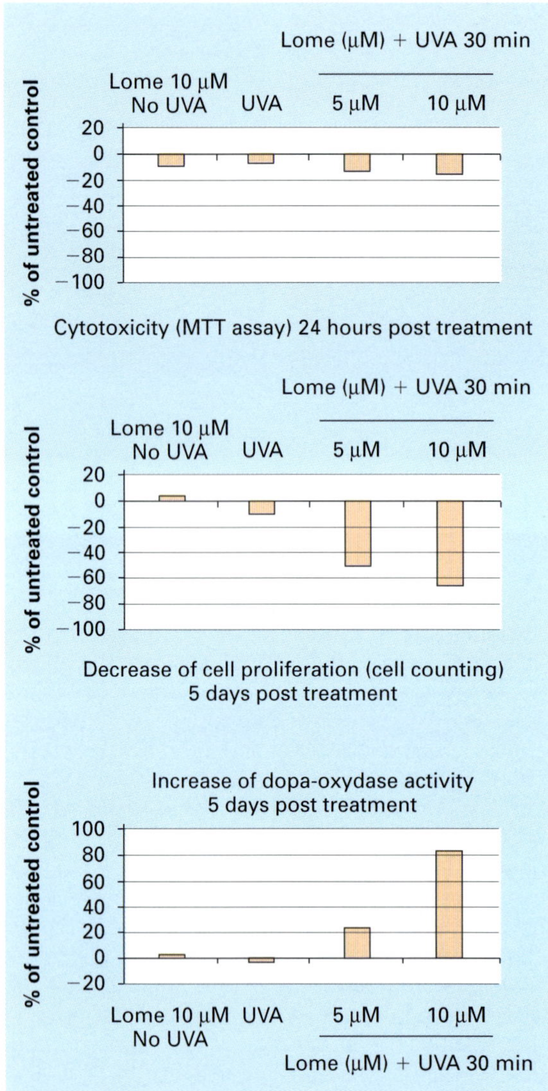

Figure 23.11

Effects of lomefloxacin exposed to UVA on cell survival (MTT assay), cell proliferation and dopa-oxidase of endogenous tyrosinase.

ent UVA protection factors, demonstrate that it is essential to broadly cover the whole UV range of sunlight and this must be done with 'adequately balanced' formulations to avoid a situation where high efficacy in the UVB region (erythema prevention) would allow longer exposure to unfiltered UVA. Our results also underline the necessity of photostability: product A can be compared to a non-photostable sunscreen which would lose its effectiveness after few hours of exposure. We suggest being particularly careful when the skin tanning process is stimulated, especially for light skin phototypes, since development of pigmentation might be associated with an increased photooxidative potential in melanocytes. Some epidemiological studies have suggested that a positive association exists between sunscreen use and melanoma incidence. Among the possible bias, it could be interesting to consider the fact that some people stop using sunscreen as soon as their tanning starts: such behaviour could significantly influence photomutagenesis in skin.

Finally, the impact of any photoreactive exogenous chemical in photosensitization of melanocytes can also be questioned, and the contribution of drug-induced sunburns in cutaneous melanoma cannot be excluded. The results presented here with the fluoroquinolone lomefloxacin also suggest that cultured melanocytes could constitute an interesting model to assess the safety of any product likely to undergo sunlight exposure.

Acknowledgements

Dr Averbeck (Institut Curie, Paris France) is gratefully acknowledged for critical reading of the manuscript and helpful discussions. Drs Candau, Forestier and Réfrégier (L'OREAL Applied Research, Centre Zviak, Clichy, France) are acknowledged for providing sunscreens with all the related data (spectra, SPF) and helpful discussions.

References

1. Tice RR, The single cell gel/comet assay: a microgel electrophoretic technique for the detection of DNA damage and repair in individual cells. In: Phillips DH, Venett S, eds, *Environmental Mutagenesis* (Bios: Oxford, 1995) 315–39.
2. Arlett CF, Lowe JE, Harcourt SA et al., Hypersensitivity of human lymphocytes to UV-B and solar irradiation, *Cancer Res* (1993) **53**:609–14.
3. Alapetite C, Moustacchi E, Wachter T, Sage E, Use of the alkaline comet assay to detect DNA repair

deficiencies in human fibroblasts exposed to UVC, UVB, UVA and -rays, *Int J Radiat Biol* (1996) **69**: 359–69.

4. Marrot L, Belaïdi JP, Chaubo C et al., An in vitro strategy to evaluate the phototoxicity of solar UV at the molecular and cellular level: application to photoprotection assessment, *Eur J Dermatol* (1998) **8**:403–12.
5. Marrot L, Belaïdi JP, Meunier JR et al., The human melanocyte as a particular target for UVA radiation and an endpoint for photoprotection assessment, *Photochem Photobiol* (1999) **69**:686–93.
6. Reavy HJ, Traynor NJ, Gibbs NK, Photogenotoxicity of skin: phototumorigenic Fluoroquinolone antibiotics detected using the comet assay, *Photochem Photobiol* (1997) **66**:368–73.
7. Kidd S, Meunier JR, Traynor NS et al., The photomutagenic fluoroquinolone Lomefloxacin photosensitizes p53 accumulation and transcriptional activity in human skin cells, *J Photochem Photobiol* (2000) **58**:26–31.
8. Im S, Moro O, Peng F et al., Activation of the cyclic AMP pathway by melanotropin mediates the response of human melanocytes to ultraviolet B radiation, *Cancer Res* (1998) **58**:47–54.
9 Lin Y, Benchimol S, Cytokines inhibit p53-mediated apoptosis but not p53-mediated G1 arrest, *Mol Cell Biol* (1995) **15**:6045–54.
10. Smit NPM, Van Der Meulen H, Koerten HK et al., Melanogenesis in cultured melanocytes can be substantially influenced by L-tyrosine and L-cysteine, *J Invest Dermatol* (1997) **109**:796–800.
11. Barker D, Dixon K, Medrano EE et al., Comparison of the response of human melanocytes with ultraviolet B irradiation, *Cancer Res* (1995) **55**:4041–6.
12. Eller MS, Ostrom K, Gilchrest BA, DNA damage enhances melanogenesis, *Proc Nati Acad Sci U S A* (1996) **93**:1087–92.
13. Hearing VJ, The melanosome: the perfect model for cellular responses to the environment, *Pigment Cell Res* (2000) **13**:2334.
14. Nylander K, Dourdon JC, Bray SE et al., Transcriptional activation of tyrosinase and TRP-1 by p53 links UV irradiation to the protective tanning response, *J Pathol* (2000) **190**:39–46.
15. Noz KC, Bauwens M, Van Buul PPW et al., Comet assay demonstrates a higher ultraviolet B sensitivity to DNA damage in dysplastic nevus cells than in common melanocytic nevus cells and foreskin melanocytes, *J Invest Dermatol* (1996) **106**: 1198–202.
16. Wenczl E, Van der Schans GP, Roza L et al. (Pheo)Melanin photosensitizes UVA-induced DNA damage in cultured human melanocytes, *J Invest Dermatol* (1998) **111**:678–82.
17. Menon IA, Persad S, Ranadive NS et al., Effects of ultraviolet–visible irradiation in the presence of melanin isolated from human black or red hair upon Ehrlich ascites carcinoma cells, *Cancer Res* (1983) **43**:3165–9.

24
Ultraviolet radiation and apoptosis

Thomas Schwarz and Dagmar Kulms

Introduction

One of the major consequences of exposing skin to ultraviolet (UV) radiation is the generation of sunburn cells (SC). SC were originally described in H&E sections on the basis of their characteristic appearance as isolated epidermal cells, with a pyknotic nucleus and a shrunken eosinophilic cytoplasm.[1] The major action spectrum responsible for inducing SC is in the UVB range (290–320 nm), although UVC (200–290 nm) or high doses of UVA (320–400 nm) also result in SC formation.[2,3] SC are detectable as early as 8-hours after UV exposure, maximally expressed at 24–48 hours and lost by 60–72 hours.[4] Although the phenomenon of SC formation has been appreciated for several decades, the functional relevance of these cells remained mostly unclear until recently.

UV radiation induces apoptosis of keratinocytes

The morphological features of SC are typical for apoptosis, which starts with cell shrinkage, blebbing of the cytoplasmic membrane, followed by condensation of the chromatin and fragmentation of the genomic DNA.[5] Cells die either by apoptosis or necrosis. Necrosis is a passive response to a severe external insult, and is characterized by cytoplasmic swelling and cell membrane disruption, with the release of lysosomal enzymes. Therefore, necrosis is usually associated with an inflammatory infiltrate. In contrast, apoptosis is an active process, in which a single cell initiates an inherent suicide program, resulting in the successive fragmentation of the cell. The membrane-enclosed fragments, also called apoptotic bodies, are phagocytosed by macrophages, without causing an inflammatory reaction. Therefore, SC are always single-standing cells and not accompanied by an inflammatory reaction.[6]

Execution of apoptosis is a highly complex process which involves a variety of biochemical pathways, including the activation of catabolic proteases, called caspases (see below).[7] Among the many stimuli which induce apoptosis, the most important ones are cell aging, cell damage (*e.g.* by ionizing or non-ionizing radiation, chemicals, growth-factor withdrawal), or activation of one of the various death receptors which are ubiquitously expressed on the cell surface.

DNA damage and UV-induced apoptosis

Genomic DNA is certainly the major chromophore for UVB radiation within the cell. UVB radiation induces two types of lesions in chromosomal DNA: (6–4) photoproducts and cyclobutane pyrimidine dimers, the latter being the predominant ones.[8] Most of these photoproducts are removed in normal cells by DNA nucleotide excision repair.[9,10] The importance and efficacy of nucleotide excision repair is impressively demonstrated by the drastically enhanced rate of skin cancer in patients suffering from xeroderma pigmentosum, which is based on defects in various components of the nucleotide excision repair.[11] But UV-induced DNA damage also plays an important role in mediating various biological effects of UVB radiation. UVB-induced immunosuppression, surface molecule expression and cytokine release can be reduced upon enhancement of repair of cyclobutane pyrimidine dimers by the topical application of the repair enzyme, T4 endonuclease V.[12–14] Similar findings were obtained when using photolyase, another repair enzyme, which reduces the numbers of pyrimidine dimers following illumination with photoreactivating light, a process called photoreactivation.[15]

The discovery of the link between SC formation and the tumor suppressor gene *p53* led to fundamental progress in the understanding of the functional role of SC. *p53*-knockout mice produce fewer SC when compared to UV-irradiated wild-type mice, demonstrating an important role for *p53* in SC formation.[16] Since *p53* is induced by DNA damage, it was suggested that *p53* eliminates, irretrievably, UV-damaged keratinocytes via induction of apoptosis, thereby preventing malignant transformation. Based on this observation, SC formation is regarded as an actively controlled cell suicide mechanism, protecting from malignant transformation.[17] Accordingly, UV-exposed *p53*-knockout mice are more prone to UV-induced skin tumors than wild-type control mice,[18] supporting the hypothesis that formation of SC protects against skin cancer. UV radiation, however, preferentially mutates *p53*;[19] thus, it may exert a selective pressure for the *p53*-mutated, and therefore damage-resistant, keratinocytes, thereby allowing these cells to clonally expand and form actinic keratosis, the pre-stage of skin cancer.[16]

The crucial role of *p53* for UV-induced apoptosis indicated that DNA damage is the major determinant of whether a cell undergoes apoptosis following UV exposure. This was further substantiated by a variety of *in vitro* studies. If DNA damage is causally related to UV-mediated apoptosis, an increase in DNA repair should result in reduction of the apoptotic response. To prove this hypothesis, we exposed the epithelial cell line HeLa to UV radiation.[20] Immediately thereafter, DNA repair was induced by addition of the bacterial repair enzyme photolyase via liposome delivery. Subsequent exposure to photoreactivating light caused a significant reduction in cyclobutane pyrimidine dimers. Accordingly, the rate of apoptosis was remarkably, but not completely, reduced.[20] Similar observations were made *in vivo*. Enhancement of DNA repair by topical application of the repair enzymes T4 endonuclease V or photolyase in liposomes reduced the number of SC.[15,21] Activation of endogenous photolyase in opossums also resulted in a decrease of SC.[22] Taken together, all these data clearly suggested that DNA damage is critically involved in UV-induced apoptosis. These findings were also in perfect accordance with the conventional photobiological concept that any biologcial effect of UVB radiation has to be mediated via DNA damage.

However, there is also increasing evidence that non-DNA pathways may be involved as well. In our *in vitro* system,[20] we could not prevent UV-induced apoptosis completely, even by increasing the concentration of photolyase, indicating that DNA damage may not be the only factor initiating the apoptosis program. This is also supported by a clinical observation: up to 4% of keratinocytes of normal-appearing sun-exposed skin cells carry *p53* mutations, and, thus, should be protected from apoptosis, but nothing like this number develop into actinic keratoses or squamous cell carcinomas. Consequently, the vast majority of *p53*-mutated cells have to undergo apoptosis induced by pathways independent of *p53* and DNA damage.[23,24] This is in accordance with the observation that *p53*-mutated cells, like the spontaneously transformed human keratinocyte cell line HaCaT,[25,26] undergo apoptosis following UV exposure.[27,28]

UV-induced apoptosis and activation of death receptors

Death receptors belong to the tumor necrosis factor (TNF) receptor gene superfamily, which is characterized by similar, cysteine-rich extracellular domains and a homologous cytoplasmic sequence termed 'death domain'.[29] Among the many death receptors, including TNF-receptor-1, TRAIL-receptor-1, TRAIL-receptor-2 and death-receptor-3 (DR-3), CD95, also called Fas or Apo-1, is one of the most potent transducers of apoptosis.[30] Activation of CD95, either by agonistic antibodies or by its natural ligand (CD95L, also called FasL) induces apoptosis. Binding of the ligand results in trimerization and clustering of CD95. Subsequently, the trimerized cytoplasmic region transduces the signal by recruiting a molecule called FADD (Fas-associating protein with death domain).[31] FADD then binds to and activates procaspase-8,[32,33] which is the initial step of a proteolytic cascade triggering the activation of other downstream caspases, such as caspases-3, -6, -7, and -9,[34] which ultimately execute apoptosis.

Rosette and Karin[35] observed that UV radiation activates multiple growth factor and cytokine receptors, consequently activating the Jun-kinase cascade. Confocal laser scanning microscopy studies revealed that exposure of HeLa cells to UV radiation induced clustering and internalization of the cell-surface receptors for epidermal growth factor, TNF and interleukin-1.[35] Since the initial events during activation of CD95 are its trimerization and clustering, we addressed whether UV radiation directly causes CD95 clustering.[27] Therefore, the transformed human keratinocyte cell line HaCaT was exposed to UVB radiation, stained with an antibody against CD95, and subsequently analyzed by confocal laser scanning microscopy. While only a very weak and diffuse CD95 staining was detectable on the surface of untreated HaCaT cells, UV-exposed HaCaT cells revealed a marked patchy staining, compatible with receptor clustering. A similar staining pattern was found upon treatment of cells with CD95L. These data provided strong evidence that UVB radiation triggers the CD95 pathway by directly activating the CD95 receptor.[27] Accordingly, by performing immunoprecipitation, we were able to detect FADD recruitment to the CD95 receptor following UV exposure. Similar findings were obtained by Rehemtulla et al.,[36] who observed that UVC induces CD95 clustering in the breast carcinoma cell line MCF7. In addition, Sheikh et al.[37] showed that the TNF receptor-1, another death receptor, becomes aggregated by UV but not by drugs, which damage DNA only.

To prove whether UV-induced clustering of CD95 is also functionally relevant, HaCaT cells were exposed to UV radiation at 10°C. Rosette and Karin[35] observed that exposing HeLa cells to UV radiation at such a low temperature, which is below the transition temperature of the membrane, prevents receptor clustering. Confocal laser scanning microscopy revealed that exposing HaCaT cells to UV at 10°C almost completely prevented CD95 aggregation. Accordingly, under these conditions, the apoptosis rate was significantly, but not completely, reduced.[27] Taken together, these data indicated that UV-induced clustering of CD95 is functionally relevant for UV-mediated apoptosis. This conclusion was also confirmed by the observation that HaCaT cells transfected with an FADD dominant-negative mutant construct were less susceptible to UV-induced apoptosis than mock transfected cells. However, since neither UV exposure at 10°C nor elimination of the FADD pathway completely prevented UV-induced apoptosis, additional pathways have to be involved (see below).

But there is additional evidence that UV radiation may also utilize the respective death ligands to activate the death receptors. UVC radiation upregulates both CD95 and CD95L in primary keratinocytes.[38] In addition, application of a neutralizing antibody against CD95L to the cells *in vitro* reduced the UVC-induced apoptosis rate. Simliar observations were obtained with freshly isolated peripheral blood lymphocytes or lymphocyte cell lines exposed to UV.[39]

UVA-1 (340–400 nm) also seems to utilize the CD95 system to induce apoptosis. T helper cells show upregulated CD95L but not CD95 after UVA-1 exposure, and apoptosis is partially reduced after addition of a neutralizing antibody against CD95.[40] The singlet oxygen scavenger sodium azide partially inhibits induction of CD95L by UVA-1, implying that reactive oxygen species are involved in the upregulation of CD95L. TUNEL staining of skin samples obtained from atopic patients treated successfully with UVA-1 phototherapy revealed T-cell apoptosis.[40] This observation gives rise to the speculation that the beneficial effect of UVA-1 in atopic dermatitis may be a consequence of apoptotic killing of T-lymphocytes.[41] The therapeutic effect of 312 nm UVB in the treatment of psoriasis also seems to depend on T-cell apoptosis.[42]

In vivo involvement of the CD95/CD95L system in UVB-induced apoptosis was demonstrated recently. UVB exposure of mice induces CD95 and CD95L expression in the skin.[43] *gld*-Mice, which lack functional CD95L, exhibited significantly fewer SC after UV exposure, suggesting that UV-induced apoptosis depends on the expression of CD95L. *p53* mutations were detected with increased frequency in chronically UVB-exposed *gld*-mice, implying that CD95L is required to eradicate keratinocytes with UV-induced DNA damage. Thus, perturbation of CD95/CD95L interactions may contribute to the development of UV-induced skin cancer.[43]

But the CD95/CD95L system does not appear to be the only death receptor/ligand system involved in UV-induced apoptosis. Autocrine secretion of TNF seems to be of relevance for UV-mediated apoptosis, since inhibition of TNF activity by neutralizing antibodies, or pentoxifylline, which inhibits the release of TNF, reduced UV-mediated cell death.[28,44] Taken together, the observations that UV radiation can activate death receptors severely challenged the concept that UV-induced apoptosis is exclusively dependent on DNA damage.

Both nuclear and membrane events contribute to UV-induced apoptosis

According to the observations that UV can induce apoptosis, either by inducing DNA damage or by activating death receptors, we recently attempted to measure the relative contribution of nuclear and membrane events in UV-induced apoptosis.[20] As mentioned above, UV irradiation of HeLa cells at 4°C, which prevents death-receptor clustering, caused partial reduction of apoptosis. Enhancement of DNA repair by photoreactivation resulted in a more pronounced inhibition of UV-induced apoptosis. However, neither of these approaches alone was able to prevent apoptosis completely. Only when receptor clustering was blocked (by keeping the cells at a low temperature) followed by photoreactivation (removing DNA damage) was almost complete reduction of apoptosis observed. Although under these experimental conditions activation of death receptors and DNA damage are induced by the same stimulus, *i.e.* UV radiation, they represent independent events and are not biochemically linked. Since inhibition of both events results in an additive reduction of apoptosis, this observation indicated that death-receptor activation and DNA damage contribute independently to UV-induced apoptosis. In addition, inhibition of caspase-3, the downstream protease in the CD95-signaling pathway, blocked both CD95L- and UV-induced apoptosis, while blockade of caspase-8, the most proximal caspase, inhibited CD95L-mediated apoptosis completely, but UV-induced apoptosis only partially. This implies that apoptosis induced by UV-mediated DNA damage is independent of caspase-8. Although nuclear effects appeared to be more effective in mediating UV-induced apoptosis than membrane events, both seem to be necessary for the complete apoptotic response. Thus, this study showed that nuclear and membrane effects are not mutually exclusive, and that both components can contribute independently to certain biological effects of UV.

Mitochondria, cytochrome *c* release and UV-induced apoptosis

Other important cellular components involved in apoptosis are the mitochondria. Initiation of cell death leads to mitochondrial permeability transition, resulting in 'megapore' formation followed by release of cytochrome *c* into the cytosol.[45] Cytosolic cytochrome *c* associates with Apaf-1 and procaspase-9, causing ATP-dependent activation of caspase-9, followed by activation of downstream caspases, consequently executing apoptosis.[46]

As observed for other apoptotic stimuli, mitochondria appear to be involved in UV-mediated apoptosis as well. Cytochrome *c* release seems to be an early event in UV-induced cell death. UV-induced cytochrome *c* release could not be prevented by caspase inhibitors, thus, it was supposed to occur upstream of caspase activation.[47] This assumption was recently confirmed by immunohistochemistry and time-lapse confocal microscopy in HeLa cells, revealing that on a single-cell level, UV-induced cytochrome *c* release is an event of a few minutes that occurs prior to phosphatidylserin exposure at the outer cell membrane and prior to the loss of plasma membrane integrity.[48] Nevertheless, it still remains to be determined how death receptor activation, DNA damage and cytochrome *c* release relate to each other in UV-induced apoptosis.

Conclusions

Major advances have been achieved over the last few years in understanding the pathomechanisms and biological role of SC. There is unanimous agreement that UV-induced apoptosis of keratinocytes is a DNA-protective phenomenon to eliminate DNA-damaged cells which are predisposed to malignant transformation. Hence, disturbances in the apoptotic machinery would be expected to confer an increased risk of UV-induced skin cancer. UV-induced apoptosis is a highly complex process in which different pathways are involved, including DNA damage, activation of death receptors on the cell surface, and release of death ligands. It remains to be determined in the future how these processes relate to each other. Further elucidation of the interplay between the different pathways will significantly increase our understanding of apoptosis in general, but also of photocarcinogenesis.

Acknowledgements

This work was supported by grants from the Federal Ministery of Education and Research (07UVB63A/5) and the European Community (ENV4-CT97-0556).

References

1. Daniels F, Brophy D, Lobitz WC, Histochemical responses of human skin following ultraviolet irradiation, *J Invest Dermatol* (1961) **37**:351–7.
2. Kumakiri M, Hashimoto K, Willis I, Biologic changes due to long-wave ultraviolet irradiation on human skin: ultrastructural study, *J Invest Dermatol* (1977) **69**:392–400.
3. Young AR, The sunburn cell, *Photodermatology* (1987) **4**:127–34.
4. Danno K, Horio T, Sunburn cell: Factors involved in its formation, *Photochem Photobiol* (1987) **45**:683–90.
5. Cohen JJ, Apoptosis, *Immunol Today* (1993) **14**: 126–30.
6. Teraki Y, Shiohara T, Apoptosis and the skin, *Eur J Dermatol* (1999) **9**:413–26.
7. Alnemri ES, Livingston DJ, Nicholson DW et al., Human ICE/CED-3 protease nomenclature, *Cell* (1996) **87**:171.
8. Patrick MH, Studies on thymine-derived UV photoproducts in DNA—I. Formation and biological role of pyrimidine adducts in DNA, *Photochem Photobiol* (1977) **25**:357–72.
9. de Laat WL, Appeldoorn E, Sugasawa K et al., DNA-binding polarity of human replication protein A positions nucleases in nucleotide excision repair, *Genes Dev* (1998) **12**:2598–609.
10. Sancar A, DNA repair in humans, *Annu Rev Genet* (1995) **29**:69–105.
11. Kraemer KH, Lee MM, Andrews AD et al., The role of sunlight and DNA repair in melanoma and nonmelanoma skin cancer. The xeroderma pigmentosum paradigm, *Arch Dermatol* (1994) **130**:1018–21.
12. Kripke ML, Cox PA, Alas LG et al., Pyrimidine dimers in DNA initiate systemic immunosuppression in UV-irradiated mice, *Proc Natl Acad Sci U S A* (1992) **89**:7516–20.
13. Kibitel J, Hejmadi V, Alas L et al., UV-DNA damage in mouse and human cells induces the expression of tumor necrosis factor alpha, *Photochem Photobiol* (1998) **67**:541–6.
14. Nishigori C, Yarosh DB, Ullrich SE et al., Evidence that DNA damage triggers interleukin 10 cytokine production in UV-irradiated murine keratinocytes, *Proc Natl Acad Sci U S A* (1996) **93**:10354–9.
15. Stege H, Roza L, Vink AA et al., Enzyme plus light therapy to repair DNA damage in ultraviolet-B-irradiated human skin, *Proc Natl Acad Sci U S A* (2000) **97**:1790–5.
16. Ziegler A, Jonason JS, Leffel DW et al., Sunburn and p53 in the onset of skin cancer, *Nature* (1994) **372**:773–6.
17. Brash DE, Ziegler A, Jonason AS et al., Sunlight and sunburn in human skin cancer: p53, apoptosis, and tumor promotion, *J Invest Dermatol Symp Proc* (1996) **1**:136–42.
18. Jiang W, Ananthaswamy HN, Muller HK et al., p53 protects against skin cancer induction by UV-B radiation, *Oncogene* (1999) **18**: 4247–53.
19. Brash DE, Rudolph JA, Simon JA et al., A role for sunlight in skin cancer: UV-induced p53 mutations in squamous cell carcinoma, *Proc Natl Acad Sci U S A* (1991) **88**:10124–8.
20. Kulms D, Pöppelmann B, Yarosh D et al., Nuclear and cell membrane effects contribute independently to the induction of apoptosis in human cells exposed to UVB radiation, *Proc Natl Acad Sci U S A* (1999) **96**:7974–9.
21. Wolf P, Cox P, Yarosh DB et al., Sunscreens and T4N5 liposomes differ in their ability to protect against ultraviolet-induced sunburn cell formation, alterations of dendritic epidermal cells, and local suppression of contact hypersensitivity, *J Invest Dermatol* (1995) **104**:287–92.
22. Ley RD, Applegate LA, Ultraviolet radiation-induced histopathologic changes in the skin of the marsupial Monodelphis domestica. II. Quantitative studies of the photoreactivation of induced hyperplasia and sunburn cell formation, *J Invest Dermatol* (1985) **85**:365–7.
23. Kraemer KH, Sunlight and skin cancer: another link revealed, *Proc Natl Acad Sci U S A* (1997) **94**: 1–14.
24. Jonason AS, Kunala S, Price GJ et al., Frequent clones of p53-mutated keratinocytes in normal

human skin, *Proc Natl Acad Sci USA* (1996) **93**:14025–9.

25. Boukamp P, Petrussevska RT, Breitkreutz D et al., Normal keratinization in a spontaneously immortalized aneuploid human keratinocyte cell line, *J Cell Biol* (1988) **106**:761–71.
26. Lehman TA, Modali R, Boukamp P et al., p53 mutations in human immortalized epithelial cell lines, *Carcinogenesis* (1993) **14**:833–9.
27. Aragane Y, Kulms D, Metze D et al., Ultraviolet light induces apoptosis via direct activation of CD95 (Fas/APO-1) independently of its ligand CD95L, *J Cell Biol* (1998) **140**:171–82.
28. Schwarz A, Bhardwaj R, Aragane Y et al., Ultraviolet-B-induced apoptosis of keratinocytes: evidence for partial involvement of tumor necrosis factor-alpha in the formation of sunburn cells, *J Invest Dermatol* (1995) **104**:922–7.
29. Ashkenazi A, Dixit VM, Death receptors: Signaling and modulation, *Science* (1998) **281**:1305–8.
30. Peter ME, Krammer PH, Mechanisms of CD95 (APO-1/Fas)-mediated apoptosis, *Curr Opin Immunol* (1998) **10**: 545–51.
31. Chinnaiyan AM, O'Rourke K, Tewari M et al., FADD, a novel death domain-containing protein, interacts with death domain of Fas and initiates apoptosis, *Cell* (1995) **81**:505–12.
32. Boldin MP, Goncharov TM, Goltsev YV et al., Involvement of MACH, a novel MORT1/FADD-interacting protease, in Fas/APO-1- and TNF receptor-induced cell death, *Cell* (1996) **85**:803–15.
33. Muzio M, Chinnaiyan AM, Kischkel FC et al., FLICE, a novel FADD-homologous ICE/CED-3 like protease, is recruited to the CD95 (Fas/APO-1) death-inducing signaling complex, *Cell* (1996) **85**:817–27.
34. Salvesen GS, Dixit VM, Caspases: intracellular signaling by proteolysis, *Cell* (1997) **91**:443–6.
35. Rosette C, Karin M, Ultraviolet light and osmotic stress: activation of the JNK cascade through multiple growth factor and cytokine receptors, *Science* (1996) **274**:1194–7.
36. Rehemtulla A, Hamilton CA, Chinnaiyan AM et al., Ultraviolet radiation-induced apoptosis is mediated by activation of CD-95 (Fas/APO-1), *J Biol Chem* (1997) **272**:25738–86.
37. Sheikh MS, Antinore MJ, Huang Y et al., Ultraviolet-irradiation-induced apoptosis is mediated via ligand independent activation of tumor necrosis factor receptor 1, *Oncogene* (1998) **17**:2555–63.
38. Leverkus M, Yaar M, Gilchrest BA, Fas/Fas ligand interaction contributes to UV-induced apoptosis in human keratinocytes, *Exp Cell Res* (1997) **232**:255–62.
39. Caricchio R, Reap EA, Cohen PL, Fas/Fas ligand interactions are involved in ultraviolet-B-induced human lymphocyte apoptosis, *J Immunol* (1998) **161**:241–51.
40. Morita A, Werfel T, Stege H et al., Evidence that singlet oxygen-induced human T helper cell apoptosis is the basic mechanism of ultraviolet-A radiation phototherapy, *J Exp Med* (1997) **186**:1763–8.
41. Krutmann J, Diepgen TL, Luger TA et al., High-dose UVA1 therapy for atopic dermatitis: results of a multicenter trial, *J Am Acad Dermatol* (1998) **38**:589–93.
42. Ozawa M, Ferenczi K, Kikuchi T et al., 312-nanometer ultraviolet B light (narrow-band UVB) induces apoptosis of T cells within psoriatic lesions, *J Exp Med* (1999) **189**:711–18.
43. Hill LL, Ouhtit A, Loughlin SM et al., Fas ligand: a sensor for DNA damage critical in skin cancer etiology, *Science* (1999) **285**:898–900.
44. Schwarz A, Mahnke K, Luger TA et al., Pentoxifylline reduces the formation of sunburn cells, *Exp Dermatol* (1997) **6**:1–5.
45. Reed JC, Double identity for proteins of the Bcl-2 family, *Nature* (1997) **387**:773–6.
46. Hu Y, Benedict MA, Ding L et al., Role of cytochrome c and dATP/ATP hydrolysis in Apaf-1-mediated caspase-9 activation and apoptosis, *EMBO J* (1999) **18**:3586–95.
47. Bossy-Wetzel E, Newmeyer DD, Green DR, Mitochondrial cytochrome c release in apoptosis occurs upstream of DEVD-specific caspase activation and independently of mitochondrial transmembrane depolarization, *EMBO J* (1998) **17**:37–49.
48. Goldstein JC, Waterhouse NJ, Juin P et al., The coordinate release of cytochrome c during apoptosis is rapid, complete and kinetically invariant, *Nat Cell Biol* (2000) **2**:156–62.

Section VII

EVALUATION SYSTEM OF MELANOGENESIS

25

Objective methods to assess pigmentation

Luc Duteil

Introduction

The color of the skin depends mainly on its pigment content, on the spectrum of the illuminating light and on the quality of its surface. When light impinges on the skin, a small percentage of light is directly reflected by the surface whereas entering photons are either absorbed or scattered by different molecules and structures present in the cutaneous layers. The pigments of the skin, also called chromophores, are mainly represented by melanin in the epidermis and by hemoglobin and bilirubin in the dermis. Other molecules such as amino acids, nucleic acids, porphyrins and carotenoids (endogenously produced) may participate at different levels in the process of absorbing the light. The pigmentation of the skin is related to the amount of melanin in the keratinocytes. The varied content of melanin in the keratinocytes produce the wide spectrum of human skin color found in the different human races. Two classes of melanins are found in humans: the eumelanins which are brown to black pigments and the phaeomelanins which are yellow to reddish-brown.[1] Melanin absorbs in a decreasing manner from ultraviolet (UV) (highest absorption) to the visible light domain. On the other hand, hemoglobin in the dermal microvasculature contributes to the overall skin color with a dominant red for oxygenated hemoglobin and bluish red for reduced hemoglobin. Here again, the hemoglobin contribution to the skin color depends on the amount of melanin in the keratinocytes which acts as a neutral filter; it is readily visible in fair-skinned people, and hardly observable at all in deeply melanized skin.[2]

Examples of different types of UV-induced skin pigmentation are illustrated in Figures 25.1a (weak daily doses of UV sun-simulated irradiations) and 25.1b (Immediate Pigment Darkening (IPD) after UVA irradiation).

The need for assessment of the skin pigmentation extends from the dermato-cosmetology domain (including sunscreens, skin pigmenting or depigmenting products and make-up evaluations) to clinical dermatology for the characterization of the various types of pigmented skin lesions. The evaluation of skin pigmentation by visual examination depends not only on the subjective perception of colors by the observer but also on the nature of the illuminant and on the geometric position of the observer relative to the skin surface. Although the human eye is able to distinguish between hundreds of colors, the results of visual assessment remain subjective and qualitative with a poor reproducibility in time.

Several objective methods have been developed[3–5] to measure skin color and were proposed as commercially available devices. These are based on different approaches to the analysis of light reflected by the skin. One is the reflectance tristimulus CIE colorimetry[6,7] where the color of the skin can be expressed in a three-dimensional coordinate space. Other techniques are based on reflectance spectrophotometry. One, scanning reflectance spectrophotometry,[8,9] analyses the spectrum of light reflected by the skin, typically between 400 nm and 700 nm, and allows the obtaining of information on chromophore content. On the other hand, the narrow-band reflectance spectrophotometry[10,11] measures the reflected light only in the specific narrow-bands of absorption of melanin and hemoglobin in order to provide melanin and erythema indexes. Beside these methods which give an average color measurement of a 0.5–1 cm^2 skin area, other techniques are based on image analysis of the skin. Some of

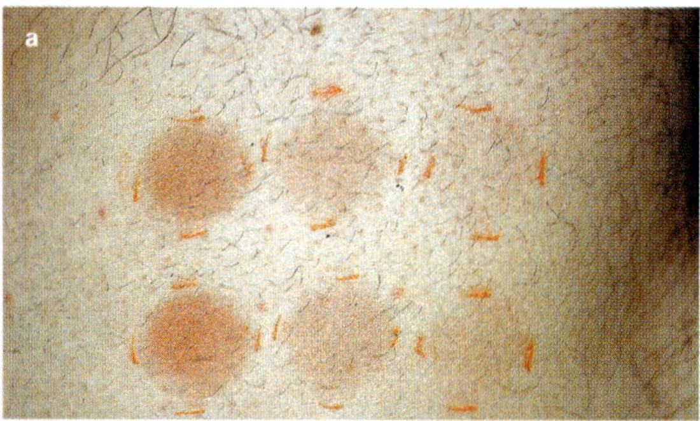

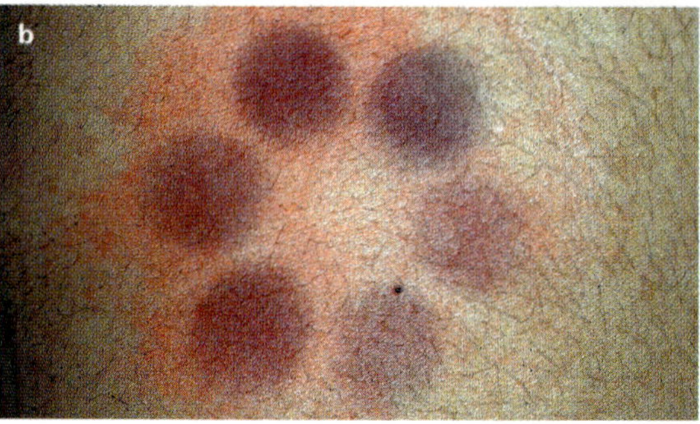

Figure 25.1

(a) Skin pigmentation induced after 10 days of daily infra MED UV sun-simulated doses (0.75, 0.5 and 0.25 MED). (b) IPD observed just after irradiation; UVA doses (from 22 to 67 J/cm^2) administered in a circular manne). MED, minimal erythema dose; IPD, immediate pigment darkening.

these techniques, taking into account the skin color heterogeneity, aim to determine the color of a very specific skin surface on digitized images.[12,13] Finally, thanks to the improvement of digital image processing technology and to the high quality of the available video camera, the technique of epiluminescence microscopy, e.g. dermatoscopy,[14,15] offers a very promising tool to allow the dermatologist to perform a very accurate non invasive diagnosis of pigmented skin lesions.

Visual assessment of skin pigmentation

The eye is the first diagnostic tool of the dermatologist. Color perception is the result of radiant electromagnetic radiations in the 'visible' wavelength range, 400–700 nm, collected by the eye and interpreted by the brain. Thus, color perception includes physical and psychophysiological aspects. The human eye is known to have a high power of discrimination between colors including shades and hues.[16,17] Factors which can produce errors in the visual color evaluation are the spectrum of ambient light, the color of surrounding objects and background. Moreover, visual memory concerning colors is not time predictable making repetitive evaluations not reliable.

Nevertheless, using a standardized environment and grading skin color with either standard color references such as Munsell standards or very precise rating scales may lead to a reliable visual color assessments. Results are particularly interesting in the case of comparative studies where multiple zones are assessed simultaneously.

As an example, Figure 25.2 illustrates the results of a study[18] in which the Persistent Pigment Darkening (PPD) induced by UVA (100 J/cm^2) was used to compare the protection afforded by ten commercially available sunscreens containing different UVA filtration systems. The products were applied 15 minutes before UVA exposure from a solar simulator at a rate of 2 mg/cm^2 on a group of ten subjects and at 1 mg/cm^2 on a second group of ten subjects. Two hours after UVA exposure, the pigmentation intensity was assessed by a trained observer using a 0 to 10-point grading scale and also by colorimetry (Chromameter CR200, Minolta, Osaka, Japan) in the L*, a*, b* mode. The results indicated a good correlation between both methods of evaluation (correlation coefficient = 0.82) which produced a similar product ranking.

Reflectance tristimulus CIE colorimetry

The colorimetry tristimulus system is based on the following two principles: the first is that each color can be matched by a suitable mixture of three selected light radiations, the second is that if two colors are matched by three radiations, the mixture of these two colors is found additive by suitable optical means. In 1931, the 'Commission Internationale de l'Eclairage (CIE)' standardized the color mixture characteristics of an 'average observer' and developed a standard framework for

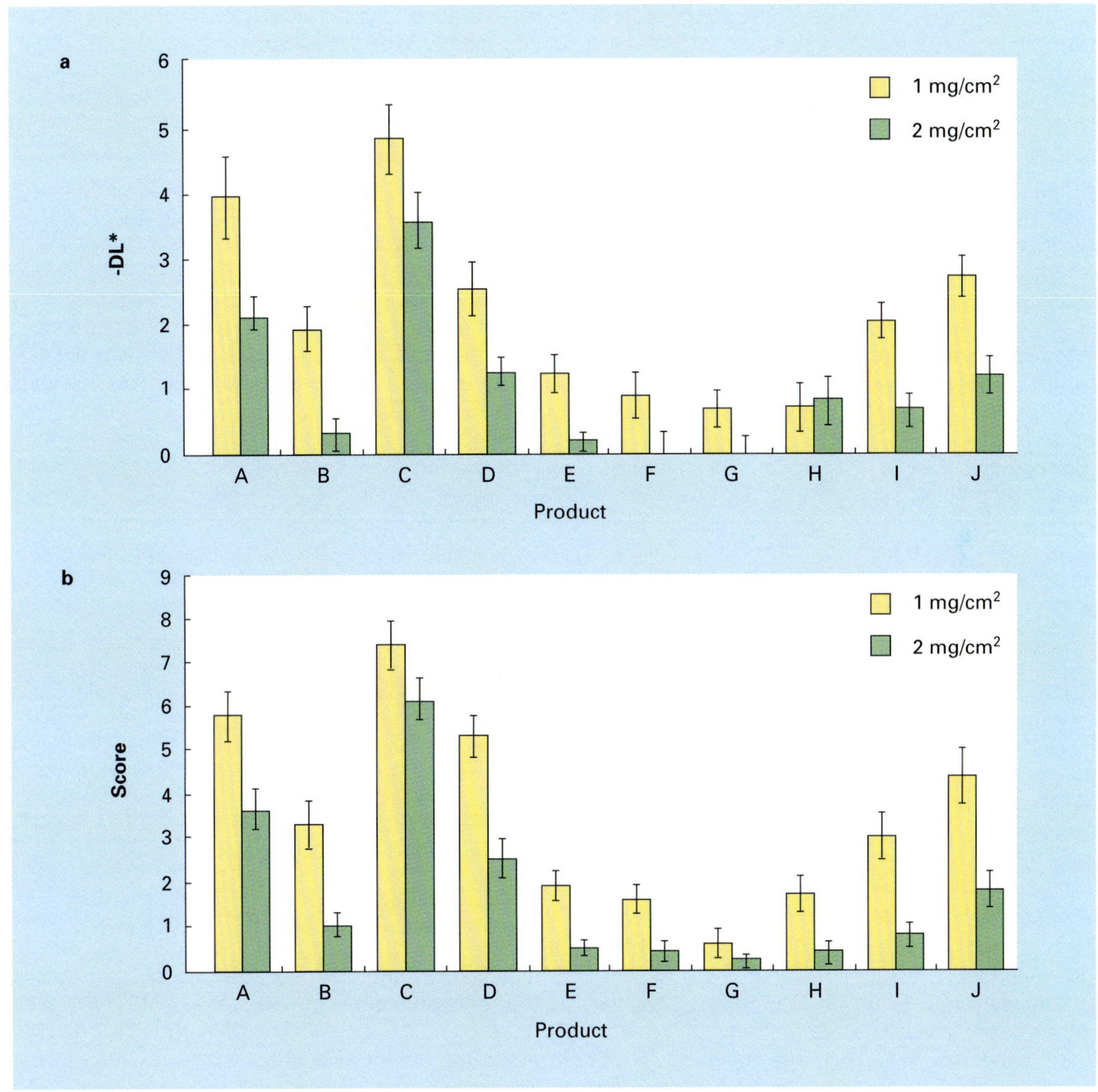

Figure 25.2

Colorimetric (a) and visual (b) evaluations of pigmentation intensity (persistent pigment darkening induced by UVA) for comparison of UVA protection activity of sunscreens (mean ± SEM).

a color specification. The standard observer is represented by functions which were determined from data obtained from series of observers matching the color at each wavelength from 400 to 700 nm with appropriate mixtures from three primary light sources. In this system, each color is defined with a set of three tristimulus primary values (X: red content, Y: green content, Z: blue content). From these values, the YXY color system is calculated, where Y is the lightness factor expressed as a percentage based on a perfect reflectance = 100% (perfect white surface) and the X and Y values are the chromaticity coordinates whose combination gives hue and chroma (saturation). The drawback of the CIE 1931 YXY system is that equal distances in the chromaticity X,Y diagram do not represent equal differences in color as perceived by the human eye. This was corrected in the CIE 1976 L* a* b* color system which more closely represents the human eye sensitivity to color. The L*, a*, b* coordinates are also calculated from the X, Y, and Z tristimulus primary values. In the L*a*b* color space, L* is the lightness ranging from 0 (black) to 100 (white), a* is the balance between red (positive values) and green (negative values) and b* is the balance between yellow (positive values) and blue (negative values).

Based on the accumulation of numerous measurements of skin color using colorimetry (Minolta chromameters CR200 and CR300) Chardon and coworkers[19,20] have shown that all the different types of basal skin color (stable state) for a selected body site (the back for example) are located inside a very determined volume in the L*a*b* color space. The volume of skin color has a vertical arched shape as shown in Figure 25.3. In this volume, the points of color are distributed from top to bottom as a function of the natural melanic pigmentation intensity with the nonmelanized skin (albino) at the top and very dark skin at the bottom. The points constitute the melanization axis which structures the volume along its longer axis and are distributed in its section as a function of the hue and chroma afforded by the natural skin pigment mixing (melanin, hemoglobin, carotenoids, etc.). Figure 25.3 indicates also that the direction of color changes in the volume depends of the skin pigment involved in the reaction related to the skin color variation. For example, following a UVA irradiation (Fig. 25.1b), the induced IPD does not follow the melanization axis but a different direction due to the fact that IPD is the bluish coloration generated by photo-oxidized melanins already present in the skin. This bluish color is expressed by a decrease of the b* component. On the other hand, the induction of an erythema translates the skin color point outside the melanization axis towards the colorimetric coordinate of hemoglobins ($L^* \approx 45$, $a^* \approx 45$, $b^* \approx 18$). Finally, the UV-induced neomelanization process translates the skin color point along the melanization axis towards the colorimetric coordinates of melanins ($L^* \approx 20$, $a^* \approx 0.2$, $b^* \approx 0.5$).

The vectorial representation of skin color points in the L*a*b* volume allows the analysis of the tanning pathways after UV irradiation. Following ultraviolet irradiation, the change of skin color induced by the variation of the pigment(s) involved in the phenomenon is expressed by the shift of the basal color point towards the color coordinates of the target pigment(s). It is interesting to note that the tanning pathways can be differentiated in intensity, hue, kinetics and lasting effects according to the nature of the UV spectrum (UVA or UVB or UVB + UVA).[21]

Since Caucasian skin has a yellow/orange aspect, the constitutional pigmentation is well described in the L* vs. b* plane. Thus, sectors of skin color categories have been delineated[19] to correspond roughly to the skin phototypes.[22] The sectors are delimited by radii originating from $L^* = 50$ and $b^* = 0$ and constitute defined angles with the b* axis (Fig. 25.4). Therefore, a subject can be characterized by the so-called individual typology angle (ITA°) which is calculated by:

$$\text{ITA}° = \text{Arctangent}\,((L^*-50)/b^*) \times 180/\pi$$

The values proposed for the angles of skin categories boundaries were:

Very light skin > 55° > Light skin > 41°
> Intermediate skin > 28° > Tanned skin > 10°

It has been shown[23] that the use of ITA° allows the determination of the range of UV doses needed to induce a minimal erythema (minimal erythema dose (MED) determination without prior irradiation).

Colorimetry has been extensively used to assess the process of UV-induced hyperpigmentation,[5,24] skin typology[25,26] and photoprotection factors.[27,28] Figure 25.5 illustrates the effects of cumulated suberythemal UV doses (sun-simulated spectrum) on skin pigmentation. Even very weak daily UV doses as low as 0.25 MED are able to induce detectable photopigmentation (decrease of L*) after ten exposures. This technique was proposed as an objective method to assess the UVA protection factor of sunscreens based on the measurement of the intensity of PPD induced by UVA.[29]

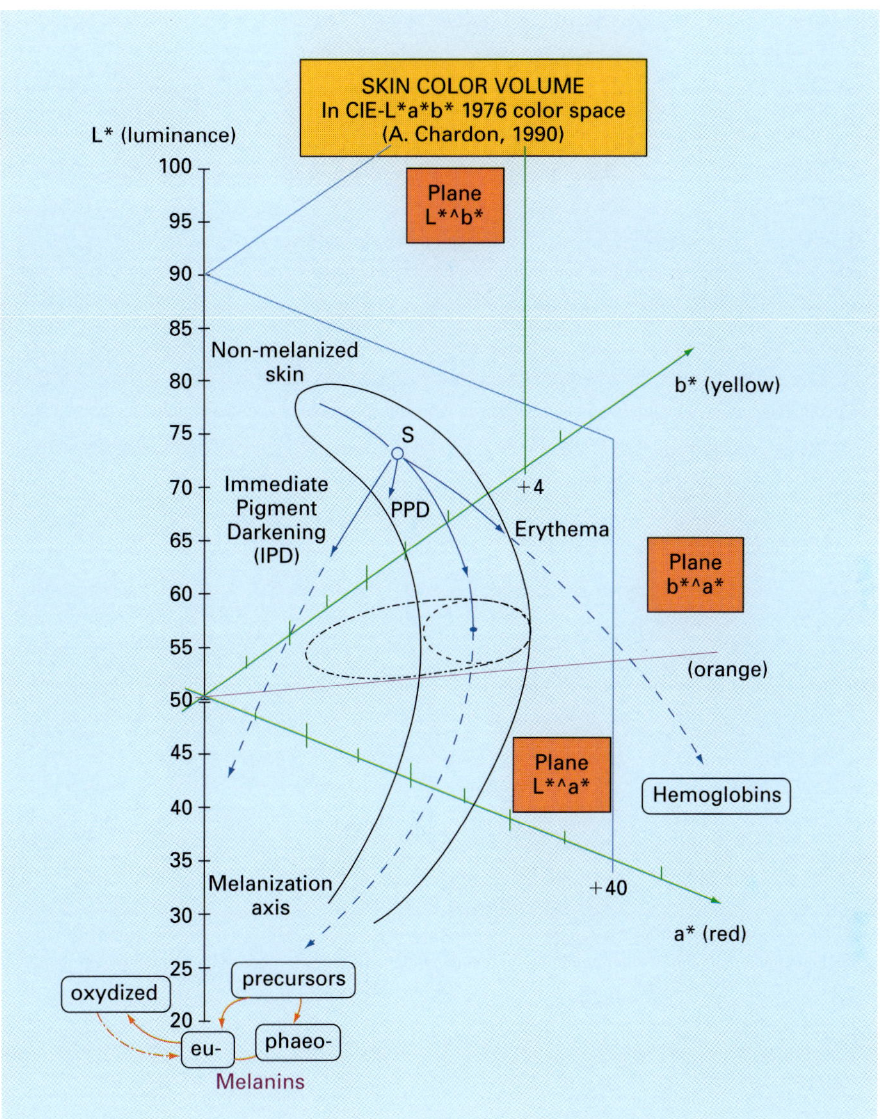

Figure 25.3

The skin color volume in the CIE L*, a*, b* color space (with permission of A. Chardon[22]).

Reflectance spectrophotometry

Reflectance spectroscopy

The scanning reflectance spectroscopy[8,9] analyses the spectrum of light reflected by the skin, typically between 400 nm and 700 nm, and allows the investigator to measure skin color and to obtain information on skin chromophore content. The optical properties of the skin are determined by the spectral absorption, reflection and scattering of the light as it strikes and penetrates the different cutaneous structures. The scanning reflectance spectrometer is built to measure the

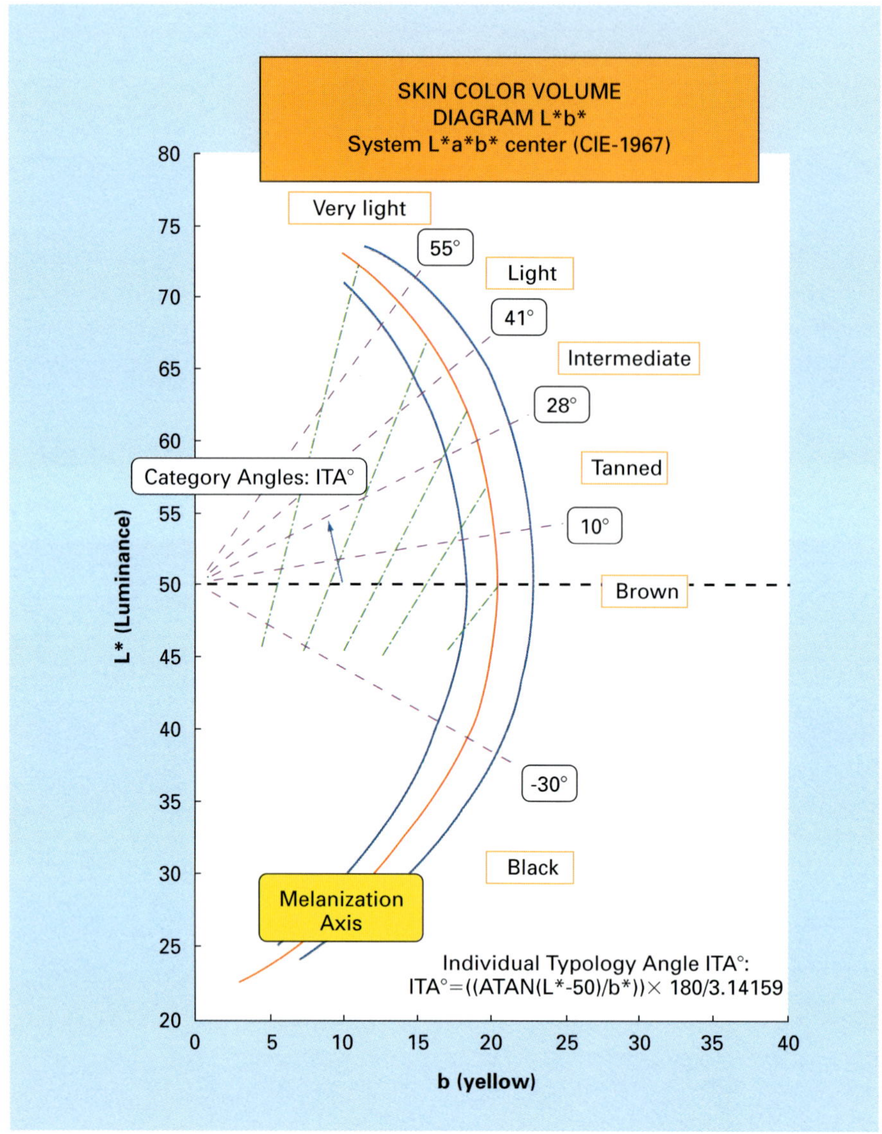

Figure 25.4

Skin color domain in the L* vs. b* plane. Sectors of skin color category are delimited by category angles (with permission of A. Chardon[22]).

diffuse reflectance of the light, i.e. the part of the light that was modified by the absorption, reflection and scattering processes inside the skin, and that was re-emitted from the skin. This technique is also called diffuse reflectance spectroscopy.[30] The instrumental setup consists of: a light source, such as a xenon short arc lamp or a tungsten halogen lamp; a measuring head which is an integrating sphere; an optical system (monochromator or equivalent) to decompose and analyse the light re-emitted by the skin; and a photodetector to measure the light intensity in the different bands of wavelength. A system of optical guides (bundles of optical fibers) conducts the light from the

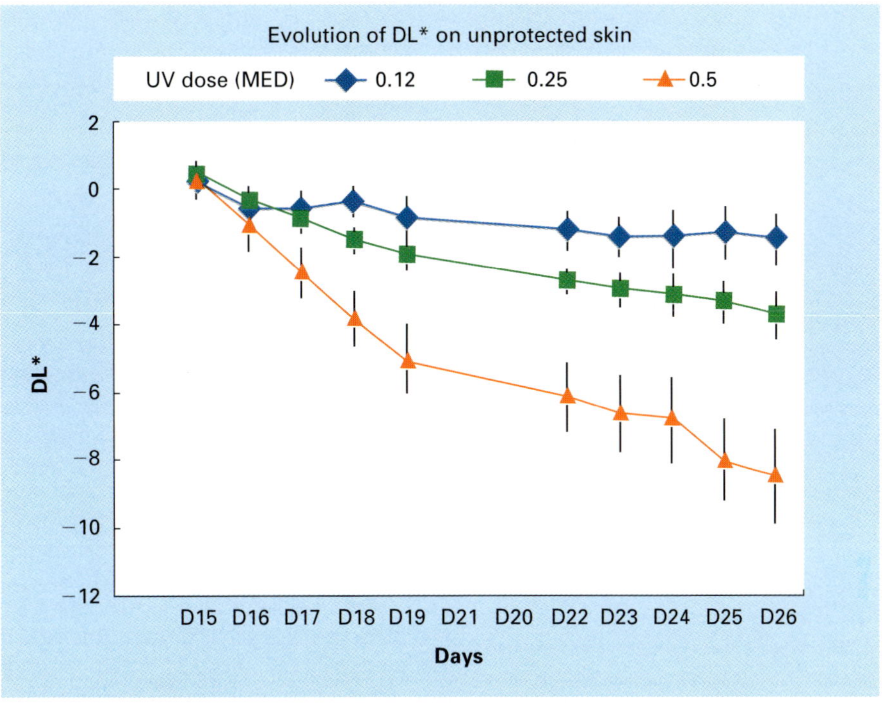

Figure 25.5

Effect of daily suberythemal UV doses (0.12, 0.25 and 0.5 MED) on skin pigmentation measured by DL* (L* on exposed skin – L* on control skin). Bars represent SEM. MED, minimal erythema dose.

source to the skin and from the skin to the monochromator and the photodetector. In some handheld instruments (Minolta 508, Osaka, Japan), the distance between the light source and the skin surface is short (about 10 cm) and the reflected light is measured by a photodiode array covered by a wedge filter.

Generally, a three-layer model is used to describe the optical properties of the skin in mathematical calculations.[31–33] The first layer, the stratum corneum, which induces mainly forward scattering, involves only a very small percentage of the total skin reflectance (at normal incidence) and thus is neglected to simplify the calculations. Light that penetrates the epidermis is mainly absorbed by melanin with the strongest absorption in the near UV range. In the dermis, both oxygenized and deoxygenized hemoglobins absorb in the ranges 405–430 nm and 540–575 nm. *In vivo*, the hemoglobin content is most easily evaluated in the range 540–575 nm where melanin affects the light absorption to a lesser extent. Light scattering by the dermal collagen matrix (without absorption) can be added in the model. Thus, the light scattered and reflected by the dermal structures goes back to the surface, passing through hemoglobin and melanin-containing layers twice. An example of skin reflectance spectra (presented as absorption spectra) is illustrated in the Figure 25.6. On this figure, compared to the normal skin spectrum, the differences of a heavily pigmented skin lesion (lentigo) spectrum and a deeply vascularized lesion (raised red spot) are clearly observable.

The methods of calculation are based on the use of pigment indexes to describe changes in skin color. A method was proposed[8] to calculate the relative amounts of the different chromophores present in the skin by using a multiple regression method to calculate reflectance spectroscopic data and taking into account the *in vitro* absorbance spectra of the skin pigments determined by prior analysis. Thus, reflectance spectroscopy, using a computerized method, allows transcutaneous analysis of the relative amount of

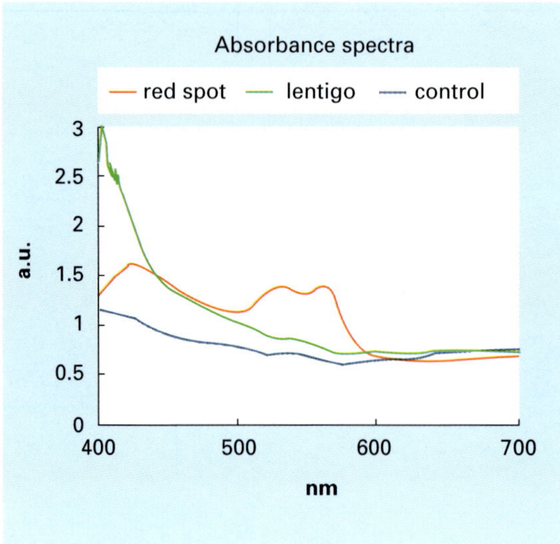

Figure 25.6

Absorbance spectra (arbitrary unit) of three types of skin area: a pigmented lentigo (shape of typical melanin absorbance curve), a raised red spot (shape of typical hemoglobin absorbance curve, absorption peaks of oxyhemoglobin visible at 542 and 577 nm) and a control skin area. Measurements performed with a Diffuse Reflectance Spectrometer (Canfield Scientific system, Fairfield, NJ, USA).

oxygenized and deoxygenized hemoglobins and melanin in the skin. However, the interpretation of the results requires expertise and the results may be influenced when there is a high quantity of one chromophore compared to the others. A study[34] has shown that spectroscopic patterns are influenced by probe application pressure and body location indicating that highly standardized conditions are needed to obtain reliable data.

Nevertheless, a recent study[35] aimed to document the optical reflectance (range 320–1100 nm) characteristics of pigmented skin lesions and to evaluate their potential for improving the differential diagnosis of malignant melanoma from benign pigmented skin lesions. Characteristic differences in spectra from benign and malignant lesions were studied and showed significant differences between lesion groups classified by histology. This simple objective technique appeared to perform as well as the expert dermatologist and could improve the diagnostic accuracy of non-specialists such as trainees and general practitioners (GPs).

Finally, in order to describe relevant clinical parameters, analysis of some specific absorption bands or peaks of the absorption spectra allow the calculation of very reliable erythema and melanin indexes.[8,30]

Narrow band reflectance spectroscopy

The reflectance spectrophotometers are known to be expensive, cumbersome and not well adapted for the routine clinical uses. Since the spectrophotometric measurements result often in the analysis of some specific narrow bands or peaks of spectra corresponding to the absorption bands of the main chromophores of the skin, the use of simpler and cheaper devices based on narrowband analysis was developed.

The Mexameter MX16® (Courage-Khazaka, Elelectronik, Köln, Germany) is equipped with 16 light-emitting diodes (LED) arranged circularly and emitting at 568 nm (green), 660 nm (red) and 880 nm (infrared). The positions of emitter and receiver (Fig. 25.7) guarantee that only diffuse and scattered light is measured. As the quantity of emitted light is defined, the quantity of light absorbed by the skin can be calculated. The system is based on the principles described by Diffey et al.[36] The melanin index (mx) is measured at two wavelengths (660 and 880 nm). These wavelengths have been chosen in order to achieve different absorption rates by the melanin pigments. For the erythema index (ex), two different wavelengths are used to measure the absorption capacity of the skin. One of these wavelengths corresponds to the spectral absorption peak of hemoglobin (568 nm) and the other wavelength (660 nm) has been chosen to avoid other color influences (e.g. bilirubin).

The intensities of the different wavelengths are electronically processed in real time and the indexes are shown on two clear digital displays:

$$mx = \frac{500}{\log 5}\left(\log \frac{\text{Infrared} - \text{Reflection}}{\text{Red} - \text{Reflection}} + \log 5\right)$$

$$ex = \frac{500}{\log 5}\left(\log \frac{\text{Red} - \text{Reflection}}{\text{Green} - \text{Reflection}} + \log 5\right)$$

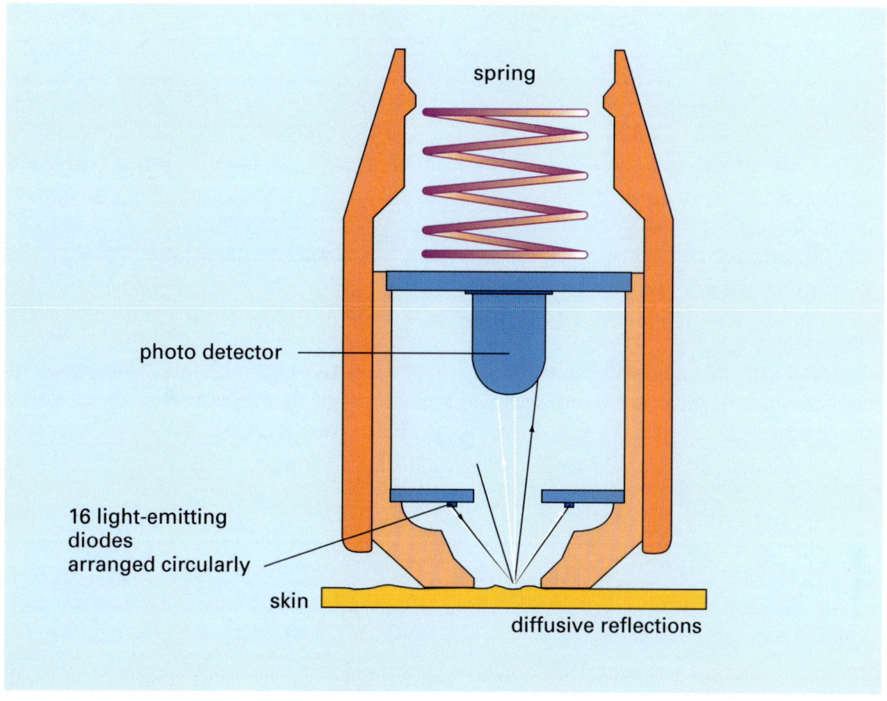

Figure 25.7

Cross-section of the measuring head of the Mexameter 16®. A spring in the measuring head provides constant pressure on the skin. The low weight (55 g) of the probe supports the easy handling.

The maximum ratio between each color is 1: 5. Thus, the range is 0–1000 with 500 being the value which corresponds to a ratio of 1:1. The higher the values the more melanin or erythema is detected. A spring in the measuring head provides constant pressure on the skin. The measuring area is 5 mm in diameter (0.2 cm^2).

Other types of narrow-band spectrophotometers such as the DermaSpectrometer (Cortex Technology, Hadsund Denmark) are based on two LEDs whose bands are centered in the green (568 nm) and in the red (655 nm). The erythema index is also calculated from the ratio of red to green reflected light intensities. The melanin index is obtained from the inverse of reflected light intensity.

Several studies[3,37] have been performed to compare narrow-band spectrophotometers to tristimulus colorimeter. The results showed that both types of instruments are able to detect very small changes in skin color. The correlation between the instruments were found to be moderately good between L* and the melanin indexes, and good between a* and the erythema indexes.

Various type applications of assessment of the cutaneous pigmentation by narrow-band spectrophotometers were performed including, for example, UV-induced pigmentation,[38,39] efficacy of depigmenting agent[40] and protection of vitiligo.[41] Skin typology[42,43] and epidemiology[44] produced numerous subjects of works. In the retrospective skin cancer case–control studies, there are major difficulties in estimating sun exposure during the lifetime of subjects because no suitable objective measurements are available.

Skin reflectance spectroscopy was recently[44] used to investigate age and gender trends in facultative and constitutive skin pigmentation in 653 Caucasians who were not using artificial tanning devices. Constitutive pigmentation at the buttocks was highest in the first years of life and then decreased substantially during the first two decades of life. After the age of 25 years, buttock pigmentation remained at a constant level. There was no gender difference in constitutive pigmentation. Facultative skin pigmentation increased with age for all the measured sites with the highest levels found at the lateral aspect of the upper arm. Based on objective measurements of skin pigmentation in this study, the authors proposed the concept of a 'sun exposure index' (SEI) which is calculated as the increase in facultative pigmentation above the constitutive level and is expressed as a percentage of the constitutive level. The SEI appeared to be related to cumulative lifetime UV exposure and may be used in epidemiological research as an objective estimate of UV exposure at different body sites in Caucasians. In another study,[45] the same authors found that the SEI was not significantly different between basal cell carcinoma patients and controls, whereas male cutaneous malignant melanoma patients had higher estimates for the lateral side of the upper arm, the chest and the back.

Dermatoscopy and skin imaging systems

Dermatoscopy (dermoscopy, epiluminescence microscopy, incident light microscopy, skin surface microscopy) is an *in vivo* noninvasive diagnostic technique allowing the observation of pigmented skin lesions.[15,46] With the progress of both hand-held optics and digital imaging techniques, recent developments of dermatoscopy have been shown to improve the diagnostic accuracy of pigmented skin lesions.

The technical set-up consists of a magnifying optical system (surface microscope, stereomicroscope, hand-held scope) allowing magnification of the lesion image. The lesion is covered with an immersion oil or any kind of liquid including water and alcohol in order to eliminate surface reflections of the illuminating light. This makes the stratum corneum translucent, enabling the visualization of pigmented structures of the epidermis and of the dermal–epidermal junction and superficial papillary dermis which are impossible to observe with the naked eye. The vessels of the superficial vascular plexus can be also observed. Most of the instruments allow 10-fold magnification, but magnifications of up to 100-fold are possible. The most advanced systems are equipped with a high-resolution video camera incorporated directly in the probe and connected to a microcomputer where digitized images are stored and processed with dedicated software.

Figure 25.8 illustrates the comparison of classical macrophotography and dermatoscopy. Reflections at the surface are now more visible with dermatosocopy and the fine structures of the lesion can be readily observed. On this figure, the classical image of melanoma can be observed showing an irregular pigment network with abrupt limits on a part of the periphery of the lesion and also with an irregular distribution of pseudopods. This figure displays the evolution of a melanoma from time zero (T0) (top) to T0 + 6 months as well.

Various diagnostic systems have been proposed for assessing dermatoscopic images. All systems take into account local and global features. For example, in the ABCD system, the investigator has to score asymmetry (A), borders (B), colors (C) and number of different dermatoscopic structures (D). For all the diagnostic systems, the color aspect of the pigmentation of the lesion is crucial, including the number of different colors, aspect of pigment networks, distribution of pigments and shape margin of pigmented areas. It is probable that color analysis performed directly on the different pigmented structures of the lesion image using one of the techniques described above would improve the potential of dermatoscopy to accurately diagnose pigmented skin lesions. This implies the resolution of technical problems such as the use a very stable illuminating system (in intensity and spectrum) associated with a constant color reference.

Some works have been performed in that way. A new imaging colorimeter (Visi-Chroma VC-100, Biophotonics, Lessines, Belgium) based on a charge coupled device (CCD) camera with tristimulus color analysis has been developed in order to measure the color in any part of a digitized image.[13] The measuring head of this instrument is equivalent to the head of a dermatoscope. Another similar system developed by Takiwaki et al.[12] was based on the analysis of brightness intensity of any picture element in the bands of red, green and blue color. After deriving absorbance indexes from the mean brightness of each band, the results showed good correlation with *in vivo* UV-induced erythema and pigmentation and also with *in vitro*

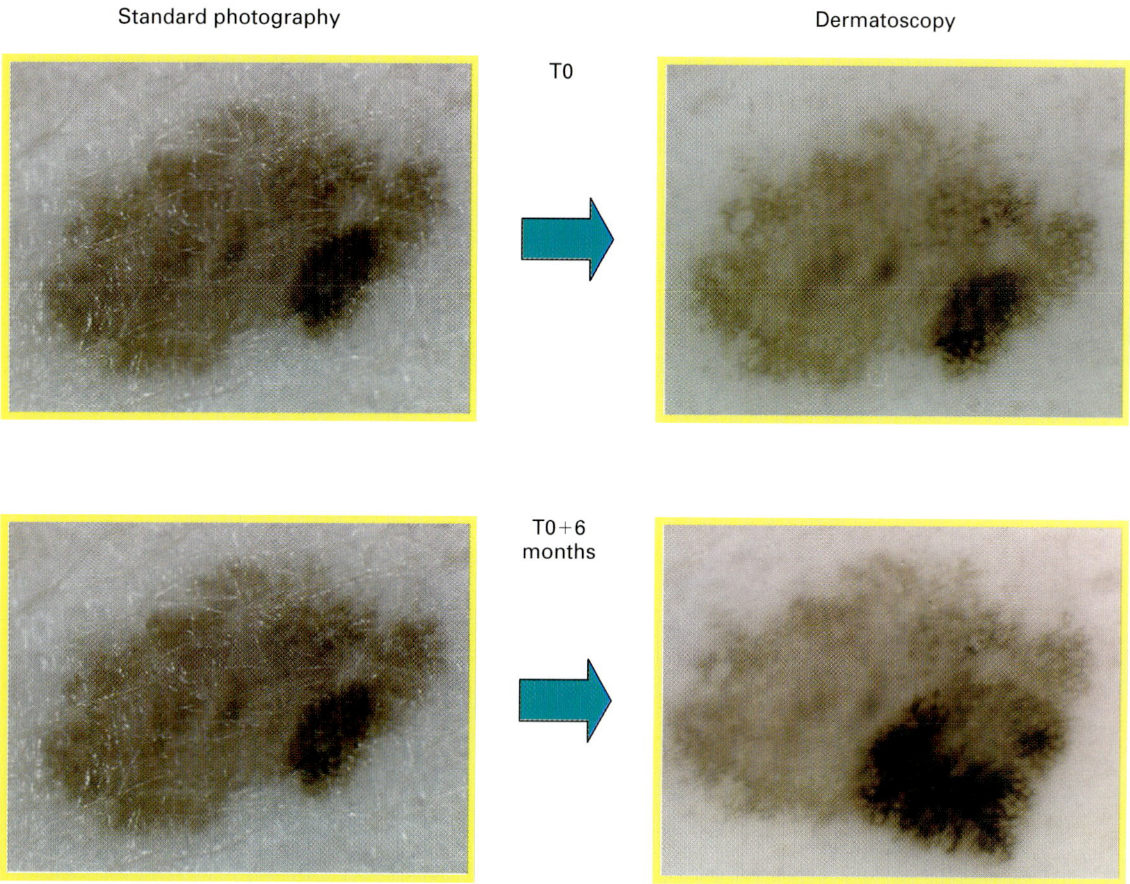

Figure 25.8

Comparison of classical macrophotography and dermatoscopy. There was a 6–month time interval between top and bottom photos (Dr. P. Bahadoran, dermatology Dept, Hôpital L'Archet, Nice, France). T0, time zero.

measurements on different concentrations of melanin and hemoglobin.

Finally, the classical photography technique performed in Wood's light is also a useful method to visualize skin pigmentation.[47,48] This technique, using UV transparent silica optical lens, is based on the filtering of the light emitted by the flash using a UVA band pass filter. The hyperpigmented skin areas such as solar lentigos (Fig. 25.10) appear darker on the black and white image compared to 'normal skin' because of the fact that melanin absorbs heavily in the UVA domain. On the other hand, depigmented lesions, such as vitiligo macules (Fig. 25.11) are displayed as white areas on the skin. Here again, the processing of these kinds of images by dedicated grey-level analysis software could increase the objective quantification level of this technique.

Conclusion

Skin pigmentation can be assessed using a wide variety of techniques. The choice depends on the objectives of the investigator. Two kinds of measurements can be identified; the first is related to the measure of skin pigmentation as a whole, i.e. as is needed in skin UV interaction

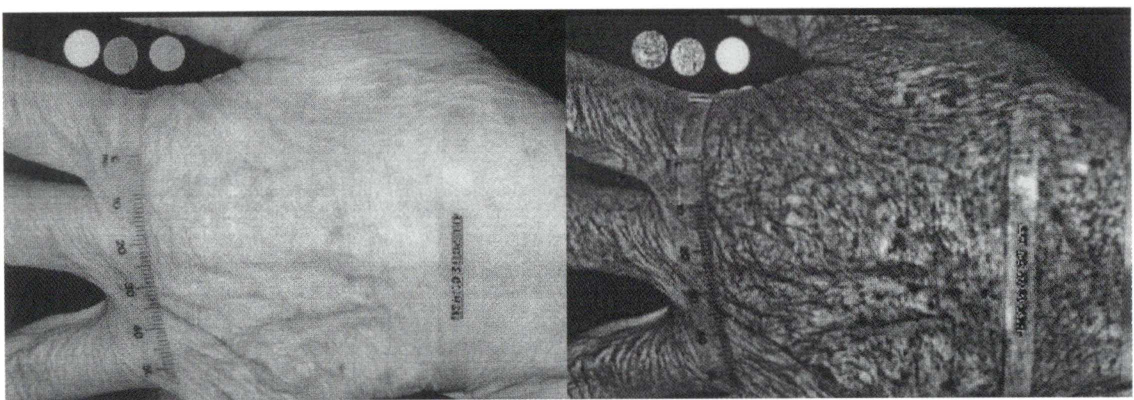

Figure 25.9

Skin lentigos (right) are enhanced by Wood's light photography (Canfield system, Fairfield, NJ, USA) compared to classical 'white light' photography (left).

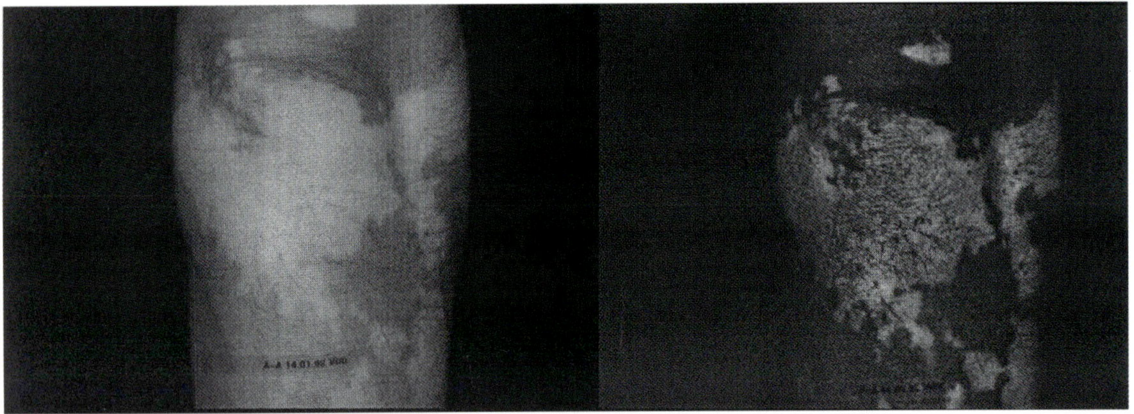

Figure 25.10

Contrast of vitiligo macules (right) is increased using Wood's light photography (Canfield system, Fairfield, NJ, USA).

studies (photoprotection, phototherapy) or skin typology and epidemiology studies; the second refers to the diagnostic assessments of pigmented skin lesion in which the accurate measurement of hue and chroma of the substructures of the pigmented lesion are very important. Nonspecific optical methods such as tristimulus colorimetry and reflectance spectroscopy are quite suitable for the first type of studies whereas techniques based on dermoscopic image analysis (descriptive or computerized) such as dermatoscopy are more appropriate for the second.

References

1. Fitzpatrick TB, Szabo G, Seiji M, et al. Biology of the melanin pigmentary system. In: *Dermatology in general medicine* (McGraw Hill: 1979) 131.
2. Diffey BL, Robson J, The influence of pigmentation and illumination on the perception of erythema, *Photodermatol Photoimmunol Photomed* (1992) **9**:45–7.
3. Takiwaki H, Overgaard L, Serup J, Comparison of narrow-band reflectance spectrophotometric and tristimulus colorimetric measurements of skin color, *Skin Pharmacol* (1994) **7**:217–55.

4. Fullerton A, Fischer T, Lahti A et al., Guidelines for measurements of skin colour and erythema, *Contact Dermatitis* (1996) **31**:1–10.
5. Seitz JC, Whitmore CG, Measurement of erythema and tanning responses in human skin using a tristimulus colorimeter, *Dermatological* (1988) **177**:70–5.
6. Weatherall IL, Coombs BD, Skin color measurements in terms of CIELAB color space values, *J Invest Dermatol* (1992) **99**:468–73.
7. Piérard GE, EEMCO guidance for the assessment of skin colour, *J Eur Acad Dermatol Venerol* (1998) **10**:1–11.
8. Andersen PH, Bjerring P, Nonivasive computerized analysis of skin chromophores *in vivo* by reflectance spectroscopy, *Photodermatol Photoimmunol Photomed* (1990) **7**:249–57.
9. Lock-Andersen J, Gniadecka M, de Fine Olivarius F et al., Skin temperature of UV-induced erythema correlated to laser Doppler flowmetry and skin reflectance measured redness, *Skin Res Technol* (1998) **4**:41–8.
10. Lock-Andersen J, Therkildsen P, de Fine Olivarius F et al., Epidermal thickness, skin pigmentation and constitutive photosensitivity, *Photodermatol Photoimmunol Photomed* (1997) **13**:153–8.
11. Feather J, Ellis DJ, Leslie G, A portable reflectometer for the rapid quantification of cutaneous haemoglobin and melanin, *Phys Med Biol* (1988) **33**:711–22.
12. Takiwaki H, Shirai S, Kanno Y et al., Quantification of erythema and pigmentation using a videomicroscope and a computer, *Br J Dermtol* (1994) **131**:85–92.
13. Barel AO, Clarys P, Alewaeters K et al., The Visi-Chroma VC-100®: a new imaging colorimeter for dermatocosmetic research, *Skin Res Technol* (2001) **7**:24–31.
14. Hofmann-Wellenhof R, Soyer HP, Wolf IH et al., Ultraviolet radiation of melanocytic nevi: a dermoscopic study, *Arch Dermatol* (1998) **134**:845–50.
15. Soyer HP, Argenziano G, Chimenti S et al., Dermoscopy of pigmented skin lesions. *Eur J Dermatol* (2001) **11**:270–6.
16. Wassermann HP, The colour of human skin. Spectral reflectance versus skin colour, *Dermatologica* (1971) **143**:166–73.
17. Bornstein M, Color and its measurements, *J Soc Cosmetic Chemists* (1968) **19**:649–67.
18. Moyal D, Duteil L, Queille-Roussel C et al., Comparison of UVA protection afforded by sunscreens with high sun protection factor. Poster, 10th Congress, Euro Acad Dermatol Venereol Munich (2001).
19. Chardon A, Cretois I, Hourseau C, Skin colour typology and suntanning pathways, *Int J Cosmet Sci* (1991) **13**:191–208.
20. Chardon A, Moyal D, Bories MF et al., Comparing suntans from actual sun using various SPF sunscreens, *Cosm and toilet* (1993) **79**:9.
21. Chardon A, Cretois I, Hourseau C, Color changes induced on various skin categories by repeated exposures to UV rays, *Biological Responses to UVA Radiation* (1992) 159–75.
22. Fitzpatrick TB, The validity and practicality of sun-reactive skin type I through VI (Editorial), *Arch Dermatol* (1988) **77**:219–21.
23. Masson P, Mérot F, Phototype and ITA° parameters as predictive for determination of MED and SPF in tanned or untanned subjects, Poster; Preprints 17th IFSCC Congress, Yokohama, October 1992.
24. Park SB, Suh DH, Youn JI, A long-term time course of colorimetric evaluation of ultraviolet light-induced skin reactions, *Clin Exp Dermatol* (1999) **24**:315–20.
25. Roh K-Y, Kim D, Ha S-J et al., Pigmentation in Koreans: study of the differences from Caucasians in age, gender and seasonal variations, *Br J Dermatol* (2001) **144**:94–9.
26. Andreassi L, Casini L, Simoni S et al., Measurement of cutaneous colour and assessment of skin type, *Photodermatol Photoimmunol Photomed* (1990) **7**:20–4.
27. Ferguson J, Brown M, Alert D et al., Collaborative development of a sun protection factor test method: a proposed European standard, *Int J Cosmet Sci* (1996) **18**:203–18.
28. Chardon A, Dupont G, Hourseau C et al., Colorimetric determination of sun-protection-factor. Poster. 15th IFSCC Congress. London, Preprints A/A24;1988, 313–22,9.
29. Moyal D, Chardon A, Kollias N, UVA protection efficacy of sunscreens can be determined by the persistent pigment darkening (PPD) method (Part 2), *Photodermatol Photoimmunol Photomed* (2000) **16**:250–5.
30. Kollias N, Baquer A, Sadiq I, Minimum erythema dose determination in individuals of skin type V and VI with diffuse reflectance spectroscopy, *Photoimmunol Photomed* (1994) **10**:249–54.
31. Bjerring P, Andersen PH, Skin reflectance spectrophotometry, *Photodermatol Photoimmunol Photomed* (1987) **4**:167–71.
32. Andersen PH, Bjerring P, A comparative evaluation of sun protective properties of a shea butter by reflectance spectroscopy, laser Doppler flowmetry

and visual scoring, *Skin Pharmacol Toxicol* (1990) **181**:267–76.

33. Anderson RR, Parrish JA, Optical properties of human skin, In: Reagen JD, Parrish JA, eds. *The science of photomedecine*; (Plenum Press: New York, 1982) 147–93.
34. Karamfilov T, Weichold S, Karte K et al., Remittance spectroscopy mapping of human skin *in vivo*. *Skin Res Technol* (1999) **5**:49–52.
35. Wallace VP, Crawford DC, Mortimer PS et al., Spectrophotometric assessment of pigmented skin lesions: methods and feature selection for evaluation of diagnostic performance, *Phys Med Biol* (2000) **45**:735–51.
36. Diffey BL, Oliver RJ, Farr PM, A portable instrument for quantifying erythema induced by ultraviolet radiation, *Br J Dermatol* (1984) **111**:663–72.
37. Clarys P, Alewaeters K, Lambrecht R et al., Skin color measurements: comparison between three instruments: the Chromameter®, the DermaSpectrometer® and the Mexameter®, *Skin Res Technol* (2000) **6**:230–8.
38. Farr PM, Besag BL, Diffey BL, The time course of UVB and UVC erythema, *J Invest Dermatol* (1988) **91**:454–7.
39. Seitz JC, Withmore CG, Measurement of erythema and tanning responses in human skin using a tristimulus colorimeter, *Dermatologica* (1988) **177**:70–5.
40. Poli F, Lakhdar H, Souissi R et al., Evaluation clinique de l'efficacité dépigmentante d'une crème: TRIO-D dans les melasma du visage, *Nouv Dermatol* (1997) **16**:1–7.
41. Gniadecka M, Wulf HC, Mortensen N et al., Photoprotection in vitiligo and normal skin *Acta Derm Venereol* (1996) **76**:429–32.
42. Hermanns JF, Petit L, Hermanns-Lê T et al., Analytic quantification of phototype-related regional skin complexion, *Skin Res Technol* (2001) **7**:168–71.
43. Lock-Andersen J, Wulf HC, Knudstorp ND, Skin pigmentation in Caucasian babies is high and evenly distributed throughout the body, *Photodermatol Photoimmunol Photomed* (1998) **14**:74–6.
44. Lock-Andersen J, Knudstorp ND, Wulf HC, Facultative skin pigmentation in caucasians: an objective biological indicator of lifetime exposure to ultraviolet radiation? *J Med Invest* (1998) **44**:121–6.
45. Lock-Andersen J, Drzewiecki KT, Wulf HC, The measurement of constitutive and facultative skin pigmentation and estimation of sun exposure in Caucasians with basal cell carcinoma and cutaneous malignant melanoma, *Br J Dermatol* (1998) **139**:610–17.
46. Carli P, De Giorgi V, Soyer HP, Dermatoscopy in the diagnosis of pigmented skin lesions: a new semiology for the dermatologist, *J Eur Acad Dermatol Venerol* (2000) **14**:353–69.
47. Fulton JE, Utilizing the ultraviolet (UV Detect) camera to enhance the appearance of photodamage and other skin conditions, *Dermatol Surg* (1997) **23**:163–9.
48. Garcia A, Fulton JE, The combination of glycolic acid and hydroquinone or kojic acid for the treatment of melasma and related conditions, *Dermatol Surg* (1996) **22**:443–7.

26

In vitro systems to study melanogenesis and its modulation

Rainer Schmidt, Christine Duval and Marcelle Régnier

Epidermal melanin is produced by highly specialized cells, which are located in the basal layer of the epidermis. These dendritic cells, called melanocytes, are continuously in close contact with their neighboring keratinocytes into which they transfer newly synthesized melanin and form the so-called epidermal melanin unit.[1] One unit is composed of one melanocyte and about 40 keratinocytes, the majority of which have left the basal layer to undergo terminal differentiation during their migration to the cell surface. The tight contact between melanocytes and keratinocytes is not only essential for the melanin transfer, but also for an intensive crosstalk occurring between the two cell types. It is known that growth and differentiation of melanocytes are largely controlled by keratinocyte-derived factors,[2,3] and that the transcription of the melanogenic enzymes tyrosinase, TRP1 and TRP2, is affected by keratinocytes.[4] Melanocytes adhere to keratinocytes through E-cadherin, allowing the formation of gap-junction-mediated channels between the two cell types.[5] It seems that, in this type of symbiosis, keratinocytes control melanocyte growth, activity and proliferation, and a loss of this control might be considered as a first step in melanocyte transformation.[5,6]

Exposure of the skin to UV radiation results in a stimulation of melanin production and, thus, an increased pigmentation, generally described as tanning. This increase in pigmentation, which is normally homogenous, can also be irregular and result in the formation of pigmentary lesions, *e.g.* melasma, a widespread facial hyperpigmented lesion with a particularly high incidence rate in woman of Asian and Hispanic origin.[7] Besides UV, many other factors are described in the pathophysiology of the pigmentary system to cause skin lesions.[8] The need to cure and correct these pigmentary disorders prompted us and others to develop *in vitro* models to study epidermal melanin production and to screen for new, efficient, and safe modulators of melanogenesis.

Based on the documented importance of keratinocyte–melanocyte interaction, we created an *in vitro* screening system composed of both cell types.[9] Briefly, normal human melanocytes and keratinocytes obtained from skin biopsies were amplifed in their respective culture media and co-seeded at a ratio of 3:10, respectively, into 96-well culture dishes, to screen potentially active modulators of melanogenesis. Figure 26.1 shows the homogeneous distribution of dopa-positive, dendritic melanocytes among the keratinocyte layer. Under these culture conditions, melanocytes synthesize and transfer melanin into the neighboring keratinocytes. For the screening assay (see Fig. 26.2), the co-cultures are exposed to the compounds under investigation in the presence of ^{14}C-thiouracil and ^{3}H-leucine. Variations in the rate of melanin synthesis are calculated on the basis of ^{14}C-thiouracil incorporation into newly synthesized melanin.[10] A reduction or increase in ^{3}H-leucine incorporation is taken as a sign of cytotoxicity or induction of abnormal proliferation, respectively. This keratinocyte–melanocyte co-culture-screening system provided not only a useful tool to compare the activity of known modulators of melanogenesis, but also allowed the performance of structure–activity studies with newly identified modulators to improve their activity.[9]

Being able to detect not only variations in the rate of melanin synthesis, but also the cytotoxicity of a molecule under investigation, revealed that the large majority of compounds that stimulated melanogenesis were, at the same time, cytotoxic. It seems as if, in response to an aggression, UV irradiation included, melanocytes increase their

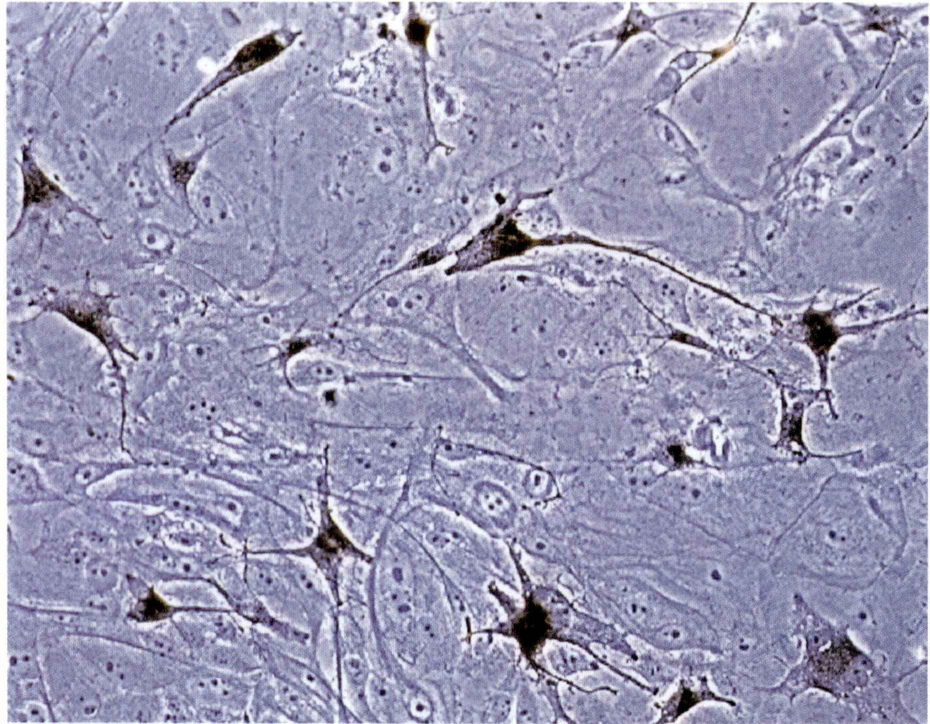

Figure 26.1

Keratinocyte–melanocyte co-cultures. dopa-Stained, dendritic melanocytes are perfectly integrated in the monolayer of keratinocytes.

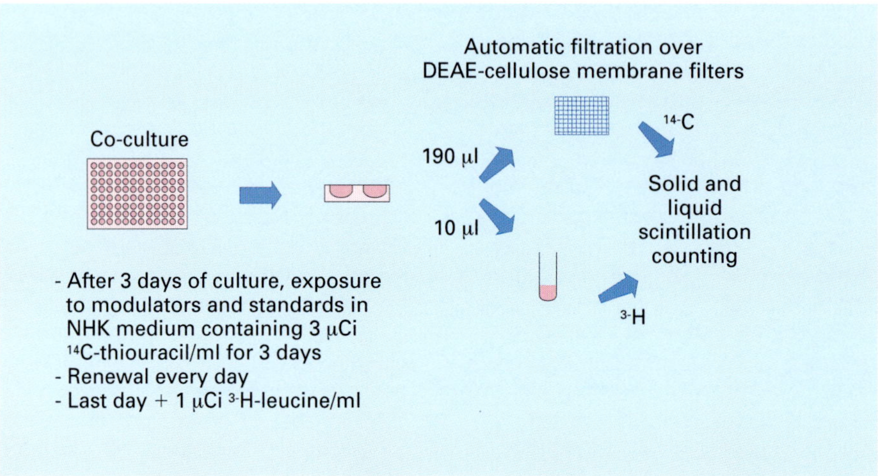

Figure 26.2

Screening assay to evaluate the efficacy of new compounds to induce or reduce the rate of melanin synthesis in NHK-NHM co-cultures.

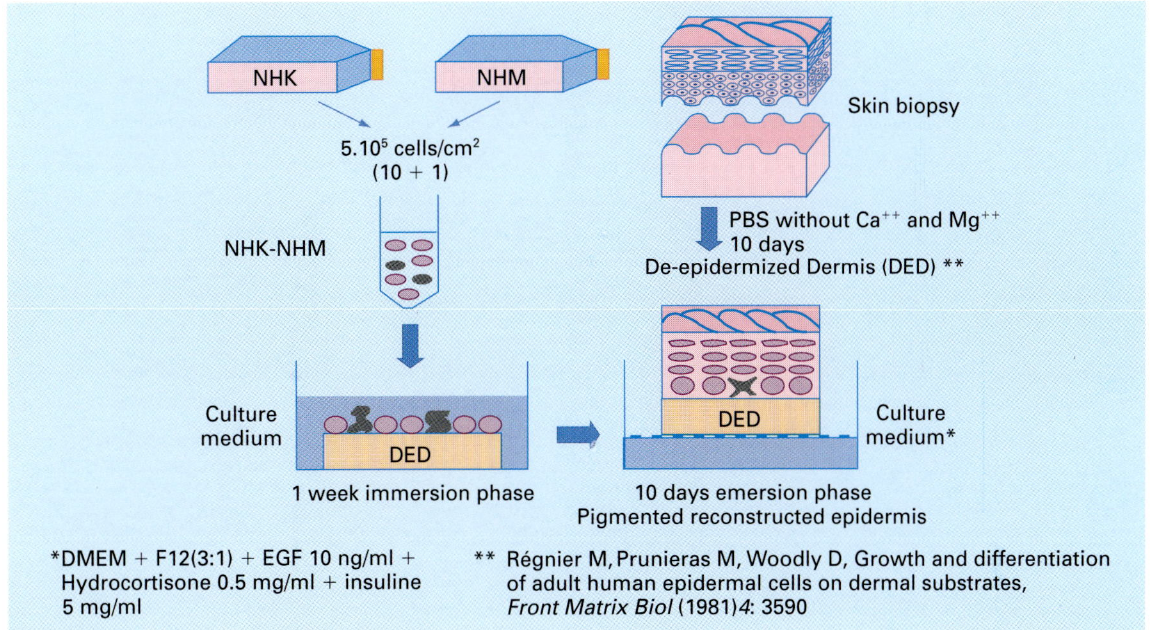

Figure 26.3

Reconstruction of a pigmented human epidermis.

production of melanin. Exceptions to this rule were compounds that exert their melanogenic activity via modulation of the cAMP level, like isobutyl-methyl xanthine.[11]

The successful integration of melanocytes into reconstructed human epidermis resulted in a further improvement of the possibilities to study pigmentation *in vitro*.[12–14] The reconstruction of a pigmented epidermis is summarized in Figure 26.3. Briefly, normal human keratinocytes and melanocytes, obtained from a skin biopsy, are amplifed separately in their appropriate, respective culture media and seeded at a ratio of 10:1 on the dermal support. After 1 week, the culture is exposed to the air–liquid interface to induce complete keratinocyte differentiation and the formation of a stratum corneum. The histological analysis after Fontana–Masson staining of the pigmented reconstructed epidermis reveals a well-stratified epithelium, with melanocytes in the basal layer which synthesize and transfer melanin to the neighboring keratinocytes (Fig. 26.4).

By culturing normal human melanocytes of different ethnic origin, we observed distinct morphologies of the cells. We, and others,[15] realized that, after integration into a reconstructed epidermis, these ethnic melanocytes preserve their characteristics and give rise to reconstructed pigmented epidermis, reflecting the phototype of the donor. These ethnic *in vitro* models are actually under investigation to study pigmentary particularities of different skin phototypes. In our hands, they provided an excellent means to assess the safety and efficacy of formulated modulators of melanogenesis after topical application. Figure 26.5 shows the depigmenting effect of kojic acid, a known inhibitor of melanin synthesis, on reconstructed Asian epidermis.

To study the melanogenic response of co-cultures and pigmented reconstructed epidermis to UV exposure, the different sources (UVA, UVB, and solar simulated radiation, SSR) were calibrated before each irradiation experiment and recorded by an Oriel spectroradiometer to guarantee reproducibility. The spectra of the respective irradiation sources are presented in Figure 26.6.

UVB irradiation was performed using BLE-1T158 fluorescent tubes with a Kodacel filter. For UVA irradiation, we used a 1000 W Xenon Solar simulator equipped with a dichroic mirror, a Schott WG 335/3 mm filter, and a UG5 2 mm filter in case of a single exposure. The reconstructed

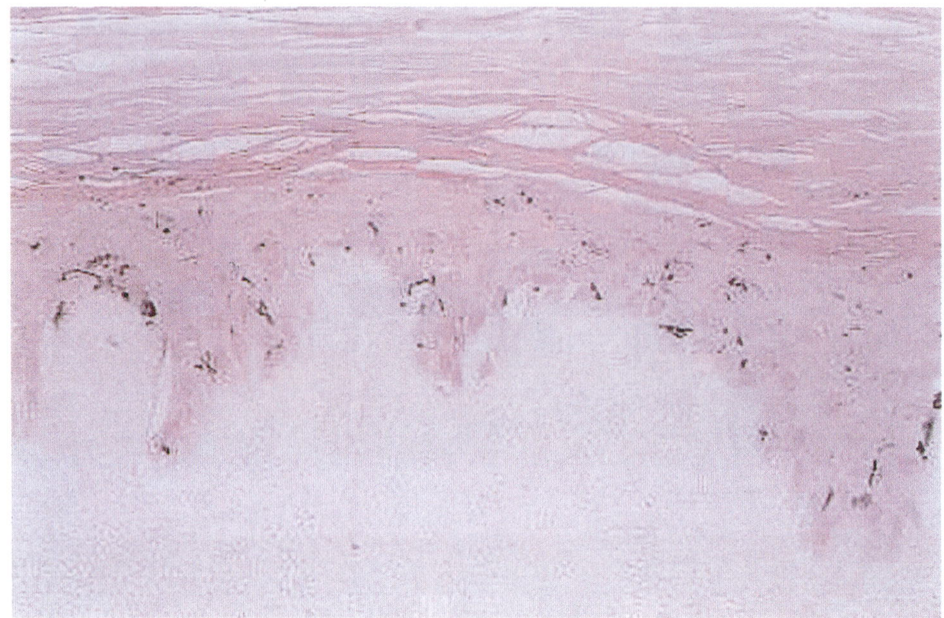

Figure 26.4

Histology of reconstructed pigmented epidermis after Fontana–Masson staining.

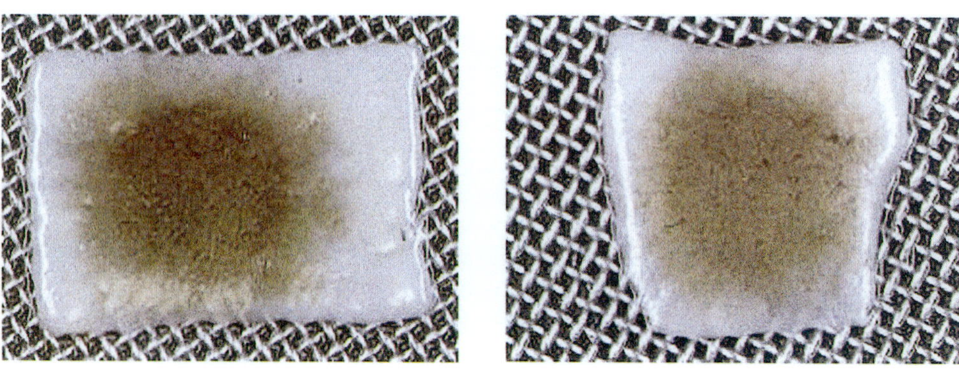

Figure 26.5

The depigmenting effect of kojic acid (500 μM) after its topical application on reconstructed pigmented human epidermis containing Asian melanocytes.

pigmented epidermis was exposed to UVB and UVA only 7 days after its air exposure, a delay necessary for the keratinocytes to form a compact stratum corneum. For SSR, reconstructed pigmented epidermis was irradiated (2.8 J/cm^2) once a day for 4 days (1000 W Xenon, Oriel Corp., equipped with a dichroic mirror and a Schott WG 320/1.5 mm filter, removing wavelengths below 290 nm). Comparing the minimal UVB doses required to induce pigmentation in

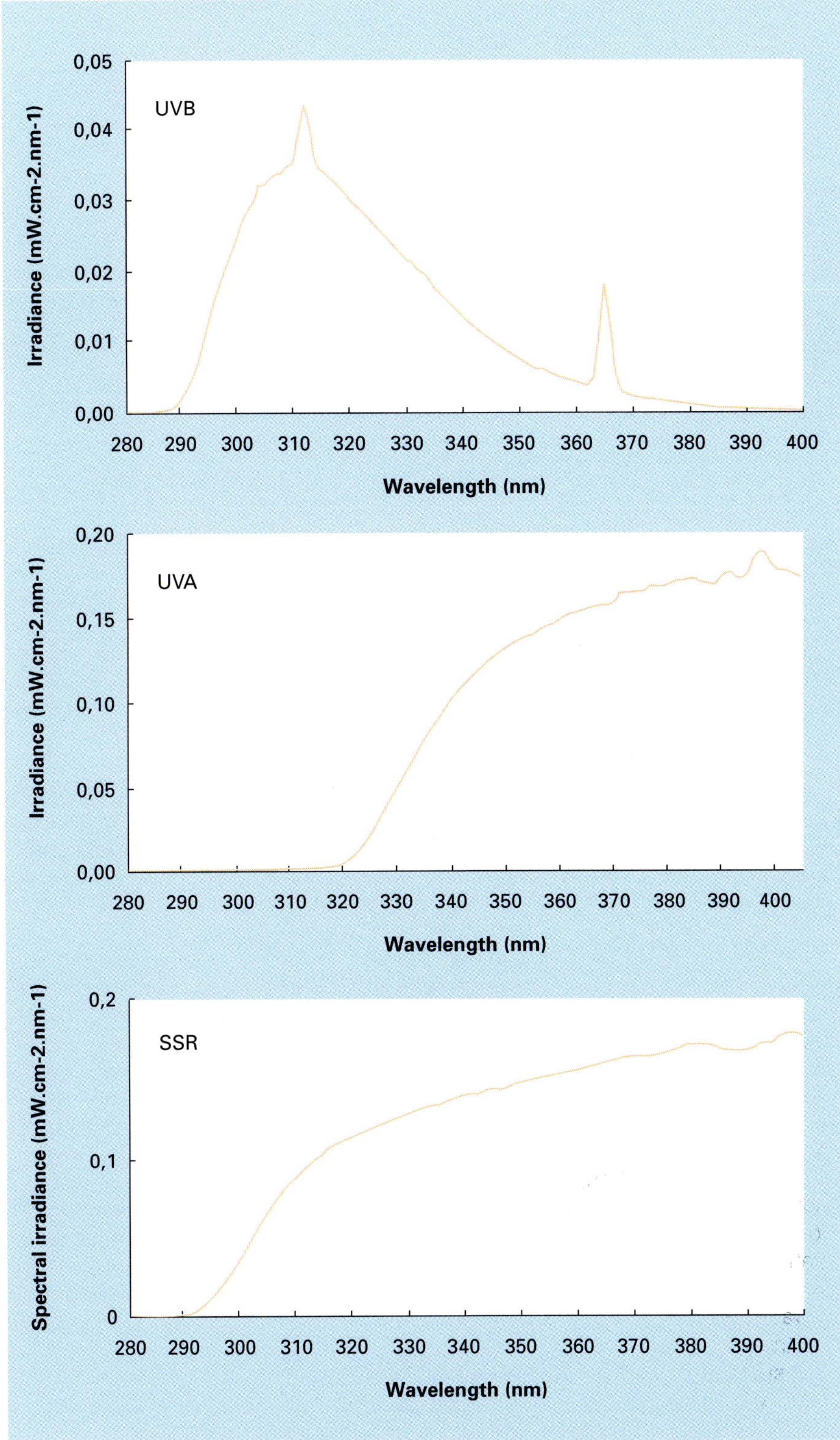

Figure 26.6

The spectra of the different UV sources used to induce a melanogenic response in NHK–NHM co-cultures and reconstructed pigmented epidermis.

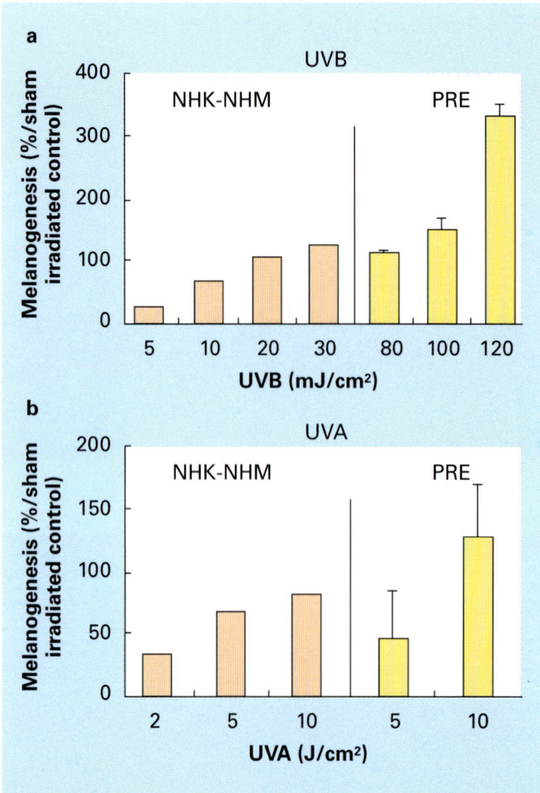

Figure 26.7

Melanogenic dose-response of NHK–NHM co-cultures and reconstructed pigmented epidermis to UVB (a) and UVA (b) irradiation.

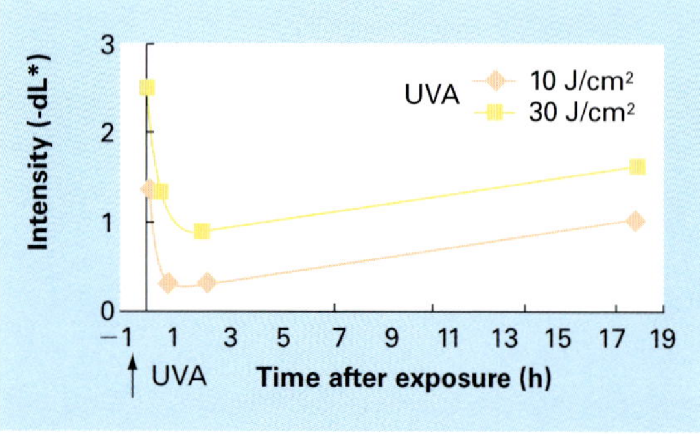

Figure 26.8

UVA-induced transient immediate pigmentation darkening in reconstructed human epidermis.

melanocyte–keratinocyte co-cultures and reconstructed pigmented epidermis revealed that an almost 10× higher dose has to be applied on the reconstructed epidermis to obtain a comparable melanogenic response, reflecting the efficacy of the stratum corneum to act as a UVB filter (Fig. 26.7). UVA irradiation triggered a melanogenic response at comparable doses in NHK–NHM co-cultures and reconstructed epidermis (Fig. 26.7), confirming the high penetration rate of longer UV radiation.

Another interesting observation was made after exposing pigmented reconstructed epidermis to UVA radiation. As *in vivo*, transient immediate pigmentation darkening, or IPD, was observed (Fig. 26.8), a phenomenon related to the reversible photo-oxidation of pre-existing, reduced melanin and its precursors, described in detail by Chardon and co-workers.[16] Exposure to 10 J/cm^2 UVA induced an immediate tanning, as revealed by a decrease in the luminance, L*, which disappeared within the next 2 hours. Exposure to a higher UV-A dose (30 J/cm^2) resulted in a more intense, immediate tanning effect, which did not completely fade (persistent tanning).

The inhibition of UV-induced pigmentation by a topically applied sunscreen reflects its capacity to absorb UV radiation and, thus, its potential photoprotection. Colleagues in our institute used reconstructed human skin to evaluate the protective effect of sunscreens against UVB- and UVA-induced damage, looking at the formation of sunburn cells after UVB exposure and the viability of fibroblasts after UVA irradiation.[17] Knowing that UV radiation is responsible for the manifestation of many hyperpigmentary disorders,[18] we had a closer look at the anti-pigmenting capacity of sunscreens after exposure of the pigmented reconstructed epidermis to SSR, matching the best the solar radiation. The sunscreen-related reduction of SSR-induced pigmentation was quantified with a spectrocolorimeter, and expressed by a reduction in L*. Figure 26.9 shows the strong reduction in L* after exposure of the pigmented reconstructed epidermis to 4 × 2.8 J/cm^2 SSR radiation, and the strong anti-pigmenting effect of a topically applied sunscreen (MEXORYL® XL, 4%).

In conclusion, these different *in vitro* models, with increasing complexity, provide, in our hands,

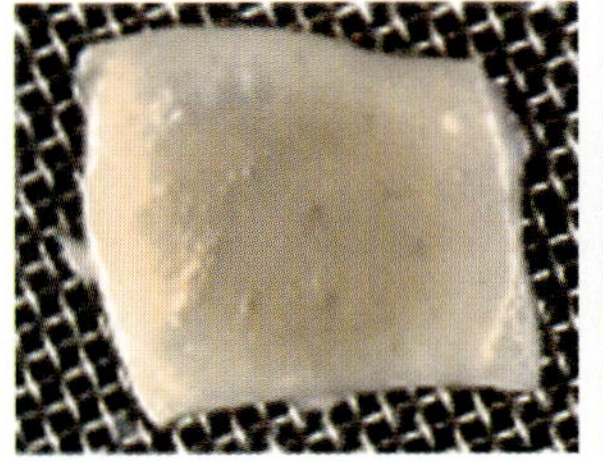

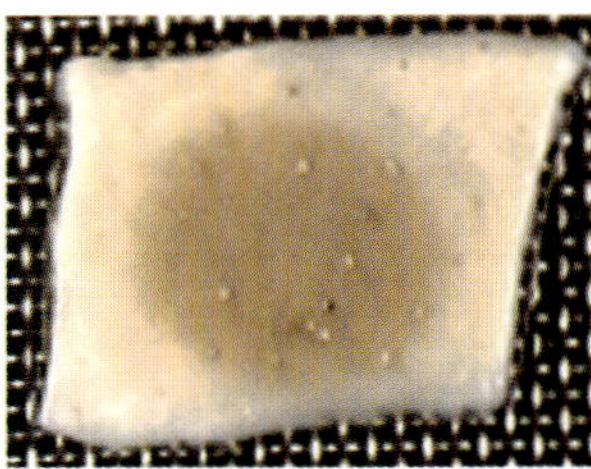

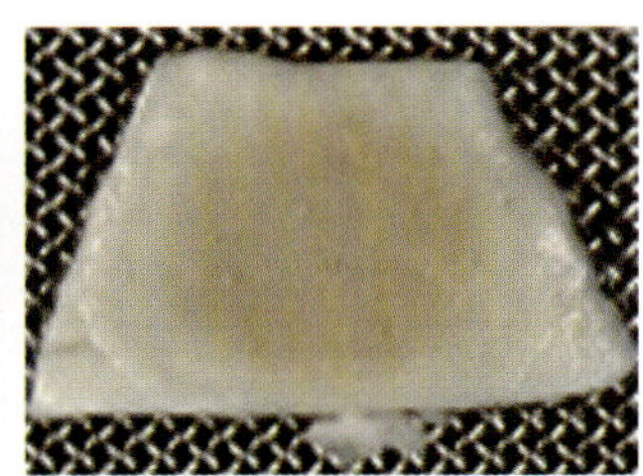

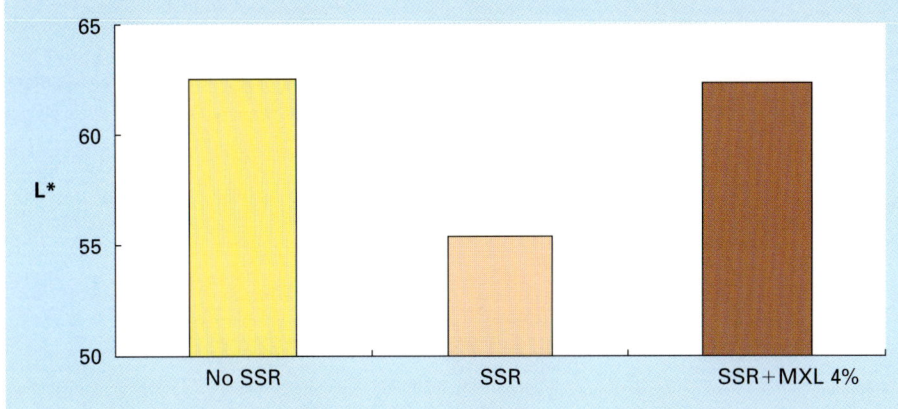

Figure 26.9

Solar simulated radiation (SSR)-induced pigmentation in reconstructed human epidermis and the anti-pigmenting effect of a sunscreen (MEXORYL® XL, 4%). Pigmentation was measured with a spectrocolorimeter and expressed in luminance, L*.

excellent models to study: (i) keratinocyte–melanocyte interaction within the epidermal melanin unit, (ii) the safety and efficacy of newly identified modulators of melanogenesis, (iii) UV-induced pigmentation, and (iv) the efficacy of sunscreens as protecting and anti-pigmenting agents.

References

1. Fitzpatrick TB, Breathnach AS, Das epidermale Melanin-Einheit System, *Dermatol Wochenschr* (1963) **147**:481–9.
2. Gordon PR, Mansur CP, Gilchrest BA, Regulation of human melanocyte growth, dendricity, and melanization by keratinocyte derived factors, *J Invest Dermatol* (1989) **92**:565–72.
3. DeLuca M, Anna FD et al., Human epithelial cells induce human melanocyte growth in vitro but only keratinocytes regulate its proper differentiation in the absence of dermis, *J Cell Biol* (1988) **107**:1919–26.
4. Kippenberger S, Bernd A et al., Transcription of melanogenesis enzymes in melanocytes: dependence upon culture conditions and co-cultivation with keratinocytes, *Pigment Cell Res* (1996) **9**:179–84.
5. Herlyn M, Crosstalk between human melanocytes and keratinocytes, *Pigment Cell Res* (2000) **13**:29.
6. Jouneau A, Yu YQ, Pasdar M, Plasticity of cadherin-catenin expression in the melanocyte lineage, *Pigment Cell Res* (2000) **13**:260–72.
7. Sanchez NP, Pathak MA et al., Melasma: A clinical, light microscopic, ultrastructural and immunofluorescence study, *J Am Acad Dermatol* (1981) **4**: 698–710.
8. Halder R, Nordlund JJ, Topical treatment of pigmentary disorders. In: Nordlund JJ, Boissy RE, Hearing VJ et al., eds, *Pigmentary System: Physiology and Pathophysiology* (Oxford University Press: Oxford, 1998) 969–75.
9. Régnier M, Duval C et al., Keratinocyte–melanocyte co-cultures and pigmented reconstructed human epidermis: Models to study modulation of melanogenesis, *Cell Mol Biol* (1999) **45**:969–80.
10. Schmidt R, Krien P, Régnier M, The use of diethylaminoethyl-cellulose membrane filters in a bioassay to quantify melanin synthesis, *Anal Biochem* (1996) **235**:113–18.
11. Friedmann PS, Gilchrest BA, Ultraviolet radiation directly induces pigment production in cultured melanocytes, *J Cell Phys* (1987) **133**:88–94.
12. Valyi-Nagy IT, Murphy GF et al., Phenotypes and interactions of human melanocytes and keratinocytes

in an epidermal reconstruction model, *Lab Invest* (1990) **62**:314–24.

13. Todd C, Hewitt SD et al., Co-culture of human melanocytes and keratinocytes in a skin equivalent model: effect of ultraviolet radiation, *Arch Dermatol Res* (1993) **285**:455–9.
14. Régnier M, Schmidt R, Reconstruction of an epidermal melanin unit by co-cultures of normal human keratinocytes (NHK) and normal human melanocytes (NHM), *J Invest Dermatol* (1994) **102**:596.
15. Bessou S, Surlève-Bazeille JE et al., Ex vivo studies of skin phototypes, *J Invest Dermatol* (1996) **107**: 684–8.
16. Chardon A, Moyal D, Hourseau C, Persistent pigment darkening response as a method for the evaluation of ultraviolet A protection assays. In: Lowe NJ, Shaath NA, Pathak MA, eds, *Sunscreen: Development Evaluation and Regulatory Aspects* (Marcel Dekker Inc, 1997) 559–81.
17. Bernerd F, Vioux C, Asselineau D, Evaluation of the protective effect of sunscreens on in vitro reconstructed human skin to UVA and UVB irradiation, *Photochem Photobiol* (2000) **71**:314–20.
18. Ortonne JP, Nordlund JJ, Mechanisms that cause abnormal skin color. In: Nordlund JJ, Boissy RE, Hearing VJ et al., eds, *The Pigmentary System: Physiology and Pathophysiology* (Oxford University Press: Oxford, 1998) 489–502.

27 Animal models for the study of ultraviolet-induced skin pigmentation

Isabelle Pélisson, Hélène Dessauvages and André Jomard

Introduction

Delayed tanning results from melanin synthesis in melanocytes and distribution to surrounding keratinocytes as a response to UV irradiation. Many of the molecular mechanisms that govern tanning have been elucidated by analyzing the melanocyte response to UV irradiation *in vitro*. However, skin irradiation stimulates the synthesis of a variety of hormones, growth factors and cytokines, and it is now clear that many keratinocyte-derived factors affect melanin synthesis in melanocytes in response to UV.[1–3] Therefore, keratinocyte–melanocyte cocultures and pigmented reconstructed epidermis are useful tools to study UV-induced pigmentation *in vitro*.[4–6]

However, UV-induced skin responses, such as erythema and inflammation, may influence tanning and cannot be addressed properly *in vitro*. Moreover, there has been an interest in the development of pre-clinical *in vivo* models for the screening of potential therapeutic agents to treat pigmentation disorders in human. Therefore, animal models of UV-induced delayed pigmentation were developed.

This chapter focuses on the description of the three animal models that are commonly used to study UV-induced pigmentation and its modulation *in vivo*: hairless pigmented mice, guinea pigs and the Yucatan miniature swine. The source of UVR and detailed irradiation protocol used to induce tanning in the different models are crucial information.[7] However, their description was voluntarily omitted in this review of the literature because the materials are not always properly described and, most of the time, at variance with each other. Therefore, the comparisons of biological responses to UVR should be made with caution and the irradiation protocols used in each study should be taken into account.

Slightly pigmented hairless mice

For many years, the study of UV-induced skin pigmentation *in vivo* was hampered by the lack of a proper mouse model: in the skin of hairy mice, epidermal melanocytes are almost entirely located in the follicular epidermis and, therefore, inaccessible to UV. Early work was undertaken in order to understand the effect of UV radiation on epidermal melanocytes by irradiating the ear, tail or plantar skin, which are devoid of hair and, therefore, easily accessible to radiations.[8–13]

Several strains of slightly pigmented hairless mice are now available for skin pigmentation studies. The hairless phenotype is of particular interest for convenient testing of the effect of UVR and/or topical agents on skin pigmentation. Moreover, when working with hairy animals, the irritation due to hair removal may affect the pigmentary response. The most commonly used strain is the Skh:HR2 one, developed by Temple University (Philadelphia, USA),[14–19] but other strains have been developed on other genetic backgrounds.[20–25]

All these strains of hairless pigmented mice have in common darkly pigmented ears and tail, whereas the back skin is not pigmented. Upon repeated UV irradiation, pigmentation is increased on the ears and tail, and a freckle-like, mottled pigmentation appears on the back. The kinetics of UV-induced pigmentation have been described by several groups: depending on the mouse strain, UV source, and irradiation protocol, the responses might differ slightly. Small brown macules typically appear on the back after 2 weeks of irradiation, and gradually become bigger and merge. They usually remain partially confluent,[14,23,24] but may evolve towards an even tan.[15] UVR dose dependently induces pigmentation on the back (Fig. 27.1);[14,23] however, it is important to remain within a dose range that induces limited inflammation for the animals' well-being, and because inflammation may affect the pigmentary response.[24]

Pigmentary changes induced by UV irradiation in the skin of hairless pigmented mice can be quantified by various means:

Visual scoring is easy to perform on the back, whereas pigmentary changes are more difficult to visualize on naturally pigmented body sites, which require the use of *ex vivo* quantification to evaluate the effects of modulators of skin pigmentation.

Fontana–Masson silver staining is routinely used on sections of paraffin-embedded skin samples. The amount of pigment can be quantified by image analysis, to reflect both melanin synthesis in melanocytes and transfer to neighboring keratinocytes. However, quantification has to be restricted to the living layers of the epidermis, because processing of the sections affects the integrity of the stratum corneum, which can be partially detached and lost. Therefore, the pigment present in corneocytes is excluded from the quantification. Nevertheless, measurement of the amount of melanin on Fontana–Masson-stained skin sections clearly shows the dose-dependent induction of pigment by UVR in the epidermis (Fig. 27.2).[14]

L-DOPA staining is applied on epidermal sheets to reveal active melanocytes in which the functional tyrosinase transforms the L-DOPA substrate into dopaquinone and subsequent dark melanins. Active dendritic melanocytes are, therefore, easily visualized by microscopic observation. This technique revealed that the interfollicular epidermis of the back of hairless pigmented mice contains few DOPA-positive melanocytes. Upon activation by UVR, the number of DOPA-positive cells dramatically increases: melanocytes become more dendritic and progressively cover the interfollicular epidermis.[24] However, some areas remain devoid of DOPA-positive melanocytes, which explains the freckle-like appearance of pigmentation. The increase in DOPA-positive melanocytes after UV

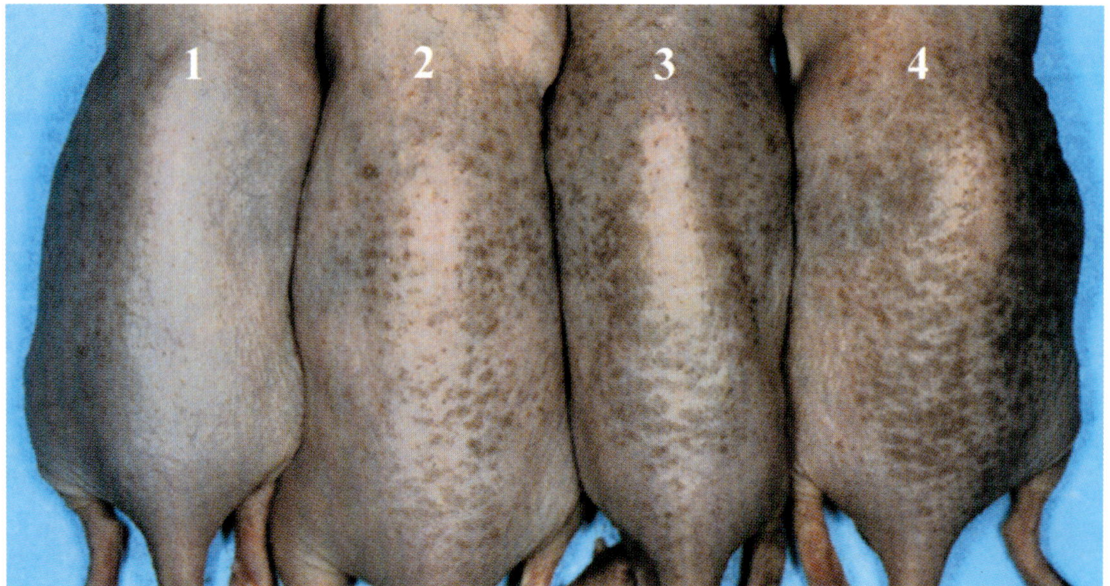

Figure 27.1

Dose-dependent induction of freckle-like mottled pigmentation on the back of Skh:HR2 mice. Animals were irradiated three times per week for 4 weeks from broad-spectrum sunlamps, with a maximum emission peak at 312 nm in the UVB. The dose received by the animals at each irradiation was estimated by the energy delivered by the lamps at 312 nm (maximum emission peak). 1 = Non-irradiated; 2 = 60 mJ/cm^2; 3 = 120 mJ/cm^2; 4 = 160 mJ/cm^2.

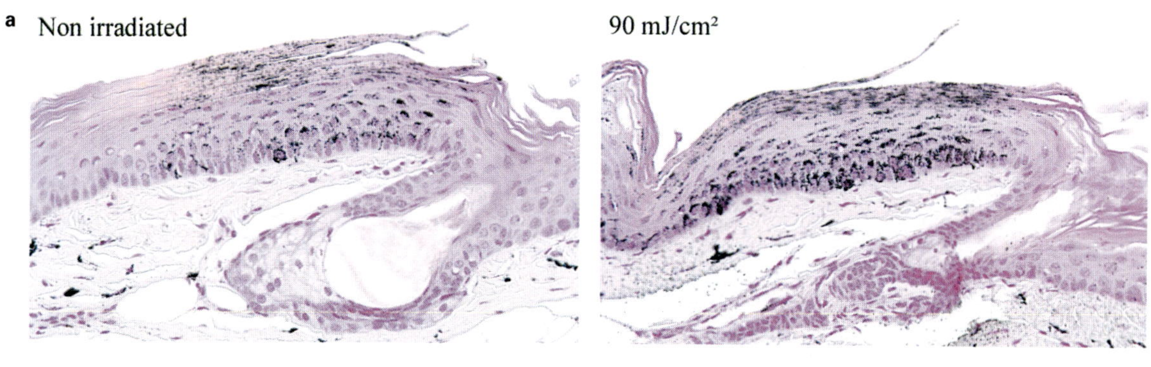

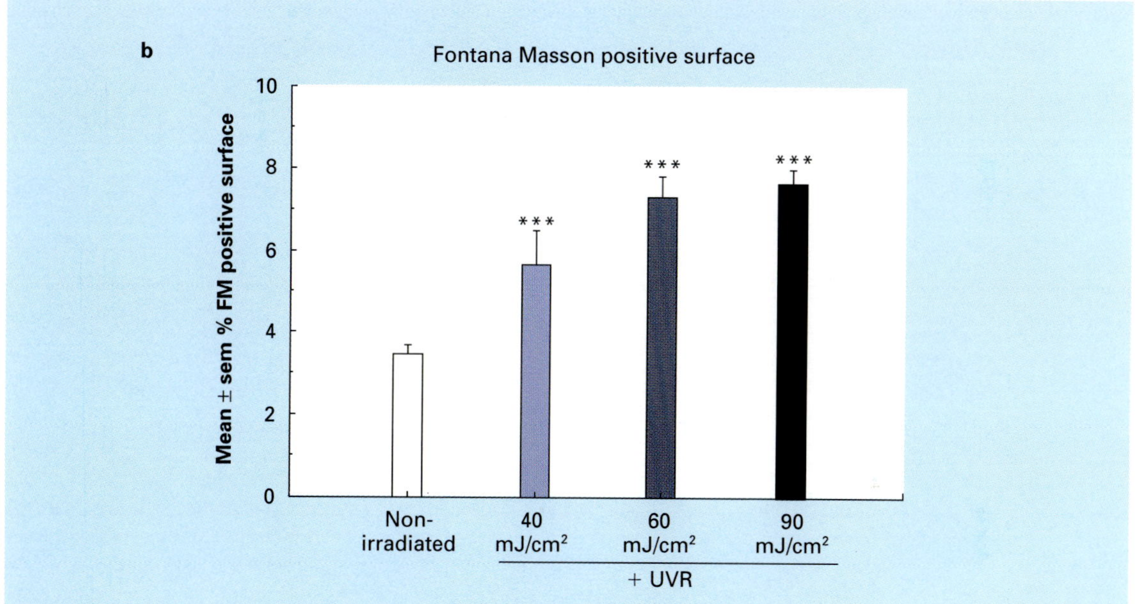

Figure 27.2

Quantification of UVR-induced pigmentation on the tail of Skh:HR2 mice using Fontana–Masson (FM) staining. Skh:HR2 mice were repeatedly irradiated with increasing doses of UVR (see Fig. 27.1) and sections were stained by the Fontana–Masson silver stain to reveal melanin. (a) Note the difference in the quantity of pigment between non-irradiated skin and skin of animals that were irradiated at 90 mJ/cm^2. (b) The amount of pigment in the living layers of the epidermis was quantified by image analysis in groups of five mice. It shows the dose-dependent induction of melanogenesis in the tail skin by UVR. Statistical analysis: comparisons between non-irradiated and irradiated animals were made using the Student's *t* test (***: $p<0.001$).

irradiation probably results both from proliferation and activation. Early work clearly showed an increase in the mitotic index of melanocytes after UV irradiation of mouse skin,[8,9] but other data support concomitant activation events.[11,14,26] The surface of L-DOPA-positive areas can be measured by image analysis from a standardized surface of irradiated back skin. This parameter reflects both the melanogenic activity and the extent of dendricity, and allows visualization of the dose-dependent effect of UVR on melanocytes (Fig. 27.3). Tail-skin epidermis, where active melanocytes are arranged in a brick-like pattern, can also be stained by L-DOPA.[10] Upon UV stimulation, the

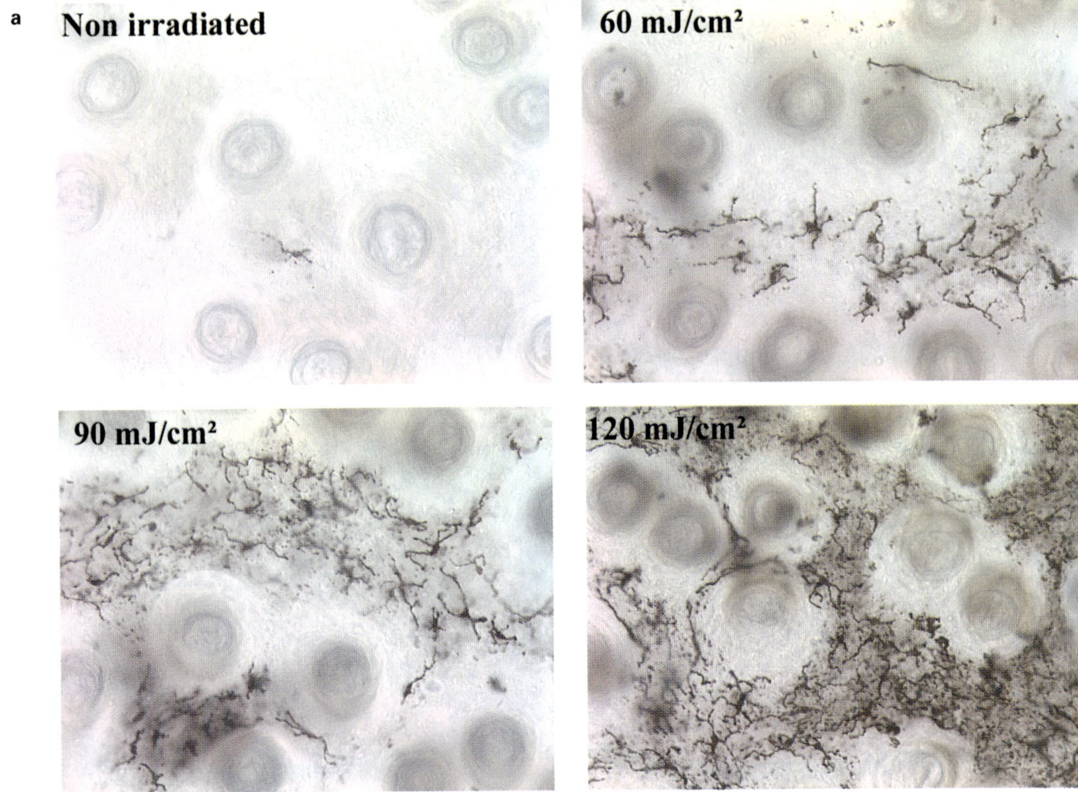

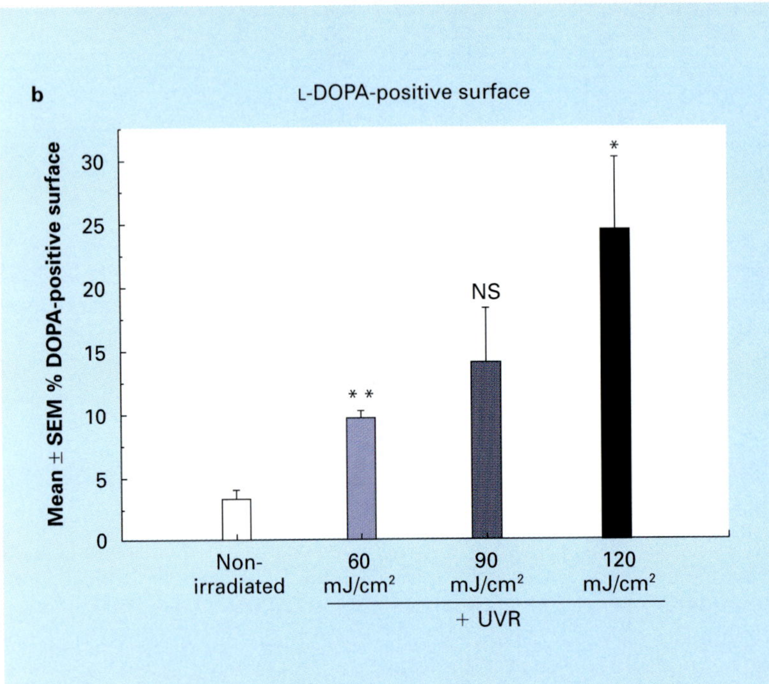

Figure 27.3

Quantification of UVR-induced pigmentation on the back of Skh:HR2 after L-DOPA staining. Skh:HR2 mice were repeatedly irradiated with increasing doses of UVR (see Fig. 27.1) and epidermal sheets from back skin were incubated with L-DOPA to identify melanogenically active cells. (a) Note the difference in the density of active melanocytes between animals that were irradiated at 60, 90 and 120 mJ/cm^2. (b) Quantification of the surface occupied by DOPA-positive melanocytes by image analysis in groups of five mice shows the dose-dependent induction of melanogenesis by UVR. Statistical analysis: comparisons between non-irradiated and irradiated animals were made using the Student's *t* test (NS: $p>0.05$; *: $p<0.05$; **: $p<0.01$).

increase in number and dendricity of active melanocytes is clearly visualized; however, the quantification of the L-DOPA reaction on the tail of UV-irradiated Skh:HR2 mice is hampered by large amounts of melanin accumulated in keratinocytes, which interferes with the proper visualization of individual cells.

The tyrosine hydroxylase activity of tyrosinase can be assessed quantitatively by measuring the conversion of [^{3}H]tyrosine to ^3H_2O.[27] Using this technique, the dose-dependent activation of tyrosinase by UVR was demonstrated in the back skin of Skh:HR2 mice.[14] However, because this technique is long and complicated when working with many samples, most authors prefer to assess tyrosinase activity by L-DOPA staining.

The total melanin content of hairless pigmented mouse skin can be assessed after UV irradiation by measuring the optical density of alkali-soluble melanins,[19] or the fluorescence emission of bleached or oxidized melanins.[28] The amount of melanin in the skin can also be quantified after filtration of protease-digested epidermis on DEAE-cellulose filters.[29]

All the above techniques have been used to study the ability of various chemical agents to modulate UV-induced pigmentation in hairless pigmented mice. For example, classical depigmenting chemicals, such as hydroquinone and 4-hydroxyanisole, are able to inhibit UV-induced pigmentation in this model.[15] Other agents, such as topical calmodulin antagonists,[18] vitamins C and E,[24] and oral selenium,[20] are also shown to prevent pigmentation in UV-irradiated hairless pigmented mice. Propigmenting activities can also be identified in this model: it was first used to confirm that MSH is involved in UV-induced pigmentation *in vivo*,[21] and applied to the identification of new furocoumarins for PUVA therapy.[22] Other agents, such as topical diacylglycerol[16] and retinoic acid,[19] have been shown to potentiate UV-induced pigmentation.

Guinea pigs

Although hairless pigmented mice are widely used in pigmentation research because of convenient testing and low cost, their pigmentary system differs significantly from that of human skin: because of the low basal amount of active melanocytes in the interfollicular epidermis, the pigmentary response to UV irradiation is mottled rather than uniform, and melanin isn't evenly distributed to all keratinocytes. In this respect, guinea pigs serve as a good animal model as their skin contains active melanocytes in the interfollicular epidermis and they develop an even tan in response to UV. Unfortunately, it is difficult to obtain pigmented guinea pigs from animal providers, and most of the published work has been done on small colonies of animals of different genetic backgrounds. The pigmentary responses may differ, depending on which type of animal is used. Indeed, the activity of interfollicular melanocytes depends on the surrounding hair color, which may vary from red to brown/black.

Most of the published work on UV-induced pigmentation in guinea pigs was done on shaved or depilated brownish[30–32] or red-haired[21,33] animals, whereas darkly pigmented animals are used to evaluate the activity of depigmenting agents.[34,35] Although it is difficult to compare results because of different strains, UV sources and irradiation protocols, it is clear that UV-induced pigmentation in guinea pigs is rather fast: a distinct tan is clearly visible and measurable 1 week after irradiation; the tan becomes darker during the following weeks,[21,30,36] and remains visible for about 10 weeks after cessation of UV.[33] UV-induced pigmentation is uniform, which permits measurement of the visible skin darkening by colorimetry.[31,32,36] Techniques described earlier are available to quantify pigmentation in guinea pigs: the increase in DOPA-positive melanocytes parallels the development of the tan.[30] Fontana–Masson staining reveals that the most prominent increase in melanin content after UV irradiation occurs in the basal layer, but keratinocytes throughout the epidermis contain more melanin,[33] with the typical accumulation of pigment on top of nuclei referred to as supranuclear caps. Because UVR induces a dark and long-lasting tan in guinea pigs, pigmented skin was used to evaluate the skin-lightening activity of compounds such as unsaturated fatty acids.[31] But, in most cases, the guinea-pig model was used to identify agents that prevent UV-induced pigmentation, such as sunscreens, tyrosinase inhibitors,[30] a plasmin inhibitor[36] or the NO synthase inhibitor L-NAME.[32] Guinea-pig skin responds to PUVA therapy by producing a dark tan,[30] and may develop a dark pigmentation in the absence of UV when treated with diacylglycerol[33] or diols.[37]

The main concern when working with guinea pigs is that the animals must be shaved, otherwise UV and test compounds cannot access the skin surface. To avoid the non-specific effect of irritation due to hair removal, hairless pigmented guinea pigs have been developed, by mating commercially available hairless albino females with either red-haired or black males.[38] The resulting F3 generation of hairless pigmented animals displayed either light red-brown skin, that responded to UV irradiation by a visible increase in pigmentation and DOPA-positive melanocytes,[38] or dark skin, that could be significantly depigmented by a combination of hydroquinone and gluthathione synthesis inhibitors.[39]

The Yucatan miniature swine

Miniature pigs are considered to be a model of choice for dermatological research because of close morphologic and functional similarities between pig skin and human skin, which have been reviewed previously.[40–42] Moreover, the size of the animal allows the demarcation of multiple test sites on the same animal, which is interesting when evaluating the activity of compounds on skin function, especially because of the elevated cost of such investigations. The use of miniature pigs for photodermatology has shown that their response to UV irradiation is close to the response of human skin in terms of erythema, sunburn cell formation,[40] and photoaging.[41]

The Yucatan miniature pig is a naturally occurring breed of swine in which skin color ranges from light to dark brown. Fontana–Masson staining shows that the distribution of pigment is very similar in Yucatan and human skin, with a concentration of melanin in the basal layer, decreased amounts in suprabasal keratinocytes, and no pigment in the dermis.[42] Repeated UV irradiation of lightly pigmented Yucatan skin rapidly induces a uniform pigmentary response; this UV-induced tan protects the skin from erythema and sunburn cell formation in subsequent irradiations.[40,43] A dose-related delayed tanning is also induced after a single UV irradiation: the pigmentation is visible after 7 days, increases until 3 weeks, and may remain visible over 8 weeks after irradiation, depending on the inducing UV dose.[44,45] An increase in the number and dendricity of DOPA-positive melanocytes precedes the onset of a visible UV-induced tan by several days.[44] This model of UV-induced pigmentation in the Yucatan miniature swine was used to confirm that sunscreens can prevent delayed tanning,[43] and that a combination of 4-hydroxyanisole and retinoic acid reverses hyperpigmentation induced by UV irradiation.[45] More recently, natural soybean extracts were shown to prevent UV-induced pigmentation by inhibition of the PAR-2 pathway involved in melanosome transfer.[46]

Because some animals present naturally dark skin in the absence of UV stimulation, the Yucatan miniature swine has also been used as a model to test the depigmenting activity of various agents. Compounds with known depigmenting efficacy in human clinical trials were shown to lighten naturally dark skin in Yucatan pigs: for example, hydroquinone and 4-hydroxyanisole (either alone or in combination with retinoic acid) depigment dark skin, as shown by visible lightening and the absence of pigment on Fontana–Masson-stained sections.[42,45] Other depigmenting agents are able to lighten dark Yucatan skin, such as phenolic compounds that are toxic to the melanocyte,[47] or a synthetic serine protease inhibitor that prevents melanosome transfer.[48]

Conclusions

The three models described above can be used to induce a visible skin pigmentation after UV irradiation. Tanning results from an increase in the number of DOPA-positive melanocytes and an accumulation of pigment in the epidermis, comparable to the response of human skin to UV irradiation.

Although UV-induced skin pigmentation is clinically different in hairless pigmented mice and humans, this model is widely used because of its low cost and because it allows convenient testing of several compounds, thus making it a useful tool for screening purposes.

Guinea pigs respond to UV irradiation with an even and long-lasting pigmentation which is closer to human tanning. The main difficulty when working with guinea pigs is that hair removal is necessary for convenient application of topical agents and monitoring of skin responses. Repeated shaving may affect the pigmentary response because it produces limited local inflammation. Therefore, the hairless pigmented guinea pigs described by Bolognia et al.[38] may represent an interesting model to study UV-induced skin pigmentation, since they combine the convenience of a small rodent with hairless skin with a pigmentary system close to that of humans.

As for Yucatan miniature swine, their pigmentary response to UVR resembles human tanning in terms of kinetic and clinical aspects. Because their skin presents many morphological and functional similarities with human skin, this model may be preferred for validation of the cutaneous pharmacological activity of pigmentation modulators, despite elevated cost. However, it should be pointed out that these animals have a variety of skin colors from light to dark brown, and that baseline pigmentation may affect the response to UV and pharmacological agents.

A few compounds with known depigmenting or propigmenting activities in humans have been evaluated in the three models. Despite different treatment protocols, which make comparisons difficult, the reported activities were globally similar, thus confirming the relevance of the models for identifying new modulators of skin pigmentation. For example, hydroquinone prevents UV-induced pigmentation in the mouse and guinea pig,[15,30] and lightens dark guinea-pig and Yucatan skin.[34,42] As for propigmenting agents, diacylglycerol induces melanogenesis in mouse and guinea-pig skin,[16,33] and both models respond to PUVA therapy with a strong tanning response.[22,30] In conclusion, the three models represent reliable tools to study the modulation of UV-induced skin pigmentation *in vivo*: they have all proved useful for detection of compounds capable of preventing or potentiating tanning responses, as well as depigmenting skin. The choice of which model to use must be guided by the investigator's requirements and facilities.

References

1. Gilchrest BA, Park HY, Eller MS et al., Mechanisms of ultraviolet light-induced pigmentation, *Photochem Photobiol* (1996) **63**:1–10.
2. Abdel-Malek Z, Regulation of human pigmentation by ultraviolet light and by endocrine, paracrine, and autocrine hormones. In: Nordlund JJ, Boissy RE, Hearing VJ et al., eds, *The Pigmentary System: Physiology and Pathophysiology* (Oxford University Press: Oxford, 1998) 115–22.
3. Ortonne JP, Ballotti R, Melanocyte biology and melanogenesis: what's new?, *J Dermatol Treat* (2000) **11; (Suppl 1)**:S15–S26.
4. Bessou S, Surleve-Bazeille JE, Sorbier E et al., Ex vivo reconstruction of the epidermis with melanocytes and the influence of UVB, *Pigment Cell Res* (1995) **8**:241–9.
5. Bessou-Touya S, Picardo M, Maresca V et al., Chimeric human epidermal reconstructs to study the role of melanocytes and keratinocytes in pigmentation and photoprotection, *J Invest Dermatol* (1998) **111**:1103–8.
6. Regnier M, Duval C, Galey JB et al., Keratinocyte–melanocyte co-cultures and pigmented reconstructed human epidermis: models to study modulation of melanogenesis, *Cell Mol Biol (Noisy-le-grand)* (1999) **45**:969–80.
7. Gasparro FP, Brown DB, Photobiology 102: UV sources and dosimetry—the proper use and measurement of 'photons as a reagent', *J Invest Dermatol* (2000) **114**:613–15.
8. Rosdahl IK, Szabo G, Mitotic activity of epidermal melanocytes in UV-irradiated mouse skin, *J Invest Dermatol* (1978) **70**:143–8.
9. Rosdahl IK, Local and systemic effects on the epidermal melanocyte population in UV-irradiated mouse skin, *J Invest Dermatol* (1979) **73**:306–9.
10. Blog FB, Szabo G, The effects of UVB and 7, 12, dimethylbenz(alpha)anthracene (DMBA) on epidermal melanocytes of the tail in C57BL mice, *J Invest Dermatol* (1979) **73**:538–44.
11. Jimbow K, Uesugi T, New melanogenesis and photobiological processes in activation and proliferation of precursor melanocytes after UV-exposure: ultrastructural differentiation of precursor melanocytes from Langerhans cells, *J Invest Dermatol* (1982) **78**:108–15.
12. Nordlund JJ, Ackles AE, Traynor FF, The proliferative and toxic effects of ultraviolet light and inflammation on epidermal pigment cells, *J Invest Dermatol* (1981) **77**:361–8.
13. Nordlund JJ, Collins CE, Rheins LA, Prostaglandin E2 and D2 but not MSH stimulate the proliferation of pigment cells in the pinnal epidermis of the DBA/2 mouse, *J Invest Dermatol* (1986) **86**:433–7.
14. Warren R, Sensitivity of mouse Skh-HR-2 to ultraviolet light: mouse pigmentation model, *Photochem Photobiol* (1986) **43**:41–7.
15. Nair X, Tramposch KM, UVB-induced pigmentation in hairless mice as an in vivo assay for topical

skin-depigmenting activity, *Skin Pharmacol* (1989) **2**:187–97.

16. Agin PP, Dowdy JC, Costlow ME, Diacylglycerol-induced melanogenesis in Skh-2 pigmented hairless mice, *Photodermatol Photoimmunol Photomed* (1991) **8**:51–6.
17. Ho KK, Halliday GM, Barnetson RS, Topical retinoic acid augments ultraviolet light-induced melanogenesis, *Melanoma Res* (1992) **2**:41–5.
18. Dowdy JC, Anthony FA, Costlow ME, Topical W-7 inhibits ultraviolet radiation-induced melanogenesis in Skh:HR2 pigmented hairless mice, *Photodermatol Photoimmunol Photomed* (1995) **11**:143–8.
19. Welsh BM, Mason RS, Halliday GM, Topical all-trans retinoic acid augments ultraviolet radiation-induced increases in activated melanocyte numbers in mice, *J Invest Dermatol* (1999) **112**:271–8.
20. Thorling EB, Overvad K, Bjerring P, Oral selenium inhibits skin reactions to UV light in hairless mice, *Acta Pathol Microbiol Immunol Scand [A]* (1983) **91**:81–3.
21. Bolognia J, Murray M, Pawelek J, UVB-induced melanogenesis may be mediated through the MSH-receptor system, *J Invest Dermatol* (1989) **92**:651–6.
22. Kinley JS, Moan J, Dall'Aqua F et al., Quantitative assessment of epidermal melanogenesis in C3H/Tif hr/hr mice treated with topical furocoumarins and UVA radiation, *J Invest Dermatol* (1994) **103**:97–103.
23. Hansen AB, Bech-Thomsen N, Wulf HC, In vivo estimation of pigmentation in ultraviolet-exposed hairless mice, *Photodermatol Photoimmunol Photomed* (1995) **11**:14–17.
24. Quevedo WC Jr, Holstein TJ, Dyckman J et al., Inhibition of UVR-induced tanning and immunosuppression by topical applications of vitamins C and E to the skin of hairless (hr/hr) mice, *Pigment Cell Res* (2000) **13**:89–98.
25. Naganumaa M, Yagi E, Fukuda M, Delayed induction of pigmented spots on UVB-irradiated hairless mice, *J Dermatol Sci* (2001) **25**:29–35.
26. Sato T, Kawada A, Uptake of tritiated thymidine by epidermal melanocytes of hairless mice during ultraviolet light radiation, *J Invest Dermatol* (1972) **58**:71–3.
27. Pomerantz SH, Tyrosine hydroxylation catalyzed by mammalian tyrosinase: an improved method of assay, *Biochem Biophys Res Commun* (1964) **16**:188–94.
28. Warren R, Gardner PA, Reed JC, Sensitivity of mouse Skh:HR-2 to ultraviolet radiation: melanocyte inactivation, *J Invest Dermatol* (1987) **88**:266–70.
29. Schmidt R, Krien P, Regnier M, The use of diethylaminoethyl-cellulose-membrane filters in a bioassay to quantify melanin synthesis, *Anal Biochem* (1996) **235**:113–18.
30. Imokawa G, Kawai M, Mishima Y et al., Differential analysis of experimental hypermelanosis induced by UVB, PUVA, and allergic contact dermatitis using a brownish guinea pig model, *Arch Dermatol Res* (1986) **278**:352–62.
31. Ando H, Ryu A, Hashimoto A et al., Linoleic acid and alpha-linolenic acid lightens ultraviolet-induced hyperpigmentation of the skin, *Arch Dermatol Res* (1998) **290**: 375–81.
32. Horikoshi T, Nakahara M, Kaminaga H et al., Involvement of nitric oxide in UVB-induced pigmentation in guinea pig skin, *Pigment Cell Res* (2000) **13**:358–63.
33. Allan AE, Archambault M, Messana E et al., Topically applied diacylglycerols increase pigmentation in guinea pig skin, *J Invest Dermatol* (1995) **105**:687–92.
34. Pathak MA, Ciganek ER, Wick M et al., An evaluation of the effectiveness of azelaic acid as a depigmenting and chemotherapeutic agent, *J Invest Dermatol* (1985) **85**:222–8.
35. Ito Y, Jimbow K, Ito S, Depigmentation of black guinea pig skin by topical application of cysteaminylphenol, cysteinylphenol, and related compounds, *J Invest Dermatol* (1987) **88**:77–82.
36. Maeda K, Naganuma M, Topical trans-4-aminomethylcyclohexanecarboxylic acid prevents ultraviolet radiation-induced pigmentation, *J Photochem Photobiol B* (1998) **47**:136–41.
37. Brown DA, Ren WY, Khorlin A et al., Aliphatic and alicyclic diols induce melanogenesis in cultured cells and guinea pig skin, *J Invest Dermatol* (1998) **110**:428–37.
38. Bolognia JL, Murray MS, Pawelek JM, Hairless pigmented guinea pigs: a new model for the study of mammalian pigmentation, *Pigment Cell Res* (1990) **3**:150–6.
39. Bolognia JL, Sodi SA, Osber MP et al., Enhancement of the depigmenting effect of hydroquinone by cystamine and buthionine sulfoximine, *Br J Dermatol* (1995) **133**:349–57.
40. Sambuco CP, Miniature swine as an animal model in photodermatology: factors influencing sunburn cell formation, *Photodermatol* (1985) **2**:144–50.
41. Fourtanier A, Berrebi C, Miniature pig as an animal model to study photoaging, *Photochem Photobiol* (1989) **50**:771–84.
42. Nair X, Tranposch K, The Yucatan miniature swine as an in vivo model for screening skin depigmentation, *J Dermatol Sci* (1991) **2**:428–33.

43. Sambuco CP, Forbes PD, Davies RE et al., Protective value of skin tanning induced by ultraviolet radiation plus a sunscreen containing bergamot oil, *J Soc Cosmet Chem* (1987) **38**:11–19.
44. Nair X, Tramposch KM, Effect of single UVR exposure on skin pigmentation and melanocyte morphology in the Yucatan miniature swine, *J Invest Dermatol* (1990) **94**:558 (abst).
45. Nair X, Parab P, Suhr L et al., Combination of 4-hydroxyanisole and all-trans retinoic acid produces synergistic skin depigmentation in swine, *J Invest Dermatol* (1993) **101**:145–9.
46. Paine C, Sharlow E, Liebel F et al., An alternative approach to depigmentation by soybean extracts via inhibition of the PAR-2 pathway, *J Invest Dermatol* (2001) **116**:587–95.
47. Jimbow M, Marusyk H, Jimbow K, The in vivo melanocytotoxicity and depigmenting potency of N-2,4-acetoxyphenyl thioethyl acetamide in the skin and hair, *Br J Dermatol* (1995) **133**:526–36.
48. Seiberg M, Paine C, Sharlow E et al., Inhibition of melanosome transfer results in skin lightening, *J Invest Dermatol* (2000) **115**:162–7.

28
Light sources for UV-induced melanogenesis studies

François J. Christiaens

Introduction

Sun is the main source of ultraviolet radiation (UVR) we are exposed to at ground level. The sun's spectrum includes ultraviolet (UV, 280–400 nm), visible (400–700 nm) and infrared (700–2500 nm) light. Although solar UV irradiance represents less than 7% of the total irradiance (280–2500 nm) received on earth,[1] UV photons and, to a lesser extent, visible photons have enough energy per quantum to induce electronic transitions. This energy makes them the most biologically effective photons. Visible biological effects are reflected by erythema and pigmentation. Melanogenesis is the biological process responsible for darkening and tanning of the skin.

Action spectra

From a clinical point of view, UVR produces at least two different melanogenic responses of the skin: immediate pigmentation and delayed pigmentation, the latter being commonly referred to as tanning. These two effects require different UV doses, depend on the wavelength range the skin is exposed to, obey different kinetic rules, may be mediated by different pathways, etc. Immediate pigment darkening is a transient phenomenon that eventually results in a stable, lasting component called persistent pigment darkening (PPD). It is thought to be due to oxidation of existing melanin. Delayed pigmentation is associated with the synthesis of new melanin. The wavelength dependence of delayed pigmentation in fair-skinned individuals[2] and of PPD[3] are shown in Figure 28.1, together with that of minimal erythema in fair-skinned individuals.[4] Minimal erythema is defined as the minimal perceptible reddening of skin after one single exposure to UVR.

Figure 28.2 shows the same action spectra with a Y-axis logarithmic scale highlighting the relative contribution of UVA (320–400 nm), especially for delayed pigmentation and minimal erythema.

These action spectra emphasize the high efficiency of UV radiation in inducing skin pigmentation. Thus, a reliable and relevant light source that emits energy in the UV range is a prime requisite to study melanogenesis.

To elucidate some of the mechanisms involved in cellular functions, and most particularly those related to UV-induced melanogenesis, it may seem that any UV light source could be used. However, if sources emitting monochromatic light, such as Philips TL01 or TL/10R fluorescent tubes, or those whose spectrum is contaminated by UVC (200–280 nm) are used, no extrapolation to melanogenesis produced by natural irradiation conditions would be possible.

Solar radiation and solar simulator spectra

Solar radiation

Solar UV irradiance received at earth level is highly variable. It depends on many parameters, such as latitude (geographical location between equator and pole), hemisphere, season of the year, time of day, thickness of the ozone layer, clouds, altitude, aerosols and albedo (light reflected by surroundings). Clouds provide the best known examples of giving significant decreases in UVR exposure. The stratospheric ozone layer has a dramatic influence

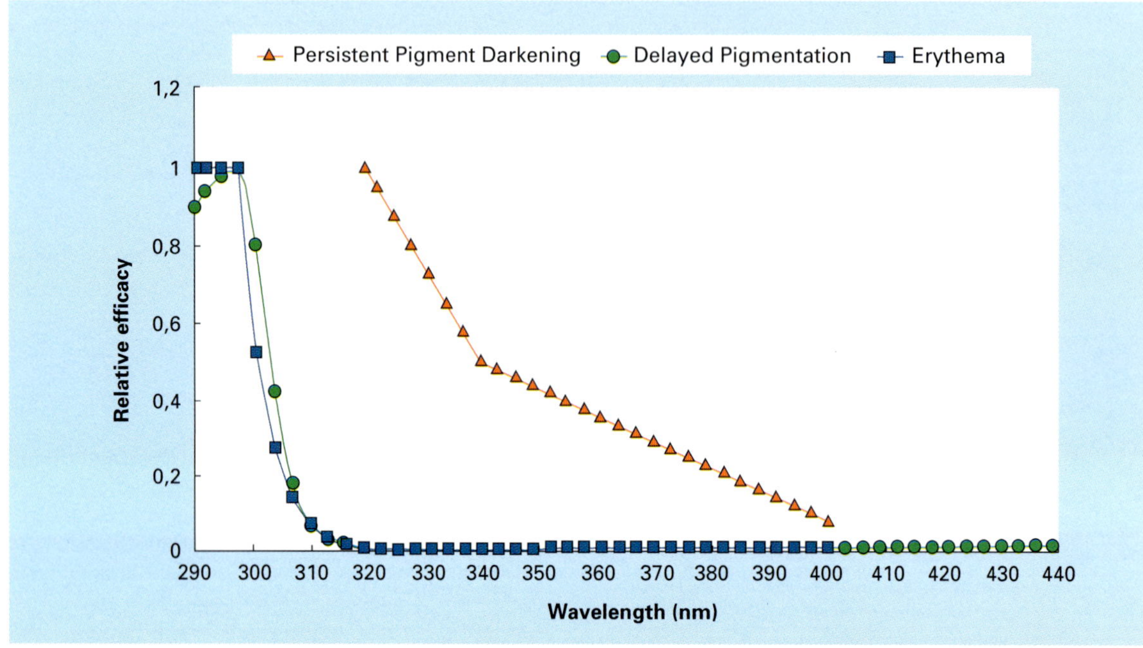

Figure 28.1

Action spectra of UV-induced pigmentation and erythema (linear scale).

on the amount of UVB (280–320 nm) reaching earth level. A slight decrease in the thickness of the ozone layer results in a significant increase in UVB irradiance and dose. The action spectrum of delayed pigmentation shows a sharp dependence on UVB. Therefore, slight changes in the ozone layer are likely to cause significant alterations in the sun's radiation, and thus in it's ability to trigger melanogenesis.

From all different solar UV spectra recorded worldwide throughout the year, a zenithal spectrum at earth level can be defined to represent a worst-case situation. This reference spectrum provides a basis for evaluating melanogenesis induced by solar exposure. Human skin exposed to such a spectrum is likely to undergo intense biological effects if a relevant dose is applied. The worst-case scenario happens in summer under clear sky conditions when the sun is overhead (zenithal). The zenithal sunlight spectrum published by the Deutsches Institut für Normung has been taken as reference in this chapter.[5]

Artificial UV sources offer significant advantages compared with natural sun exposure, which has unpredictable variations and limited availability. Because of their superior output and stability, these sources are used for conducting robust laboratory experiments.

Solar simulators

Commercially available UV sources have been classified into four categories according to the type of bulb they use: short-arc xenon, long-arc xenon, metal halide arc and fluorescent tubes. Additional filters may be inserted into the output beam to modify the emission spectrum. Sources including an incandescent filament bulb emit very low UV irradiance; therefore, they were excluded from this study.

- Various models of solar simulators equipped with a short-arc xenon bulb are provided by suppliers including the Solar Light Company, Thermo Oriel, Kratos Analytical (now Spectral Energy Corp.), Schoeffel Optical and others. The lamp input power ranges from 150 W to at

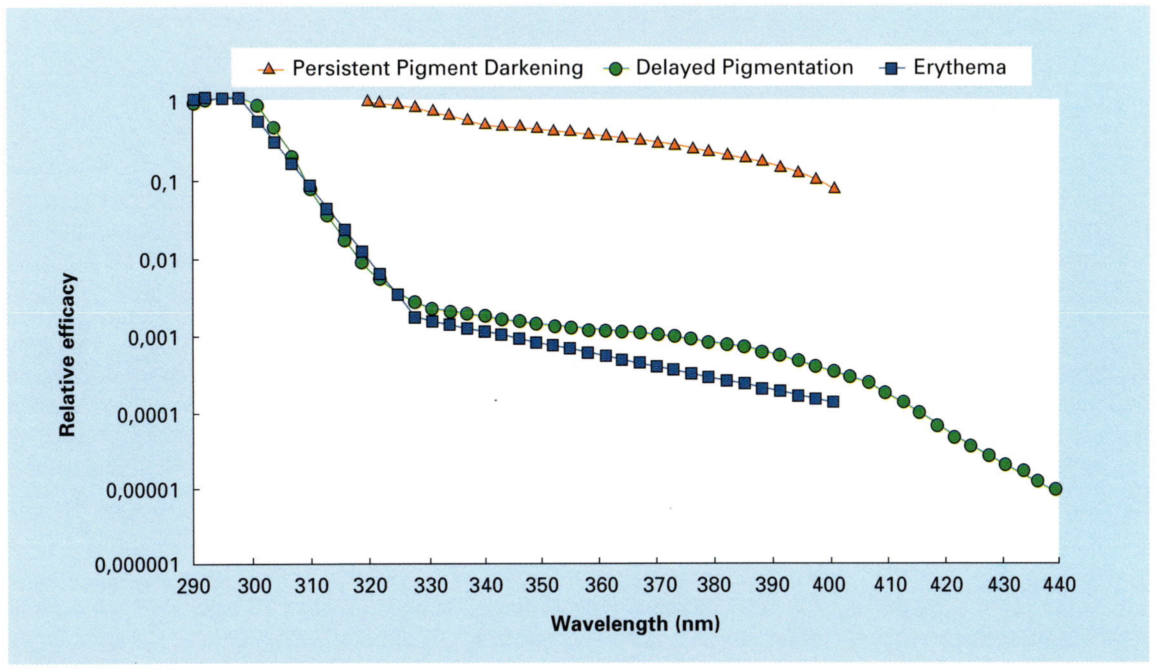

Figure 28.2

Action spectra of UV-induced pigmentation and erythema (logarithmic scale).

least 6 kW, which is the highest level for research purposes. Filters and dichroic mirrors are added to tailor the spectrum. In most cases, a 1-mm Schott WG-320 filter is used to control the short wavelength cut-off, absorbing all UVC and a significant amount of short UVB photons. In addition, the Solar Light and Oriel devices mostly use a 1-mm Schott UG-11 filter to remove visible and infrared radiation. Other devices use either the same filter or others (such as a Schott UG-5, 2-mm thick), or multiple dichroic mirrors to remove the longer wavelengths.

- Long-arc xenon simulators are brand-named Suntest or Xenotest lamps (previously supplied by Heraeus, now by Atlas Electric Devices Co., Chicago, IL, USA). The special UV filter provided with the simulator shapes the spectrum to mimic that of the sun.
- Metal halide lamps can be purchased from Dr K. Hönle GmbH (Martinsried, Germany) and filtered with an H2 filter. Another type of metal halide lamp is sold by Atlas. It can be equipped with Solar Simulated Radiation (SSR) filtration.
- The fluorescent tube category encompasses UVB tubes, UVA tubes and UVA-340 tubes. TL12 fluorescent UVB tubes are manufactured by Philips (Philips Eclairage, Boulogne, France). Westinghouse FS-40 tubes, Wolff Helarium tubes and Vilber-Lourmat UVB tubes deliver similar spectra. For biological assays, these tubes may be filtered with a Kodacel sheet (cellulose triacetate) to remove any radiation below 290 nm. To our knowledge, they have never been associated with UVA tubes for studying melanogenesis. Fluorescent UVA-340 tubes are manufactured by QPanel Co., Cleveland, OH, USA. Their brand name suggests that they have maximal irradiance at 340 nm; however, they emit significant radiation from 300 nm up to more than 400 nm. It should be noted that Philips 'Cleo Natural Light' fluorescent tubes deliver a radiation spectrum similar to that of QPanel UVA-340 tubes. A description of fluorescent UVA tubes is given later in this chapter.

In the present chapter, six types of lamp have been investigated:

1. A short-arc xenon 1000 W Oriel solar UV simulator, 4″ × 4″ type, equipped with a dichroic mirror and a Schott WG-320 filter, 1.5 mm thick. No short-pass filter (Schott UG-11-like filter) was added, so that visible light was removed only by the dichroic mirror.
2. A long-arc xenon Atlas Suntest lamp, CPS type, equipped with the standard special UV filter.
3. A 400 W metal halide lamp from Dr K. Hönle GmbH, UVASpot type, equipped with an H2 filter.
4. A metal halide lamp, SolarConstant 4000 type, provided by Atlas.
5. A Philips TL12 UVB fluorescent tube (20 W).
6. A Q-Panel UVA-340 fluorescent tube.

The respective spectral irradiances have been measured with a Bentham DM150 spectroradiometer (Bentham Instruments Limited, Reading, UK). Spectral calibration of the spectroradiometer was performed using a mercury pen lamp, and irradiance calibration was achieved using a calibrated Quartz Tungsten Halogen lamp traceable to the National Physics Laboratory (Teddington, UK).

Artificial UV sources selected for this study show a wide range of irradiances. Irradiance emitted by fluorescent tubes is much lower than that of xenon-arc or metal halide lamps. For an easier graphical comparison of the sources, their spectral irradiance has been divided by their respective UV irradiance. Relative spectral irradiance of the selected sources is shown in Figures 28.3–28.5, with the spectrum of reference sunlight. Zenithal sun irradiance is 3.45 W m^{-2} for UVB and 60.3 W m^{-2} for UVA.[5] Oriel solar simulators (equipped with a short-arc xenon bulb) commonly emit UVB irradiance as high as 20 W m^{-2} and UVA irradiance as high as 200 W m^{-2}. Irradiances delivered by metal halide lamps may be much higher, depending on the distance between the source and the exposed area, e.g. at 30 cm, 20 W m^{-2} for UVB irradiance and 600 W m^{-2} for UVA irradiance.

From relative spectral irradiances measured in this study, it appears that short-arc xenon sources provide the most suitable solution when the aim is to simulate solar light received at the ground level. Moreover, a long-arc xenon lamp equipped with a

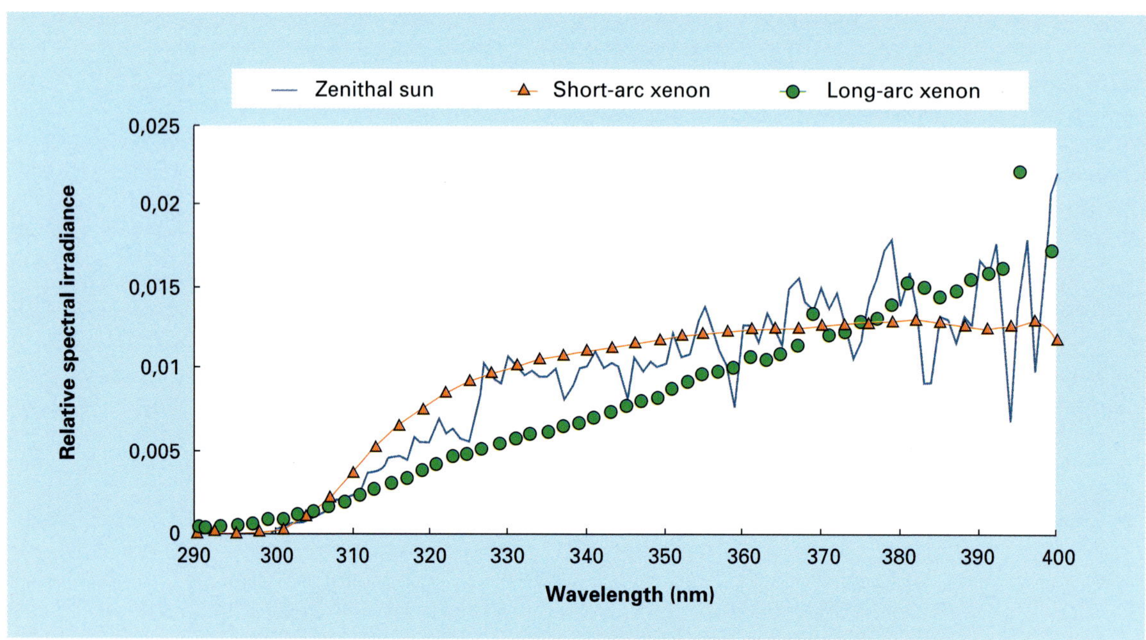

Figure 28.3

Zenithal sun and xenon sources spectra.

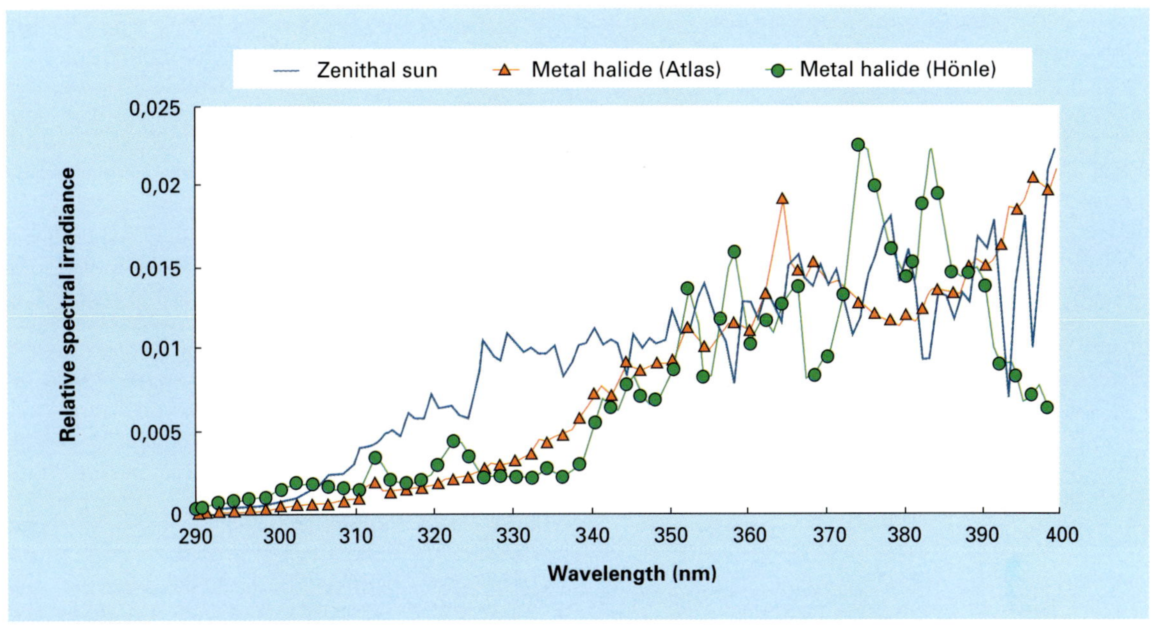

Figure 28.4

Zenithal sun and metal halide lamp spectra.

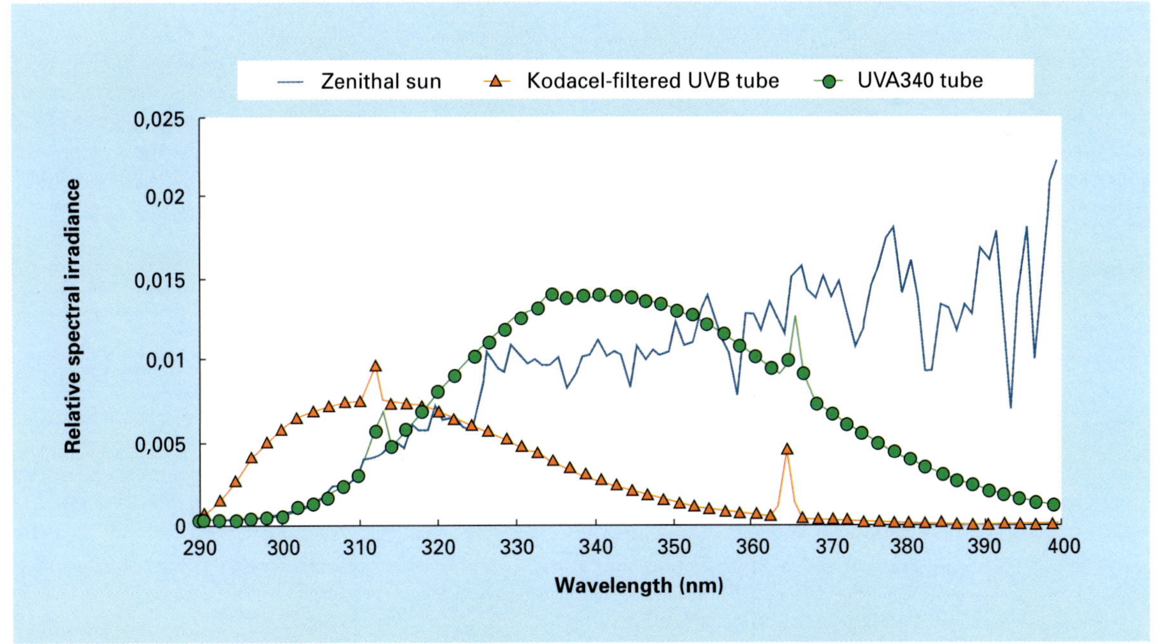

Figure 28.5

Zenithal sun and fluorescent tube spectra.

Schott WG-320 filter would emit a spectrum very similar to the zenithal sun spectrum delivered by short-arc xenon solar simulators.[6] Using an accurately filtered xenon-arc solar simulator guarantees the relevance of experimental exposure conditions. From our experience, both short-arc and long-arc xenon simulators equipped with a WG-320 filter thicker than 1 mm may eliminate the right amount of radiation (all UVC and short UVB) and provide a correct spectrum. However, because of the variability between various batches of WG-320 filters, the filter thickness cannot be reliable enough to predict its transmittance. Only the measurement of the spectral irradiance of a solar simulator can guarantee its relevance.

UVA sources

Outdoor

UVA radiation definitely stimulates melanogenesis.[2,3] By far the most common source of UVA is sunlight. UVA represent at least 95% of the solar UV irradiance received at earth level at a low altitude.[1] In a first approach, the shape of solar UVA irradiance does not depend on parameters such as clouds, ozone, etc. In contrast, the level of solar UVA irradiance depends on fewer parameters than solar UVB. For example, the thickness of the ozone layer hardly affects UVA irradiance. Furthermore, solar UVA irradiance shows little variation with season and latitude as compared to solar UVB. UVA radiation is not filtered by common glass.

Artificial UVA sources

The following typical commercial sources, emitting a broad spectrum of radiation, have been investigated in this study:

- Oriel short-arc xenon solar UV simulator (Oriel, Stratford, CT, USA), equipped with a dichroic mirror and a Schott WG-335 3-mm filter. No short-pass filter such as Schott UG-11-like filter was added to remove visible light.
- Long-arc xenon lamp Suntest (Atlas Electric Devices Co., Chicago, IL, USA). The standard glass filter provided by the manufacturer replaced the standard special UV filter in order to get only the UVA part of the spectrum.
- Metal halide lamps from Dr K. Hönle GmbH (Martinsried, Germany), filtered with the special filter 'H1', which blocks UVB but not UVA rays. This kind of lamp has been used extensively in sunbeds.[7,8]
- Fluorescent UVA tubes manufactured by Philips (model TL09) and provided by Vilber-Lourmat, Marne-la-Vallée, France. This type of source is used in most sunbeds designed for tanning.[7,8] Wolff Belarium fluorescent tubes gave similar spectra according to our measurements.

Spectral irradiances have been measured with a Bentham DM150 spectroradiometer, as indicated above. Oriel solar simulators commonly emit UVA irradiance as high as 200 W m^{-2}. UVA irradiance delivered by metal halide lamps may be much higher, depending on the distance between the source and the exposed area, e.g. 500 W m^{-2} at 30 cm.

Spectral irradiances have been divided by their respective UV irradiance to allow a clear representation. They are expressed as relative irradiance and are shown in Figures 28.6 and 28.7. The spectrum of zenithal sunlight filtered by a glass window has been added.

No direct comparison with the sun's spectrum can be made, since it always includes UVB radiation. Even so, people may be exposed to UVA merely through window glass. Therefore, a source emitting UVA is likely to be partially representative of the UV radiation received from the sun in real life. Studies involving UVA sources most often imply repeated exposure.

Discussion

Important considerations on the quality and relevance of sources and measurement devices can be drawn from data shown above.

Short-wavelength filtration

The action spectrum of delayed pigmentation depends highly on wavelength. When studying the effects related to delayed pigmentation, the rough resemblance between the source spectrum and

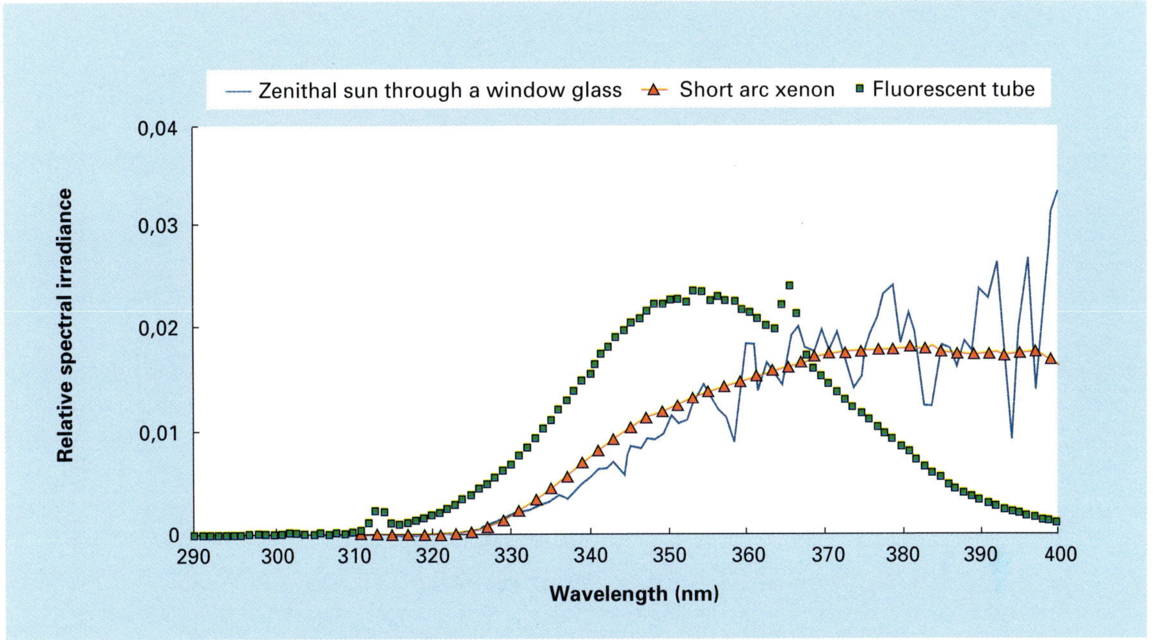

Figure 28.6

Spectra of UVA-filtered by a short-arc xenon source and a fluorescent UVA tube, compared with the zenithal spectrum though a window glass.

the zenithal sun spectrum may fail to guarantee the relevance of the source. The source is considered as relevant when it produces similar biological effects outdoors and indoors. To ensure that the source spectrum matches that of sun, compliance criteria have to be used. Such criteria are proposed in the Colipa Sun Protection Factor (SPF) test method.[9] This method is based on the minimal erythema action spectrum and criteria are defined using calculations involving this action spectrum. By extension, the proposed criteria can also be used to assess the relevance of a source used for melanogenesis studies, because minimal erythema and delayed pigmentation action spectra are closely similar in the UVB range. The CIE erythema action spectrum[4] is a widely used surrogate to estimate other biological effects.[10,11]

Furthermore, melanogenesis may be studied along with other biological effects. Gilchrest and colleagues showed that DNA photodamage enhanced melanogenesis.[12,13] DNA photodamage is highly variable with wavelength[14–18] and its action spectrum is quite similar to that of minimal erythema, which suggests that using a source whose spectrum complies with the Colipa SPF test method criteria is appropriate.

Coohill et al.[19] emphasized the need to pay attention to the filtration of the source, reporting that the presence of any contaminating wavelengths shorter than those intended for the study alter the measured melanogenesis. Although numerous studies carried out on the wavelength range between 220 and 290 nm have been useful to elucidate some of the mechanisms of cellular functions, these wavelengths are environmentally and physiologically irrelevant. The nature of primary and secondary chromophores, photoproducts, and mechanisms for cellular response involved in sun exposure, appear to be clearly different from those reported for wavelengths shorter than about 300 nm. Thus, studies involving unrealistic wavelengths[20–26] need to be scrutinized to determine whether the interpretations can be extrapolated to real-life conditions. Recently, Gasparro and colleagues determined that the source spectrum is an essential parameter in photobiological studies,[27,28] and it should be considered at an early design stage of a study protocol.

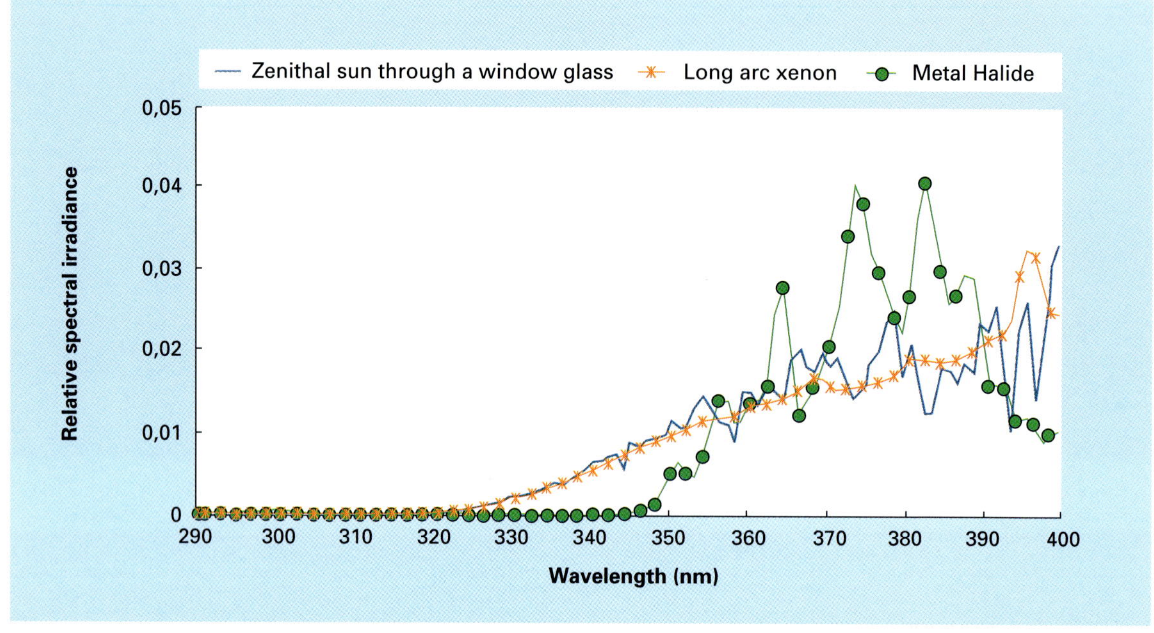

Figure 28.7

Spectra of UVA-filtered by a long-arc xenon source and a metal halide lamp, compared with the zenithal spectrum through a window glass.

So, much care should be given to filter out the shorter UVB wavelengths.

Shielding in *in vitro* studies

For *in vitro* irradiation, shielding must be addressed. The spectral transmission of any lid covering irradiated cells should be measured precisely. Most plastic materials absorb UV, so that the transmitted spectrum of the source through the lid differs from the source spectrum in both level and shape. Recently, Gasparro and colleagues measured the transmission of commonly available plastic lids, highlighting the dramatic alteration of the radiation spectrum received by the cells and its consequences on the results and interpretations.[29] Plastic materials generally absorb more UVB than UVA; consequently, melanogenesis may be prevented or significantly altered when irradiating through a lid.

Basal cells are naturally shielded by epidermis *in vivo*. Bruls et al.[30] published transmission measurements in Caucasian human skin. The epidermis absorbs UVB more efficiently than UVA, which alters the spectrum of solar light reaching basal cells. The proportion of UVA relative to total UV is higher than at the skin surface. Therefore, when irradiating cultured cells in a monolayer, the spectral output of solar UV simulators may need to be fine-tuned in order to get relevant data.

So-called UVA sources

Ninety-eight percent (98%) of the energy emitted by Philips TL09 fluorescent tubes lies in the UVA and 2% in the UVB range (see spectrum in Fig. 28.6). To calculate the biological effectiveness of the source, the product of the emission spectrum by the delayed pigmentation action spectrum has been considered. Resulting data show that UVB radiation accounts for two-thirds of induced pigmentation. It thus appears clear that such a source should not be labeled 'UVA source' when used in melanogenesis studies. Furthermore, accurate spectroradiometry is required to measure accurately low irradiances in order to do correct calculations.

Gilchrest and Eller[13] showed that UV-induced pyrimidine dimers are related to UV-induced melanogenesis. Moreover, 75% of pyrimidine dimers can be induced by the 0.8% UVB content of an UVA sunlamp.[31] Therefore, the term 'ultraviolet A sunlamp' is not reliable for the purpose of melanogenesis studies. In addition, the study made by Woollons et al.[31] highlights that only accurate spectroradiometers (equipped with a double monochromator) can provide reliable irradiance measurements leading to proper interpretations.

Doses

A comparison of indoor- and outdoor-received doses is only relevant when both spectra are very similar. As an example, results derived from experiments conducted with unfiltered UVB fluorescent tubes cannot be extrapolated to real-life conditions; the emission spectra of the two sources are far too different. When artificial UV sources used differ widely from the sun's spectrum, subsequent huge discrepancies in the doses have been recorded.[32] Outdoor irradiance measurements give information on available UV coming from direct sunlight and diffuse skylight. Measured doses may be compared to those received by a static sunbather lying horizontally, with no shading. In this situation, the maximal UV dose that may be received is 150 J cm^{-2} in 1 day. However, whenever activity differs from sunbathing, specific anatomical areas, such as cheeks or the back, may receive different doses. Thus, comparisons between doses received in laboratory and outdoor conditions are only representative of sunbathing.

A frequently asked question is which dose, UVB dose or total UV dose, should be chosen as a relevant parameter? Indicating only UVB dose means taking into account UVB only, i.e. the effects of UVA rays are taken as being negligible. This assumption is not valid for melanogenesis studies, as shown by action spectra.[2,3] Numerous studies involving UVA sources confirmed the role of UVA in melanogenesis both *in vivo*[33,34] and *in vitro*.[35,36] Therefore, a proper way to reflect the contribution of UVA radiation to melanogenesis is to report both UVB and total UV doses.

It is assumed that melanogenesis depends on the UV dose received and not on the irradiation rate. When this hypothesis holds, melanogenesis is said to follow the reciprocity law. The stable component (PPD) of immediate pigmentation obeys the reciprocity law[34] while full immediate pigmentation does not.

When skin cells are irradiated at a high dose rate, defense and repair functions may be overwhelmed. For instance, melanin would not scavenge UV-induced free radicals.[37] When a more realistic dose rate (closer to that of solar UV) is applied, other events, *e.g.* mutagenesis, may have time to develop, and are more likely to represent what really happens. These events are far more insidious because they can lead to skin cancer. Therefore, whenever experimental conditions allow it, the irradiance level of the UV source should be as close as possible to the sun's irradiance level, i.e. 64 W m^{-2} or lower.

Conclusions and recommendations

The spectral output of UV sources must be considered at an early design stage of a study. Photons are active 'reagents'; thus, they need to be controlled experimentally as carefully as other parameters. A regular check of sources spectra is a prime requisite to achieve reliable results and helps draw relevant interpretations. The most relevant studies include fully characterized experimental conditions.

The following recommendations include and add to those previously made by Gasparro and Brown.[27]

- The source used, the manufacturer and the spectral output obtained should at least be described. The type and thickness of filters should also be described.
- Authors should not rely on manufacturer's data sheets for source characteristics, they should be considered only as a rough guideline. There can be variations from one batch to another. Therefore, to ensure rigorous and best conditions for reliability, spectroradiometry should be employed to determine the spectral output of the lamps used to perform the experiments.

- The radiometer or spectroradiometer should be calibrated against standards traceable to the National Institute of Standards Technology (Gaithersburg, USA) or an equivalent national bureau of standards.
- The lamps need a minimal warm-up period of at least 20 minutes prior to proceeding to irradiance readings through any filter or lid that might be covering the irradiated sample or cells.
- The plastic used to make tissue culture dishes may attenuate strongly the UVB range of the spectrum and/or have an effect in the UVA range. Thus, the meter probe must be placed at the very place where the cells are irradiated, under the same conditions.
- While spectroradiometric measurements need only be performed at relatively infrequent intervals (when a new lamp is installed or after 200 hours or 6 months of use), radiometric measurements need to be performed in each experiment. Variations in electric voltage from day to day cause changes in the energy output of the lamps.
- Irradiation of cells must be performed in a colorless, transparent medium (e.g. PBS or Hank buffer) devoid of organic compounds that could act as photosensitizers.
- Both UVB and UVA (as well as UVC and visible when present) irradiances and/or doses should be recorded and reported.
- If a comparison with real-life conditions is intended:
  - The source should not emit wavelengths below 290 nm. At least a graphical comparison between the source spectrum and the spectrum of zenithal sunlight is strongly encouraged. Please remember that whatever the studied effect, the state-of-the-art solar UV simulator includes a correctly filtered xenon bulb.
  - The UV dose delivered for acute exposure must be lower than 150 J cm^{-2}, which is the highest UV dose that can be received from sunlight at earth level in 1 day.
  - Comparisons with real life apply only to a sunbathing situation.
  - A dose rate lower than or close to the zenithal sun dose rate (6.37 mW cm^{-2} = 0.38 J cm^{-2} s^{-1}) should be used whenever possible, otherwise the assumption that the reciprocity law applies must be made explicitly.

Acknowledgements

The author would like to thank C. Bouillon, A. Chardon, C. Duval, A. Fourtanier, P. Krien, L. Marrot, S. Seité and M. Verschoore for reviewing the manuscript and providing constructive comments.

References

1. Commission Internationale de l'Éclairage (CIE), Solar spectral irradiance, *Publ. CIE N° 85*, 1989.
2. Parrish JA, Jaenicke KF, Anderson RR, Erythema and melanogenesis action spectra of normal human skin, *Photochem Photobiol* (1982) **36**:187–91.
3. Chardon AM, Moyal D, Hourseau C, Persistent pigment darkening response as a method for evaluation of UVA protection assays. In: (Lowe NJ, Shaath NA, Pathak MA eds) *Sunscreens Development, Evaluation, and Regulatory Aspects* (Marcel Dekker, Inc.: New York, 1997) 559–82.
4. Commission Internationale de l'Éclairage (CIE), Erythema reference action spectrum and standard erythema dose, *Publ. CIE N° S 007/E*, 1998.
5. Deutsches Institut für Normung e.V.(DIN), Experimentelle Bewertung des Erythemschutzes von externen Sonnenschutzmitteln für die menschliche Haut (Experimental evaluation of the protection from erythema by external sunscreen products for the human skin), *DIN 67501*, Berlin (1999).
6. Christiaens FJ, Fourtanier A, Choosing a solar ultraviolet simulator with an appropriate spectrum. *Programme and Book of Abstracts*. International Conference on Photobiology, San Francisco, 1–6 July 2000 (Abstract).
7. McGinley J, Martin CJ, Mackie RM, Sunbeds in current use in Scotland: a survey of their output and patterns of use, *Br J Dermatol* (1998) **139**:428–38.
8. Moseley H, Davidson M, Ferguson J, A hazard assessment of artificial tanning units, *Photodermatol Photoimmunol Photomed* (1998) **14**:79–87.
9. The European Cosmetic and Toiletry Association (Colipa), Sun Protection Factor test method. *Report 94/289*, 1994.
10. Kligman LH, Sayre RM, An action spectrum for ultraviolet induced elastosis in hairless mice: quantification of elastosis by image analysis, *Photochem Photobiol* (1991) **53**:237–42.

11. Bech-Thomsen N, Wulf HC, Carcinogenic potential of fluorescent UV tanning sources can be estimated using the CIE erythema action spectrum, *Int J Radiat Biol* (1993) **64**:445–50.
12. Eller MS, Ostrom K, Gilchrest BA, DNA damage enhances melanogenesis, *Proc Natl Acad Sci USA* (1996) **93**:1087–92.
13. Gilchrest BA, Eller MS, DNA photodamage stimulates melanogenesis and other photoprotective responses, *J Invest Dermatol* (1999) **4**:35–40.
14. Setlow RB, The wavelengths in sunlight effective in producing skin cancer: a theoretical analysis, *Proc Natl Acad Sci USA* (1974) **71**:3363–6.
15. Freeman SE, Hacham H, Gange RW et al., Wavelength dependence of pyrimidine dimer formation in DNA of human skin irradiated *in situ* with UV light, *Proc Natl Acad Sci USA* (1989) **86**:5605–9.
16. Garcés F, Dávila CA, Alterations in DNA irradiated with ultraviolet radiation. I- The formation process of cyclobutylpyrimidine dimers: cross sections, action spectra and quantum yields, *Photochem Photobiol* (1982) **35**:9–16.
17. Kuluncsics Z, Perdiz D, Brulay E et al., Wavelength dependence of ultraviolet-induced DNA damage distribution: involvement of direct or indirect mechanisms and possible artefacts, *J Photochem Photobiol B* (1999) **49**:71–80.
18. Ley RD, Peak MJ, Lyon LL, Induction of pyrimidine dimers in epidermal DNA of hairless mice by UVB: an action spectrum, *J Invest Dermatol* (1983) **80**:188–91.
19. Coohill TP, Peak MJ, Peak JG, The effects of the ultraviolet wavelengths of radiation present in sunlight on human cells *in vitro*, *Photochem Photobiol* (1987) **46**:1043–50.
20. Bech-Thomsen N, Poulsen T, Christensen DH et al., UVA tanning devices interact with solar-simulated UV radiation in skin tumor development in hairless mice, *Arch Dermatol Res* (1992) **284**:353–7.
21. Abdel-Malek ZA, Swope VB, Smalara D et al., Analysis of the UV-induced melanogenesis and growth arrest of human melanocytes, *Pigment Cell Res* (1994) **7**:326–32.
22. Barker D, Dixon K, Medrano EE et al., Comparison of the responses of human melanocytes with different melanin contents to ultraviolet B irradiation, *Cancer Res* (1995) **55**:4041–6.
23. Medrano EE, Im S, Yang F, Abdel-Malek, ZA, Ultraviolet B light induces G1 arrest in human melanocytes by prolonged inhibition of retinoblastoma protein phosphorylation associated with long-term expression of the p21Waf-1/SDI-1/Cip-1 protein, *Cancer Res* (1995) **55**:4047–52.
24. Im S, Moro O, Peng F et al., Activation of the cyclic AMP pathway by alpha-melanotropin mediates the response of human melanocytes to ultraviolet B radiation, *Cancer Res* (1998) **58**:47–54.
25. Suzuki M, Protective effect of fine-particle titanium dioxide on UVB-induced DNA damage in hairless mouse skin, *Photodermatology* (1987) **4**:209–11.
26. Sauter ER, Klein-Szanto AJP, Atillasoy ES et al., Ultraviolet B-induced squamous epithelial and melanocytic cell changes in a xenograft model of cancer development in human skin, *Mol Carcinogen* (1998) **23**:168–74.
27. Gasparro FG, Brown DB, Photobiology 102: UV sources and dosimetry – the proper use and measurement of 'Photons as a reagent', *J Invest Dermatol* (2000) **114**:613–16.
28. Brown DB, Peritz AE, Mitchell DL et al., Common fluorescent sunlamps are an inappropriate substitute for sunlight, *Photochem Photobiol* (2000) **72**:340–4.
29. Brown DB, Peritz AE, Uitto J, Gasparro FG, Ultraviolet-filtering properties of commonly used tissue cell culture plasticware, *Photodermatol Photoimmunol Photomed* (2001) **17**:126–9.
30. Bruls WAG, Slaper H, van der Leun J, Berrens L, Transmission of human epidermis and stratum corneum as a function of thickness in the UV and visible wavelengths, *Photochem Photobiol* (1984) **40**:485–94.
31. Woollons A, Kipp C, Young AR et al., The 0.8% ultraviolet B content of an ultraviolet A sunlamp induces 75% of cyclobutane pyrimidine dimers in human keratinocytes *in vitro*, *Br J Dermatol* (1999) **140**:1023–30.
32. Niggli HJ, Röthlisberger R, Sunlight-induced pyrimidine dimers in human skin fibroblasts in comparison with dimerization after artificial UV-irradiation, *Photochem Photobiol* (1988) **48**:353–6.
33. Margolis RJ, Sherwood ME, Maytum DJ et al., Longwave ultraviolet radiation (UVA 320–400 nm)-induced tan protects human skin against further UVA injury, *J Invest Dermatol* (1989) **93**:713–18.
34. Moyal D, Chardon AM, Kollias N, Determination of UVA protection factors using the persistent pigment darkening (PPD) as the end point. 1. Calibration of the method, *Photodermatol Photoimmunol Photomed* (2000) **16**:245–9.

35. Duval C, Régnier M, Schmidt R, Distinct melanogenic response of human melanocytes in mono-culture, in co-culture with keratinocytes and in reconstructed epidermis, to UV exposure, *Pigment Cell Res* (2001) **14**:348–55.
36. Marrot L, Belaidi J-P, Chaubo C et al., An *in vitro* strategy to evaluate the phototoxicity of solar UV at the molecular and cellular level: application to photoprotection assessment, *Eur J Dermatol* (1998) **8**:403–12.
37. Hill HZ, The function of melanin or six blind people examine an elephant, *BioEssays* (1992) **14**:49–56.

Section VIII

MELANOMAGENESIS AND PHOTOPROTECTION

29

Immediate and delayed pigmentary responses to solar UVA radiation (320–400 nm)

Alain Chardon and Dominique Moyal

Introduction

What the main components of UVA suntanning are is still being debated among photobiologists and dermatologists. What are the precise characteristics of the UVA-induced pigmentary phenomena currently named immediate pigment darkening (IPD), IPD residue, lasting pigmentation, PPD, delayed pigmentation, facultative pigmentation, true melanization, direct or indirect pigmentation, neo-melanization, etc? Do some of these denominations cover the same phenomenon?

The colour of human skin derives from the impact of light on it and is influenced by several constitutive factors, including, principally, melanin quality[1–3] and content, and the number, size and distribution of melanosomes in the epidermis.[4–11] The resultant skin colour is thus influenced by the constitutive or intrinsic skin colour and the facultative or inducible skin pigmentation. The facultative skin colour is commonly referred to as "suntan". This can be obtained from exposures to actual sun or to sunbeds.

In this Chapter, we will mainly discuss the tanning effects of UVA radiation (320–400 nm) as it can been observed visually and quantified by colorimetric measurements. Let us notice that UVA suntanning can be obtained either with artificial UVA light from sunbeds or in actual sun, using an efficient UVB-filtering system.[17] The various skin reactions induced by repeated UVB, UVA, and UVB+UVA exposures under artificial sources on the backs of volunteers have been followed for several weeks by colorimetry in the CIE 1976 L*a*b* colour space,[13,14] in order to describe the characteristics of the respective "suntanning pathways". Using a vectorial analysis technique[17] built on databases, including their respective colour previously characterized, it was possible to separate the components of suntanning. The plotted respective kinetics obtained after UVA-radiation stimulation[15,16] confirmed many results from previous studies[4–11] and also clarified some points hardly detectable and quantifiable by visual evaluation. The conclusions of these studies were verified along subsequent similar suntanning pathways,[18] followed in actual sun or with artificial UV sources, on skin protected or not by sunscreens. Sunscreens generally intervene in reducing short-wavelength erythema, thus favouring long-wavelength suntanning.

UVA suntanning includes four main visible photobiologic phenomena, resulting from different photobiologic processes and distinguishable by their specific colour, hue, intensity and stability (kinetics). Three of them are linked to the skin's melanic components: immediate transient pigmentation (immediate pigment darkening, or IPD), lasting immediate pigmentation (persistent pigment darkening, or PPD), and delayed pigmentation (neo-melanization). The fourth, linked to the haemoglobin pigments, are the vasodilatory actinic and thermal erythemas.

Immediate pigment darkening

During short, single exposure to long UVA rays of skin types II to IV, a dark-bluish pigmentation ($\Delta L^* << 0$, $\Delta b^* < 0$, $\Delta a^* > 0$) develops, with practically no dose threshold and with UVA doses smaller than about 6 J.cm^{-2}.[19–22] This phenomenon is transient and fades out about 2 hours after the end of exposure, which means that, though dose-dependent, it saturates very fast: it is what is called IPD. This immediate pigmenting reaction has been attributed to the photo-oxidation of pre-existing melanins and melanin precursors. This reaction was better seen in pigmented individuals of skin phototypes III and IV.[7,8]

The IPD phenomenon was first observed in 1902 by Meirowsky. The dependence of IPD on oxygen concentration was first described by Henschke and Schulze in 1939.[23] Later, Auletta et al described the effects of hypoxia upon erythema and pigment responses[24] and Rorsman and Teigner confirmed a hypopigmentation due to ischæmia on compressed zones of subjects exposed on sunbeds.[25] IPD inhibition in the absence of oxygen suggests the oxidative nature of the reactions involved.[8] The skin is able to show IPD when it is exposed to UVA doses as low as 2 J.cm^{-2} to 10 J.cm^{-2}. During UVA exposure, a bluish-grey coloration develops (Fig. 29.1), reaching its maximum at the end of the UVA exposure. IPD reaction indicates that a photo-oxidation takes place that converts uncoloured, partially polymerized melanins, or melanin precursors, into coloured pigments.[21,27] Then, IPD gradually fades out. The transient aspect of this pigmentation, as well as its fast saturation in intensity, are attributed to the reversible oxidative reaction. This process is limited by the pre-existing amount of oxidable materials enclosed in the melanosomes. This would imply that there is a stronger IPD reaction in persons with a higher level of native melanic pigments (skin types III and IV).[8]

Persistent pigment darkening

For UVA doses higher than about 10 J.cm^{-2}, a stable residual pigmentation (persistent pigment darkening) is observed after the transient part of IPD has faded out.[20,21] The immediate pigmentation, while fading out after UVA exposure, loses a part of its blue component so that a grey residue is remaining about 2 hours post exposure and beyond (Fig. 29.1). Although induced with different dose ranges, both IPD and PPD phenomena result from an immediate UVA effect. It could be inferred that PPD cannot occur without an IPD response,

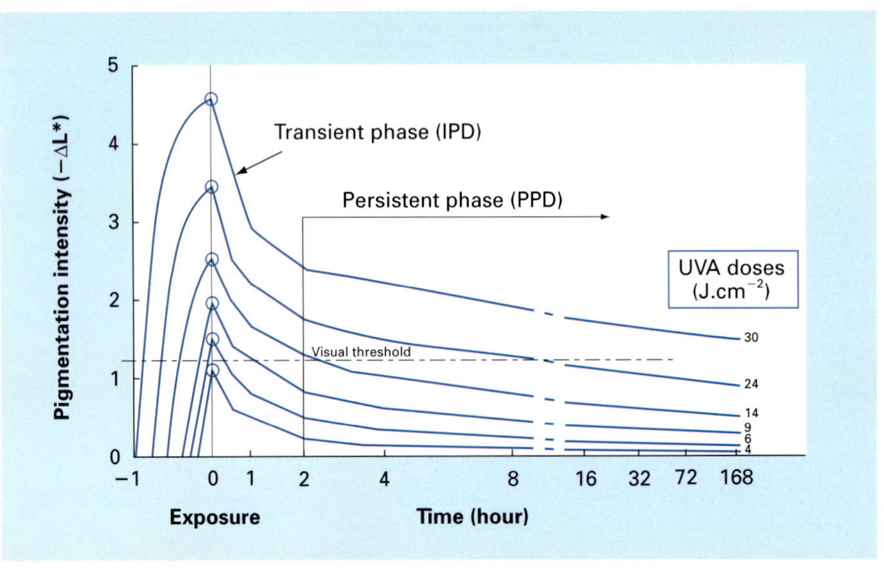

Figure 29.1

While various UVA doses are applied to skin (phototypes II to IV), an immediate grey-blue pigmentation develops, reaching its maximum at the end of exposure. Then, the transient part of this pigmentation (IPD) quickly fades away. If the UVA dose was sufficient, a persistent part (PPD) may last for several hours or days.

and IPD seems to constitute a substrate in the formation of PPD, at least for pigmented skins, but this hypothesis is controversial. The UVA dose required to induce PPD is about 15 $J.cm^{-2}$, and represents a little less than the amount received in 1 hour of exposure to a quasi-zenithal sun.

Both colorimetric measurements performed on skin types II to IV[20] and spectrocolorimetric measurements on types IV and V[21,22] showed that the PPD colour change due to a single, high dose of UVA stabilizes between dark blue "IPD" colour and brown (dark yellow) neo-melanization colour (Fig. 29.2). It is, however, difficult to conclude whether this intermediate colour is due to specific intermediate pigments, to a mixture of dark/blue and brown pigments, or to physical changes in the structure of the skin or of the pigments involved. The plateau observed in the colorimetric kinetics of the lasting immediate pigmentation over 7 days (Fig. 29.1) would suggest that there is no actual, induced neo-melanization in the range of UVA doses lower than 50 $J.cm^{-2}$ (single exposure). The intermediate stable colour (PPD) would rather be due to intermediate pigments, distinct from basic melanins and from photo-oxidized melanins (IPD). This hypothesis seems to be confirmed by studies based on confocal microscopy analysis (unpublished) and electron microscopy,[8,27] which could not show any specific granule distribution or morphological alteration of melanocytes in these conditions.

Another important, and surprising, typical characteristic of PPD pigmentation is that, contrary to that often said about the IPD response, it has, so far not been possible, for a given range of applied UVA doses, to find a significant correlation between PPD intensity (or its dose–response slope) and subject phototype (or its skin colour typing as per the Individual Typology Angle, ITA°).[15,20] Actually, IPD and PPD are distinguished by their dose–response curves, since IPD response increases quickly with low UVA doses but saturates quickly too, mainly at longer UVA wavelengths, while PPD needs higher doses and its dose–response curve is more linear (Fig. 29.3). All these findings suggest that IPD and PPD

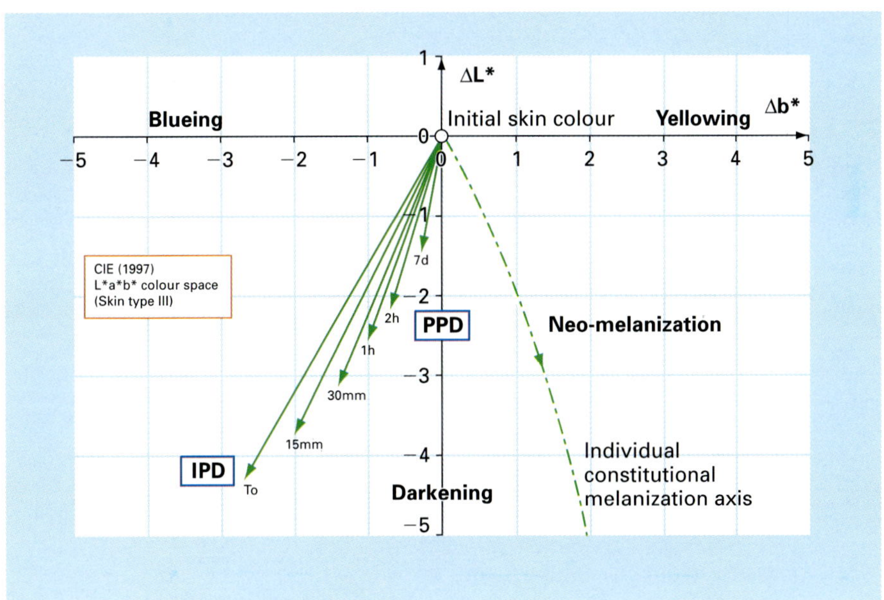

Figure 29.2

After the end of a sufficient UVA exposure, the transient immediate skin pigmentation (IPD) induced quickly decreases, while its grey-blue hue rotates towards a grey hue, that of the stable component (PPD). For each individual, this hue is clearly distinct from the brown (dark yellow) hue of both constitutive melanization and neo-melanization, which suggests that they are from distinct origins.

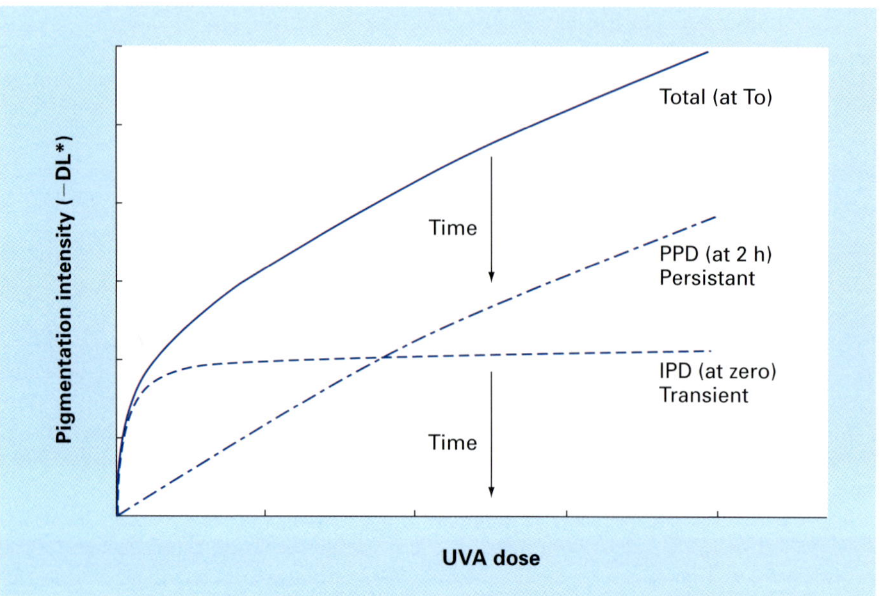

Figure 29.3

The total pigmentation as observed immediately after skin exposure to a sufficient dose of UVA would be the sum of two phenomena, distinct by their dose–response curves: IPD, inducible with a small UVA dose, transient and quickly saturating, and PPD, more persistant and linearly dose-dependent, and needing higher UVA doses. Two hours post exposure, only PPD remains perceptible.

phenomena, though concomitant, are from clearly distinct origins: reversible photo-oxidation of melanins and/or precursors for transient IPD, and irreversible, non-enzymatic polymerization of precursors for PPD. This could explain why PPD needs high UVA doses and may be induced on some phototype-I or "very light" skins, sometimes with high visual contrast (high colorimetric dose–response slope). According to this hypothesis, it would not be necessary for high levels of visible melanins (types III and IV) to be present in the skin to be able to produce PPD. Uncoloured/ invisible melanin precursors (immature melanins in skin type I) would be sufficient to produce specific visible pigments, provided high UVA doses are applied. It has be noticed that, in this case, the pigmentation present just after UVA exposure is no longer so unstable, because it is then due to PPD rather than to IPD.

To summarize with immediate pigmentations, we can say that if a single dose of UVA exposure of between 10 and 50 $J.cm^{-2}$ is applied, the pigmentation visible at the end of exposure is the sum of both previous phenomena. The first one, IPD or transient pigmentation, disappears within 2 hours and the second one, PPD or lasting immediate pigmentation, would only remain detectable for about 2 weeks, depending on the UVA dose applied. For high or repeated UVA doses, the induction of IPD and PPD could generate an imbalance in the melanosomes, which may be a signal to the cells to produce more melanin precursors and metabolites to start or accelerate the process of neo-melanogenesis or delayed pigmentation.

Neo-melanization

Through instrumental follow-up, the colour of the residual PPD pigmentation cannot be confused with that of the delayed pigmentation resulting from neo-melanization, because the latter occurs with a typical brown (dark yellow) colour, similar to basic melanins, and only in certain conditions: after induction of a UVA erythema on dark skin (phototypes III, IV and V) with UVA doses higher than 60 $J.cm^{-2}$, on very fair skin (phototype I) with UVA doses higher than 15 $J.cm^{-2}$, or after successive UVA exposures on all phototypes, even by suberythemogenic doses,[28,29] but cumulating a sufficient dose, similar to that needed with single exposure. Colorimetric follow-up clearly confirmed that neo-melanization starts with a 2-day delay after UVA exposure. A recent, unpublished suntanning pathway resulting from repeated exposures to UVA on light skins during a 13-week schedule clearly showed a marked increase in skin pigmentation resulting from a delayed pigmentary response, and a slight increase in red hue consistent with the development of a slight erythema. An increment in the size of the melanosomes synthetized by melanocytes was also observed.

It is noticeable that the time courses of UVA and UVB erythema differ markedly from each other, as developed below. UVA exposure seems to give rise to immediate erythema, whereas UVB induces delayed erythema, peaking approximately at 24 hours after exposure. However, the time courses of UVA- and UVB-delayed tanning, though induced with very different UV energetic doses, are similar and finally lead to the same type of melanins.[15] Melanocytes are activated by cumulated exposures to UVA, as well as to UVB, rays and melanogenesis involves increased formation of melanins and transfer of new melanosomes. In both cases, the acquired melanic pigmentations, after the specific transient colour change due to a variable mixture of erythema, IPD and PPD, always end in joining the individual "melanization axis" in the skin colour volume.[15] In such a way, they are individually predictable by the initial skin colour. This would mean that the final, new melanins induced by UVA, as well as by UVB, are issued from enzymatic (delayed) reactions of the same type as for the basic melanins already present in the skin before UV exposure, and are similarly genetically programmed (Fig. 29.4). However, it has been reported that the UVA-induced melanization would be less protective against subsequent UVB-induced erythema than UVB-induced melanization.[30–32] This might be attributed to the additional protective effect of the hyperkeratose accompanying the UVB melanization and following the initial UVB inflammation.

Finally, it has been shown that exposures of Caucasian skins to cumulative UVA and UVB doses applied together induce a pigmentation response that is practically additive, both in intensity and colour, as compared with that respectively obtained with the same, separate UVA and UVB cumulated energetic doses.[15] UVA melanization acquired by cumulative UVA exposures appeared much more lasting than that acquired with UVB exposures. UVA melanization continued to increase after the end of the exposure sequence, to reach a plateau and then slowly decrease over several weeks (Fig. 29.4). Contrarily, UVB melanization immediately starts decreasing, to return in one week to about 50% of the maximum acquired at the end of the exposure sequence.[15] However, due to the gap in erythemal efficacy between UVA and UVB, at similar tanning intensity, the energetic UVA doses applied could, in practice, be much higher than with UVB. Comparison of intrinsic tanning efficacy and durability should be performed at similar doses.

UVA erythema

Pigmentary responses cannot be evoked without also mentioning the characteristics of the UVA erythema, which often accompanies them. UVA erythema contributes towards at least 15% of the whole sun erythema. UVA erythema appears very quickly during exposure and lasts much longer than UVB erythema. According to spectrophotometric measurements, which guarantees that we are dealing with a haemoglobin response (absorption peaks at 542 and 564 nm) and not simply a reddish, melanic hue, UVA erythema may last, to a small extent in any persistent pigmentation[21,22] observed on fair skins. This mixed response at 24 hours is used in the erythema/pigmentation UVA-PF (UVA protection factor) test method.[33,34] However, care should be taken by appropriate means not to confuse the actinic UVA erythema with the immediate erythema induced by heat load due to the global spectrum, including infrared and visible rays, which are always more or less present in UV sources. The vessels concerned are not at the same depth in the skin and the kinetics and colour aspects are distinct: thermal erythema is marbled and short lasting while actinic UVA erythema is more uniform and longer lasting.[35] The hypothesis of a possible reddish pigmentation

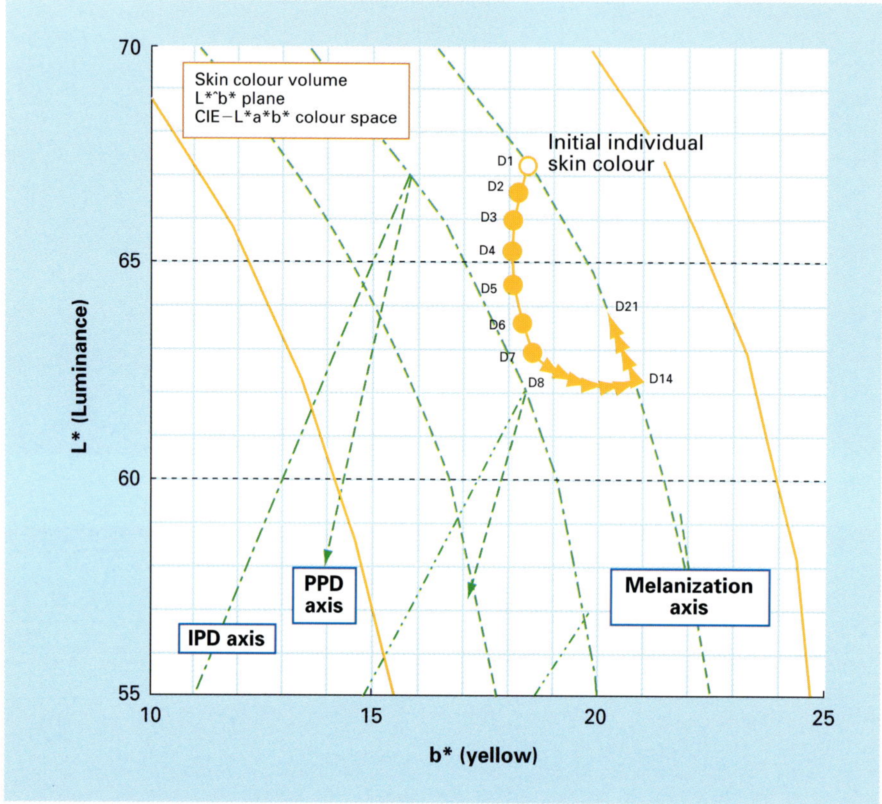

Figure 29.4

The distribution of skin colours in the CIE-L*a*b* colour space constitutes the "skin colour volume", the total of all individual melanization axes. For each subject S of a given constitutive skin colour, the various skin pigmentations inducible under UVA and/or UVB exposures are characterized by their proper axes, directed toward the basic colours of the pigments involved: erythema (haemoglobins), IPD photo-oxidized melanins), PPD (polymerized melanin precursors?) and neo-melanization (eu-/phaeo-melanins).

on fair skin with high pheomelanin content[1] was also mentioned.[15]

Reciprocity law

The question of the reciprocity law (Scharzschild's law) has mainly arisen in consideration of the skin response application for the development of protection factors for sunscreen testing: global-UV erythema for SPF (sun protection factor) testing,[37–40] UVA erythema,[41,42] IPD,[43,45] PPD,[19,20] or mixed erythema/PPD response[33,34] for UVA-PF testing. Reciprocity law relies on the equivalence of exposure time and UV source irradiance in inducing a given response intensity, generally the threshold response: this implies that the threshold dose is independent of the UV source irradiance. A pre-requisite for reciprocity law validation is that the response concerned was relatively stable after exposure. Otherwise, there is competition between formation speed (higher with higher irradiance) and fading speed (independent of irradiance). The resultant speed of the formation depends on the source irradiance, and the response intensity quickly saturates at variable levels when an equilibrium results between formation and fading kinetics. Reciprocity law is a fundamental need for the validation of a protection factor test method.[46,47]

Because UV-induced erythema at 24 hours is a stable response in a reasonable time frame, it was demonstrated as fully complying with the reciprocity law for the SPF application[37–39] in a wide range of exposure times (from a few seconds to more than 2 hours). However, to our knowledge, reciprocity of pure UVA erythema has never been published.

As for the IPD/PPD skin response, studies show that the unstable IPD does not comply with the reciprocity law,[20,21,26] while its stable PPD part does.[20,46–48] It is noteworthy that IPD cannot be obtained at very low irradiance levels, such as those encountered by skin under very efficient, photostable UVA sunscreens. Indeed, when the source irradiance is too low or strongly reduced by the sunscreen layer, the fading speed of the induced pigmentation widely exceeds the formation speed, and no pigmentation is obtained. Thus, the UVA dose applied must be strongly increased to give a visible (stable) response at the end of exposure, actually reaching the (stable) PPD threshold dose. The consequence is that comparing the threshold pigmenting dose (PPD) on protected skin to the threshold pigmenting dose (IPD) on unprotected skin to calculate an IPD UVA-PF would result in an inconsistent protection factor with mixed endpoints, variable with the protective efficacy to be measured. This phenomenon explains why IPD UVA-PFs diverge in a non-linear manner, with no relation to the actual UVA protection level of the sunscreen when UVA increases[20,48] and that a single PPD response at 2–24 hours must be obtained on both protected and unprotected areas to ensure reliable UVA-PFs.[46,47] There are fundamental reasons why PPD was preferred to IPD as an end-point for an in-vivo UVA-PF test method.[49, 50]

In our knowledge, no specific study has been dedicated to the reciprocity of neo-melanization, for example at 7 days, probably because of lack of specific application or because of the difficulty of the task, linked to a weak and mixed response (neo-melanization and PPD) after a single UVA exposure. However, considering the dose–response curves of both PPD and neo-melanization and their stability, it may be expected that the law would hold.

Action spectra

An important characteristic of pigmented skin response is the action spectrum, *ie* the sensitivity of the skin in relation to the incident-light wavelength in the UVA waveband. Indeed, every skin response above mentioned, erythema included, has been considered, separately or in combination, as an end-point for the implementation of an in-vivo UVA-PF in unsensitized human skin. With the emission spectrum of the UV source, the action spectrum of the response(s) selected defines the specific sensitivity of the UVA test method along the UVA spectrum.

Fig. 29.5 gives the relative action spectra of erythema at 24 hours post exposure, according to the CIE-1987 standard, IPD as observed immediately at the end of exposure, PPD as observed 2 hours post exposure, and melanization at 7 days.[52–59] A common aspect of these spectra is that they present a higher response in the short UVA, except for IPD, which would show less sensitivity at the shortest UVA wavelengths. However, it must be taken into account that, in the experiment from which this IPD spectrum was drawn,[52] the spectral UV xenon source used was not of constant irradiance along the UVA spectrum (lower irradiance at lower wavelengths); coupled with the non-validity of the reciprocity law for the transient IPD, this may lead to some bias. Anyway, because the reciprocity law does not hold for IPD, its action spectrum is intrinsically irradiance dependent. Another remark concerning the UVA action spectra of pigmentary responses is that on sensitive skins, the spectral doses needed to induce the pigmentary responses are close to the erythema threshold dose. It is thus difficult, while studying the pigment response action spectra, to induce a single pigmentary response without inducing a correlative, lasting erythemal response, particularly in the short UVA wavelength (around 320–330 nm), where the erythema action spectrum steeply increases. It is also difficult to distinguish, at 7 days after a single exposure, the part assignable to neo-melanization and that due to residual PPD. It must be noted that these action spectra extend into the short visible waveband (blue light), which thus also participates in the suntanning process, particularly when efficient UVB+UVA sunscreens are used during sun exposures.

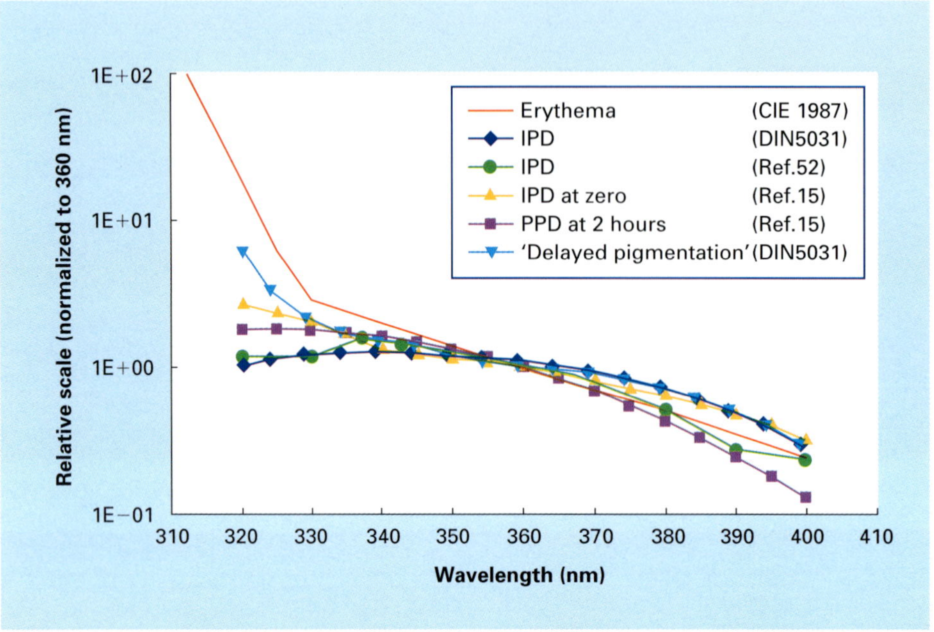

Figure 29.5

Action spectra of the various responses of the skin to UVA exposures: erythema, transient immediate pigment darkening (IPD), persistent pigment darkening (PPD) and delayed pigmentation (neo-melanization). All of them present similar shapes and more sensitivity to short UVA. They also extend into the short visible (blue) light.

Conclusion

Facultative skin pigmentation is commonly opposed to constitutive pigmentation. If facultative pigmentation covers what is not basic or intrinsic pigmentation, this term involves any colour changes that may be observed, simultaneously or successively, during or following a sequence of repeated exposures to UVA, *ie* during a suntanning pathway: erythema, IPD, PPD and neo-melanization, all phenomena inducible by UVA rays in variable intensity and duration, depending on the doses applied and their schedule. It was possible to colorimetrically separate these respective components because they are fortunately distinguished by their colour and hue (direction) in the tridimensional colour space (Fig. 29.6). Constitutive and facultative pigmentations are not so opposed, since colorimetric measurements showed that the suntans acquired either under UVB, UVA or whole UV rays, present the same predictable final aspects in terms of colour, unique to each individual, after the various transient phenomena have faded away. This suggests that whatever the mode and mechanisms of induction, the final pigmentations acquired during a suntanning process would respond to the same genetic program.

References

1. Thody A, Higgins E, Wakamatsu K, Ito S, et al, Pheomelanin as well as eumelanin is present in human epidermis, *J Invest Dermatol* (1991) **97**: 340–4.
2. Little M, Wolff M, Skin and hair reflectance in women with red hair, *Annals of Human Biology* (1981) **8**:231–41.
3. Edwards E, Duntley Q, The pigments and color of living skin, *Am J Anatomy* (1939) **65**:1–33.
4. Caswell M, The kinetics of the tanning response to tanning bed exposures, *Photodermatol Photoimmunol Photomed* (2000) **16**:10–14.

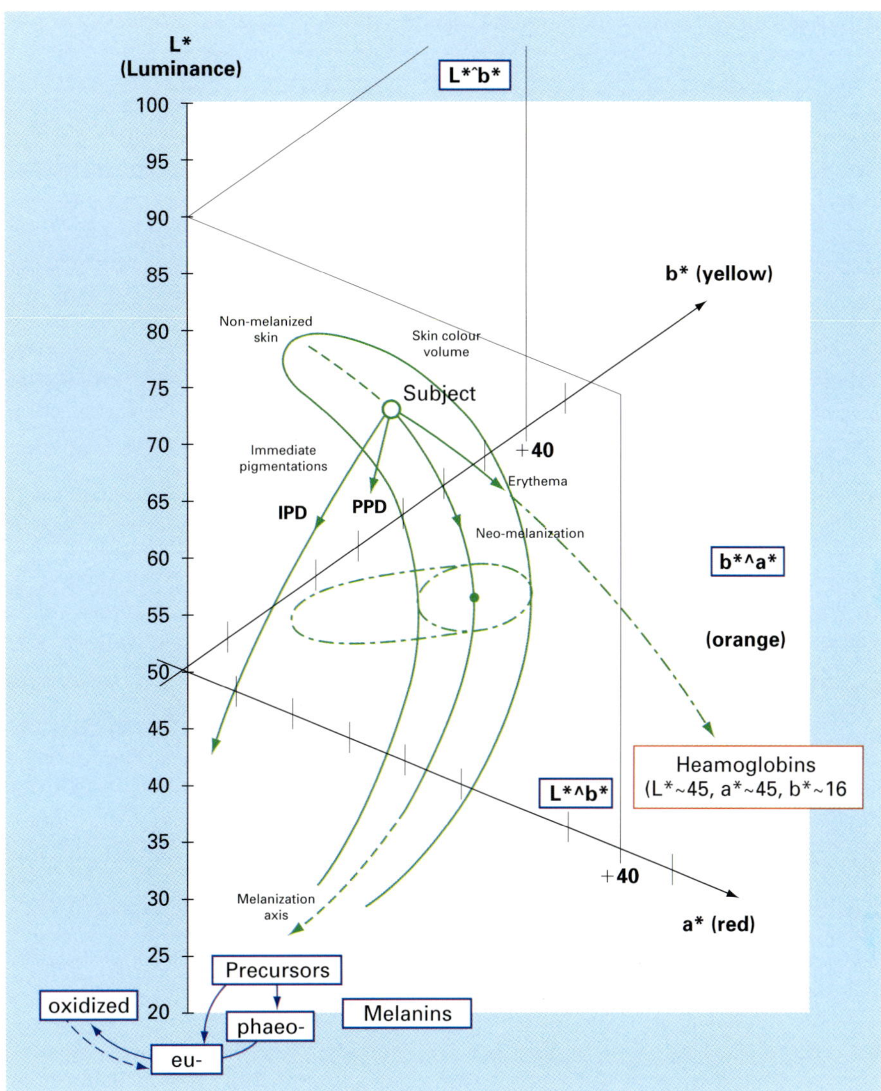

Figure 29.6

Typical colorimetric suntanning pathway induced on type III ("intermediate" skin colour category[15,37]) skins by cumulative UVA exposures applied over 7 days and followed for three weeks in the L*^b* plane (CIE-L*a*b* colour space). The influence of the blue-hue PPD pigmentation is clearly perceptible during the exposure phase and 1 week after, until the pathway reaches the individual melanization axis. Note that, unlike UVB, with UVA the pigmentation continues to increase even after the end of exposure, and the return to the initial, individual colour along the melanization axis is slow. No erythema was actually perceptible (suberythemal UVA doses, phototype III).

5. Pathak MA, Riley FC, Fitzpatrick TB, Melanogenesis in human skin following to long wave ultraviolet and visible light, *J Invest Dermatol* (1962) **39**:435–43.

6. Olson R, Gaylor J, Everett M, Skin color, melanin and erythema, *Arch Dermatol* (1973) **108**:541–4.

7. Jimbow K, Fitzpatrick T, Changes in distribution pattern of cytoplasmic filaments in human

melanocytes during ultraviolet-mediated melanin pigmentation, *J Cell Biology* (1975) **65**:481–8.

8. Kaidbey K, Kligman A, The acute effects of long-wave ultraviolet radiation on human skin, *J Invest Dermatol* (1978) **72**:253–6.
9. Pathak M, Immediate and delayed pigmentary and other cutaneous responses to solar UVA radiation (320–400nm). In: Urbach F, Gange R, eds, *The Biological Effects of UVA Radiation* (Praeger Publ: New York, 1986) 156–67.
10. Breit R, Endres L, The erythemal and pigmentary responses to UVA. In: Urbach F, Gange R, eds, *The Biological Effects of UVA Radiation* (Praeger Publ: New York, 1986) 156–67.
11. Breit R, Delayed pigmentation by UV-A. In: Urbach F, ed, *Biological Responses to Ultraviolet A Radiation* (Valdenmar: Overland, Kansas, 1992) 145–50.
12. Kawada A, UVB-induced erythema, delayed tanning, and UVA-induced immediate tanning in Japanese skin, *Photodermatol* (1986) **3**:327–33.
13. Commission Internationale de l'Eclairage, *Colorimetry*, 2nd edn (Publication CIE No. 15-2. 1986).
14. Chardon A, Mesures de la pigmentation cutanée – Essai de méthode pour l'interprétation de la couleur de la peau dans l'espace CIE-L*a*b* 1976. In: Imbert P, Zahouani H, eds, *Actualités en Ingénierie cutanée* (Editions Eska: Paris, 2001) 197–207.
15. Chardon A, Crétois I, Hourseau C, Skin colour typology and suntanning pathways, *Int J Cosm Sci* (1991) **13**:191–208.
16. Chardon A, Colorimetric vectorial decomposition of the suntanning components (erythema, pigmention, melanisation) in the CIE-L*a*b* colour space (unpublished, 1992).
17. Chardon A, Moyal D, Bories MF, et al, Comparing suntans from actual sun using various SPF sunscreens, *Cosmetics and Toiletries* (1993) **79**.
18. Park S, Suh D, J Youn, A long-term time course of colorimetric evaluation of ultraviolet light-induced skin reactions, *Clin Experiment Dermatol* (1999) **24**: 315–20.
19. Moyal D, Chardon A, Hourseau C, Colorimetric definition of the skin immediate pigment darkening: its application for the UVA protection assessment (Poster, preprint), 16th IFSCC Congress, New York. October 1990.
20. Chardon A, Moyal D, Hourseau C, Persistent Pigment Darkening response as a method for evaluation of UVA protection assays. In: Lowe N, Shath N, Pathak M, eds, *Sunscreens: Development, Evaluation and Regulatory Aspects*, 2nd edn (Marcel Dekker Inc, 1996) 559–82.
21. Kollias N, UVA melanogenesis – Spectral observations. In: Urbach F, ed, *Biological Responses to Ultraviolet A Radiation* (Valdenmar: Overland, Kansas, 1992) 151–7.
22. Sakamaki T, Dong Tian W, Moyal D, et al, The reactions of human skin to UVA radiation (320–400 nm). (Abstract 101), 29th Annual Meeting of the ASP, Chicago IL, USA, July 7–12, 2001.
23. Henschke U, Schulze R, Uber pigmentierung durch langwelliges ultraviolett, *Strahlentherapie* (1939) **64**: 14–43.
24. Auletta M, Gange W, Tan O Matzinger B, Effect of cutaneous hypoxia upon erythema and pigment responses to UVA, UVB and PUVA (8-MPO + UVA) in human skin, *J Invest Dermatol* (1986) **6**:649–52.
25. Rorsman H, Tegner E, Biochemical observations in UV-induced pigmentation, *Photodermatol* (1988) **5**: 30–8.
26. Kollias N, Bykowski JL, Immediate pigment darkening thresholds of human skin to monochromatic (362nm) ultraviolet A radiation are fluence rate dependent, *Photodermatol Photoimmunol Photomed* (1999) **15**:175–8.
27. Hönigsmann H, Schuler G, Aberer W, et al, Immediate pigment darkening phenomenon. A reevaluation of its mechanisms, *J Invest Dermatol* (1986) **87**: 648–52.
28. Seité S, Moyal D, Richard S, et al, Effects of repeated suberythemal doses of UVA in human skin, *Eur J Dermatol* (1997) **7**:203–9.
29. Bech-Thomsen N, Ravnborg L, Wulf HC, A quantitative study of the melanogenesis effect of multiple suberythemal doses of different ultraviolet radiation sources, *Photodermatol Photoimmunol Photomed* (1994) **10**:53–6.
30. Margolis R, Sherwood M, Maytum D, et al, Longwave ultraviolet radiation (UVA, 320–400nm)-induced tan protects human skin against further UVA injury, *J Invest Dermatol* (1989) **93**: 713–18.
31. Kaidbey K, Kligman A, Sunburn protection by long-wave ultraviolet-induced pigmentation, *Arch Dermatol* (1978) **114**:46–8.
32. Montpoint S, Peyron JL, Meynadier J, et al, Etude coopérative du 'Club d'études et de recherche en photobiologie cutanée': la pigmentation tardive en UVA protège-t-elle contre l'érythème UVB? *Nouv Dermatol* (1990) **9**:408.
33. Sakamaki T, Dong Tian W, Moyal D, et al, The reactions of human skin to UVA radiation (320–400 nm). (Abstract 101), 29th Annual Meeting of the ASP, Chicago, IL, USA, July 7–12, 2001.

34. Cole C, van Fossen R, Measurement of sunscren UVA protection: an unsensitized human model, *J Am Acad Dermatol* (1992) **26**:178–84.
35. Cole C, Multicenter evaluation of sunscreens UVA protectiveness with the protection factor test method, *J Am Acad Dermatol* (1994) **30**:729–36.
36. Moyal D, Chardon A, Hourseau C, Infra-red erythema and the part it plays in actinic erythema, *Eur J Dermatol* (1993) **3**:64–7.
37. Colipa Task Force "Sun Protection Measurement": Colipa SPF Test Method. Colipa 94/289, October 1994.
38. Colipa Task Force "Sun Protection Measurement": Collaborative development of a sun protection factor test method: a proposed European Standard, *Int J Cosmet Sci* (1996) **18**:203–18.
39. Sayre RM, Kaidbey KH, Reciprocity for solar simulators used in sunscreen testing, *Photodermatol Photoimmunol Photomed* (1990) **7**:198–210.
40. Meanwhell E, Diffey B: Reciprocity of ultraviolet erythema in human skin. Photoimmunol. 1989; 6: 146–8.
41. Stanfield J, Stewart S, Krochmal, UVA protection factors. In: Urbach F, Gange R, eds, *The Biological Effects of UVA Radiation* (Praeger Publ: New York, 1986) 469–79.
42. Mark R, Gabriel KL, Affrime A, et al, A method for evaluating the UVA protection of sunscreens in human volunteers (Poster) (Dermal Clinical Evaluation Society: Elisabeth, NJ, USA, 1990).
43. Poelman MC, Cesarini JP, Ruse F, et al, A non phototoxic method for testing in vivo the UVA photoprotection. XIVth IFSCC Congress, Barcelona,1986. Preprints, **2**:811–13.
44. Kaidbey K, Barnes A, Determination of UVA protection factors by means of immediate pigment darkening in normal skin, *J Am Acad Dermatol* (1991) **25**:262–6.
45. Kollias N, IPD reciprocity and optical methods for the evaluation of sunscreens, FDA workshop (Minutes of the meeting), Rockville, USA, May 12, 1994.
46. Moyal D, Chardon A, Kollias N, Determination of UVA protection factors using the persistent pigment darkening (PPD) as the end point – (Part 1) Calibration of the method, *Photodermatol Photoimmunol Photomed* (2000) **16**:245–9.
47. Moyal D, Chardon A, Kollias N, UVA protection efficacy of sunscreens can be determined by the persistent pigment darkening (PPD) method (Part 2), *Photodermatol Photoimmunol Photomed* (2000) **16**:250–5.
48. Chardon A, Moyal D, Hourseau C, Méthode d'évaluation de la protection UVA des écrans solaires par la pigmentation immédiate persistante (PPD), VIIlemes Journées de la Société Française de Photobiologie, Clermont-Ferrand, 2&-23 September 1995.
49. Japan Cosmetic Industry Association (JCIA): Measurement standards for UVA protection efficacy (Effective January 1, 1996), 11/21/1995.
50. Lim H, Naylor M, Hönigsman H, et al, American Academy of Dermatology consensus conference on UVA protection of sunscreens: summary and recommendations, *J Am Acad Dermatol* (2001) **44**: 505–8.
51. CIE: A reference action spectrum for ultraviolet induced erythema in human skin. Cie Research note, 6, 17–22, 1987.
52. Irwin C, Barnes A, Veres D, et al, An ultraviolet radiation action spectrum for immediate pigment darkening, *Photochem Photobiol* (1993) **57**:504–7.
53. Park Y, Gange R, Levins P, et al, Action spectra for erythema and melanogenesis of skin types III and IV (1982).
54. Parrish J, Jaenicke K, Anderson R, Erythema and melonogenesis action spectra of normal human skin, *Photochem Photobiol* (1982) **36**:187–91.
55. Gange R, Park Y-K, Auletta M, et al, Action spectra for cutaneous responses to ultraviolet radiation. In: Urbach F, Gange R, eds, *The Biological Effects of UVA Radiations* (Praeger Publ: New York, 1986) 57–66.
56. Satoh Y, Akira Kawada, Action spectrum for melanin pigmentation to ultraviolet light, and Japanese skin typing. In: Fitzpatrick T, Wick M, eds, *Brown meloderma* (University of Tokyo Press, 1986).
57. Kollias N, Malallah Y, Al-Ajmi H, et al, Erythema and melanogenesis action spectra in heavily pigmented individuals as compared to fair-skinned Caucasians, *Photodermatol Photoimmunol Photomed* (1996) **12**: 183–8.
58. Ortel B, Gange R, UV-A action spectra for erythema and pigmentation. In: Urbach F, ed, *Biological Responses to Ultraviolet A Radiation* (Valdenmar: Overland, Kansas, 1992) 79–82.
59. Deutsche Norm, Strahlungsphysik im optischen Bereich und Lichttechnik – Teil 10: Photobiologisch wirksame Strahlung, Grösen, Kurzziechen und Wirkungsspektrum, DIN 5031-10, 1996.

30 The role of ultraviolet light in melanomagenesis

Carola Berking and Meenhard Herlyn

Epidemiology, animal models and UV effects on skin

Exposure to sunlight has consistently been shown to be the most important environmental risk factor for the development of melanoma and its precursor lesions.[1] Intense, intermittent sun exposure resulting in sunburns, particularly in childhood, has been associated with increased risk of melanoma.[2–5] Deleterious effects of the ultraviolet (UV) wavelengths of the sunlight spectrum, UVB (290–320 nm) and UVA (320–400 nm), have been suggested to be responsible for melanoma induction. However, the precise contributions of specific wavelengths in the UVA and UVB range are unknown.

In few animal models, UV light could be linked to melanomagenesis. In *Xiphophorus* hybrid fish,[6] melanoma could be induced by wavelengths in the UVA region, but these animals also develop spontaneous melanomas, harboring a predisposing proto-oncogene XMRK.[7] In the South American opossums, UV light has been shown to induce melanocytic lesions, including melanoma, when activation of the light-dependent photolyase enzyme was prevented.[8] When irradiated as sucklings, progression to melanomas including metastasis, could be observed in adult opossums.[9] In this model, the potency of UVA for melanoma induction was found to be negligible when compared to UVB.[10] More recently, a transgenic mouse model has been introduced with promising results of melanoma induction by UV irradiation.[11] Inappropriate expression of hepatocyte growth factor (HGF) in the skin leads to extrafollicular localization and accumulation of melanocytes in the murine dermis and epidermis. Upon a single dose of erythrogenic UV irradiation of neonates, nevus-like lesions and melanomas developed in high frequencies, whereas chronic suberythemal UV doses led preferentially to non-melanocytic tumors.[12]

Experimental animal models can help to understand UV-associated etiology and pathobiology of melanoma, but they do not necessarily mirror the biology of human melanoma development. They may be based on genetic susceptibilities of certain animal strains that are not found in humans. More importantly, the skin architecture in animals shows substantial differences from that in humans. Whereas in mice the epidermis is only a few layers thin, human epidermis is composed of multiple layers. Murine melanocytes are primarily found in the hair follicles, whereas human melanocytes are located in the basal layer of the epidermis in close contact to keratinocytes. Human keratinocytes are thought to play a crucial role in directing localization and survival of melanocytes in the epidermis through the expression of the c-kit ligand SCF (stem cell factor).[13] A homeostatic interaction between keratinocytes and melanocytes is maintained through adhesion molecules, such as E-cadherin, and keratinocytes are believed to be the regulatory masters over melanocytes.[14–16] During melanocyte transformation, this homeostatic balance between epidermal keratinocytes and melanocytes gets disrupted.[15] The cause of this disruption remains speculative, but UV light likely plays an essential role. Based on extensive photocarcinogenesis studies of non-melanoma skin cancer and UV-irradiation studies of keratinocytes, fibroblasts, and melanocytes *in vitro*,[17–19] different routes of action of UV light on melanocytes and the surrounding skin cells can be proposed. UV light could directly act on melanocytes through DNA damage and induction of mutations.[1] Melanocytes, unlike keratinocytes, do not easily undergo apoptosis after UV exposure, but survive despite possibly considerable UV-light-mediated DNA damage. This phenomenon may be due to the constitutive expression of anti-apoptotic proteins, such as Bcl-2, in melanocytes.[20] It has been hypothesized that the photodamaged melanocytes are at high risk for incorporating mutations into the DNA, which may lead, over time, to clonal expansion of these cells.[1] High intermittent doses of UV radiation hereby would result in more mutated melanocytes than low chronic doses of UV radiation because of the lack of photoprotective tanning of acutely, in contrast to chronically, UV-light-exposed skin. This mutation hypothesis conforms with the epidemiological association of sunburn, *i.e.* acute intermittent sun exposure, and melanoma risk.

UV light, on the other hand, can also activate melanocytes indirectly by the induction or suppression of growth factors and cytokines in the skin. This activation, in turn, could render the melanocytes more susceptible to mutagenic effects of UV light or of other, yet unknown, carcinogens. It has been shown that UVB can stimulate the expression of IL-1, IL-3, IL-6, tumor necrosis factor (TNF-α), GM-CSF,[21] ET-1,[22] IL-8,[23] IL-12,[24] and VEGF[25] in keratinocytes, and IL-1α and bFGF expression in HeLa cells.[26] UVA was found to induce IL-6 and TNF-α expression in keratinocytes and dermal fibroblasts.[27] UVA, but not UVB light can induce HGF expression in skin fibroblasts. HGF, in turn, has been shown to downregulate E-cadherin, which is a prerequisite for decoupling of melanocytes from keratinocytes before they can undergo proliferation and migration—two hallmarks of cancer.[28,29]

Taken together, UV light can have different hypothetical contributions to melanocyte transformation, which are, however, far from being understood and which may be unique to the human system.

Experimental models of UV-induced human melanoma

To study UV-mediated melanocyte transformation in human skin, our laboratory has developed a chimeric human skin/immunodeficient mouse model, which enables long-term UV irradiation studies of up to 2 years.[30,31] Normal human skin is grafted to severe combined immunodeficiency disease (SCID) or recombinase activating gene-1 (Rag-1) knockout mice and can be used after a healing period of 3–4 weeks. The combined treatment of skin with one topical application of dimethyl(a)benzanthracene (DMBA) and with UVB irradiations at 500 J/m^2 three times weekly led to hyperplastic lentiginous melanocyte changes in 77% after a median of 12 months.[32] After 15 months, a nodular pigmented melanoma developed. This was the first report of an experimentally induced human melanoma *in vivo* and the first evidence that UVB indeed can promote melanomagenesis in humans. Follow-up studies with modifications of this model demonstrated that melanocytic lesions were much less easily inducible in adult skin than in neonatal foreskin, suggesting that melanocytes from young donors were more susceptible for transformation by DMBA and UVB than melanocytes from adults.[33] This may be due to the statistically higher number of proliferating melanocytes in non-adult skin versus primarily quiescent melanocytes in adult skin. These data support the epidemiological observation that sunburns in childhood are of higher risk for melanoma development than in adulthood.[2] However, they stand in contrast to the hypothesis of accumulating light-induced mutations in melanocytes over time, which would have resulted in a higher incidence of melanoma lesions in adult skin when compared to young skin that has never been exposed to sun before.

The incidence of melanoma in the described human skin graft model is relatively low and the induction period long, considering the relatively short lifespan of mice. Moreover, DMBA is a chemical carcinogen, which is normally not found in the environment. We have, therefore, recently developed an alternative model of melanomagenesis in human skin grafts.[34]

We hypothesized that the first critical step in tumor formation, *i.e.* the uncontrolled proliferation of melanocytes, may be induced by a combination of UV damage and an imbalance of growth factor production by cells in the immediate area of the melanocyte. Increased expression of select growth factors known to be mitogenic for melanocytes was achieved by intradermal injection of adenoviral vectors carrying the respective gene of the growth factor. This led to transduction of fibroblasts and consequent production of the growth factor in the skin. Figure 30.1a demonstrates

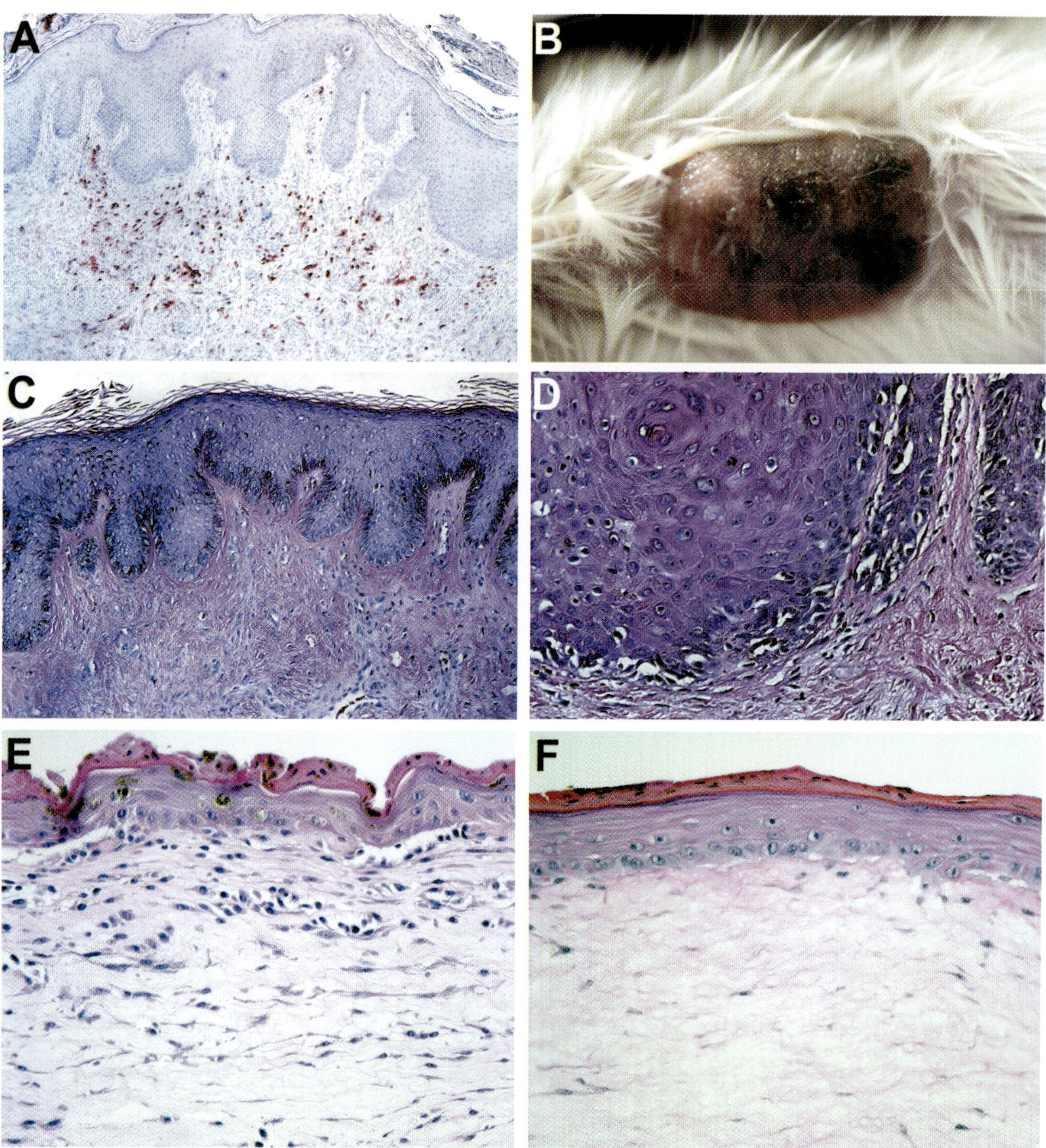

Figure 30.1

(a) Immunohistochemical detection of bFGF protein (in red) in a foreskin graft injected with adenoviral vectors carrying the gene for the 18 kDa bFGF protein. Fibroblasts are positively stained in the upper dermis (100×). (b) Human abdominal skin graft on SCID mouse after four intradermal injections of 100 μl of bFGF adenovirus in PBS and 10 irradiations with 40 mJ/cm^2 UVB. Note the development of black macules. (c) Foreskin graft after six injections of bFGF adenovirus and 18 UVB irradiations (week 7), showing pathological hyperpigmentation of the entire epidermis and hypercellularity of the thickened dermis (H&E, 400×). (d) Lentiginous form of malignant melanoma in an abdominal skin graft after seven injections of bFGF adenovirus and 26 UVB irradiations (week 9) (H&E, 200×). (e, f) Human skin reconstructs with bFGF- (e) or LacZ- (f) transduced melanocytes mixed with normal human keratinocytes at a ratio of 1:2. Note the brown pigmented clusters in and on top of the epidermis as well as the increased number of fibroblasts in the dermis (H&E, 200×).

the immunohistochemical detection of bFGF expression in fibroblasts in the dermis after adenoviral transduction. Weekly injections ensured a stable expression over several weeks to months. Concomitantly, skin grafts were irradiated three times weekly with 30–50 mJ/cm^2 of UVB and 100–200 mJ/cm^2 of UVA. Among the tested growth factors, bFGF, HGF, IGF-1, and PDGF-A, the strongest effects on melanocytes were observed with bFGF. Black-pigmented macules developed within 2–3 weeks of treatment (Fig. 30.1b), and histological analyses demonstrated pathological hyperpigmentation, proliferation and hyperplasia of activated melanocytes (Fig. 30.1c). In one skin graft, a lentiginous form of malignant melanoma developed within 2 months of treatment (Fig. 30.1d). This study demonstrated that melanocytes could be transformed *in vivo* by the aberrant expression of a physiologically occurring growth factor, bFGF, in combination with UV light. Exposure of human skin grafted to immunodeficient RAG-1 mice without any other treatment does not induce malignant transformation. The success for transformation of the combined treatment is potentially due to: (a) bFGF is released by the dermal fibroblasts and induces proliferation of melanocytes. Only then are they susceptible to transformation; (b) bFGF stimulates human fibroblasts to produce additional factors that are mitogenic for melanocytes; and (c) murine inflammatory and stromal cells are attracted and activated to stimulate the melanocytes. Our reconstruct data (Figs 30.1e and 30.1f) suggest that bFGF can act as a paracrine factor, despite the lack of a signal sequence. It remains to be investigated how UVB irradiation induces effects in the skin that synergize with the activity of bFGF.

Future perspectives

It has become possible to engineer human skin in organotypic culture *in vitro* and to include either melanocytes or melanoma cells in this system.[35] In this model, each cell type can be genetically modified before reconstruction of the skin.

For *in vivo* studies, skin reconstructs can be grafted to immunodeficient animals. This transfer onto a living host leads to vascularization of the reconstructed dermis and maturation of the basement membrane of the reconstructed epidermis, rendering the engineered skin grafts almost indistinguishable from real skin. Successfully engrafted skin reconstructs survive throughout the lifetime of the animal, making *in vivo* UV irradiation studies possible.[36]

The model will allow systematic analysis of genes that are associated with melanoma and can play a role in UV-induced melanomagenesis. Our laboratory is testing the roles of a variety of genes by overexpression in melanocytes, keratinocytes, and fibroblasts. We are also suppressing the biological activity of selected genes by constructing dominant-negative mutants or antisense molecules. For consistent results within experimental groups, we plan to use melanocytes from individuals who have a high susceptibility for melanoma development. This combined *in vitro*/*in vivo* model should help us to address some questions that we cannot address in mouse skin, because the architecture of murine skin differs widely from that of human skin.

Acknowledgements

Much of this work was supported by the outstanding technical assistance of E. DeJesus, R. Finko, R. Takemoto, E. Aglow, and K. Chruma.

References

1. Gilchrest BA, Eller MS, Geller AC et al., The pathogenesis of melanoma induced by ultraviolet radiation, *N Engl J Med* (1999) **340**:1341–8.
2. Zanetti R, Franceschi S, Rosso S et al., Cutaneous melanoma and sunburns in childhood in a southern European population, *Eur J Cancer* (1992) **28A**:1172–6.
3. Elwood JM, Jopson J, Melanoma and sun exposure: an overview of published studies, *Int J Cancer* (1997) **73**:198–203.
4. Green A, Whiteman D, Frost C et al., Sun exposure, skin cancers and related skin conditions, *J Epidemiol* (1999) **9**:S7–S131.
5. Marks R, Epidemiology of melanoma, *Clin Exp Dermatol* (2000) **25**:459–63.
6. Setlow RB, Grist E, Thompson K et al., Wavelengths effective in induction of malignant melanoma, *Proc Natl Acad Sci U S A* (1993) **90**:6666–70.

7. Adam D, Maueler W, Schartl M, Transcriptional activation of the melanoma inducing Xmrk oncogene in Xiphophorus, *Oncogene* (1991) **6**:73–80.
8. Ley RD, Applegate LA, Padilla RS et al., Ultraviolet radiation-induced malignant melanoma in Monodelphis domestica, *Photochem Photobiol* (1989) **50**:1–5.
9. Robinson ES, VandeBerg JL, Hubbard GB et al., Malignant melanoma in ultraviolet irradiated laboratory opossums: initiation in suckling young, metastasis in adults, and xenograft behavior in nude mice, *Cancer Res* (1994) **54**:5986–91.
10. Robinson ES, Hill RH Jr, Kripke ML et al., The Monodelphis melanoma model: initial report on large ultraviolet A exposures of suckling young, *Photochem Photobiol* (2000) **71**:743–6.
11. Noonan FP, Otsuka T, Bang S et al., Accelerated ultraviolet radiation-induced carcinogenesis in hepatocyte growth factor/scatter factor transgenic mice, *Cancer Res* (2000) **60**:3738–43.
12. Noonan FP, Recio JA, Takayama H et al., Neonatal sunburn and melanoma in mice, *Nature* (2001) **413**:217–2.
13. Kunisada T, Lu SZ, Yoshida H et al., Murine cutaneous mastocytosis and epidermal melanocytosis induced by keratinocyte expression of transgenic stem cell factor, *J Exp Med* (1998) **187**:1565–73.
14. Valyi-Nagy IT, Hirka G, Jensen PJ et al., Undifferentiated keratinocytes control growth, morphology, and antigen expression of normal melanocytes through cell–cell contact, *Lab Invest* (1993) **69**:152–9.
15. Hsu MY, Meier FE, Nesbit M et al., E-cadherin expression in melanoma cells restores keratinocyte-mediated growth control and down-regulates expression of invasion-related adhesion receptors, *Am J Pathol* (2000) **156**:1515–25.
16. Hsu MY, Andl T, Li G et al., Cadherin repertoire determines partner-specific gap junctional communication during melanoma progression, *J Cell Sci* (2000) **113**:1535–42.
17. Wikonkal NM, Brash DE, Ultraviolet radiation induced signature mutations in photocarcinogenesis, *J Invest Dermatol Symp Proc* (1999) **4**:6–10.
18. Krutmann J, Grewe M, Involvement of cytokines, DNA damage, and reactive oxygen intermediates in ultraviolet radiation-induced modulation of intercellular adhesion molecule-1 expression, *J Invest Dermatol* (1995) **105**:67S–70S.
19. Chakraborty AK, Funasaka Y, Slominski A et al., UV light and MSH receptors, *Ann N Y Acad Sci* (1999) **885**:100–16.
20. Klein-Parker HA, Warshawski L, Tron VA, Melanocytes in human skin express bcl-2 protein, *J Cutan Pathol* (1994) **21**:297–301.
21. Schwarz T, Luger TA, Effect of UV irradiation on epidermal cell cytokine production, *J Photochem Photobiol B* (1989) **4**:1–13.
22. Imokawa G, Yada Y, Miyagishi M, Endothelins secreted from human keratinocytes are intrinsic mitogens for human melanocytes, *J Biol Chem* (1992) **267**:24675–80.
23. Kondo S, Kono T, Sauder DN et al., IL-8 gene expression and production in human keratinocytes and their modulation by UVB, *J Invest Dermatol* (1993) **101**:690–4.
24. Enk CD, Mahanty S, Blauvelt A et al., UVB induces IL-12 transcription in human keratinocytes in vivo and in vitro, *Photochem Photobiol* (1996) **63**:854–9.
25. Brauchle M, Funk JO, Kind P et al., Ultraviolet B and H_2O_2 are potent inducers of vascular endothelial growth factor expression in cultured keratinocytes, *J Biol Chem* (1996) **271**:21793–7.
26. Kramer M, Sachsenmaier C, Herrlich P et al., UV irradiation-induced interleukin-1 and basic fibroblast growth factor synthesis and release mediate part of the UV response, *J Biol Chem* (1993) **268**:6734–41.
27. Avalos-Diaz E, Alvarado-Flores E, Herrera-Esparza R, UV-A irradiation induces transcription of IL-6 and TNF-alpha genes in human keratinocytes and dermal fibroblasts, *Rev Rheum Engl Ed* (1999) **66**:13–19.
28. Kunisada T, Yamazaki H, Hirobe T et al., Keratinocyte expression of transgenic hepatocyte growth factor affects melanocyte development, leading to dermal melanocytosis, *Mech Dev* (2000) **94**:67–78.
29. Herlyn M, Berking C, Li G et al., Lessons from melanocyte development for understanding the biological events in naevus and melanoma formation, *Melanoma Res* (2000) **10**:1–10.
30. Soballe PW, Montone KT, Satyamoorthy K et al., Carcinogenesis in human skin grafted to SCID mice, *Cancer Res* (1996) **56**:757–64.
31. Atillasoy ES, Elenitsas R, Sauter ER et al., UVB induction of epithelial tumors in human skin using a RAG-1 mouse xenograft model, *J Invest Dermatol* (1997) **109**:704–9.
32. Atillasoy ES, Seykora JT, Soballe PW et al., UVB induces atypical melanocytic lesions and melanoma in human skin, *Am J Pathol* (1998) **152**:1179–86.

33. Berking C, Takemoto R, Binder RL, Photocarcinogenesis in human adult skin grafts, *Carcinogenesis* (2002) **23**:181–7.
34. Berking C, Takemoto R, Satyamoorthy K et al., Basic fibroblast growth factor and ultraviolet b transform melanocytes in human skin, *Am J Pathol* (2001) **158**:943–53.
35. Meier F, Nesbit M, Hsu MY et al., Human melanoma progression in skin reconstructs: Biological significance of bFGF, *Am J Pathol* (2000) **156**:193–200.
36. Berking C, Herlyn M, Human skin reconstruct models: A new application for studies of melanocyte and melanoma biology, *Histol Histopathol* (2001) **16**.

31 Molecular phototypes

Jonathan L. Rees

Introduction

This review will concentrate on what we know of the genetics of the melanocortin-1 receptor (MC1R) in humans and the role of the MC1R in determining human hair colour, skin colour and the skin's response to ultraviolet radiation (UVR). The reason for this emphasis on the MC1R is straightforward; if rare Mendelian disorders, such as albinism, are ignored, the MC1R is the only gene so far identified that plays a major role in the determination of phototype in humans.

Whilst emphasizing what we know, I also want to discuss a little of what we don't know. In particular, I will try to clarify the concept of phototype, seeking to answer the following sorts of questions: what is a phototype; can one individual have more than one phototype; is there a gold-standard phototype; is there a single molecular *basis* for phototype or are there just molecular *bases*?

Second, I want to say a little about the sorts of experimental approaches my own group is pursuing in order to understand the relation between genotype and phenotype. This emphasis on genetics is not meant to diminish the contribution of environmental factors in the cutaneous response to UVR, a neglected topic which deserves greater interest.

The review will naturally fall into three sections. First, a discussion about definitions, and what we might hope to achieve from the various operational definitions that might be suggested for phototype. Second, following the identification of the MC1R as a key control point in murine coat colour pigmentation, an account of the role of the MC1R in human pigmentation. And third, some details of our ongoing work on trying to quantify human phototypes.

Phototype: one or many, and what do we mean?

Humans vary enormously in their response to UVR. The magnitude of this variation depends on the assay and, hence, the end-point chosen. For instance, if one examines the acute erythemal response to UVR B (UVB), Northern Europeans vary somewhere between five- and 10-fold. If the study group is broadened to include other world populations, such as Asians and Africans, then the variation would be even greater (although precise estimates are not available). Similarly, if cancer was chosen as an end-point, then large differences in age-specific incidence rates would be found. The ratio of absolute rates between populations would vary, however, on the tumour type selected. Ratios for squamous cell carcinoma and actinic keratoses would be larger than those for melanoma or basal cell carcinoma. The point is simply stated: comparisons between different groups of humans or between different humans will produce different numerical scores, depending on the assay chosen. There is no *one* phototype scale, merely a *variety* of phototype scales.

A large number of end-points have been chosen to try and capture some of the variation in the cutaneous response to UVR. Simple assessment of erythema has been widely used and has much to commend it.[1] It has the virtue of simplicity, has a clear biological and medical meaning in terms of burning, can be measured objectively using simple equipment,[2] and, because of the congruent action spectrum with that of DNA damage, has a good deal of intellectual coherence.[1] There are, however, many other alternative end-points. For instance, one might choose DNA damage directly. In reality, of course, such an assay, like erythema, is a snapshot of the skin's response to UVR and, because we have no quantitative model that links DNA repair with cancer and integrates the various roles of mutation, tumour promotion or even cutaneous immunosuppression, it is perhaps naive to expect that any individual assay end-point may capture or mirror precisely acute or long-term effects. Cutaneous immunosuppression provides an example.

There is a widely-held view that UVR-induced cutaneous immunosuppression is important in the pathogenesis of skin cancer.[3] The evidence appears quite clear in the mouse, whereas in humans, in the view of this author, enthusiasm exceeds any hard evidence. Pharmacologically-induced systemic immunosuppression in humans, of course, has been noted to have profound effects but this is not the same as UVR-induced local immunosuppression. Of the various assay systems used, frequently involving inhibition of contact sensitivity by UVR, there is an implicit view that, somehow, these assays will usefully predict the effects of UVR in the chronic state, or the reaction of the immune system to malignant clones.[3] There is little reason for such enthusiasm.

A second critique, and a neglected one, is that a large number of papers claim to show that there are discrepancies between the various operational end-points that may be chosen (such as erythema and immunosuppression).[3,4] Should we be surprised by this?

If one was to take an extreme case, say an albino in Tanzania, then it would not be surprising if the various assays, such as erythemal response or cutaneous immunosuppression, were not grossly abnormal in the same individual. At the extremes, therefore, there would be significant covariance between the different measures used. However, within the main body of what one might imagine a Gaussian distribution of variability, individual assay systems may well show different dose–response kinetics. In practice, this may mean that, for instance, in an individual with heavily pigmented skin, it may be possible to produce effects on the cutaneous immune system without apparent effects on erythema. Much of these apparent discrepancies can be explained by simple methodological inadequacies. If you examine the kinetics of skin to UVR, a sigmoid curve is seen.[1] The ratio of this assay system readout to any other depends on the point chosen. Most experiments comparing the various end-points (*e.g.* erythema, inhibition of contact sensitivity) have neglected this aspect. The production of 'sun protection ratios' (as has become a veritable industry in recent years) is also open to the same criticism. One should, therefore, not be surprised that differences are found in the response to UVR between the various proposed assay systems, indeed, quite the opposite. In reality, the failure to link short-term with long-term effects vitiates the pseudo-precision of most of these claims.

In conclusion, the concept of phototype reflects the attempt to capture some of the population variation in the cutaneous response to UVR. Claims for a gold-standard phototype could only be accepted when acute and long-term effects are shown to be correlated, and when there is an adequate quantitative model linking, for example, cutaneous immunosuppression, mutagenesis, tumour promotion and inflammation. Even with all these caveats, the phototype would refer to a specific end-point, such as squamous cell carcinogenesis or photoaging. At present, such a quantitative model does not exist.

Genetic determinations of phototype

The realization of the importance of genetic factors in determining phototype may be as old as genetics itself. Modern interest in the genetics of human pigmentation trace back to the nineteenth century and Francis Galton, and to the eugenics movement, particularly in North America, in the early twentieth century (especially studies by Davenport and others on red hair at the Cold Spring Harbour Laboratory[5]). The first twin study utilizing the concepts of identical and non-identical twins, was performed by Siemens on melanocytic nevi in the early part of the twentieth century,[6] and skin colour and hair colour have been used as a method of trying to distinguish monozygotic from dizygotic twins until comparatively recent times.

The facility and speed with which modern genetic approaches have been wedded to the identification of factors important in human pigmentation owe much to the development of the 'mouse fancy' over the last two centuries.[5] The collection of mice with different coat colours, and exchange of animals between enthusiasts, allowed the development of the resource of a large variety of naturally-occurring mutants. Subsequently, this resource has allowed experimental crosses to be made and, more recently, positional cloning of loci important in determining mouse coat colour to be undertaken.

One particular locus, the *extension* locus, is of relevance to the current chapter. Extension-mutant mice are characterized by both loss-of-function and gain-of-function mutations.[7,8] Loss of function results in yellow hair (*e-/e-*), characterized by an increased phaeomelanin-to-eumelanin ratio, whereas, by contrast, dominant, or gain-of-function, mutations (*E+/E+*) result in animals with black hair with a diminished ratio of eumelanin to phaeomelanin.[6] In the early 1990s, Roger Cone's group, based on a strategy of screening for G-coupled receptors in melanoma cells, identified the product of the *extension* locus as the MC1R.[9,10] They showed that various coat-colour mutants could be accounted for by mutation of the MC1R.[9,10]

The MC1R—a key control point in melanin pigmentation

The MC1R is a 317 amino acid gene that encodes a G-coupled 7-pass transmembrane receptor.[9] The receptor is a member of a large family of G-coupled receptors, but is found within a sub-class of melanocortin receptors, now numbered MC1R, MC2R, MC3R, MC4R and MC5R.[12] The MC2R is the receptor for ACTH; the MC3R and MC4R are both widely distributed within the central nervous system, with the latter playing a key role in the control of body weight and energy homeostasis. The MC5R is distributed throughout a large number of tissues but knockout experiments in the mouse suggest that it plays a rate-limiting role in the control of sebogenesis in skin.[13]

By definition, the various receptors show similarities in primary structure but differ significantly in their pharmacological properties. There are also significant differences between the mouse and human receptor of each type in terms of binding and activation characteristics.[10,12]

It is widely assumed that the endogenous ligand for the MC1R is α-melanocyte-stimulating hormone (α MSH). However, it has been pointed out that ACTH is also active at this receptor (conversely, MC2R is primarily responsive to ACTH).[14,15] Intracellular coupling is with cyclic AMP, although there is continued debate about which other pathways may be important in mediating any effects from the membrane on melanogenesis. For the present, the evidence implicating cyclic AMP seems convincing and cyclic AMP seems to form an experimentally useful end-point with which to examine receptor characteristics.

The MC1R: A gene for red hair

Following the cloning of the mouse and human MC1R by Cone and others,[16] it became clear that the MC1R was a clear candidate gene for red hair and (potentially) sun sensitivity in humans. An initial case control study confirmed the importance of the MC1R in humans, showing that coding sequence variants of the MC1R were far more common in individuals with red hair than in those without red hair.[17] Nevertheless, there were surprises. First, and importantly, the mode of inheritance appeared unclear. Some individuals with red hair had one sequence variant, other individuals had two variants (on different alleles), whereas some further individuals had more than one change upon each allele. Red hair has traditionally been thought of as *approximating* to a Mendelian recessive, although alternative modes of inheritance have been proposed, but the evidence for them was not decisive. The change in hair colour with age and incomplete penetrance depending on age, may provide uncertainty about phenotype definition in many individuals.

The second surprise was that there was not just one or two sequence changes identified but a large number of sequence variants.[17] To date, we have identified over 30 coding region sequence variants within a region of under 1 kilobase.[17–19] Many of these changes in Northern European populations are non-synonymous.[18] Thirdly, whereas some of the sequence changes could be imagined to disrupt the receptor (based on what was already known about this family of receptors), a putative role for some of the others was less convincing.

Thus, whereas within a year it was possible to suspect that this gene played a role in the production of red hair in humans, clarifying the mode of inheritance and determining which alleles may be functionally important has taken various groups, particularly my own laboratory, the last 5 years.[18–23]

Common variants of the MC1R are strongly associated with red hair

In order to clarify the above issues, we initially carried out a population study based in Ireland, relating changes at the MC1R to the hair phenotype.[19,20] Possession of one of the common sequence variants that we suspected may play an etiological role in red hair (at codons 151, 160 and 294) conferred an odds ratio of ~5 for the possession of red hair; compound heterozygotes conferred an odds ratio of >30. Although other alleles, such as the codon 60, are common, their role has been harder to pin down.[20]

Subsequently, we have been able to confirm these associations in other populations and in different parts of Northern Europe.[20] The 151, 160 and 294 are all important in determining red-hair status, but various frameshift mutations and variants at codon 142 also seem to be functionally significant.[20] Other missense changes may also show diminished function. These population studies, therefore, show that a number of different alleles are associated with red hair.

The mode of inheritance of red hair

In order to clarify the mode of inheritance and the relation between particular alleles and the red-hair phenotype, we have undertaken family studies. In brief, red hair, indeed, approximates to an autosomal recessive trait. If the alleles described above are treated as partial or complete loss-of-function mutations, then it is possible, within these Northern European populations, to predict hair colour at age 21, using a simple autosomal recessive model, and be correct eight or nine times out of 10.[20]

Nevertheless, not all individuals with red hair are homozygous loss-of-function mutations. Perhaps 20% of individuals with red hair carry only one putatively functionally important allele.[20] Sequencing 3 or 4 kilobases upstream and downstream of the MC1R coding region has not provided any evidence for functionally significant mutations outwith the coding region either (Amanda Ray and JLR, unpublished work). Interestingly, recent analyses of our own suggest that the particular shade of red varies between individuals who are compound heterozygote and those who carry changes on one allele only.[20] As a general rule, individuals with bright red hair, such as might be described as carrot red hair, tend to be compound heterozygotes or homozygotes, whereas individuals with strawberry blonde hair or auburn hair tend to have one wild-type or pseudo-wild-type allele. These results are interesting but ascertainment bias cannot be completely excluded, as detection of individuals with strawberry blonde or auburn hair is more problematic than identification of those individuals with bright red hair. This is because, in Northern UK populations, perhaps over 30% of the population are heterozygote for functionally significant MC1R alleles—there is, therefore, a possibility of misclassification of persons with strawberry blonde or auburn hair.

The MC1R—more than just red hair

Individuals with red hair are, in general, more sensitive to the effects of UVR, judged by a number of criteria. As a group they tend to freckle easily, they tend to burn following acute exposure and, perhaps most importantly, they fail to develop a protective tan following repeated exposure. They are, of course, also at an increased risk of skin cancer of both melanoma and squamous and basal cell carcinoma.

As hinted above, the effect of the MC1R may be dosage dependent. We have shown, for instance that there is a clear dosage effect on the number of freckling sites.[20] Individuals who have homozygote loss-of-function mutations of the MC1R have more freckling sites than those individuals who are heterozygote, who, in turn, have more freckling sites than those who are wild type or pseudo-wild-type. We can see a similar heterozygote effect on beard colour.[20] For example, some individuals with dark hair have a red beard. They are more likely to be heterozygous than those without a red beard and dark hair. We have, however, failed to see any relation between the MC1R and eye colour.[20]

Of relevance to the present chapter was to examine the relation between MC1R status and phototype and the cutaneous response to UVR. The experimental approach we took was to use a modified Fitzpatrick classification, namely to attempt to classify individuals based on their recall of their ability to tan and burn in response to the sun, and relate this classification to an individual's MC1R status. Not surprisingly, individuals who are homozygous or compound heterozygote for functionally-significant MC1R alleles show a lower Fitzpatrick score (*i.e.* they tended to burn and not tan well).[21] Conversely, and again not surprisingly, individuals who are wild type for the MC1R allele tended to lie at the other extreme, *i.e.* they tan and don't tend to burn. However, heterozygotes were clearly in between these two extremes, and these differences were all statistically significant and the magnitude of effect large.[21]

One way to summarize this would be to imagine an individual of a particular skin type classification (say, skin type 2) who was wild type and then, if you like, statistically add in a variant MC1R allele. The effect would be to make this individual four or five times more likely to be in a lower Fitzpatrick classification. The effect is, therefore, not small and in Northern European populations at least, shows that the MC1R is a key determinant of the cutaneous response to UVR.[21]

The genetic physiology of the MC1R

The description above shows that there is a relation between MC1R status and the Fitzpatrick or modified Fitzpatrick classification. Fitzpatrick classification is, of course, based on recall.[24] The classification, however useful in particular clinical situations, is known to be far from perfect.[25] There are issues about failure of being able to classify some individuals because the inverse relationship between tanning and erythema is not absolute. This is a key point. Many previous studies have suggested that the difference between skin type 1 individuals and skin type 3 individuals in acute erythemal responses is not large.[26–29] In order to investigate this further and relate the MC1R to this phenotype, we have recently irradiated individuals with a graded series of doses of UVB on a sun-protected site (the buttock) and related the dose response in erythema measured at 24 hours to MC1R status.[30] First of all, we saw little difference in the MED between individuals with red hair and those without red hair. Statistical power may be an issue but the most likely conclusion is that the differences, if present, are really rather moderate and may well be explained by the differential background pigmentation, even in sun-protected sites such as the buttock. The gradient of the erythemal dose response is, however, steeper in individuals with red hair and, again, there is a clear relation with MC1R status. In individuals who are homozygous, loss-of-function mutations have a steeper erythemal dose response than those who are wild type. Such differences can be observed even when the unit of analysis is the MC1R genotype rather than the pigmentary phenotype.

The similarities between redheads in their acute erythemal responses and the differences in the Fitzpatrick classification for such individuals with red hair and MC1R mutations may, at first, seem surprising. In reality, of course, the two assay systems are not using the same end-point. The Fitzpatrick system is an anamnestic classification which essentially relates the ability to burn during development of photoprotection (to whatever degree, and whether involving pigmentation or non-pigmentary photadaption). By contrast, the MED, and the dose response to UVR measured at 24 hours, is better thought of as an assay of cutaneous inflammation in response to UVR. If, and only if, basal pigmentation is significantly different would you expect to see some relation with pigmentary status. A thought experiment might perhaps make this clear.

Imagine a red-haired, pale-skinned, heavily-freckled individual being exposed to a dose response of UVR. Imagine the contrast of a brown-haired, Northern European individual with brown eyes undergoing a similar irradiation. Basal or constitutive differences in pigmentation may matter, but they will be small, and the erythemal response to UVR is not primarily dependent on pigment in the basal state, unless differences are large. If, however, these individuals are repeatedly exposed to UVR, say two or three times a week, then the individual with red hair will fail to pigment to the same degree as the individual with brown hair. The magnitude of the difference in response to UVR therefore develops only with recurrent exposure. When looked at this way, it can be seen that the Fitzpatrick classification is not mirroring reality in always imagining that tanning and burning are inverse characteristics. They may be, but this presupposes that repeated exposures have taken place. It follows from this work that what is required are assays based on repeated exposure to UVR rather than single exposures.

Assays of the acute response to erythema based on multiple UVR exposures

In the past, technical issues have made the study of tanning and erythemal responses in the same individual problematic. Users of the well-known reflectance instruments[2] are confounded by the overlap in the spectrum between melanin and blood. Blood flow, of course, is measurable using a laser Doppler, although some, but not all, laser Dopplers are markedly influenced by pigmentary status. Conversely, assessment of pigmentation is problematic in the presence of alterations in blood flow.

It would seem, however, that newer technology will allow these issues to be resolved. Recently, we have managed to perform pilot studies using such an approach and our results suggest that individuals who may apparently have a very similar phototype, based on acute erythemal responses, diverge markedly following two or three exposures. Such assay systems would allow far better precision to be assigned to phenotype and, in turn, allow greater study of the determinants, be they genetic or environmental, of phototype.

Conclusions

In this chapter, I have reviewed the concept of phototype. I have argued that there is no such thing as one particular phototype but that there are various operational definitions one can use. The definition of phototype and the measurement of phototype depends on the end-point(s) you choose. For our own work, we have continued to use erythema as an end-point and, in particular, have tried to develop measurement of erythema in the presence of differences in basal or facultative pigmentation.

When the rare Mendelian disorders, such as albinism, are ignored, the MC1R is the only gene we know of which plays a large role in variation in phototype in Northern European populations. Loss-of-function mutations, or mutations that lead to at least some impairment of function, are common in many European populations. The majority of individuals with red hair are compound heterozygotes or homozygotes at the MC1R, but there is clear evidence of a heterozygote effect on freckling sites, on beard colour, on sun sensitivity (measured as the Fitzpatrick classification) and shade of red hair colour. The MC1R has been an especially tractable gene with which to work because it is small, and many of the mutations involve the coding region. It seems likely that many other pigment genes identified in the murine system will also play a role in determining human variation in pigment. Areas of great future interest will be the identification of the genetic basis of blonde hair in humans and examination of the different genetic influences on acute inflammation in the skin in response to UVR and their relation with pigmentation.

Acknowledgements

It is a pleasure to acknowledge my collaborators over the last 5 years, particularly Ian Jackson in the MRC Human Genetics Unit in Edinburgh, Professor Tony Thody (now in Bradford), and Dr Eugene Healy, originally in Newcastle and now in Southampton. The unpublished human experiments referred to have been carried out in collaboration with Dr Niamh Flanagan and Dr Tom Ha in Edinburgh. I am grateful for grant support from The Wellcome Trust, a CERIES research reward and The Leech Trust.

References

1. Diffey BL, Farr PM, Quantitative aspects of ultraviolet erythema, *Clin Phys Physiol Measurement* (1991) **12**:311–25.
2. Diffey BL, Oliver RJ, Farr PM, A portable instrument for quantifying erythema induced by ultraviolet radiation, *Br J Dermatol* (1984) **111**:663–72.
3. Young AR, Walker SL, Photoprotection from UVR-

induced immunosuppresion. In: Krutmann J, Elmets CA, eds, *Photoimmunology* (Blackwell: Oxford 1995): 285–97.

4. Damian DL, Halliday GM, Barnetson RS, Broad-spectrum sunscreens provide greater protection against ultraviolet-radiation-induced suppression of contact hypersensitivity to a recall antigen in humans, *J Invest Dermatol* (1997) **109**:146–51.
5. Davenport GC, Davenport CB, Heredity of eye-colour in man. *Science* (1907) **26**:589–592.
6. Robbins LS, Nadeau JH, Johnson KR et al., Pigmentation phenotypes of variant extension locus alleles result from point mutations that alter MSH receptor function. *Cell* (1993) **72**:827–834.
7. Jackson IJ, Mouse coat colour mutations: a molecular genetic resource which spans the centuries, *Bioessays* (1991) **13**:439–46.
8. Silvers WK, *Coat Colors of Mice* (Springer-Verlag: New York, 1979).
9. Mountjoy KG, Robbins LS, Mortrud MT et al., The cloning of a family of genes that encode the melanocortin receptors, *Science* (1992) **257**: 1248–51.
10. Cone RD, Mountjoy KG, Robbins LS et al., Cloning and functional characterization of a family of receptors for the melanotropic peptides, *Ann N Y Acad Sci* (1993) **680**:342–63.
11. Healy E, Birch-Machin MA, Rees JL, The human melanocortin-1 receptor. In: Cone RD, ed, (Humana Press: New Jersey, 2000) 341–60.
12. Cone RD, Lu D, Koppula S et al., The melanocortin receptors: agonists, antagonists, and the hormonal control of pigmentation, *Rec Prog Horm Res* (1996) **51**:287–317.
13. Chen WB, Kelly MA, Opitz-Araya X et al., Exocrine gland dysfunction in MC5-R-deficient mice: Evidence for coordinated regulation of exocrine gland function by melanocortin peptides, *Cell* (1997) **91**:789–98.
14. Tsatmali M, Yukitake J, Thody AJ, ACTH1–17 is a more potent agonist at the human MC1 receptor than alpha-MSH, *Cell Mol Biol (Noisy-le-grand)* (1999) **45**:1029–34.
15. Wakamatsu K, Graham A, Cook D et al., Characterisation of ACTH peptides in human skin and their activation of the melanocortin-1 receptor, *Pigment Cell Res* (1997) **10**:288–97.
16. Spector TD, The history of twin and sibling-pair studies. In: Advances in twin and sib-pair analysis, Spector TD, Snieder H, MacGregor AJ, eds. London: Greenwich Medical Media (distributed by OUP), 1999, 2–9.
17. Valverde P, Healy E, Jackson I et al., Variants of the melanocyte-stimulating hormone receptor gene are associated with red hair and fair skin in humans, *Nat Genet* (1995) **11**:328–30.
18. Harding RM, Healy E, Ray AJ et al., Evidence for variable selective pressures at the human pigmentation locus, MC1R, *Am J Hum Genet* (2000) **66**: 1351–61.
19. Smith R, Healy E, Siddiqui S et al., Melanocortin 1 receptor variants in an Irish population, *J Invest Dermatol* (1998) **111**:119–22.
20. Flanagan N, Healy E, Ray A et al., Pleiotropic effects of the melanocortin 1 receptor (MC1R) gene on human pigmentation, *Hum Mol Genet* (2000) **9**:2531–7.
21. Healy E, Flannagan N, Ray A et al., Melanocortin-1-receptor gene and sun sensitivity in individuals without red hair, *Lancet* (2000) **355**:1072–3.
22. Schioth HB, Phillips S, Rudzish R et al., Loss of function mutations of the human melanocortin 1 receptor are common and associated with red hair, *Biochem Biophysi Res Communi* (1999) **260**:488–91.
23. Valverde P, Healy E, Sikkink S et al., The Asp84Glu variant of the melanocortin 1 receptor (MC1R) is associated with melanoma, *Hum Mol Genet* (1996) **5**:1663–6.
24. Fitzpatrick TB, The validity and practicality of sun-reactive skin types I through VI, *Arch Dermatol* (1988) **124**:869–71.
25. Rampen FH, Fleuren BA, de Boo TM et al., Unreliability of self-reported burning tendency and tanning ability, *Arch Dermatol* (1988) **124**:885–8.
26. Andreassi L, Simoni S, Fiorini P et al., Phenotypic characters related to skin type and minimal erythemal dose. *Photodermatology* (1987) **4**:43–6.
27. Baron ED, Stern RS, Taylor CR, Correlating skin type and minimum erythema dose, *Arch Dermatol* (1999) **135**:1278–9.
28. Lock-Andersen J, Wulf HC, Knudstorp ND, Interdependence of eye and hair colour, skin type and skin pigmentation in a Caucasian population, *Acta Derm Venereol (Stockh)* (1998) **78**:214–9.
29. Westerhof D, Estevez-Uscanga O, Meens J et al., The relation between constitutional skin color and photosensitivity estimated from UV-induced erythema and pigmentation dose response curves, *J Invest Dermatol* (1990) **94**:812–16.
30. Flanagan N, Ray AJ, Todd C et al., The relation between melanocortin 1 receptor genotype and experimentally assessed ultraviolet radiation sensitivity, *J Invest Dermatol* (2001) **117(5)**:1314–7.

32
The value of melanin as a sunscreen

James J. Nordlund

Introduction: The functions of melanin

Melanin is a remarkable substance. It has been synthesized and deposited in the skin, eyes and ears of almost every person who has come onto the earth. It is found in all vertebrates, many sub-vertebrates and even in plants. Its presence in large quantities makes the skin of some individuals living in Africa or Australia much darker than the skin of peoples living in Europe and North or South America (Fig. 32.1). And, over centuries, this biochemical difference in skin color has had social and political implications resulting in the subjugation of billions of peoples on six of the seven world's continents.

Melanin, obviously, is found in the skin. But melanin and melanocytes can also be found in the normal tissues of the eye (uveal tract and retinal pigment epithelium), in the ear, leptomeninges[1,2] and, at times, in ectopic sites.[3] Neuromelanin is found within the brain and likely is different in structure from that found in the skin. Certainly, its function in the brain must be different from that in the skin and eyes.

The structure of melanin, a polymer composed of indole units, is not yet known,[4–6] although its synthesis is thoroughly understood.[7,8] The function of melanin continues to be subject of interest for many scholarly individuals.[9] A partial list of the functions of melanin include the following:

- Protection against photodegradation of nutrients like folic acid.
- Protection against excessive production of potentially toxic nutrients like vitamin D.
- Heat collector.
- Camouflage.
- Oxygen scavenger.
- Energy transporter.
- Drug binder.
- Modulator of the inflammatory response.
- Sunscreen.

It seems likely that melanin probably functions in all of these ways and possibly in other ways not yet identified by anthropological or clinical studies or by laboratory investigations.

Melanin as a sunscreen

The epidermis is composed mainly of keratinocytes (Fig. 32.2). Not all keratinocytes can proliferate or serve as a source of non-melanoma skin cancer. It is thought that there are stem cells within the basilar layer of the epidermis and in the bulge area of the hair follicles that serve as a proliferating pool of keratinocytes. It is these stem cells that might be the source of most non-melanoma skin cancers.

Interspersed between the basilar keratinocytes are melanocytes (Fig. 32.2), the cellular origin of melanomas. Melanocytes are unique in their capacity to synthesize melanin. Melanin is synthesized within particulate melanosomes which subsequently are transferred into the surrounding basilar keratinocytes.[10,11] The melanosomes form an umbrella or screen (Fig. 32.2) over the nucleus of basilar keratinocytes.[12] This cap seems to be a mechanism by which melanosomes protect proliferating cells from mutations induced by sunlight. Basilar keratinocytes migrate through the epidermis to the stratum corneum, from where they are desquamated, along with their load of melanin. Once the cells leave the basilar layer, they are no longer capable of mitosis and cannot be a source for skin cancers. The melanin remains within the keratinocytes during this transit. As the cells near the upper layers of the epidermis, some of the melanin is degraded from particulate

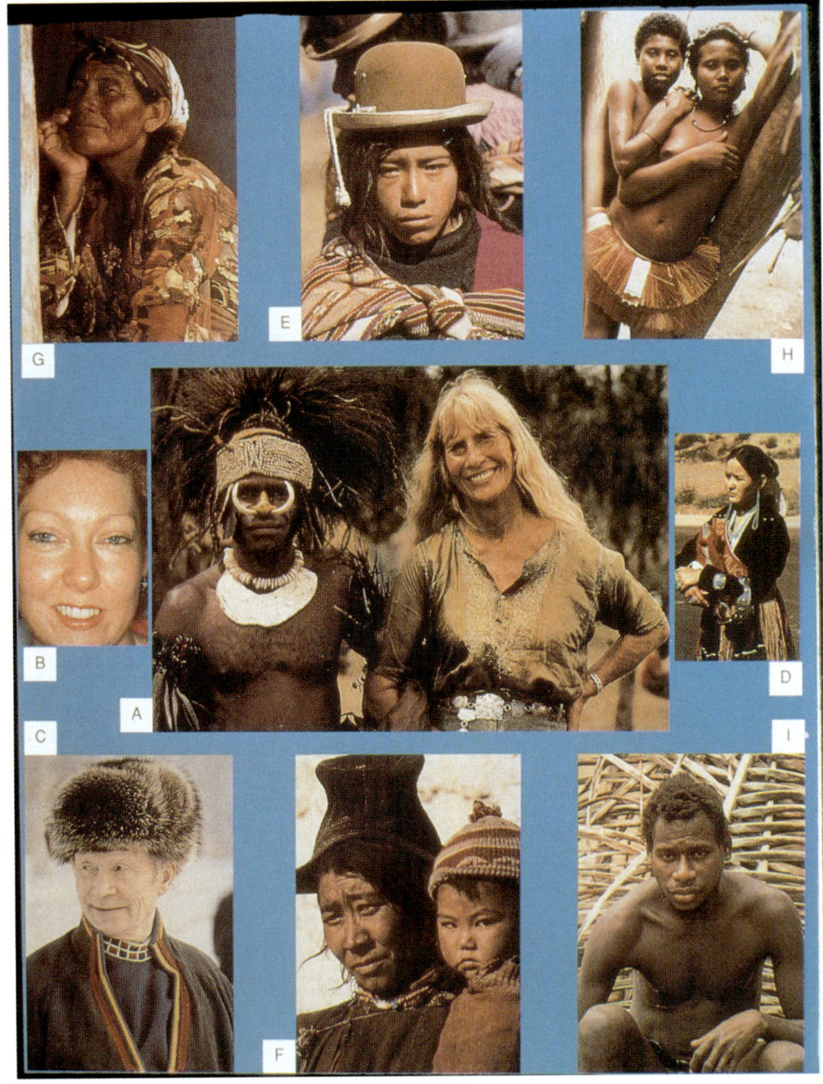

Figure 32.1

Human skin colors, from white to black with red, blond, brown and black hair. Reproduced with permission.[9]

melanosomes into a melanin dust (Fig. 32.2). The absorptive capacity of melanin dust for ultraviolet light is much greater than the absorption by particulate melanosomes.[13] Ultraviolet energy absorbed by the melanin is presumably converted into heat that is dissipated as harmless energy.

The best recognized function of melanin is that of sunscreen. The absorption spectrum of melanin for electromagnetic radiation is maximum in the ultraviolet range, *i.e.* about 290–400 nm, but extends into the spectrum of visible light (400–700 nm).[14] Measurements of the absorptive capacity of melanin, either suspended in a cream and applied to the skin surface or deposited within the epidermis, indicate that melanin has a sun protective factor (SPF) of about 2–4, *i.e.* the melanin absorbs about 50–75% of the incident sunlight.[12,15,16]

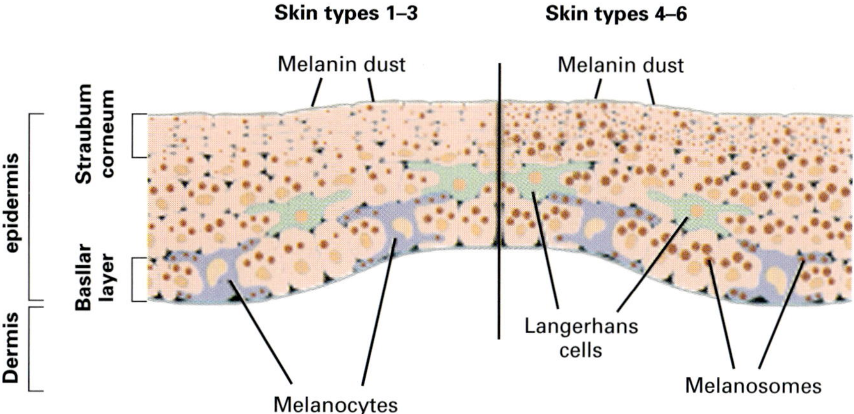

Figure 32.2

Schematic drawing of the skin illustrating the three cell types of the skin. Melanocytes are located along the basal lamina and inject melanosomes into surrounding keratinocytes, where they form an umbrella over the nucleus. Some degrade into dust as the melanosomes are carried to the stratum corneum. Note that the Langerhans cells are located in mid-epidermis, above the melanin screen.

For centuries, it has been obvious that individuals with darker skin tolerated the cutaneous effects of sunlight better than those with lighter skin.[10] In recent years, skin types have been described that are based on the probability of skin burning or tanning following exposure to sunlight.[17]

- Type 1 Always burns; never tans—Celtic individuals.
- Type 2 Always burns; tans minimally—Northern Europeans.
- Type 3 Burns moderately; tans gradually—Scandinavians.
- Type 4 Rarely burns; tans well—Southern Europeans.
- Type 5 Burns minimally; tans very well—Orientals and Hispanics.
- Type 6 Never burns; tans very well—Africans, Indians, Aborigines.[11]

Although more recent studies suggest that there are better ways to type skin color, this system exemplifies the inverse relationship between the tendency of skin to sunburn and its capacity to tan. Dark-skinned individuals might burn if exposed to excessive sunlight, but such events are uncommon. For those of Celtic inheritance, who have red hair, blue eyes and freckles (Fig. 32.3), sunburn is a daily problem. Protection against serious sunburn has survival value, since blistering burns would limit the ability of the sufferer to gather or hunt for food. Golger's rule of pigmentation notes that individuals with dark skin reside near the equator and that those with light skin inhabit areas far distant from the equator that have limited sun exposure.[12] It has been assumed that human skin color evolved as Golger described, so that those living near the equator had adequate protection against the ravages of excessive sun exposure.

Every dermatologist recognizes the evidence of cutaneous damage related to sun exposure. The skin is covered by lesions, called actinic keratoses (Figs 32.4 and 32.5), that are located exclusively within exposed skin. Some of these, possibly as

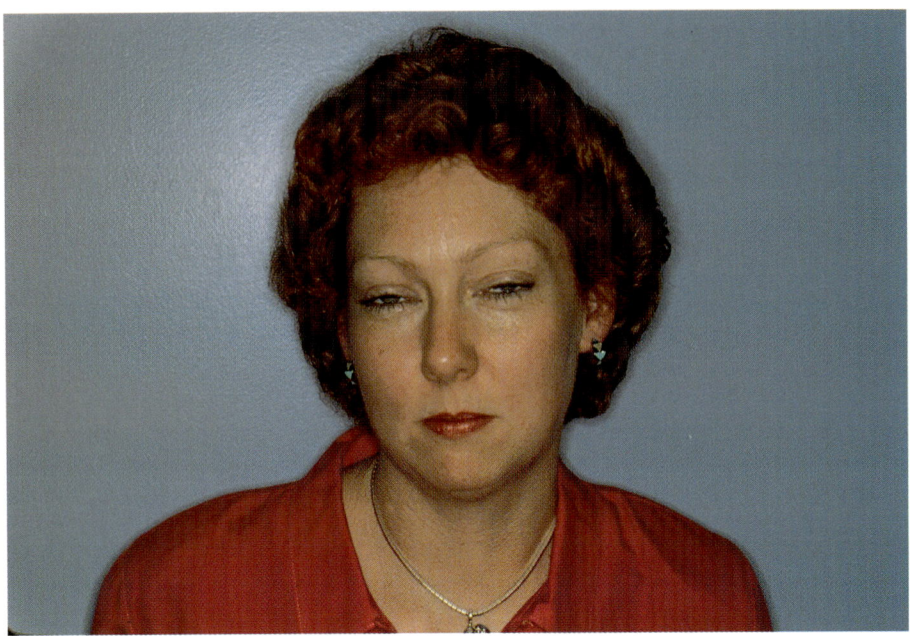

Figure 32.3

Celtic traits. This woman has red hair, blue eyes, fair type 1 skin color and freckles. She is readily sunburned.

few as 1 in 300, will convert into basal or squamous cell carcinomas (Figs 32.6–8). These latter tumors are derived from keratinocytes that are located along the basal lamina, which demarcates the epidermis from the dermis. Melanomas (Fig. 32.9), derived from melanocytes, are also associated with sun exposure, especially intense, intermittent exposures that result in blistering burns. Almost all skin cancers are observed in those individuals with skin types 1, 2 or 3. This point is emphasized by the effects of sunlight on those with a genetic abnormality that limits the ability of skin to produce melanin, *i.e.* albinism. Pigmented people (Figs 32.10 and 32.11) can develop skin cancers (see below) but such cancers are rare. In contrast, albino Africans (Fig. 32.12) and others with oculocutaneous albinism have a high risk of getting skin cancers (Fig. 32.13), probably 50% or higher.[18–21] Clearly, melanin provides some protection against the carcinogenic effects of ultraviolet light.[12,15]

The amount of photodamage in skin cells is determined by the amount of light that penetrates the skin, where it interacts with components of proliferating cells. It can have direct or indirect effects. Light that hits and is absorbed by chromosomal DNA causes formation of pyrimidine dimers and other 6–4 photoproducts.[16,22,23] Absorption of UV by melanin prevents such damage to DNA. Ultraviolet light might also produce high-energy oxygen radicals that indirectly produce imperfections in DNA, such as 8-hydroxydeoxyguanosine.[24] Melanin can detoxify oxygen radicals and prevent some secondary damage.[25]

Results of *in vitro* studies in which melanoma cells or melanocytes were used as targets for UVB (290–320 nm) ultraviolet radiation, demonstrate that the number of pyrimidine dimers and other photoproducts[16] was reduced by 20% in heavily melanized cells compared to cells with little melanin. DNA damage was significantly reduced by melanin in skin explants maintained in culture.[23] *In vivo,* the number of photoproducts was reduced by 30% in heavily melanized skin, compared to lightly colored skin.[26] It is hard to deny the importance of melanin as one method by which nature has provided humans and other animals with sun protection.

Light reflected from the surface of the skin, or stratum corneum, is harmless. Reflection is one mechanism by which the skin is protected from sunlight, and melanin appears to contribute to

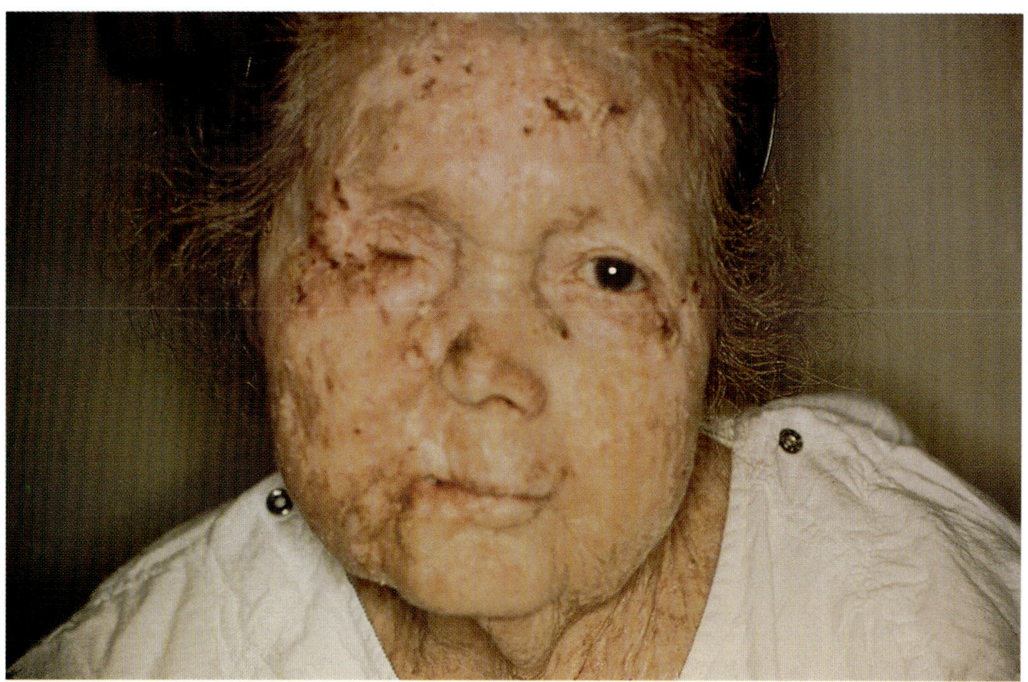

Figure 32.4

An Hispanic woman showing facial erosions and scars from sun exposure despite her darker skin color.

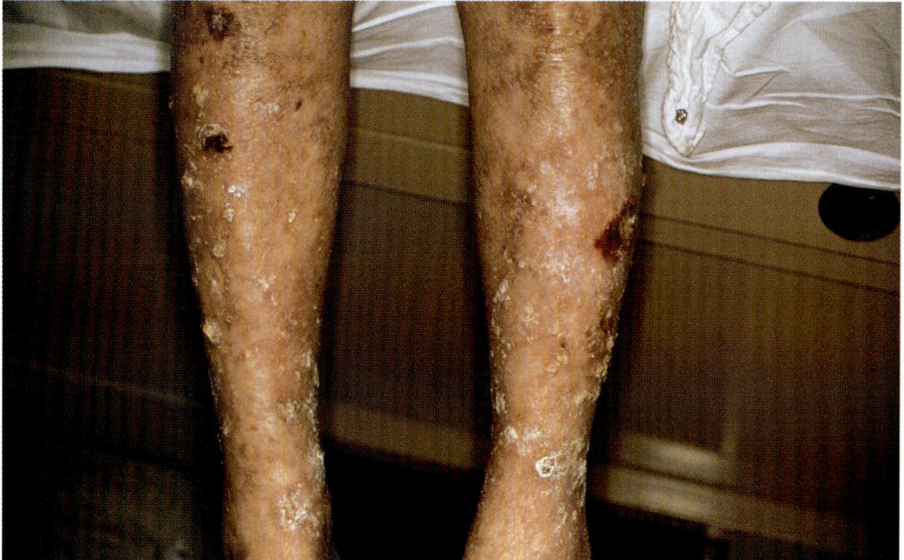

Figure 32.5

The legs of the patient in Figure 32.4. She has numerous actinic keratoses on the legs, a manifestation of moderate to severe sun damage.

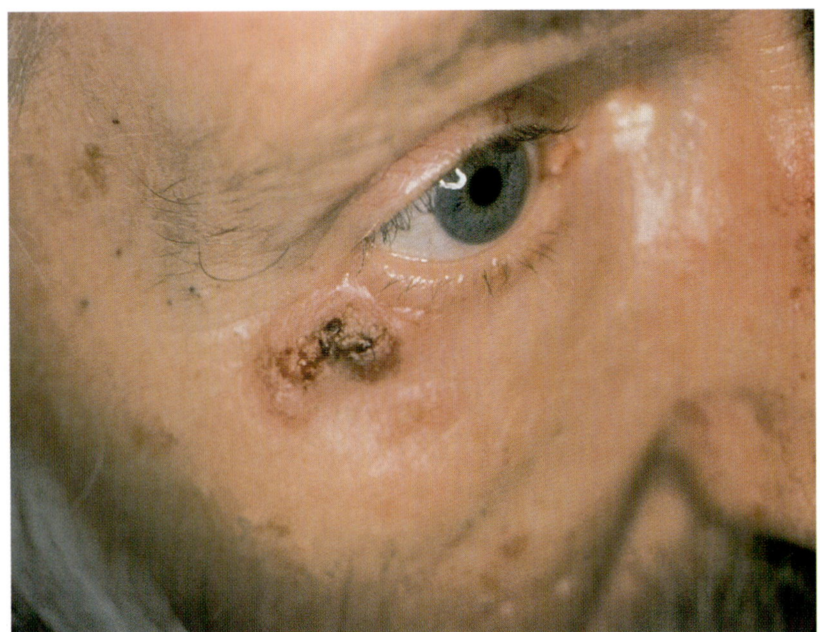

Figure 32.6

A man with blue eyes and type 1 skin color. There is a basal cell carcinoma located at the lateral angle of the eye.

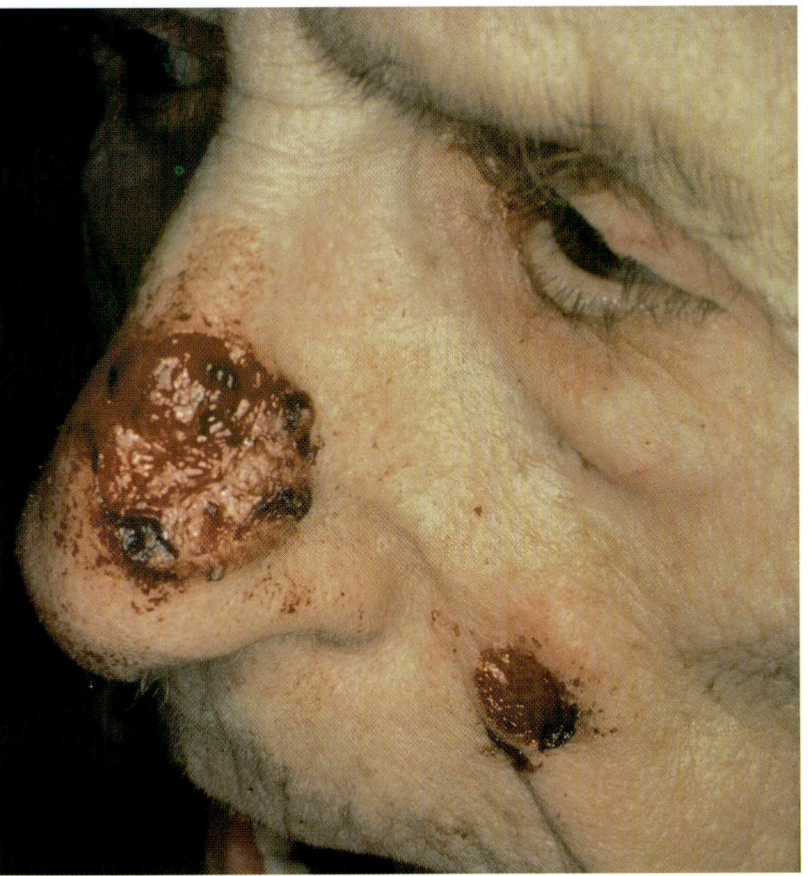

Figure 32.7

An elderly woman with a friable tumor on the tip of the nose. This is a squamous cell carcinoma.

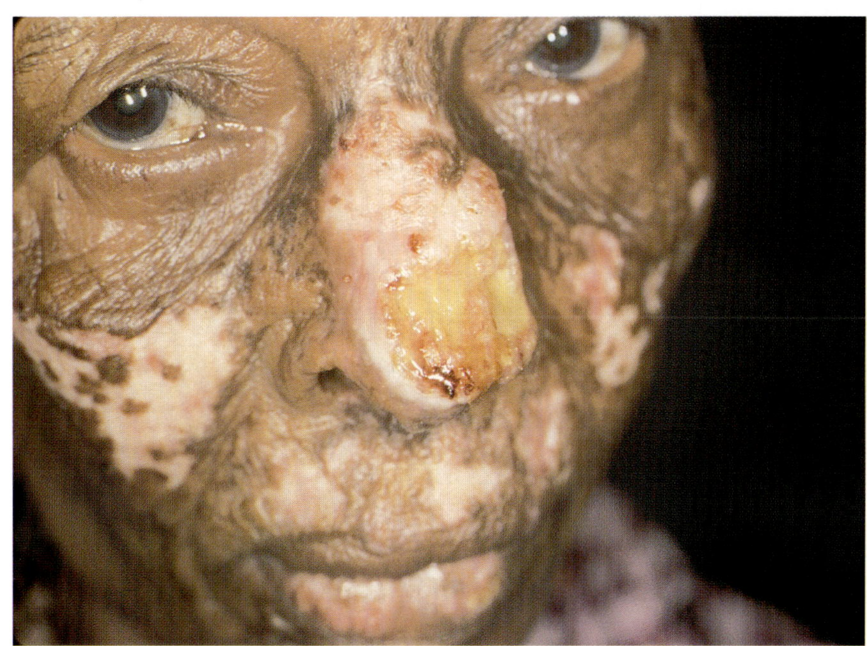

Figure 32.8

A squamous cell carcinoma on the nose of an African woman, who also has lupus erythematosus that caused depigmentation of her skin. Note the cancer arose in the depigmented skin.

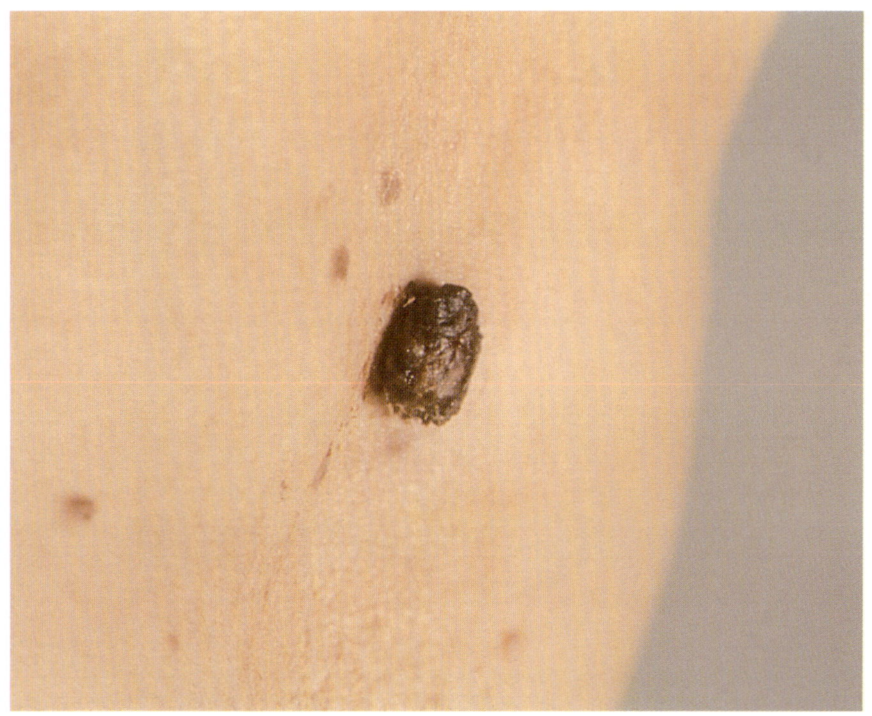

Figure 32.9

A fair-skinned man with a nodular melanoma on the back. The dark spots surrounding the tumor are satellite tumors. The patient died from the melanoma.

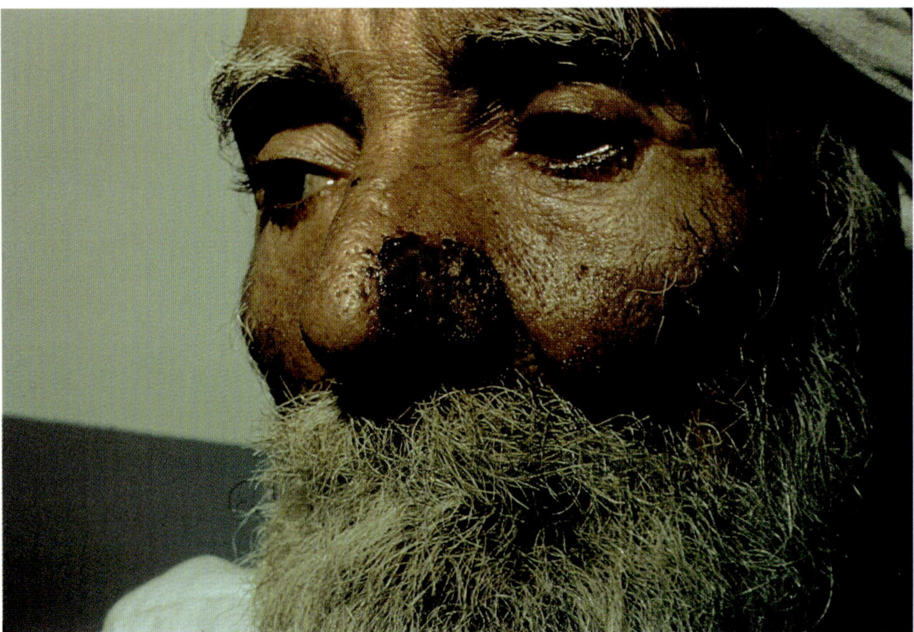

Figure 32.10

An Indian man with basal cell carcinoma on the nose, despite his dark complexion.

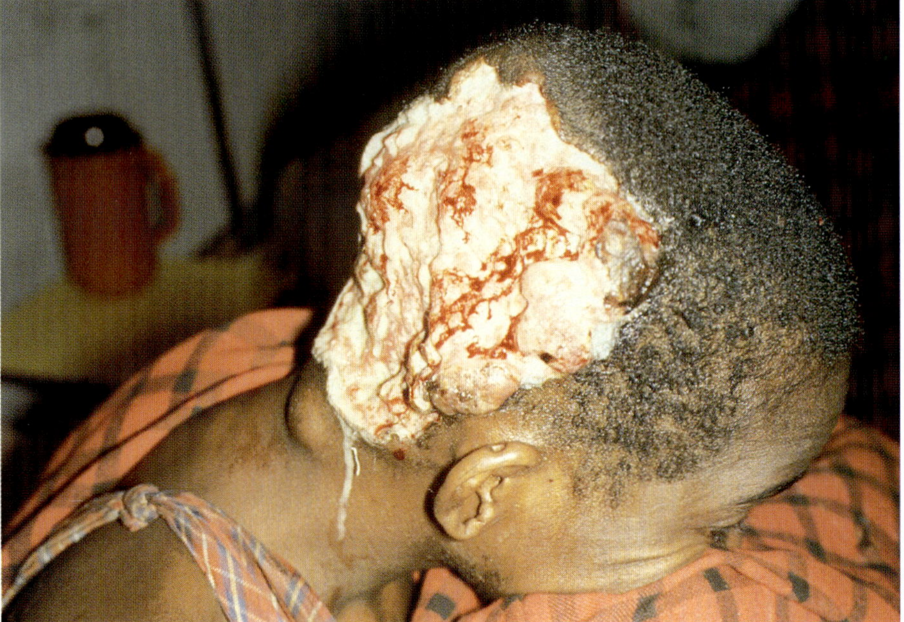

Figure 32.11

A highly malignant squamous cell carcinoma that arose on the scalp of the Masaai warrior. The patient died from the cancer.

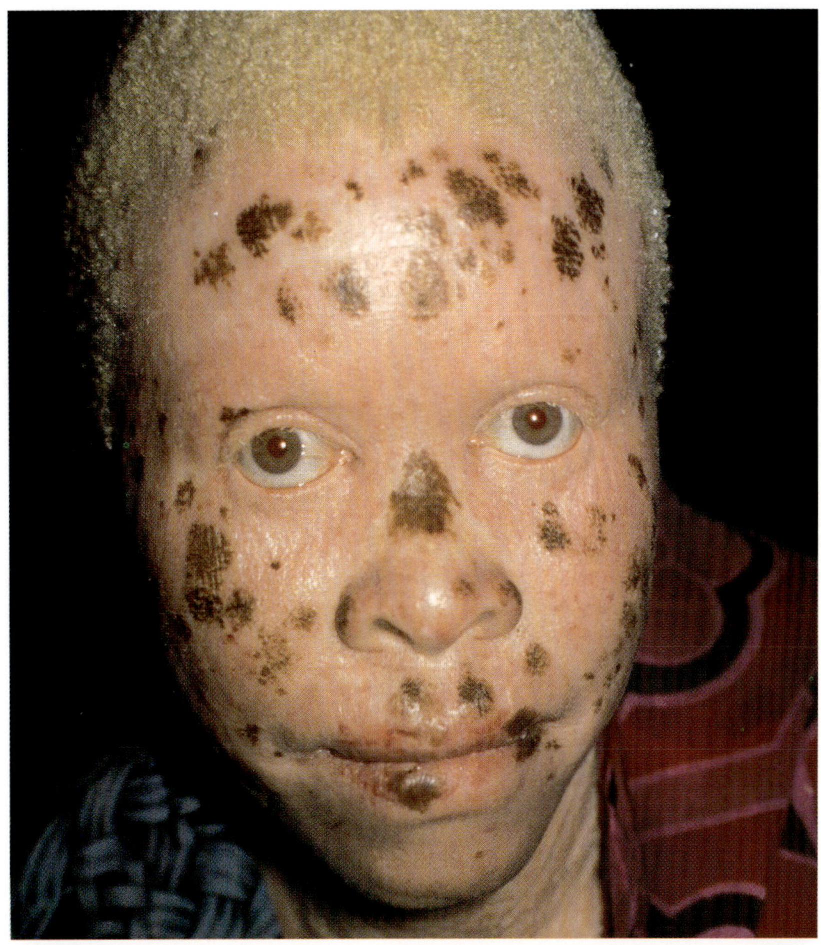

Figure 32.12

An African girl with oculocutaneous albinism (OCA 2) who has many lentigines on her face following prolonged exposure to sun. These are manifestations of sun damage.

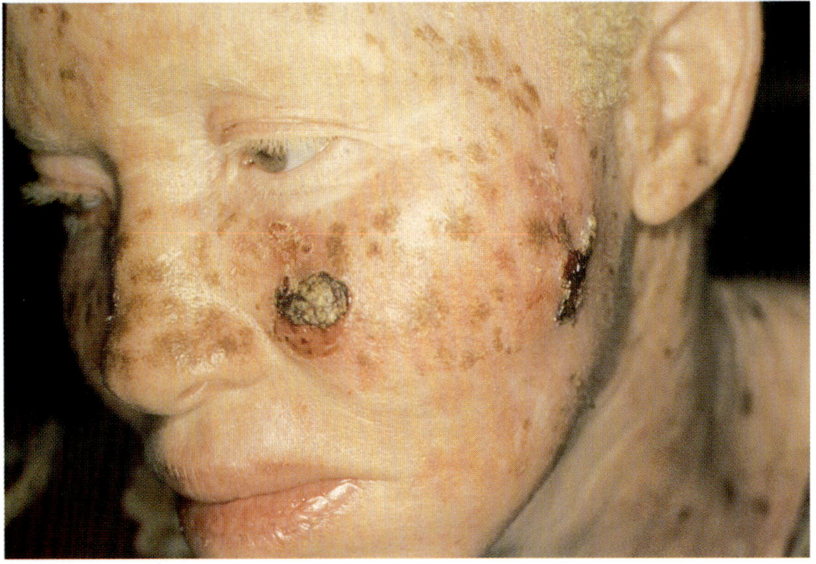

Figure 32.13

A squamous cell carcinoma on the cheek of an African albino (OCA 2).

reflection.[27,28] Moderately melanized skin, such as types 3 and 4 skin color, has a higher capacity to reflect ultraviolet light than skin with lighter or darker colors.[27]

Another mechanism employed by the skin to protect itself from sun is thickening, in particular the stratum corneum, following sun exposure (Fig. 32.14) A thick stratum corneum is a very effective way of diminishing sun damage.[25]

Despite this variety of mechanisms to prevent mutation transformation of skin cells into cancers, DNA damage occurs. Cells have a set of enzymes that can repair DNA damaged either by sunlight or chemical carcinogens. Activation of these DNA repair mechanisms seems to activate production of melanin.[29] It seems that skin utilizes tanning as a positive feedback to prevent additional damage from sunlight.

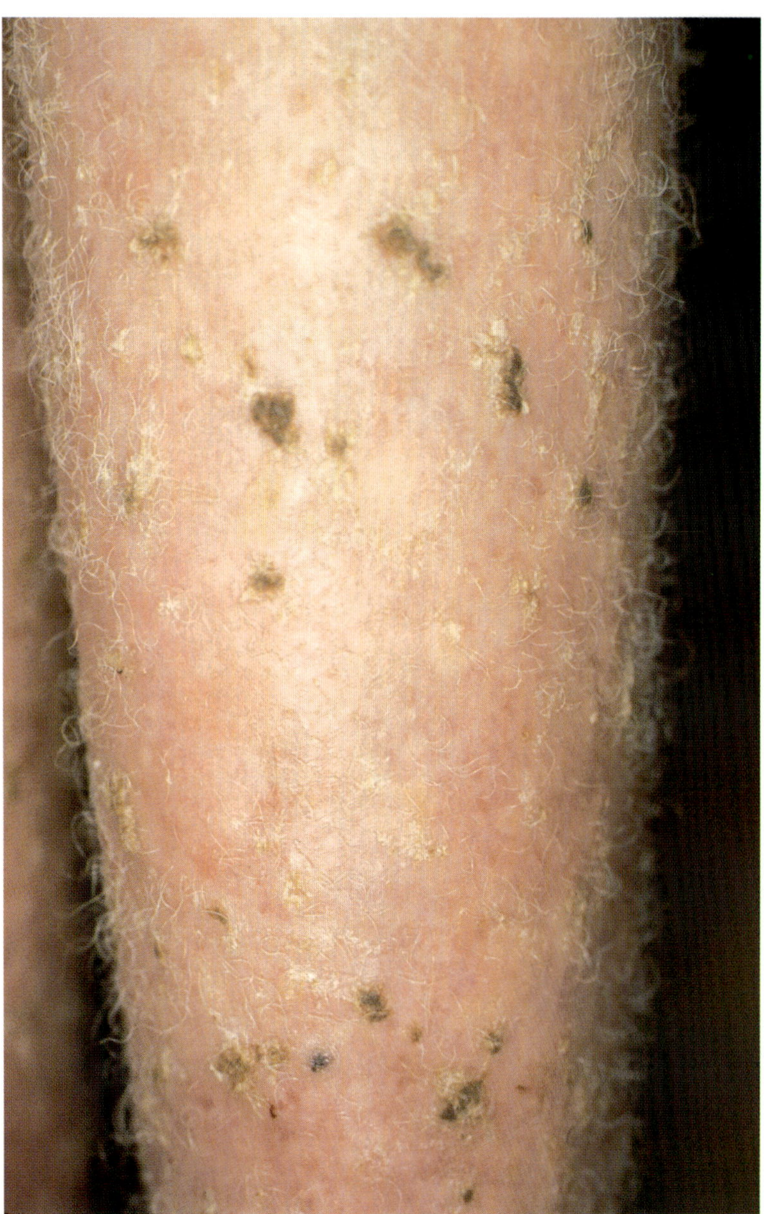

Figure 32.14

The leg of an African albino showing many actinic keratoses and thickening of the stratum corneum.

Limitations of melanin as a sunscreen: Clinical and histological data

Golger's rule of skin color seems to describe well the distribution of skin color for the denizens of Europe, the Middle East and Africa. Yet, the tribes of peoples that migrated to the Americas do not show this distribution of skin color. The American Indians in all three Americas all have similar type 3 or 4 skin color. There is no obvious color gradient between the Eskimos, who inhabit the Arctic circle, and the Aztecs and Incas, living near the equator, often at very high altitudes. Asian peoples on the Siberian plains, in Mongolia, China or Japan, have skin colors that are similar. None is very dark, mostly type 3 or 4 skin color. Yet they have very few skin cancers, fewer than might be expected from skin color alone.[15]

If melanin was an effective sun block, light-induced or aggravated disorders should be uncommon in those with very dark skins, like African-Americans. It is well documented that those with dark skin are as susceptible to light-induced disorders as those with light skin.[12,30] Lupus erythematosus, a disorder that is often aggravated by ultraviolet light, seems especially common in African-Americans (Figs 32.8 and 32.15).[31–33]

Solar elastosis is a clinical/histopathological description of alterations seen in the dermis caused by sunlight, in particular the UVA 320–400 nm spectrum (Fig. 32.16). The individual with solar elastosis has a yellowish color to the skin and thick, heavy wrinkles (Figs 32.17 and 32.18). Histologically, the elastic tissue in the dermis is degraded or destroyed (Figs 32.19 and 32.20). It is interesting that individuals with dark skin often exhibit as much solar elastosis as those with lighter skin color (Figs 32.17 and 32.18).[12] The epidermis of such individuals is normal, but the dermis shows severe degenerative changes. The significance is that the light, especially UVA, penetrated through

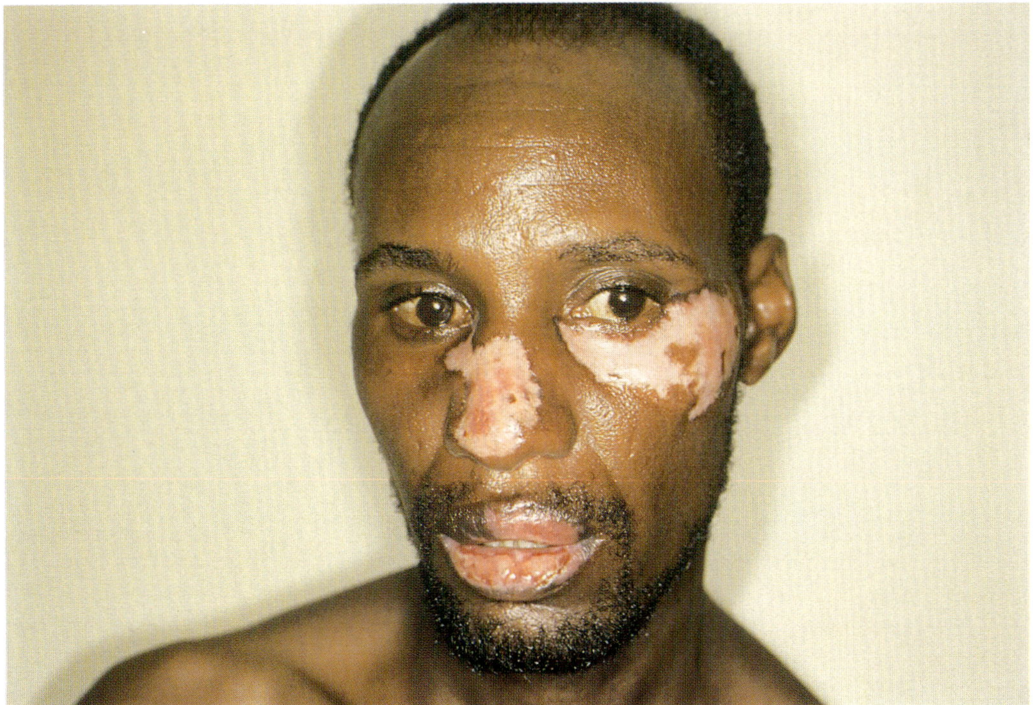

Figure 32.15

An African man with lupus erythematosus on the face. The disorder caused scarring and loss of pigmentation.

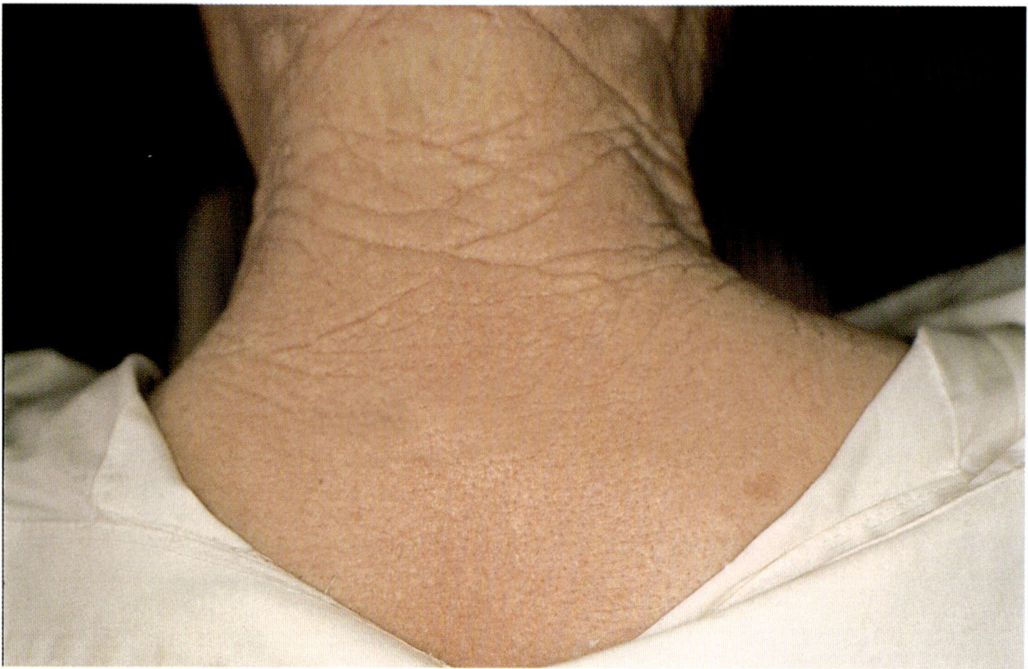

Figure 32.16

The neck of an albino showing the thick wrinkles typical of solar elastosis, a manifestation of dermal damage.

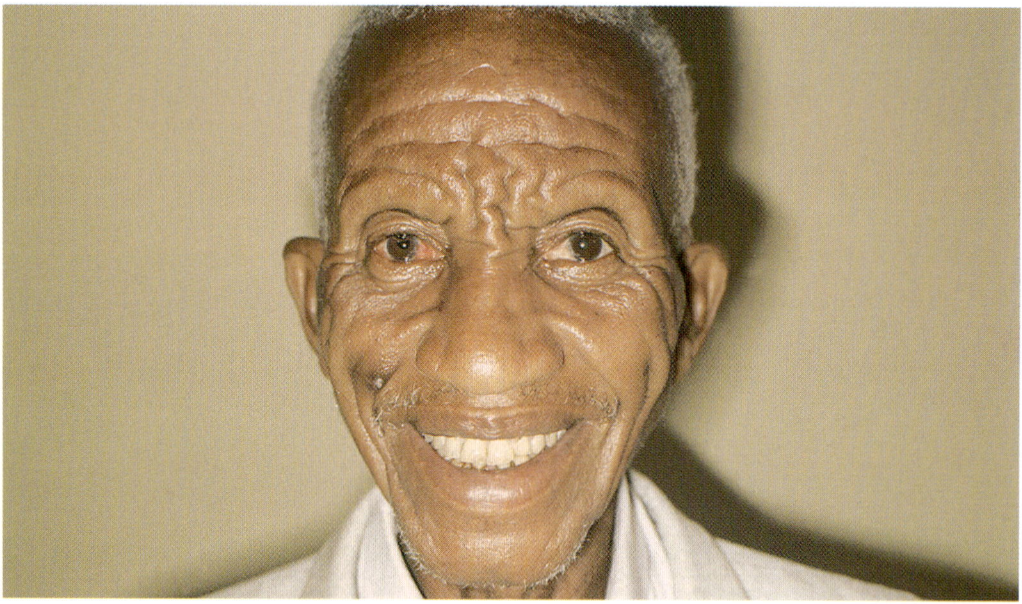

Figure 32.17

An African man with marked wrinkling of his facial skin, typical of solar elastosis.

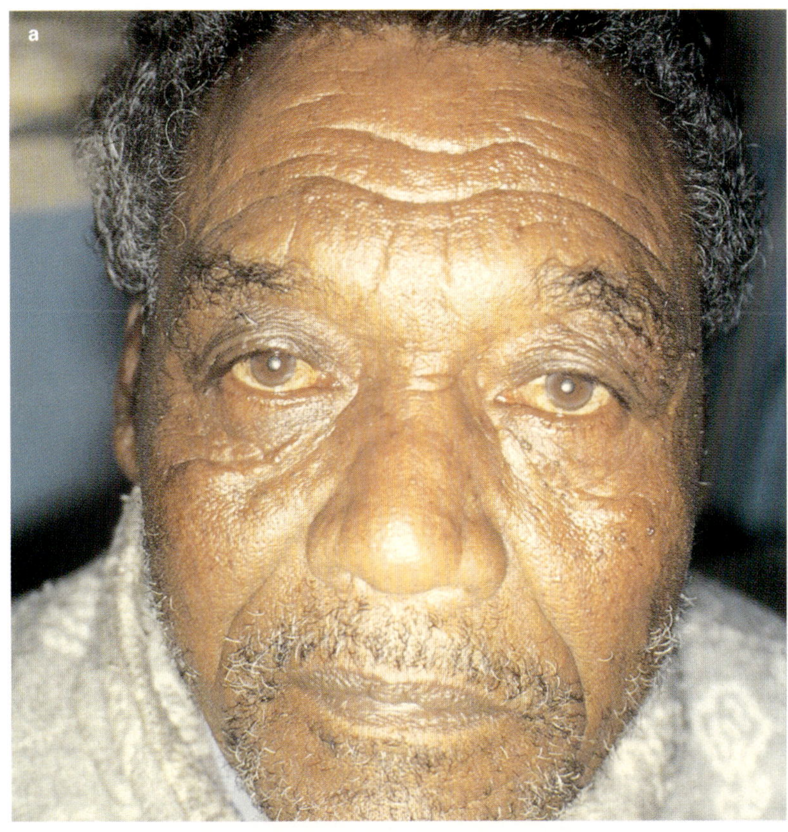

Figure 32.18 a and b

Thickened skin of an African man with solar elastosis. He also shows sebaceous hyperplasia and comedones near the eye, also signs of dermal sun damage.

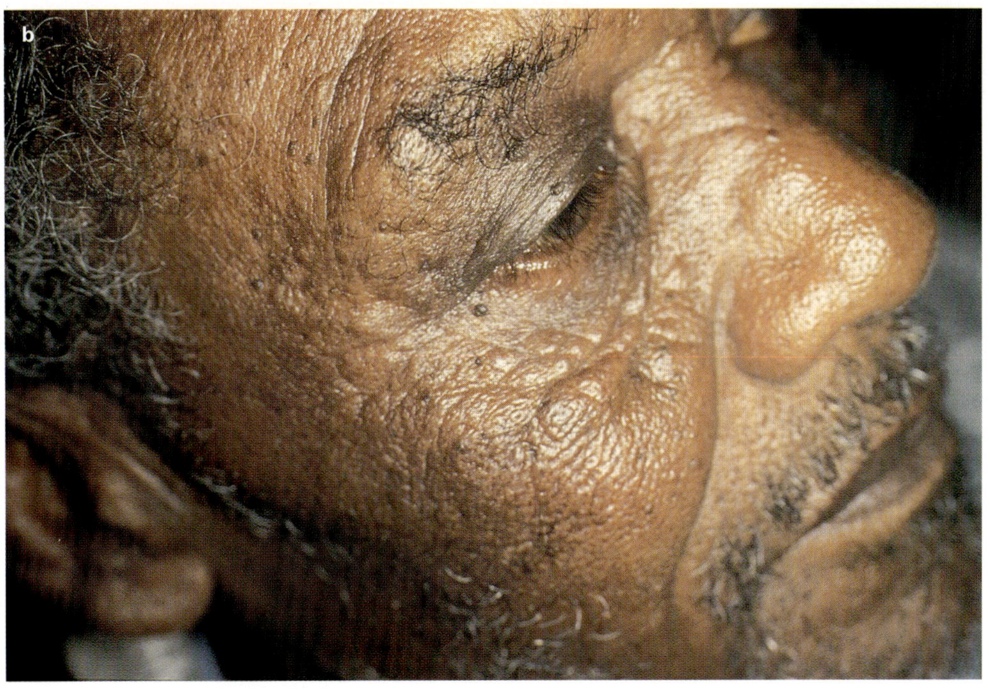

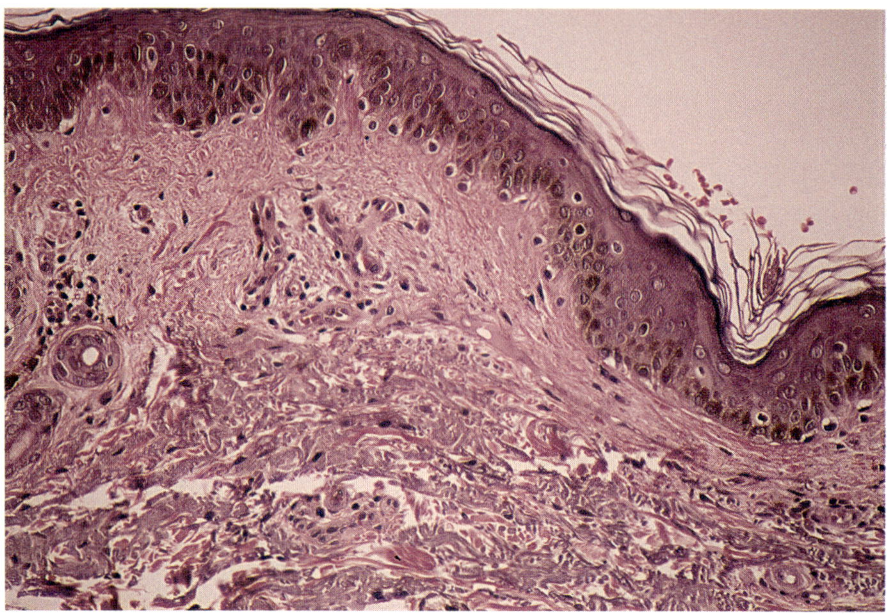

Figure 32.19

Histology of skin from an Indian man who was a farmer most of his life. The dermis shows severe solar elastosis.

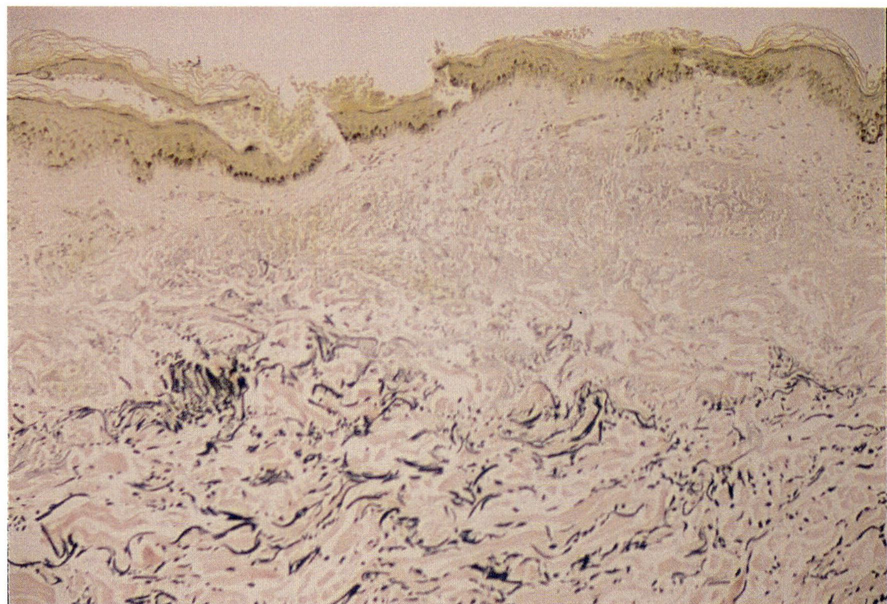

Figure 32.20

Elastic stain of tissue from the patient in Figure 32.19. Normal elastic fibers are delicate strands that stain black. Note the absence of elastic fibers from the upper dermis, a manifestation of solar elastosis.

the epidermis to the dermis but produced little or no epidermal damage. If this conclusion is correct, then the melanin barrier in the epidermis, be it dust or particulate, was not especially effective in reflecting or absorbing the UVA.

Skin cancer is common in light-skinned (type 1, 2 or 3 skin color) individuals (Figs 32.6–9). The most common type is basal cell carcinoma (Fig. 32.6) (about 75%), followed by squamous cell carcinomas (Figs 32.7 and 32.8) (20%) and melanomas (Fig. 32.9) (5%). Albinos, regardless of ethnic background, have type 1 skin color and are at risk for getting skin cancers (Fig. 32.13).[18–21,34,35] However, albinos most frequently form squamous cell carcinoma (75%) and, less commonly, basal cell cancers (25%). Melanomas are almost never observed in albinos, although they have a normal number of melanocytes in the skin. Thus, one must conclude that factors other than melanin are involved in preventing melanomas or basal cell carcinomas in type 1 or 2 skin. Skin cancers do occur even in individuals with types 4, 5 or 6 skin color, but are uncommon (Figs 32.10, 11 and 21).[15] All of these data suggest that melanin alone cannot protect the skin from mutational events caused by ultraviolet light.

Vitiligo is an acquired disorder in which melanocytes are destroyed and the skin is completely white. It has been noted that vitiligo skin does not seem to manifest more evidence of sun damage than normal-appearing skin in the same subject.[36,37] More recently, it has been noted that skin cancers are unusual, indeed rare, in vitiliginous skin, even when the individual has had depigmentation for several decades and lived in sun-drenched environments (Figs 32.22 and 32.23) (personal observation). The obvious conclusion is that the skin has mechanisms other than melanin to protect itself very effectively.

Langerhans cells are part of the immune system and are located in the epidermis (Fig. 32.2), where they can initiate or effect an immune response. Ultraviolet light has been shown to decrease the number of Langerhans cells within the epidermis.[15,38] The alteration in the number of Langerhans cells is accompanied by a diminution in the vigor of an immune response to antigens. Sun-induced immune suppression is as marked in those with dark skin as those with light skin, *i.e.* melanin has little protective effect on the skin immune response.[15,39,40] A vigorous immune

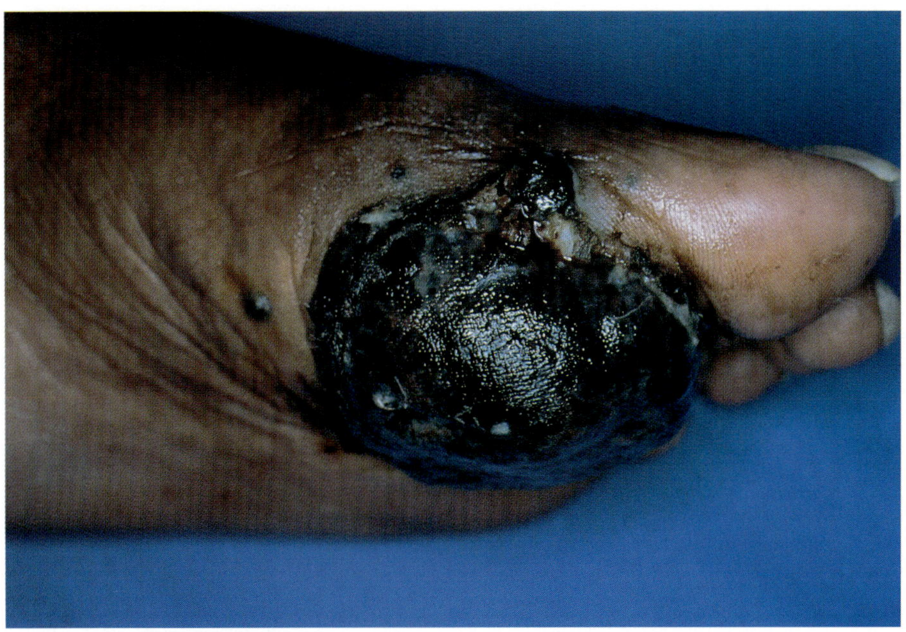

Figure 32.21

A melanoma on the foot of an African woman.

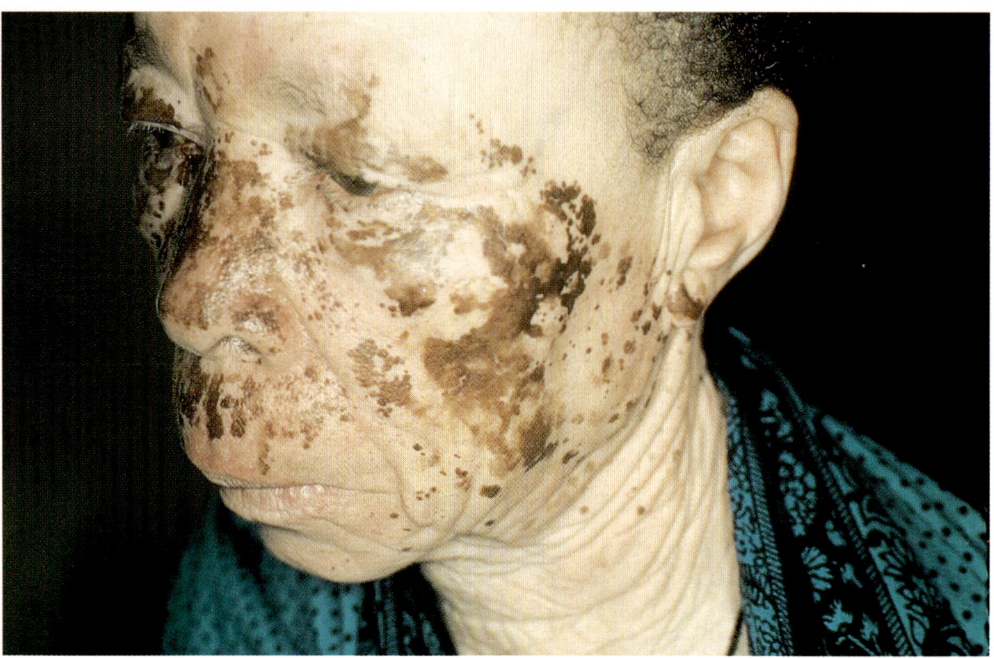

Figure 32.22

A 72-year-old woman, who worked as a farmer most of her life. She had vitiligo for about 20 years. She has some re-pigmentation on the face but she shows no keratoses or other changes of sun damage that are seen in African albinos, even by 1 year of age.

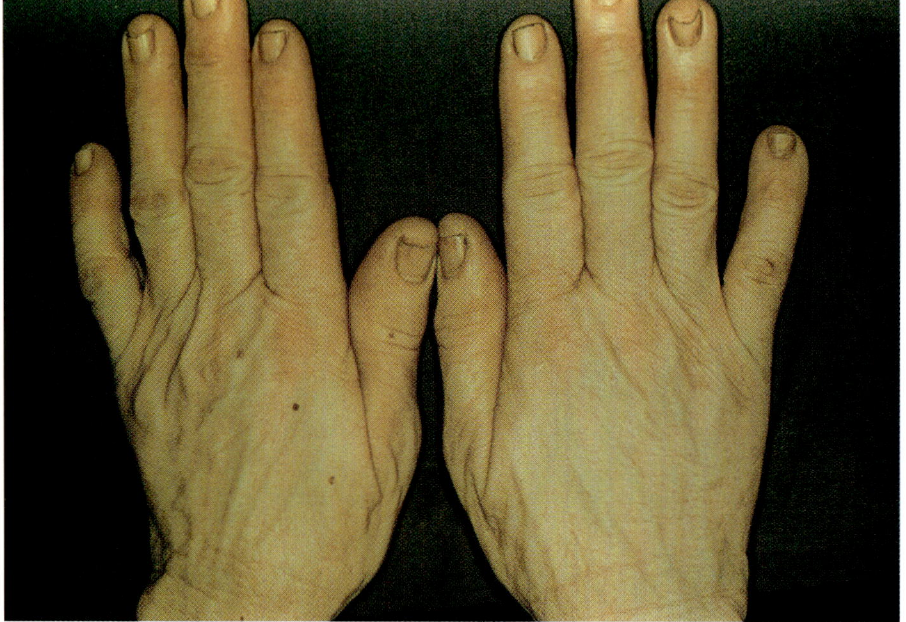

Figure 32.23

The hands of the woman in Figure 94. The epidermis was remarkably normal, although the wrinkling is typical of solar elastosis.

response in the skin seems most important in preventing skin cancers. Evidence for this are the numerous and dangerous sun-induced skin cancers observed in patients who require immunosuppressive drugs to prevent rejection of a transplanted kidney or heart. They are unable to reject the graft but also skin cancers. Thus, melanin, the majority of which is located in the lower one or two layers of the epidermis, provides poor protection for the epidermal skin-associated lymphoid tissue located in the middle of the epidermis (Fig. 32.2).

There are a number of enzymes and molecules that can quench oxygen radicals produced by sunlight. Such enzymes include catalases, superoxide dismutases or oligopeptides, such as glutathione.[41] Within the cells, there are systems of enzymes that repair mutations and damage caused by sunlight. Children with defective repair mechanisms, called Xeroderma pigmentosum, are plagued by skin cancers that eventually cause their demise. Even heavily melanized individuals with Xeroderma pigmentosum get skin cancers (Fig. 32.24).

Limitations of melanin as a sunscreen: Biochemical and cellular data

The protective effects of melanin have been studied *in vitro* in cultured melanoma cells, melanocytes and reconstituted skin. These targets have been exposed to either UVB (290–320 nm) or UVA (320–400 nm). The protective value of melanin seems to depend somewhat on the spectrum of light used. It appears to be more protective against UVB. It should be remembered, however, that, in normal sunlight, there is 1000 × more UVA than UVB.

Using murine melanoma cells, Hill[15] observed that the induction of pyrimidine dimers by UVB was similar in heavily and lightly melanized melanoma cells. Moreover, she noted that lipid peroxidation seemed to be greater in melanized cells. She also noted that UVB killed more heavily melanized murine melanoma cells than cells with a small amount of melanin. She concluded that melanin might be a two-edged sword, providing some protection but not complete protection, and that melanin might, at times, be harmful.[42]

Other investigators observed similar effects. Melanin (combination of eumelanin and pheomelanin) increased the oxidative effects of UVA on DNA. Heavily melanized cells had a twofold greater quantity of 8-hydroxydeoxyguanosine defects than lightly pigmented cells.[24] The investigator concluded that melanin seemed to sensitize melanoma cells to UVA. Results of other studies on normal melanocytes confirm these findings. For example, it was found that low doses of UVA had similar effects on white and dark cells, but large doses of UVA killed more white melanocytes than dark cells.[43] Pheomelanin or melanin intermediates seem to sensitize melanocytes to damage from UVA.[44]

Skin reconstructions containing keratinocytes with or without melanocytes can be maintained in culture. Exposure to UVB showed that DNA damage was similar in epidermal sheets, whether there were melanocytes or not. The number of pyrimidine dimers and cyclobutane dimers was similar in dark and light constructs.[45] In contrast, UVA seemed to cause more lipid peroxidation in sheets with little or no melanin. In whole epidermis, melanin seems more protective against UVA than UVB.

Hypothesis

The conclusion that seems inescapable is that melanin is not a perfect sunscreen, *i.e.* it does not provide a complete shield against sunlight, preventing all types of DNA damage. Such a conclusion should not be surprising, since it is well known that UVB penetration into the epidermis is necessary for synthesis of vitamin D, an essential factor for health and survival. Without vitamin D, individuals get rickets, characterized by low calcium absorption and soft bones. The pelvis in rachitic women is deformed and birth of viable children is often not possible. Thus, some sunlight and vitamin D are essential for good health and the survival of the human race. Clearly, sunlight is not evil and melanin must not provide a complete shield against penetration of all ultraviolet light.

It is a biological truism that Nature provides duplication or redundancy for essential processes. Redundancy indicates that Nature deals with problems in several ways. And that seems to be true for sun protection. There are many

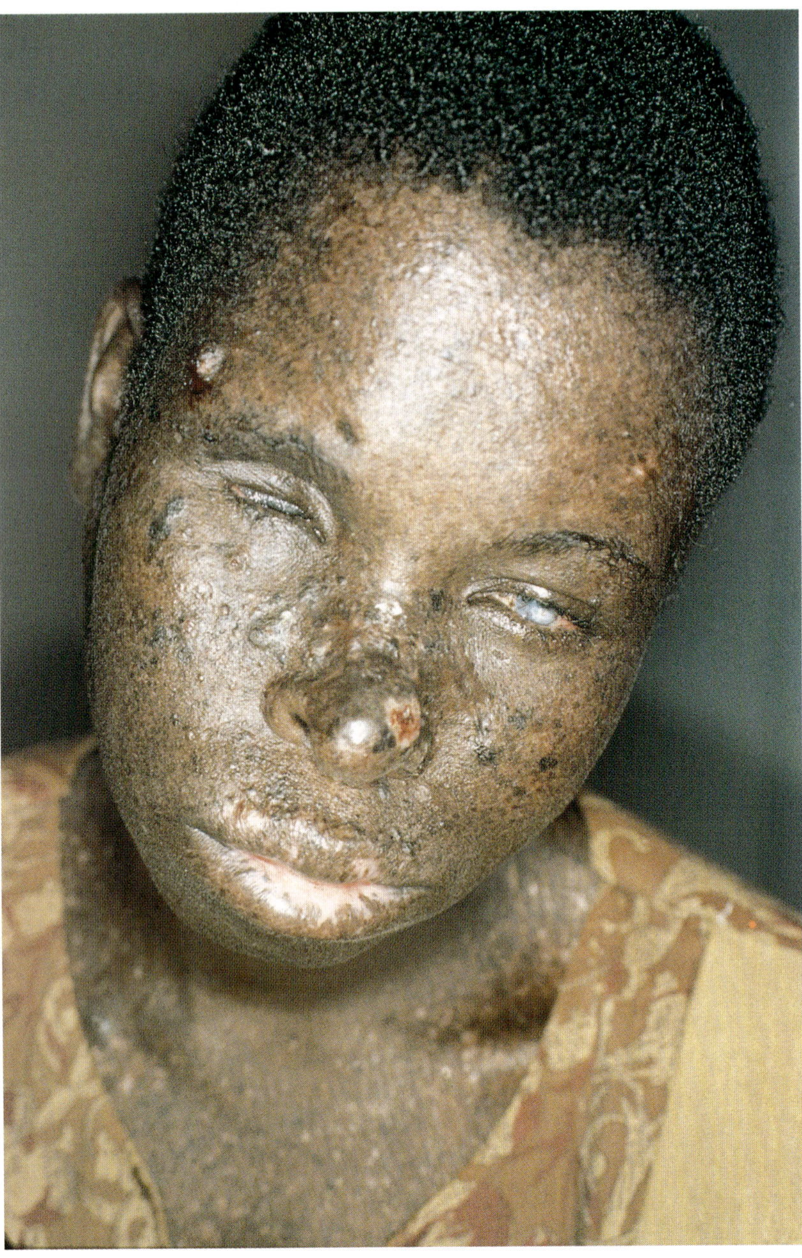

Figure 32.24

An African with Xeroderma pigmentosum. He has had numerous skin cancers, including both squamous cell carcinomas and melanomas.

chromatophores in the skin that absorb light. For example, carotenoids and flavenoids are found in the skin and are capable of absorbing some ultraviolet light. Urocanic acid is present in large amounts and, after absorbing UVB, undergoes a *cis/trans* isomerization.[25,41] The *cis* molecule is involved in immune suppression. Clearly, molecules other than melanin can absorb light that penetrates into the epidermis.[46] And the stratum corneum becomes thicker in response to sun exposure, thereby protecting the proliferating pool of stem cells in the basilar layer and hair follicles.[25]

Nature sets both lower and upper limits, within which an individual must function. Blood pressure must neither be too high nor too low, the pulse rate cannot be too fast or too slow, blood sugar must be within limits. And, similarly, human exposure to sunlight must be within limits. Enough sun is needed to produce all factors essential for human health. Too much sun leads to dangerous cancers, like melanoma or less aggressive tumors like basal and squamous cell carcinomas. The secret for biological success in sunny climates is to get enough but not too much, *i.e.* neither develop a sunburn nor get a highly malignant cancer like melanoma. The obvious conclusion, we think, is that Nature has found numerous ways to minimize sun damage, while extracting the energy necessary to photosynthesize vitamin D. We propose that melanin is an ideal sunscreen. Melanin broadens the limits within which humans can function, *i.e.* it permits humans to occupy virtually any location on earth, the equator or the Arctic. Melanin assists those in the tropics by raising the upper limits before which burning, mutations or other forms of DNA damage occur. Less melanin lowers the minimal amount of ultraviolet light necessary for good health and is advantageous to those living a far distance from the equator. In conjunction with epidermal thickening, other chromatophores and DNA repair, the skin is superbly protected to permit good health, even while ultraviolet light penetrates into the dermis to cause wrinkles. Thus, melanin manifested as skin color is one of several methods used by Nature to broaden the upper and lower limits of sun exposure consistent with good health and survival.

The current problem with sunlight relates to a cultural tendency of Western societies to push good things to excess. In Western society, it is common to believe that we have uncovered all of Nature's secrets and can manipulate them to fulfill our most extreme desires. There is a failure to respect Nature's rules. We want to lie in the sun all day without the consequences. We use sunscreens that remove UVB principally and, to some degree, UVA. Even the best sunscreens permit some UVB and UVA to penetrate, in actuality a large amount when the skin is exposed for an entire day or several days. Excessive UVA penetration causes damage to DNA and the dermis. Accelerated 'photoaging' is the result. Those with dark skins tend to avoid excessive sunlight. Those with white skin slather on sunscreens and lay out all day. One wonders why. Melanin is the ideal sunscreen, but only for those who believed the ancient Greeks, who noted that moderation in all things is a sign of wisdom.

References

1. Boissy R, Extracutaneous melanocytes. In: Nordlund JJ, Boissy RE, Hearing VJ et al., eds, *Pigmentary System: Physiology and Pathophysiology* (Oxford University Press: Oxford, 1998) 59–74.
2. Goldgeier MH, Klein LE, Klein-Angerer S et al., The distribution of melanocytes in the leptomeninges of the human brain, *J Invest Dermatol* (1984) **82**:235–8.
3. Nordlund JJ, The lives of pigment cells, *Dermatol Clin* (1986) **4**:407–18.
4. Sarna T, Swartz H, The physical properties of melanins. In: Nordlund JJ, Boissy RE, Hearing VJ et al., eds, *Pigmentary System: Physiology and Pathophysiology* (Oxford University Press: Oxford, 1998) 333–58.
5. Prota G, D'Ischia M, Napolitano A, The chemistry of melanins and related metabolites. In: Nordlund JJ, Boissy RE, Hearing VJ et al., eds, *Pigmentary System: Physiology and Pathophysiology* (Oxford University Press: Oxford, 1998) 307–32.
6. Riley P, Mechanisms of inhibition of melanin pigmentation. In: Nordlund JJ, Boissy RE, Hearing VJ et al., eds, *Pigmentary System: Physiology and Pathophysiology* (Oxford University Press: Oxford, 1998) 401–22.
7. Hearing V, Regulation of melanin formation. In: Nordlund JJ, Boissy RE, Hearing VJ et al., eds, *Pigmentary System: Physiology and Pathophysiology* (Oxford University Press: Oxford, 1998) 423–38.
8. Pawelek J, Chakraborty A, The enzymology of Melanogenesis. In: Nordlund JJ, Boissy RE, Hearing VJ et al., eds, *Pigmentary System: Physiology and Pathophysiology* (Oxford University Press: Oxford, 1998) 391–400.
9. Nordlund JJ, Boissy RE, Hearing VJ et al., eds, *The Pigmentary System: Physiology and Pathophysiology*, 1st edn (Oxford University Press: Oxford, 1998) 1–1198.
10. Quevedo W, Holstein T, General biology of mammalian pigmentation. In: Nordlund JJ, Boissy RE, Hearing VJ et al., eds, *Pigmentary System: Physiology and Pathophysiology* (Oxford University Press: Oxford, 1998).
11. Nordlund JJ, Ortonne J, The normal color of human skin. In: Nordlund JJ, Boissy RE, Hearing VJ et al., eds, *Pigmentary System: Physiology and Pathophysiology* (Oxford University Press: Oxford, 1998).
12. Kligman A, Is melanin sun-protective? Yes, with qualifications. A histologic study of facial skin of elderly black Women. In: Zeise L, Chedekel M,

Fitzpatrick T, eds, *Melanin: Its Role in Human Photoprotection* (Valdenmar Publishing Co: Overland Park, KS, 1995) 95–102.

13. Morison W, Is melanin a sunscreen? In: Zeise L, Chedekel M, Fitzpatrick T, eds, *Melanin: Its Role in Human Photoprotection* (Valdenmar Publishing Co: Overland Park, KS, 1995) 103–8.
14. Kollias N, The spectroscopy of human melanin pigmentation. In: Zeise L, Chedekel M, Fitzpatrick T, eds, *Melanin: Its Role in Human Photoprotection* (Valdenmar Publishing Co: Overland Park, KS, 1995) 31–8.
15. Hill H, Is melanin photoprotective or is it photosensitizing? In: Zeise L, Chedekel M, Fitzpatrick T, eds, *Melanin: Its Role in Human Photoprotection* (Valdenmar Publishing Co: Overland Park, KS, 1995) 81–9.
16. Kobayashi N, Muramatsu T, Yamashina Y et al., Photoprotection by melanin against photoproduct type DNA damage formation and cell killing. In: Zeise L, Chedekel M, Fitzpatrick T, eds, *Melanin: Its Role in Human Photoprotection* (Valdenmar Publishing Co: Overland Park, KS, 1995) 141–50.
17. Fitzpatrick T, The validity and practicality of sun-reactive skin types I through VI, *Arch Dermatol* (1988) **124**:869–71.
18. Kromberg JG, Castle D, Zwane EM, Jenkins T et al., Albinism and skin cancer in Southern Africa, *Clin Genet* (1989) **36**:43–52.
19. Lookingbill D, Lookingvill GL, Leppard B, Actinic damage and skin cancer in albinos in northern Tanzania: Findings in 164 patients enrolled in an outreach skin care program, *J Am Acad Dermatol* (1995) **32**:653–8.
20. Aquaron R, Oculocutaneous albinism in Cameroon. A 15–year follow-up study, *Ophthal Paediatr Genet* (1990) **11**:255–63.
21. Keeler CE, Albinism, xeroderma pigmentosum and skin cancer, *NCI Monogr* (1963) **10**:349–59.
22. Kobayashi N, Muramatsu T, Yamashina Y et al., Melanin reduces ultraviolet-induced DNA damage formation and killing rate in cultured human melanoma cells, *J Invest Dermatol* (1993) **101**: 685–9.
23. Kobayashi N, Nakagawa A, Muramatsu T et al., Supranuclear melanin caps reduce ultraviolet induced DNA photoproducts in human epidermis, *J Invest Dermatol* (1998) **110**:806–10.
24. Kvam E, Tyrrell RM, The role of melanin in the induction of oxidative DNA base damage by ultraviolet A irradiation of DNA or melanoma cells, *J Invest Dermatol* (1999) **113**:209–13.
25. Stanzl K, Zastrow L, Melanin: An effective photoprotectant against UV-A rays. In: Zeise L, Chedekel M, Fitzpatrick T, eds, *Melanin: Its Role in Human Photoprotection* (Valdenmar Publishing Co: Overland Park, KS, 1995) 59–63.
26. Bykov VJ, Marcusson JA, Hemminki K, Effect of constitutional pigmentation on ultraviolet B-induced DNA damage in fair-skinned people, *J Invest Dermatol* (2000) **114**:40–3.
27. Cader A, Jankowski J, Reflection of ultraviolet radiation from different skin types, *Health Phys* (1998) **74**:169–72.
28. Jablonski NG, Chaplin G, The evolution of human skin coloration, *J Hum Evol* (2000) **39**:57–106.
29. Gilchrest BA, Eller MS, DNA photodamage stimulates melanogenesis and other photoprotective responses, *J Invest Dermatol Symp Proc* (1999) **4**: 35–40.
30. Nordlund JJ, Melanin and melanocytes: Their function and significance from a clinicians point of view. In: Zeise L, Chedekel M, Fitzpatrick T, eds, *Melanin: Its Role in Human Photoprotection* (Valdenmar Publishing Co: Overland Park, KS, 1995) 183–94.
31. Gedalia A, Molina JF, Molina J et al., Childhood-onset systemic lupus erythematosus: a comparative study of African Americans and Latin Americans, *J Natl Med Assoc* (1999) **91**:497–501.
32. Molina JF, Molina J, Garcia C et al., Ethnic differences in the clinical expression of systemic lupus erythematosus: a comparative study between African-Americans and Latin Americans, *Lupus* (1997) **6**:63–7.
33. Willis I, Photosensitivity reactions in black skin, *Dermatol Clin* (1988) **6**:369–75.
34. Luande J, Henschke CI, Mohammed N, The Tanzanian human albino skin. Natural history, *Cancer* (1985) **55**:1823–8.
35. Yakubu A, Mabogunje OA, Skin cancer in African albinos, *Acta Oncologica* (1993) **32**:621–2.
36. Wildfang IL, Jacobsen FK, Thestrup-Pedersen K, PUVA treatment of vitiligo: a retrospective study of 59 patients, *Acta Dermato-Venereologica* (1992) **72**:305–6.
37. Calanchini-Postizzi E, Frenk E, Long-term actinic damage in sun-exposed vitiligo and normally pigmented skin, *Dermatologica* (1987) **174**:266–71.
38. Nordlund JJ, Ackles AE, Lerner AB, The effects of ultraviolet light and certain drugs on La-bearing Langerhans cells in murine epidermis, *Cell Immunol* (1981) **60**:50–63.
39. Vermeer M, Schmieder GJ, Yoshikawa T et al., Effects of ultraviolet B light on cutaneous immune

responses of humans with deeply pigmented skin, *J Invest Dermatol* (1991) **97**:729–34.

40. Young AR, Potten CS, Chadwick CA et al., Inhibition of UV radiation-induced DNA damage by a 5-methoxypsoralen tan in human skin, *Pigment Cell Res* (1988) **1**:350–4.
41. Pathak M, Functions of melanin and protection by melanin. In: Zeise L, Chedekel M, Fitzpatrick T, eds, *Melanin: Its Role in Human Photoprotection* (Valdenmar Publishing Co: Overland Park, KS, 1995) 125–40.
42. Hill HZ, Li W, Xin P, Mitchell DL et al., Melanin: a two edged sword? *Pigment Cell Res* (1997) **10**: -158–61.
43. Yohn JJ, Lyons MB, Norris DA, Cultured human melanocytes from black and white donors have different sunlight and ultraviolet A radiation sensitivities, *J Invest Dermatol* (1992) **99**:454–9.
44. Wenczl E, Van der Schans GP, Roza L et al., (Pheo)melanin photosensitizes UVA-induced DNA damage in cultured human melanocytes, *J Invest Dermatol* (1998) **111**:678–82.
45. Cario-Andre M, Pain C, Gall Y et al., Studies on epidermis reconstructed with and without melanocytes: Melanocytes prevent sunburn cell formation but not appearance of DNA damaged cells in fair-skinned Caucasians, *J Invest Dermatol* (2000) **115**:193–9.
46. Simon JD, Spectroscopic and dynamic studies of the epidermal chromophores trans-urocanic acid and eumelanin, *Am Chem Soc* (2000) **33**: 307–13.

33 The future of sunscreens

Jean Krutmann and Helger Stege

Introduction

Because of increased leasure time, the growing popularity of staying outdoors and of holidays in the sun, it has become more and more important to study the molecular and photobiological effects that ultraviolet (UV) radiation exerts on human skin. Information obtained from these studies is being used constantly to improve the quality of sunscreen preparations containing organic and inorganic filters. It is also fostering the development of active agents that can be used in combination with, or in addition to, UV filters to provide better photoprotection for human skin. These studies have also provided new test models which allow for proving or disproving the efficacy of actives.

In this review, two examples are given to illustrate these developments: (i) the use of topically applied DNA repair enzymes to prevent UVB-radiation-induced damage, and (ii) the development of a novel assay for the detection of mitochondrial (mt) DNA mutations in human skin that can be used to assess the efficacy of actives to protect against photoaging.

UVB photoprotection with topically applied DNA repair enzymes

The induction of photoproducts within the DNA of epidermal cells is detrimental to human health. Among the DNA lesions induced by UVB radiation, cyclobutane pyrimidine dimers predominate. Dimer formation is crucial for the initation of skin cancer because it is linked to the generation of mutations in tumor suppressor genes. It is now also generally believed that dimers contribute to the development of skin cancer by immunosuppression, thereby allowing transformed cells to grow unimpeded.[1–3] Conventional photoprotection by sunscreens is exclusively prophylactic in nature and of no value once DNA damage has occurred. However, in collaboration with AGI Dermatics, Freeport, NY, USA, we have recently assessed whether it is possible to repair UVB-radiation-induced DNA damage by topical application of a DNA repair enzyme.[2] In these studies, the DNA repair enzyme photolyase was used that specifically converts cyclobutane pyriminide dimers into their original DNA structure after exposure to photoreativating light. Dimer-specific photolyase is present in an active form in numerous prokaryotes and certain eukaryotes, but not in human skin. Photolyase was derived from *Anacystis nidulans* and subsequently incorporated into liposomes. The liposome component was formed from the lipids egg phopshatidylcholine, egg phosphatidylethanolamine and oleic acid, and from the membrane stabilizer cholesterol hemisuccinate. Photolyase-containing liposomes were applied immediately after UVB irradiation as a lotion onto UVB-irradiated human skin.

When a dose of UVB radiation sufficient to induce erythema was administered to the skin of healthy subjects, significant numbers of dimers were formed within epidermal cells.[2] Topical application of photolyase-containing liposomes to UVB-irradiated skin and subsequent exposure to photoreactivating light decreased the number of UVB-radiation-induced dimers by 40–45%. No reduction was observed if the liposomes were filled with the repair enzyme or if photoreactivation preceded the application of the filled liposomes. These observations indicated that it is indeed possible to repair UVB-radiation-induced DNA damage in human skin by the topical application of DNA repair enzymes encapsulated into liposomes. The partial repair that was achieved was sufficient to provide immunoprotection to UVB-irradiated human skin. The UVB dose administered suppressed the expression of intercellular adhesion molecule-1, a molecule required for immunity and inflammatory events in the skin.[1,3] Photolyase-induced dimer repair completely prevented this UVB-radiation-induced immunosuppressive effect. Similarly, in individuals hypersensitive to nickel sulfate, UVB-radiation suppressed the elicitation phase of the hypersensitivity reaction to nickel sulfate, and this immunosuppressive effect was also completely prevented by partial repair of UVB-radiation-induced dimers which could be achieved with the topical application of photolyase-containing liposomes.[2]

UVB-radiation-induced immunosuppression plays an important role in photocarcinogenesis.[3] The prevention of immunosuppression in UVB-irradiated human skin by topical application of DNA repair-enzyme-containing liposomes thus indicated the possibility that this approach could prevent skin cancer in humans. Accordingly, in a recent international multicenter trial, it has been demonstrated that topical application of DNA repair enzymes is indeed able to lower the rate of new skin cancers in patients with Xeroderma pigmentosum. Taken together, these studies suggest that topical application of exogenous DNA repair enzymes to human skin is a novel and effective approach to protect skin from detrimental effects that are caused through the generation of dimers.[4] This photoprotective approach differs from conventional photoprotection in its ability to remove damage that has already occurred. DNA repair-enzyme-containing liposomes could thus ideally be combined as an aftersun strategy with conventional sunscreens to provide photoprotection and repair at the same time. In fact, aftersun preparations, as well as sunscreen formulations containing liposomes filled with biologically active photolyase, have been made available to the public by the cosmetic industry just recently and the efficacy of these products has been proven both *in vitro* and *in vivo*.

Mitochondrial DNA mutations: a novel biomarker to evaluate protection against photoaging

Mitochondria are cell organelles whose main function is to generate energy for the cell. This is achieved by a multistep process called oxidative phosphorylation. Located at the inner mt membrane are five multiprotein complexes which generate an electrochemical protein gradient used in the last step of the process to turn ADP into ATP. This process is not completely error free and ultimately leads to the generation of reactive oxygen species (ROS). In close proximity to this site lies the mitochondrion's own genetic material, the mt DNA. The human mt DNA is a 16559-bp-long, circular and double-stranded molecule of which 4–10 copies exist per cell. Mutations of mt DNA have been found to play a causative role in a number of degenerative diseases such as Alzheimer's disease, but also in the normal aging process, where an accumulation of mt DNA mutation is accompanied by a decline of mt function. More recently, we and others have shown that mt DNA mutations are also involved in the process of photoaging.[5] Chronically sun-exposed skin showing clinical signs of photoaging has a higher mutation frequency of the mt DNA than sun-protected skin.[6] The capacity of solar UV radiation to cause the formation of mt DNA mutations has been demonstrated both *in vitro* and *in vivo*. Normal human fibroblasts, when repetitively exposed for 3 weeks to sublethal, nonapoptogenic doses of UVA radiation, exhibit a time- and dose-dependent increase in the most frequent mt DNA mutation, the so-called common deletion.[7] In a very similar manner, repetitive irradiation of normal human buttock skin also led to the induction of the common deletion (Berneburg M, Plettenberg H, Krutmann J et al., manuscript submitted for publication). In human skin, the common deletion could still be detected up to 180 months after cessation of the irradiation regimen, indicating that the common deletion serves a memory function in human skin for previously afflicted DNA damage.

By employing this combined *in vitro/in vivo* model for photoaging of human skin, it has been possible to assess the efficacy of sunscreens, antioxidants and active agents to provide protection against photoaging. Accordingly, broad-spectrum sunscreens filtering in the UVB and UVA range were found to prevent the formation of the common deletion *in vivo* in human skin. Also, *in vitro* studies have revealed a crucial role for ROS in the generation of the common deletion; several antioxidants were found to be capable of preventing the UVA-radiation-induced generation of the common deletion. Most interestingly, the formation of the common deletion could be delayed, or even completely prevented, if the irradiated cells were supplemented with creatine as an energy equivalent (Berneburg M, Kürten V, Krutmann J et al., manuscript submitted for publication). These studies show that the *in vitro*/*in vivo* model described above will be extremely useful to prove or disprove cosmetic claims concerning protection of human skin against photoaging. It will also allow a search for new actives that can help to prevent or even repair mt DNA mutations and the resulting consequences in human skin.

References

1. Ahrens C, Grewe M, Berneburg M et al., ICAM-1 expression and photocarcinogensis in DNA repair defective individuals, *Proc Natl Acad Sci USA* (1997); **94**:6837–41.
2. Stege H, Roza L, Vink AA et al., Enzyme plus light therapy to repair DNA damage in ultraviolet-B-irradiated human skin, *Proc Natl Acad Sci USA* (2000); **97**:1790–5.
3. Krutmann J, Elmets CA, *Photoimmunology.* (Blackwell: Oxford, 1995).
4. Yarosh D, Klein J, O'Connor A et al., Effect of topically applied T4 endonuclease V in liposomes on skin cancer in xeroderma pigmentosum: a randomised study, *Lancet* (2001); **357**:926–9.
5. Berneburg M, Plettenberg H, Krutmann J, Photaging of human skin, *Photodermatol Photoimmunol Photomed* (2000) **16**:239–44.
6. Berneburg M, Gattermann N, Stege H et al., Chronically ultraviolet-exposed human skin shows a higher mutation frequency of mitochondrial DNA as compared to unexposed skin and the hematopoietic system, *Photochem Photobiol* (1997) **66**:271–5.
7. Berneburg M, Grether-Beck S, Kürten V et al., Singlet oxygen mediates the UVA-induced generation of the photoaging-associated common deletion, *J Biol Chem* (1999); **274**:15345–9.

Section IX

PSYCHOSOCIOLOGY OF SUNTANNING

34
Psychological aspects of tanning

Sylvie G. Consoli

Introduction

Lengthy and repeated exposure to ultraviolet (UV) radiation in order to obtain a tan is both a short-term and a long-term health risk. A major long-term danger is skin cancer. The frequency of malignant melanoma, which mainly affects fair-skinned people, has been rising dramatically in recent years. Tanning has now become a true public health problem. An increasing number of information campaigns on the dangers of UV radiation are being targeted at fair-skinned people, yet their behavior has hardly changed. It is, therefore, important to examine the characteristics and motivations of such people in order to increase the impact of such campaigns.

The skin, like the brain, derives from the ectoderm, the outermost cell layer of the embryo. The skin is a extremely versatile sensory organ, as reflected in its complex anatomy. It acts as a protective envelope against environmental aggression, and contributes to regulating the body's metabolism and temperature. It is also an important purveyor of interpersonal signals. The skin is different from other organs, which we expect to function silently and invisibly, and repair when they dysfunction. In contrast, the skin is a visible organ of human relationships, expressing, unveiling or even betraying emotions and feelings through, for example, pallor, blushing, and excessive sweating. The skin participates in our affective and social life, including seduction and love. It is meant to be looked at, touched, caressed and smelled. It is strongly linked to pleasure.

Throughout our lives, our skin acts as an interface between ourselves and others. Visible to ourselves and others, it bears the indelible scars of life events, the effect of passing years, and physical transformations that result from, but also reflect, our identity, especially our sexual identity. This is also revealed by our head hair and body hair, and our esthetic practices, which depend on local culture and fashion. Each individual's skin is modeled by other peoples' regards, through the codes inherent in fashion, socioeconomic status and the society in which we live. Depending on the customs and fashions of each epoch and culture, people have scented, decorated, depilated, and blanched or, on the contrary, tanned their skin. The aspect of our skin, together with our hair and nails, is influenced by other peoples' innumerable and more or less explicit demands and desires: from haircuts imposed by parents on their adolescent children, to the tan imposed by fashion in our Western countries, which is a sign of social success.

Etymologically, the word 'cosmetic' implies not only adornment, but also orderliness. The main aim of cosmetology is to make the skin more beautiful. The skin—one of the most important organs in interpersonal relationships—contributes to our self-image and to the image we wish to project. To a large extent, it determines our overall attractiveness. Michel Serres, a French philosopher, said that the skin was a person's 'outpost', 'in the front line'.[1] Among the other elements that compose an individual, the skin represents the way in which an individual wishes to experience him/herself, and to be seen and experienced by others. On this basis, it is easier to understand why we all want our skin to be in harmony (or 'in orderly coherence') with the image we have of ourselves and with the image we present to others. What could be more natural, therefore, than to wish to beautify our skin?

The desire to be tanned

Tanning is an integral part of cosmetology. These days, tanned skin is considered to be more attractive in 'white' countries, but this has not always been the case.

Historical background

Until at least the First World War, elegant Western women, and men too, tried to keep their skin as white as possible, using parasols, veils, powders and ointments to do so. The word 'tan' derives from the process used to convert animal skins into leather. A tan was therefore considered as the destruction of the complexion by the sun. It was a sign of low social status, a negative consequence of working in the fields, at a time when most of the Western population were farmers. Yet, in the 1930s, and in the years following the Second World War, there was an esthetic revolution: tanning came into fashion.

As hemlines rose, hair became shorter, and bathing costumes became skimpier, there was a social obligation to be tanned, at least in summer. This cultural revolution was attributed by some to Coco Chanel, and by others to American GIs arriving in Europe in 1944 with tanned skins and tanning lotion in their napsacks. There was also the conjugated influence of the search for the exotic, practice of sports, physical culture, and paid vacations on Western women's relationships to their bodies, to the sun and to nature.

Social and economic factors also played an important role in the glorification of tanning. Indeed, after the Second World War, the hardest work shifted from the fields to the factories. Being tanned, therefore, meant having enough leisure time to get out into the open air, and to 'benefit' from sunshine by sunbathing.

All this illustrates how much the current desire to be tanned is rooted in history, culture, fashion and economic changes.

Needless to say, no sooner had the tanning mode appeared than voices were raised against it. In 1935, Alexis Carrel, a Nobel prizewinner, wrote ambiguously that the effect of exposure of our body to the sun was unknown, and that, until it was, the white race should not indulge in nudism or exaggerated darkening of the skin by natural light or UV rays.[2]

Beauty

The attitudes of today's elegant people towards tanning are therefore modeled by representations of beauty that society, through fashion, offers us in newspapers, cinema, television, and, now, the Internet. For many, beauty is a guarantee of social success, and even happiness. Men are also concerned by this mode, even if the links between beauty, virility and seduction are even more complex than those between beauty, femininity and seduction. Indeed, an elderly man with a wizened, tanned face may appear virile, and even attractive, as his appearance is interpreted as showing his socioprofessional success; he can confirm this with his intelligence and checkbook. Women are not yet equal players in this game: to remain feminine, a woman may still have to mask her intelligence, and also the effects of age and life events—often through a good tan.

But beauty also has subtle and hidden facets. It is, like a tan, ephemeral: its quest is a dream, but the dream can turn into a nightmare, reducing its follower to slavery. Beauty is often considered intangible and enigmatic. Our definition of beauty in Western societies depends partly on our social status, and also on its stereotypic representations: we are constantly bombarded with images of beautiful young women and young men. The message underlying advertisements and images conveyed by other media is the same: success belongs to the beautiful, the young and, often, the tanned.

Many studies have shown the importance of physical appearance in interpersonal relationships. A person's image is composed of a variety of signals, including height, weight, hairstyle, facial harmony, voice, odor, and factors underlying nonverbal communication. Someone with an attractive physical appearance projects success in love and work, and abundant personal qualities. It has been shown that cosmetic changes can help women to find work more easily and to achieve higher salaries. Furthermore, cosmetic improvements have often been successfully used to treat patients suffering from depression and low self-esteem.

Populations prone to tanning

Tanning is especially popular among young Westerners of both sexes between the ages of 18 and 30. Tanning, especially by young men, can be achieved through recreational activities like swimming, watersports and beach games. Note that young men rarely use sunscreens.

Sunbathing is most popular among young single women. They are more likely than young men to use sunscreens, which now resemble cosmetics, with pleasant textures and perfumes. During the last 15 years, these young women have started to be tanned all year round, or at least to prepare and then prolong their natural summer tan, by the use of tanning salons. Men also use tanning salons, albeit to a lesser extent.[3]

This very lucrative industry often promotes its goods by stating that the artificial tan is safer than the natural tan, with slogans like 'safer tan than sun'. Many consumers accept this unquestioningly, and fail to protect their skin or even their eyes. A survey of 1000 young people in Minnesota showed that 34% of them regularly used UV salons, and that only half had been informed by the salon owners of the associated risks.[4] The commercial promotion of tanning is a major factor in the public health risk.

Another study, conducted in 1993 among 1502 Swedish students aged from 14 to 19, confirms the American data: 57% of those who responded to a questionnaire on their tanning habits—70% of girls and 44% of boys—had used a UV salon at least four times in the past year. Use of UV lamps correlated with smoking (at ages 14–15 years), gender (most users were girls), age (use increasing with age), excessive exposure to the sun, and a negative self-image (weight, height, hair, and body form). This study also showed that the students best informed of the potential risks were those who used the salons most often. There was, therefore, no parallel relationship between the degree of information and the degree of prevention.[5]

Thus, natural and artificial tanning is popular among adolescents, who are still struggling to come to terms with their new, adult identity. Adolescence is a delicate period of sexual and emotional maturation, preparing for the process of separation. Adolescents begin to seek persons other than their parents to seduce, and must find different mental and physical resources from those they used in childhood to achieve this goal. For years, many adolescents are ashamed of the visible transformations their bodies are undergoing. Indeed, the body undergoes multiple visible and invisible upheavals during this period of life. Adolescents have extreme narcissic insecurity, and they lose confidence in their capacity to seduce. This narcissic insecurity can be exacerbated by the slightest imperfection of the skin of the face or body, and attenuated by a new hair color or a tan.

In addition, adolescents tend to live for the moment (they want it all, right now) and refuse to accept constraints. They undergo so many physical and mental changes that they find it difficult to project themselves into the future, especially the distant future. They prefer immediate narcissic rewards and feel unconcerned by the long-term dangers. They are in 'risk denial', or put their perceived invulnerability to the test by displaying steadfast optimism. Of course, older people can also have adolescent-like behavior towards tanning, particularly if they have a poor self-image and low self-esteem, and are suffering from anxiety and depression.

The main motivations

People of all ages can have a poor self-image, and this is often accompanied by low self-esteem. The most frequently stated motivation for tanning is to have a more pleasing physical appearance (this is true for both women and men) and, therefore, a greater power of seduction.

This is hardly surprising in Western societies, where images are all-powerful, and especially images representing individuals whose physical appearance suggests social, financial, and sexual success. As if these attributes guaranteed happiness! These images have a considerable impact, particularly on young people, who are seeking role models upon whom to reconstruct their narcissism after the mental and physical upheavals of adolescence.

This is borne out by the fact that young men tend to use sunscreens less that young women during their outdoor activities. This reflects the desire to correspond to the images of handsome, strong, sporty, muscular, tanned young men, who are hardly ever seen protecting themselves with a hat or sunscreen. Sunscreens are seen as cosmetic creams 'for girls', and applying them can be considered unmanly.

The desire to look healthy is less often quoted as the reason for tanning than it was 15 years ago.[7] But, even today, physical deterioration and old age are still shameful and must be hidden, as if they perturbed the social order.

A frequently stated reason for using UV salons is relaxation. It is true that it can be tempting, after a busy day in the office or home, to seek a moment of relaxation and daydreaming in a tanning salon. UV salons are ideal for this purpose, as they are usually immediately available and cost far less than a trip to a sunny country, which would take days or weeks to organize.[8]

Conclusions

Excessive tanning is a new risk behavior in our modern industrial societies, fascinated as we are by technology and money, and in which image and appearance are all-powerful.

This is most strongly felt by adolescents, young adults, and emotionally immature and depressive individuals of all ages. Indeed, most such people have a poor self-image and low self-esteem. They will do anything to valorize the image they have of themselves and that they present to others, in an attempt to hide their secret and imaginary weaknesses and find a little self-esteem. Tanning is a relatively easy way of improving one's self-image, even if most people are aware of the associated long-term risks. But for some, the immediate narcissic reward is more important than all other considerations.

Thus, effective prevention campaigns should not only inform people of the short- and long-term health risks of excessive UV exposure, but also convince the media—the mirror of our society—of the need to counter the influence of the advertising industry and present attractive images of men and women with untanned skin. The esthetic risks of excessive tanning—such as the risk of premature skin aging—should also be stressed.

Finally, general practitioners, gynecologists and dermatologists are no doubt the best placed to identify and treat the emotional immaturity, depression, and dysfunctional role-model identification and imagination that underlie this type of risk behavior. Only in this way can people be liberated from the dictates of fashion that place their health at risk.

References

1. Serres M, Les Cinq Sens. Grasset, Paris, 1985.
2. Ory P, L'invention du bronzage. In: Czechowski N, Nahoum-Grapp V, eds, *Fatale beauté* (Autrement: Paris, 1987) **97**:146–52.
3. Spencer JM, Amonette RA, Indoor tanning: risks, benefits, and future trends, *J Am Acad Dermatol* (1985) **33**:288–98.
4. Oliphant JA, Foster JL, McBride CM, The use of commercial tanning facilities by suburban Minnesota adolescents, *Am J Public Health* (1994) **81**: 476–8.
5. Boldeman C, Jansson B, Nilsson B et al., Sunbed use in Swedish Urban Adolescents related to behavioral characteristics, *Prev Med* (1997) **26**:114–19.
6. Hillhouse JJ, Adler CM, Drinnon J et al., Application of Azjen's theory of planned behavior to predict sunbathing, tanning salon use, and sunscreen use intentions and behaviors, *J Behav Med* (1997) **20**: 365–78.
7. Robinson JK, Rigel DS, Amonette RA, Trends in sun exposure knowledge, attitudes, and behaviors: 1986 to 1996, *J Am Acad Dermatol* (1997) **37**: 179–86.
8. Beasley TM, Kittel BS, Factors that influence health risk behaviors among tanning salon patrons, *Eval Health Prof* (1997) **20**:371–88.

35

Sociological perspectives on suntanning

Jean Jacques Bonerandi

People's attitudes about the sun have always been closely related to cultural values. The technological revolution of the twentieth century has profoundly changed our society, as well as our relationship with the natural environment. Within this context, it might be timely to recall the more balanced attitudes toward sun exposure in more traditional settings.

Physiological aspects

Are humans cut out for the sun? Are species living in sunny natural habitats better protected than humans?

According to phylogeneticians, land animals can be classified into two groups, according to whether their natural habitat is the savanna or forest. Humans are forest dwellers by nature. However, our keen adaptive powers have allowed us to leave the cover of the treetops and survive under a wide range of environmental conditions. Humans now inhabit almost every region of the earth, including zones most exposed to solar radiation.

Unfortunately, humans are one of the least protected animals against solar radiation. We have little or no body hair; our skin, including the outermost horny layer, is thin; our melanin system is largely ineffective, except in blacks. Tanning in Caucasians provides poor protection and has even been compared to scarring, since it is more of a visible proof of skin injury than an effective mechanism of skin protection.

Primitive societies

Sun worship

In primitive societies, humans had little scientific understanding of their natural environment. The sun was often worshipped as an awesome god that could either bestow life or cause destruction. The most blatant examples of deification of the sun are Amon Ra in Egyptian mythology and Apollo in the religions of the Ancient Greeks and Romans. Pre-Columbian Indians sacrificed their children as a sacrifice to their sun god.

The day of the paleface

While worshiping the sun as a god, most people in the past shunned its effects on the skin. Until recently, whiteness was a symbol of purity, virginity, and nobility. Pale skin belonged to the affluent upper classes, while bronzed skin was a visible sign of the poor working classes. In front of their mirrors, fashionable people used a variety of weird and even deadly tricks to achieve the coveted Snow-White appearance. The ideal woman had pale, translucent skin. Although the cultural values and class distinctions underlying these practices seem laughable nowadays, the resulting behavior avoided the ravages of the solar radiation. This type of behavior persisted into the twentieth century and continues in a few remote rural societies with a traditional relationship with nature.

Second half of the twentieth century: Suntan worship

A variety of factors caused the norm to change from white to dark after so many centuries in Western society.

New social organization

In traditional societies, most of the population was rural. It was not until the Industrial Revolution in the nineteenth century that people began to move into cities and a sizable proportion of people without a direct link to the natural environment developed. The Technological Revolution of the twentieth century has further changed the relationship humans have with their environment. New means of transportation have developed that enable people to move rapidly from one climate to another. Social progress has provided more time and opportunity for leisure.

Changing trends

The founding of the Scouting movement by Robert Baden-Powell at the beginning of last century was a watershed event in the modern-day triumph of sports and outdoor pursuits. At the time, public interest in nature was growing and contributed to the popularity of open-air activities, which was to explode with the institution of the paid vacation. Mass culture contributed enormously to incorporating these trends into the collective mind, through images involving jet-set icons like Coco Chanel, manly heroes such as WWII GIs and Western cowboys, movie stars in Cannes and Hollywood, and sunbathers at vacation resorts. Slowly but surely, the suntan became a symbol of beauty, health, affluence, and happiness.

Changing clothing styles

Ready-to-wear clothing became more widespread, with fashions supporting outdoor lifestyles. Although styles and hemlines fluctuate, the tendency has been to downsize coverage. Women's legs have gradually been bared. In both sexes, the practice of outdoor sports has led to regular exposure of the arms, legs, and even the trunk. In the last 50 years, there has been a significant reduction in the size of swimsuits. Coverage has now been reduced to private parts.

Decline of protective instincts

Strangely, instinct and logic no longer act as a brake on solar exposure. Few people with respiratory insufficiency would attempt to climb Mount Everest. Yet people with insufficient skin pigmentation, such as individuals with blond or red hair and individuals with freckles, regularly expose themselves at the same time of day and for as many hours as dark-skinned people. They are oblivious of the common-sense conclusion that this behavior is out of proportion with the natural protective capacity of their skin and that they should avoid excessive exposure.

A major industry feeds on the suntan cult. Travel agents, real-estate promoters, and cosmetic manufacturers have not only perpetuated but also nurtured the social norm that the suntan is an important quality of good-looking people. There are an enormous number of suntanning products on the market, ranging from tanning accelerators/ intensifiers, protection creams, and hydrating lotions recommended for use before, during, and after sunbathing. Once again, contrary to common sense, these products are usually utilized in place of, rather than in conjunction with, protective clothing. As a result, consumption of suncreens has skyrocketed but there has been no real gain in protection, since these products have served only as an excuse for longer exposure. Indoor tanning salons have proliferated by convincing consumers that artificial tanning is safer and that they can get a 'protective' base tan without sunburning.

The most important changes in sun behavior observed over the last few decades are as follows:

- Increase in the number of individuals exposed.
- Increase in mean dose of radiation/individual independently of natural protection.
- Increase in the incidence of acute sunburning.
- Exposure of children at a younger age.
- Exposure of zones that had never seen sunlight.

The suntan craze peaked in the 1970s (sea, sex and sun). In the same period, study data first confirmed the ravages of overexposure in the post-war period, and public education campaigns began in earnest.

The new millennium: A time for reflection

We now know that sunlight does not give happiness. Overexposure causes cancer, sometimes, and wrinkles, always. Is wrinkling compatible with happiness?

Modern populations consider themselves aware and well organized. They try to stay informed about benefits and dangers in their environment. Scientific data have a significant impact on their behavior.

The link between exposure to solar radiation and skin cancer is certain.

- *The cause has been identified.* It is ultraviolet (UV) light. The most deleterious component for the skin is the UVB wavelength. The UVA wavelengths are less harmful. Shorter UVC wavelengths are absorbed by the superficial layer of the atmosphere and do not reach us.
- *The mechanism is also known.* Absorption of UV radiation alters molecules called target molecules. DNA in cell nuclei is a highly sensitive target molecule. Intracellular repair mechanisms may fail and defective repair promotes development of skin cancer. In addition, UV rays impair the immune system, thus reducing the defenses of the skin against cancer cells.
- *The risk of cancer is related to individual sensitivity.* Skin color is the major risk factor but cumulative lifetime dose is also important.

For the most dangerous form of skin cancer, *i.e.* melanoma, the relationship with sun exposure is more complex. Studies have demonstrated unexplained discrepancies.

- One series of studies showed that intense exposure to sunlight over an individual's lifetime and, in particular, during childhood and adolescence, was correlated with a significant increase in the risk of melanoma.
- Other evidence indicated no correlation between cumulative sun exposure and occurrence of melanoma. One study showed that melanoma is more common in people with indoor than outdoor occupations.

Based on this finding, it has been speculated that intense, intermittent exposure may play a greater role in the induction of melanoma than cumulative dose. This would mean that melanoma is different from other forms of skin cancer in this regard.

A clear relationship has also been established between sun exposure and skin aging. Both UVB and UVA wavelengths, and even infrared wavelengths, induce dermatoheliosis, the main cause of skin aging. In many cases, premature skin aging contrasts with an otherwise youthful appearance corresponding to healthy eating habits and an active lifestyle.

Proper sun behavior is a timely topic in 2002

With respect to sun exposure, it is important to know and promulgate several basic concepts.

- *Fair-skinned Caucasians are high-risk subjects.* This is especially true for people with skin types 1 and 2, *i.e.* who always burn and never tan, for people with blond or red hair and people with many moles on their skin. Photoprotection must begin during childhood.
- *Solar radiation is most harmful* in the middle of the day, from 12 am to 4 pm, and at altitudes higher than 1000 m.
- *Protective measures must be adapted to skin type:*
    - Type 1: maximum protection. Complete avoidance of sun exposure is advisable.
    - Type 2: moderate protection allows careful exposure.
    - Type 3 and 4: moderate protection allows careful exposure.

The best sun protection strategy is to wear clothes. The value of sunscreens in preventing skin cancers has not been definitely established. This is true even for total sunblocks, and for recent formulations that have demonstrated effectiveness against UVA and good photostability. Only broad-spectrum sunscreens, with a sun protection factor >30, should be used. Sunscreen must be reapplied after swimming or sweating.

The safest approach to sun exposure would consist of calculating each individual's risk factors at birth. The person would adapt his/her behavior and use of sun protective measures in function of his/her own level of risk. Like a person with a driving license, the person could be issued a tanning license. There could be 'speed limits', 'one-way streets', 'no passing zones', and 'no parking zones'.

Without going that far, education and information campaigns seem to be having an impact. There are signs that magazine articles and television reports have been effective. Bathing suits are covering more. In fashion ads, there is a tendency toward the natural look with fair skin being naturally fair and dark skin being naturally dark. The blush has returned to cover-girl faces. Although it is still too early to be sure, a new day in sun behavior may be dawning.

Further reading

Bouissou X, Le soleil et l'homme: mythes, santé et apparences. Thèse médecine, 1986, Faculté de Médecine de Grenoble.

Ghozland F, Toulouse ed., *Cosmétiques, être et paraître* (Milan, 1987) 70–1.

Grob JJ, Bonerandi JJ, Nouveau soleil, nouvelle dermatologie, *Ann Dermatol Vénéréol* (1991) **118**:925–9.

Ory P, L'invention du bronzage. In: *Fatale Beauté* (Coll. Autrement n°91, Juin 1987) 146–52.

Perrot P, *Le travail des apparences ou les transformations du corps féminin, XVIIè–XIXè siècle* (Seuil: Paris, 1984) 145.

36
Conclusions

Jean-Paul Ortonne and Robert Ballotti

Skin colour plays a key role in the psychological and social aspects of human life. In western society, tanned skin is considered to be more attractive, while in East Africa or in South America, people prefer a fair complexion. Beyond its aesthetic role, skin pigmentation provides an efficient protection against the noxious effects of solar light. It is now clear that dark skins, with high eumelanin and low pheomelanin content, are less susceptible to solar induced photodamage. Thus, it might be dangerous for dark-skinned people, living in sunny countries, to decrease skin melanin content by lightening their complexion. Alternatively, it might be hazardous for fair-complexioned people to darken their suntans through long exposure to sunlight. These days, cosmetic sunscreens, if correctly used, provide a very efficient protection against UV induced damage, but they also interfere with skin tanning. However, the desire to be tan is deeply rooted in the behaviour of Westerners and it would be judicious to develop photoprotective agents that permit the sun to tan the skin.

UV-induced DNA damage is the main cause of the deleterious effects of solar light and is particularly incriminated in photo-induced skin carcinogenesis. Recently, it was proposed to limit UV-induced DNA damage by stimulating DNA repair. First, it was proposed to reduce DNA damage by using a topical application of the DNA-repair enzyme photolyase, derived from Anacystis nidulans, that specifically converts cyclobutane dimers into their original DNA structure after exposure to photoreactivating light. A more recent report shows that IL-12 caused a dramatic induction of DNA repair, pointing to the possibility of using this cytokine in topical application to limit UV-induced DNA damage. However, this cytokine also blocks apoptosis, a protective process which eliminates the irremediably damaged cells.

In conclusion, since Westerners want to be tanned and since eumelanin plays a key photoprotective role, it would be valuable to search for new and safe melanogenic agents that would increase skin tanning without exposure to the solar light, thereby providing protective and aesthetic benefits. The first step in reaching this aim is to dissect molecular events by identifying new molecular targets for pharmacological intervention in the modification of hair and skin colour. This monograph illustrates that basic research is currently paving the way to such strategies .

Much remains to be done to improve natural photoprotection of the skin and to prevent skin cancer. However, the amazing increase in our knowledge of melanogenesis and melanocyte biology generates great hope among patients suffering from pigmentary disorders of the skin and among their physicians who anticipate the arrival of effective new drugs in this field in the very near future.

Index